SURGERY OF THE FOOT

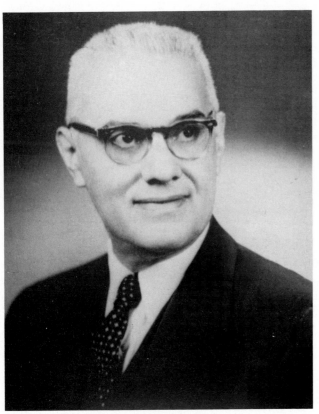

HENRI L. DuVRIES
1899-1980

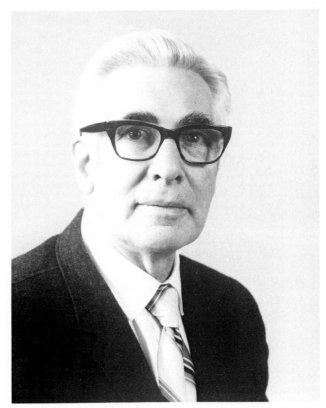

VERNE T. INMAN
1905-1980

SURGERY of the FOOT

IN MEMORY OF HENRI L. DuVRIES and VERNE T. INMAN

Edition 5

EDITOR

Roger A. Mann, M.D.

Private Practice Orthopaedic Surgery, *Oakland, California;*
Director of Foot Fellowship Program,
Chief, Foot Surgery, Children's Hospital of the East Bay, *Oakland, California;*
Chief, Foot Surgery, Samuel Merritt Hospital, *Oakland, California;*
Consultant, Gait Analysis Laboratory,
Shriner's Hospital for Crippled Children, *San Francisco, California;*
Consultant, Foot Surgery, Oak Knoll Naval Hospital, *Oakland, California;*
Consultant, Foot Surgery, Letterman General Hospital, *San Francisco, California;*
Associate Clinical Professor, Department of Orthopaedic Surgery,
San Francisco, California.

with 1584 illustrations

The C. V. Mosby Company   ST. LOUIS · TORONTO · PRINCETON   1986

MOSBY

A TRADITION OF PUBLISHING EXCELLENCE

Editor: Eugenia A. Klein
Developmental editor: Kathryn H. Falk
Editing supervisor: Elaine Steinborn
Manuscript editors: Timothy O'Brien, Marybeth Engelhardt, Melissa Neves
Book design: Gail Morey Hudson
Cover design: Suzanne Oberholtzer
Production: Carol O'Leary, Jeanne A. Gulledge

FIFTH EDITION

Printed in the United States of America

The C.V. Mosby Company
11830 Westline Industrial Drive, St. Louis, Missouri 63146

Library of Congress Cataloging in Publication Data

Main entry under title:

Surgery of the foot.

  Rev. ed. of: DuVries' Surgery of the foot. 4th ed. / editor, Roger A. Mann. 1978.
  Includes bibliographies and index.
  1. Foot—Surgery. I. Mann, Roger A., 1936-
II. DuVries, Henri L. III. Inman, Verne Thompson,
1905-   . IV. DuVries, Henri L. Surgery of the foot.
[DNLM: 1. Foot—surgery. WE 880 S961]
RD563.D94 1985   617'.585059   85-8843
ISBN 0-8016-2334-0

C/MV/MV 9 8 7 6 5 4 3 2   01/B/058

Contributors

Donald E. Baxter, M.D.

Assistant Professor of Orthopaedic Surgery and Chief, Foot Service, University of Texas at Houston and Clinical Instructor, Baylor College of Medicine, Houston, Texas.

Michael W. Chapman, M.D.

Professor and Chairman, Department of Orthopaedic Surgery, University of California, Davis, School of Medicine, Sacramento, California.

Michael J. Coughlin, M.D., P.A.

Clinical Instructor of Surgery, Division of Orthopaedics and Rehabilitation, Oregon Health Sciences University, Portland Oregon; Chief of Orthopaedic Surgery, St. Alphonsus Regional Medical Center, Boise, Idaho.

Jesse C. DeLee, M.D.

Associate Professor, Department of Orthopaedics, University of Texas Health Science Center, San Antonio, Texas.

Igor Z. Drobocky, M.D.*

Staff Diagnostic Radiologist, Doctors' Hospital, San Leandro, and Laurel Grove Hospital in Castro Valley; Consultant Radiologist, U.S. Navy, Oakland Naval Hospital, Oakland, California.

Earl N. Feiwell, M.D.

Chief, Orthopaedic Surgeon, Myelodysplasia Team, Rancho Los Amigos Hospital, Downey California; Associate Clinical Professor, Orthopaedic Surgery, University of Southern California School of Medicine, Los Angeles.

Douglas E. Garland, M.D.

Associate Clinical Professor of Orthopedic Surgery, University of Southern California, Los Angeles, California; Chief, Adult Head Trauma Service and Co-Chief, Spinal Cord Injury Service, Rancho Los Amigos Hospital, Downey, California.

M. Mark Hoffer, M.D.

Professor and Chief, Division of Orthopaedic Surgery, University of California School of Medicine, Irvine, California.

John D. Hsu, M.D., C.M., F.A.C.S.

Clinical Professor, Department of Orthopedics, University of Southern California, School of Medicine; Attending Orthopaedic Surgeon and Chief, Muscle Disease Clinics, Rancho Los Amigos Hospital, Downey, California, and Orthopaedic Hospital, Los Angeles, California.

Walter W. Huurman, M.D.

Associate Professor, Department of Orthopaedic Surgery and Rehabilitation; Assistant Professor, Department of Pediatrics, and Director of Pediatric Orthopaedics, The University of Nebraska Medical Center, Omaha, Nebraska.

James O. Johnston, M.D.

Chief of Orthopaedics, Kaiser Hospital, Oakland, California; Clinical Professor of Orthopaedics, University of California School of Medicine, San Francisco, California.

Roger A. Mann, M.D.

Associate Clinical Professor, Department of Orthopaedic Surgery, University of California School of Medicine; Director, Gait Analysis Laboratory, Shriner's Hospital for Crippled Children, San Francisco, California; Chief, Foot Surgery, Children's Hospital of the East Bay and Samuel Merritt Hospital; Consultant, Foot Surgery, Oak Knoll Naval Hospital, Oakland, California.

Landrus L. Pfeffinger, M.D.

Associate Clinical Professor, Orthopaedic Surgery, University of California School of Medicine, San Francisco, California; Attending Orthopaedic Surgeon, Highland General Hospital, Oakland, California and George Miller School of Handicapped, Richard, California.

Stanford F. Pollock, M.D.

Orthopaedic Surgeon, Active Staff, Mills Memorial Hospital, San Mateo, California.

G. James Sammarco, M.D., F.A.C.S.

Associate Clinical Professor, Director, Performing Arts Clinic, Senior Consultant, Foot and Ankle Clinic, Department of Orthopaedic Surgery, University of Cincinnati Medical Center, Cincinnati, Ohio.

Jerral S. Seibert, M.D.

Associate Clinical Professor of Dermatology, University of California School of Medicine, San Francisco, California.

Francesca M. Thompson, M.D.

Orthopaedic Surgeon and Chief, Orthopaedic Foot Clinic, Roosevelt Hospital, St. Luke's-Roosevelt Hospital Center, New York, New York

---

*Deceased.

F. William Wagner, Jr., M.D.

Clinical Professor of Orthopaedic Surgery, University of Southern California School of Medicine, Los Angeles, California; Chief Consultant, Orthopaedic Diabetic Service, Rancho Los Amigos Hospital, Downey, California; Director, Foot and Ankle Service, Los Angeles County—USC Medical Center, Los Angeles, California.

Robert L. Waters, M.D.

Chief, Surgical Services, Rancho Los Amigos Hospital, Downey, California; Clinical Professor of Orthopedic Surgery, University of Southern California School of Medicine, Los Angeles, California.

To my professors
HENRI L. DuVRIES and VERNE T. INMAN

To my parents
for the opportunities presented to me

To my wife and family
for their patience and understanding

Preface

Twenty-six years ago, Henri DuVries presented to the medical world his vast clinical experience in the first edition of *Surgery of the Foot*. Verne T. Inman assumed the role of editor with the third edition, adding to it his superb interpretations of biomechanics and functional anatomy. These two brilliant men are no longer alive, but the legacy of their lives' work lives on. Although their names are not present in the chapter headings, many of the basic principles expounded on in this text are based on their work.

It was the stimulating biomechanical and anatomic lectures of Verne T. Inman that introduced me to orthopaedics and his magnetic personality that attracted me to train in his residency program. He possessed a special interest in the function of the foot, which I acquired while working in his biomechanics laboratory. In the course of my residency I trained with Henri DuVries, who at that time had already published the first edition and was working on the second. He further stimulated my interest in the foot from a clinical standpoint. Following my formal training I spent a year of fellowship in foot surgery with him, furthering my clinical knowledge. When I was asked to edit the fourth edition by my former professors, I was greatly honored. Their input was invaluable to me in the preparation of the book. The orthopaedic world has lost two brilliant men, but much of their teaching can be found within the pages of this book, which is dedicated to them.

In preparation of the fifth edition of *Surgery of the Foot*, I have once again obtained the input of contributing authors. I feel they are important since their knowledge in their specific fields adds to the scope of the book.

Through the use of contributing authors, a textbook has been created that covers every major aspect of the foot in such a manner as to leave the reader, whether he or she is an orthopaedic surgeon, a general practitioner, or a medical student, with a clear, concise appreciation of each topic.

I look on my task as the editor of this book as one of presenting each subject in such a way that it will be meaningful to the practitioner. It is not meant to be a review of the world literature. The author's recommended treatment is to be found within each particular topic. Although the authors may present several treatment modalities, I have asked them to state specifically how they prefer to approach each particular problem.

In the clinical chapters I have written, the treatment is based on the continued review of the clinical material from my private practice. With the help of my fellows in foot surgery, every major clinical problem has been carefully assessed, and this material is what forms the basis of the recommended methods of treatment. I believe that it is through this careful, critical clinical assessment that the various treatment modalities can be compared, and in this manner the treatment of choice can be more accurately selected.

After the basic considerations of the foot in the first three chapters on biomechanics, examination of the foot, and radiographic examination, an extensive discussion of the deformities of the great toe, along with complications associated with bunion surgery, is presented. This section has been included not to discredit any particular procedure but to point out the pitfalls associated with bunion surgery. It is hoped that by being more acutely aware of the complications following bunion surgery the reader may more readily avoid these complications. The lesser toe deformities have been included in a single chapter in this edition to provide a fuller understanding of the clinical problems associated with the lesser toes and the metatarsophalangeal joints. The section on arthritis brings together our current knowledge and treatment plans for osteoarthritis as well as rheumatoid arthritis. The keratotic disorders of the plantar skin are once again approached from a clinical viewpoint that presents the reader with a clear understanding as to the differential diagnoses and treatment of these sometimes difficult problems. The neuromuscular diseases that affect the foot are presented in depth, with a presentation of the congenital neurologic disorders—such as myelodysplasia, cerebral palsy, and motor unit disease—as well as the acquired neurologic disorders such as those resulting from stroke and head trauma. The section on bones and their afflictions presents a concise review of the various soft tissue and bony tumors as well as the metabolic disorders that can affect the foot. The chapter on dermatology carefully outlines the basic dermatologic problems involving the foot and their treatments. The section on infections carefully analyzes the soft tissue and bony effects of infection, along with how to diagnose and treat the various problems. The chapter on diabetes presents a complete approach to the diabetic patient, discussing the proper technique to be used in the diagnosis, and then, in a schematic manner, a logical sequence to follow in the treatment of the disorders of the diabetic foot.

In this edition a separate section has been added for the foot in athletics, particularly running and dancing. The section on pediatric problems of the foot has been revised and updated. The book ends with an extensive, up-to-date study of fractures of the foot and ankle that presents the reader with a careful review of the literature, the diagnoses, and the preferred methods of treatment of fractures and dislocations about the foot and ankle.

Although this fifth edition has been significantly reorganized and upgraded, I still believe, as I stated in the preface to the fourth edition, that as medicine continues to progress, the information in this textbook will again need to be upgraded. The principles presented, however, are basic in their approach and will not change significantly over the years.

ROGER A. MANN

Preface to first edition

This book has been written in response to a continuing request by my students and colleagues that I draw together into one place of reference the fundamentals and the recommendations contained in my lectures and clinical demonstrations over a span of 30 years. As Frederic Wood Jones commented, "It is probably the experience of most teachers of anatomy that the student is generally better acquainted with the intimate structure of the hand than with that of the foot."* My friends among orthopaedic surgeons agree that the teaching of their specialty does not allot sufficient time to problems of the foot. They will forgive, therefore, and perhaps welcome as an adjunct to teaching, the elementary portions of the contents and the didactic approach.

Extreme disabilities of the foot, such as the talipes deformities, have received studious attention in published reports. They have on that account been given only a cursory nod of recognition here. This book is directed toward the commoner disabilities, which have been sparsely considered in medical writing and which have been widely neglected in teaching and practice.

The expanding awareness of the diversity of pathologic changes in the feet and of the complexities of treatment represents an advance since the days when all foot disabilities were always attributed to so-called fallen arches and when a prescription of arch supports satisfied the diagnostician that nothing further could be done about the patient whose feet continued to hurt.

This far from definitive effort of mine has reached the printed page through the encouragement and helpfulness, advice, and direction of so many of my friends and colleagues that I hesitate to name them lest by inadvertence one should be overlooked. If that happens, my deepest regret! Certainly I must mention my friends of long standing, Dr. August F. Daro; Dr. William M. Scholl, who turned his collection of photographs and anatomic models over to me for study and selective use and who has been otherwise helpful in so many ways; Dr. Ernest Nora, Sr., a constant friend since our medical school days, who reviewed the chapter on Tumors, Cysts, and Exostoses; so many on the Staff of Columbus Hospital; Dr. Carlo Scuderi, who reviewed the first rough material and then introduced me to my patient and cooperative publishers; Dr. Edwin Hirsch, who made the photographic facilities of St. Luke's Hospital* available to me; Dr. Karl A. Meyer, my former professor in medical school, who wrote the Foreword as a final expression of years of encouragement. Dr. Edward L. Compere crowned my effort by writing the Introduction, having first reviewed some of the material in its early stages and, later, all in its final form.

Special credit should be given to Miss Ethel H. Davis for superbly editing and organizing the manuscript.

It is tempting to list those who gave me direction in one way or another: Dr. Peter A. Rosi, Dr. Charles N. Pease, Dr. Joseph P. Cascino, Dr. Steven O. Schwartz, Dr. Caesar Portes, Dr. Abe Rubin, and Dr. Harold Wheeler. The skill of my artists, Miss Edith Hodgson, Miss Gloria Jones, and Dr. Allen Whitney, must not go unsung. And to all, mentioned or not, in the measure of their interest, my gratitude!

Only wives whose husbands have attempted the writing of books and the husbands who have known the stamina of their wives during the process can appreciate how much meaning there is in my dedication to Frances DuVries.

HENRI L. DuVRIES, D.P.M., M.D.
1959

---

*Jones, F.W.: Structure and function as seen in the foot, London, 1944, Baillière, Tindall & Cox, Ltd., p. 3.

*Now Presbyterian-St. Luke's Hospital.

Contents

1

Biomechanics of the foot and ankle

ROGER A. MANN

The initial chapters of this text on surgery will be concerned not with anatomy, as is customary, but with a discussion of the biomechanics of the foot and ankle. The specific relationships will be emphasized, and some methods for functional evaluation of the foot will be presented. These alterations were initiated for several reasons.

First, it has been assumed that the orthopaedic surgeon possesses an accurate knowledge of the anatomic aspects of the foot and ankle. If this knowledge is lacking, textbooks of anatomy are available that depict in detail the precise anatomic structures comprising this part of the human body. It seems redundant to devote space here to what can only be a superficial review of the anatomy of the foot and ankle.

Second, it seems mandatory that any textbook on surgery of the foot should begin with a discussion of the biomechanics of the foot and ankle as an integral part of the locomotor system. The human foot is an intricate mechanism that functions interdependently with other components of the locomotor system. No text is readily available to the surgeon that clearly enunciates the functional interrelationships of the various parts of the foot. Interference with the functioning of a single part may be reflected in altered functions of the remaining parts. Yet the surgeon is constantly called on to change the anatomic and structural components of the foot. When so doing, he should be fully aware of the possible consequences of his actions.

Third, wide variations are known to occur in the component parts of the foot and ankle, and these variations are reflected in the degree of contribution of each part to the behavior of the entire foot. Depending on the contributions of an individual component, the loss

or functional modification of that component by surgical intervention may result in either minor or major alterations in the functional behavior of adjacent components. An understanding of basic interrelationships may assist the surgeon in explaining to himself why the same procedure performed on the foot of one person produced a satisfactory result whereas in another person the result was unsatisfactory.

Fourth, by being alert to the mechanical behavior of the foot, the physician may find that some foot disabilities caused by malfunction of a component part can be successfully treated by nonsurgical procedures rather than attacked surgically as has been customary. Furthermore, some operative procedures that fail to achieve completely the desired result can be further improved by minor alterations in the behavior of adjacent components through shoe modification or the use of inserts. An understanding of the biomechanics of the foot and ankle should, therefore be an essential aid in surgical decision making and contribute to the success of postoperative treatment.

LOCOMOTOR SYSTEM

The human foot is too often viewed as a semirigid base whose principal function is to provide a stable support for the superincumbent body. In reality the foot is poorly designed for this purpose. Standing for prolonged periods of time can result in a feeling of fatigue or can produce actual discomfort in the feet. One always prefers to sit rather than stand. Furthermore, it is far less tiring to walk, run, jump, or dance on normally functioning feet—either barefooted or in comfortable shoes—than it is to stand. The foot, therefore, appears to have evolved as a dynamic mechanism functioning as

1

an integral part of the locomotor system and should be studied as such rather than as a static structure designed exclusively for support.

Since human locomotion involves all major segments of the body, obviously certain suprapedal movements demand specific functions from the foot and alterations in these movements from above may be reflected below by changes in the behavior of the foot. Likewise, the manner in which the foot functions may be reflected in patterns of movement in the other segments of the body. Therefore the basic functional interrelationships between the foot and the remainder of the locomotor apparatus must be clearly understood.

To begin a review of the locomotor system, one must recognize that ambulating man is both a physical machine and a biologic organism. The former makes him subject to the physical laws of motion, the latter to the laws of muscular action. All characteristics of muscular behavior are exploited in locomotion; for example, when called on to perform such external work as initiating or accelerating angular motion around joints, muscles rarely contract at lengths below their resting lengths (Bresler and Berry, 1951; Close and Inman, 1953; Ryker, 1952). When motion in the skeletal segments is decelerated or when external forces work on the body, activated muscles become efficient. Activated muscles, in fact, are approximately six times as efficient when resisting elongation as when shortening to perform external work (Abbott et al., 1952; Asmussen, 1953; Banister and Brown, 1968). In addition, noncontractile elements in muscles and specific connective tissue structures assist muscular action. Thus human locomotion is a blending of physical and biologic forces that compromise to achieve maximum efficiency at minimum cost.

Man uses a unique and characteristic orthograde bipedal mode of locomotion. This method of locomotion imposes gross similarities in the manner in which all of us walk. However, each of us exhibits minor individual differences that allow us to recognize a friend or acquaintance even when he is viewed from a distance. The causes of these individual characteristics of locomotion are many. Each of us differs somewhat in the length and distribution of mass of the various segments of the body—segments that must be moved by muscles of varying fiber lengths. Furthermore, individual differences occur in the position of axes of movement of the joints, with concomitant variations in effective lever arms. Such factors as these and many more combine to establish in each of us a final idiosyncratic manner of locomotion.

A smoothly performing locomotor system results from the harmonious integration of many components. This final integration does not require that the specific contribution of a single isolated component be identical in every individual, nor must it even be identical within the same individual. The contribution of a single component varies under different circumstances. Type of shoe, amount of fatigue, weight of load carried, and other such variables can cause diminished functioning of some components with compensatory increased functioning of others. An enormous number of variations in the behavior of individual components is possible; however, the diversely functioning components, when integrated, are found to be complementary and will produce smooth bodily progression.

Average values of single anthropometric observations are, in themselves, of little value. The surgeon should be alert to the anthropometric variations that occur within the population, but it is more important for him to understand the functional interrelationships among the various components. This is particularly true in the case of the foot, where anatomic variations are extensive. If average values are the only bases of comparison, it becomes difficult to explain why some feet function adequately and asymptomatically, although their measurements deviate from the average, whereas others function symptomatically, even though their measurements approximate the average. It appears reasonable therefore to use average values only to provide a mathematical reference for demonstrating the extent of possible deviations from these averages. Therefore emphasis will be placed on functional interrelationships and not on descriptive anatomy.

Human locomotion is a learned process; it does not develop as the result of an inborn reflex. This statement is supported by Popova (1935), who studied the changing gait in growing children. The first few steps of an infant holding onto his mother's hand exemplify the learning process necessary to achieve orthograde progression. Scott (1969) of the Canadian National Institute for the Blind noted that congenitally blind children never attempt to stand and walk spontaneously but must be carefully taught. The result of this learning process is the integration of the neuromusculoskeletal mechanisms, with their gross similarities and individual variations, into an adequately functioning system of locomotion. Once a person has learned to walk and has attained maximum growth, a built-in regulatory mechanism is a part of his physiologic makeup and works whether the person is an amputee learning to use a new prosthesis, a long distance runner, or a woman wearing high-heeled shoes.

Ralston (1958) has noted that nature's sole aim with all of us seems to be to achieve a system that will take us from one spot to another with the least expenditure of energy.

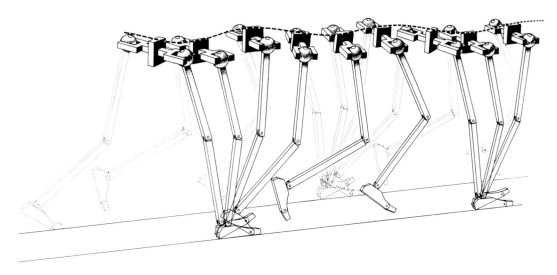

Fig. 1-1. Displacement of center of gravity of body in smooth sinusoidal path. (From Saunders, J.B.C.M., Inman, V.T., and Eberhart, H.D.: J. Bone Joint Surg. **35A:**552, 1953.)

KINEMATICS OF HUMAN LOCOMOTION

Walking is more than merely placing one foot before the other. During walking all major segments of the body are in motion and displacements of the body occur that can be accurately described.

Vertical displacements of the body

The rhythmic upward and downward displacement of the body during walking is familiar to everyone and is particularly noticeable when someone is out of step in a parade. These displacements in the vertical plane are obviously a necessary concomitant of bipedal locomotion. When the legs are separated, as during the period of transmission of the body weight from one leg to the other (double weight bearing), the distance between the trunk and the floor must be less than when it passes over a relatively extended leg as it does during mid-stance. Since the nature of bipedal locomotion demands such vertical oscillations of the body, they should occur in a smooth manner for the conservation of energies. Fig. 1-1 shows that the center of gravity of the body does displace in a smooth sinusoidal path; the amplitude of displacement is approximately 4 to 5 cm (Ryker, 1952; Saunders et al., 1953).

Although movements of the pelvis and hip modify the amplitude of the sinusoidal pathway, the knee, ankle, and foot are particularly involved in converting what would be a series of intersecting arcs into a smooth, sinusoidal curve (Saunders et al., 1953). This conversion requires both simultaneous and precise sequential motions in the knee, ankle, and foot.

The center of gravity of the body reaches its maximum elevation immediately after passage over the weight-bearing leg; it then begins to fall. This fall must be stopped at the termination of the swing phase of the other leg as the heel strikes the ground. If one were forced to walk stiff-kneed and without the foot and ankle, the downward deceleration of the center of gravity at this point would be instantaneous. The body would be subject to a severe jar and the locomotor system would lose kinetic energy. Actually the falling center of gravity of the body is smoothly decelerated, because relative shortening of the leg occurs at the time of impact against a gradually increasing resistance. The knee flexes against a graded contraction of the quadriceps muscle; the ankle plantar flexes against the resisting anterior tibial muscles. After foot-flat position is reached, further shortening is achieved by pronation of the foot to a degree permitted by the ligamentous structures within.

Although the occurrence of this pronatory movement is more important in regard to other functions of the foot, it must be mentioned here because it constitutes an additional factor to that of knee flexion and ankle plantar flexion needed to smoothly decelerate and finally to stop the downward path of the body.

After decelerating to zero, the center of gravity must now evenly accelerate upward to propel it over the opposite leg. The kinetics of this phenomenon are complex, but the kinematics are simple. The leg is relatively elongated by transitory extension of the knee; further plantar flexion of the ankle elevates the heel, and supination of the foot occurs. Elevation of the heel is the major component contributing to upward acceleration of the center of gravity at this time.

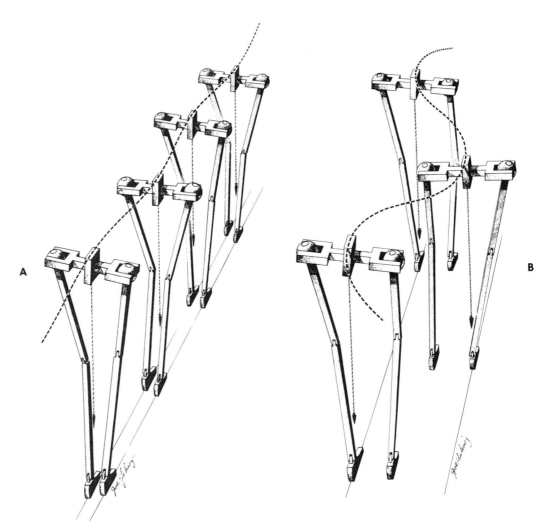

Fig. 1-2. A, Slight lateral displacement of body occurring during walking with feet close together. **B,** Increased lateral displacement of body occurring during walking with feet wide apart. (From Saunders, J.B.C.M., Inman, V.T., and Eberhart, H.D.: J. Bone Joint Surg. **35A:**552, 1953.)

Horizontal displacements of the body

In addition to vertical displacements of the body, a series of axial rotatory movements occur that can be measured in a horizontal plane. Rotations of the pelvis and the shoulder girdle are familiar to any observant person. Similar horizontal rotations occur in the femoral and tibial segments of the extremities. The tibias rotate about their long axes—internally during swing phase and into the first part of stance phase and externally during the latter part of stance. This motion continues until the toes leave the ground; the degree of these rotations is subject to marked individual variations. Levens et al. (1948), in a study of a series of 12 male subjects, recorded the minimum amount of horizontal rotation of the tibia in space at 13° and the maximum at 25° with an average of 19°. A great portion of this rotation occurs when the foot is firmly placed on the floor; the shoe normally does not slip but remains fixed. The

rotations, however, generate a torque of 7 to 8 newton-meters, which is one of considerable magnitude (Cunningham, 1950).

For these movements to occur, a mechanism must exist in the foot that will permit the rotations but will offer resistance to them of a magnitude such that they will be transmitted through the foot to the floor and will be recorded on the force plate as torques. The ankle and subtalar joints are such mechanisms and will be described.

Lateral displacements of the body

When a person is walking, his body does not remain precisely in the plane of progression but oscillates slightly from side to side to keep the center of gravity approximately over the weight-bearing foot. Everyone has experienced this lateral shift of the body with each step but may not have consciously appreciated its

Vertical force

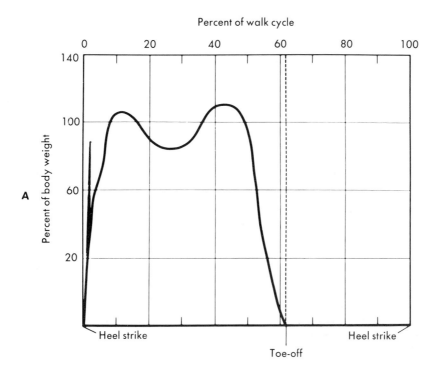

Forward-aft shear

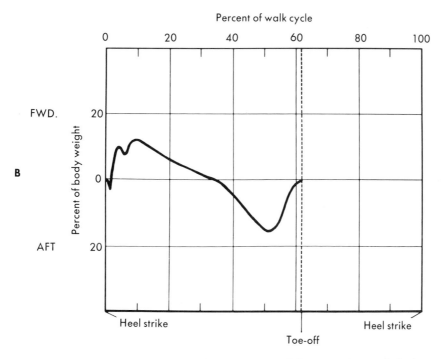

Fig. 1-3. Ground reaction to walking. A, Vertical force. B, Fore-and-aft shear.
Continued.

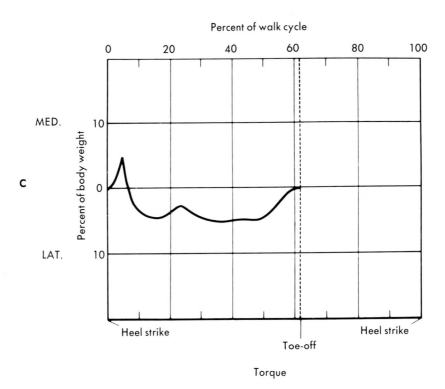

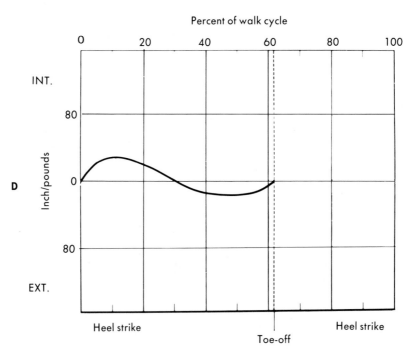

Fig. 1-3, cont'd. C, Medial and lateral shear. **D,** Torque.

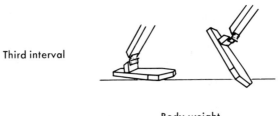

Third interval

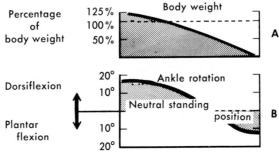

Fig. 1-8. Composite of all events of third interval of walking or period extending from foot flat to toe-off.

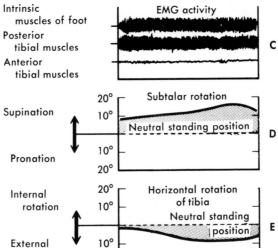

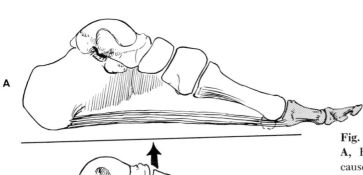

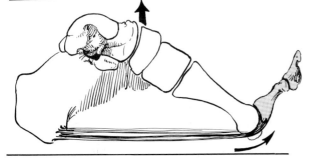

Fig. 1-9. Diagrammatic representation of "windlass action." **A,** Foot flat. **B,** Increased tension of plantar aponeurosis caused by dorsiflexion of the toes with resultant elevation of longitudinal arch.

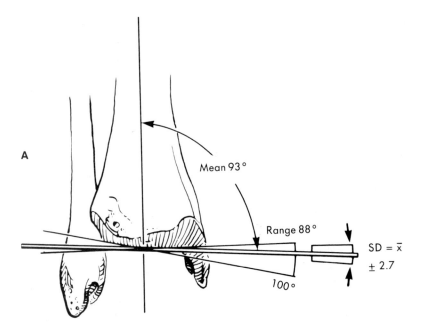

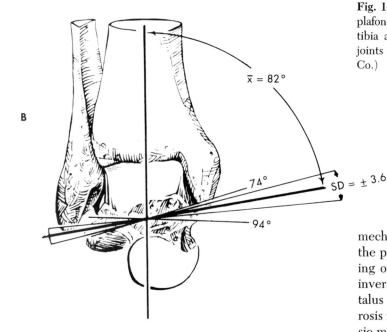

Fig. 1-10. **A,** Variations in angle between midline of tibia and plafond of mortise. **B,** Variations in angle between midline of tibia and empirical axis of ankle. (From Inman, V.T.: The joints of the ankle, Baltimore, 1976, The Williams & Wilkins Co.)

course there is muscle function occurring above, and the intrinsic muscles are likewise active, but the mechanism of the plantar aponeurosis appears to be the strongest and most dynamic mechanism bringing about stabilization of the arch.

During this third interval of the stance phase the foot is converted from the flexible structure that was present during the first interval and the partially stabilized foot that was present in the second interval into a rigid arch. The following is a summary of the mechanisms by which this stability has been achieved. Most of these mechanisms occur simultaneously to produce this stability. Starting proximally and proceeding distally, the

mechanisms comprise the external rotation of the tibia, the progressive inversion of the subtalar joint, the locking of the transverse tarsal joint brought about by the inversion of the subtalar joint, the seating of the convex talus into the concave navicular, the plantar aponeurosis functioning as a windlass, the activity of the intrinsic muscles of the foot, and the function of the extrinsic muscles of the foot.

AXES OF ROTATION
Ankle joint

It is easy to visualize that the direction of the ankle axis in the transverse plane of the leg will dictate the vertical plane in which the foot will flex and extend. In the clinical literature this plane of ankle motion in relation to the sagittal plane of the leg is referred to by orthopaedists as the degree of tibial torsion and by podiatrists as malleolar torsion. Although it is common knowledge that the ankle axis is directed laterally and posteriorly as projected on the transverse plane of the

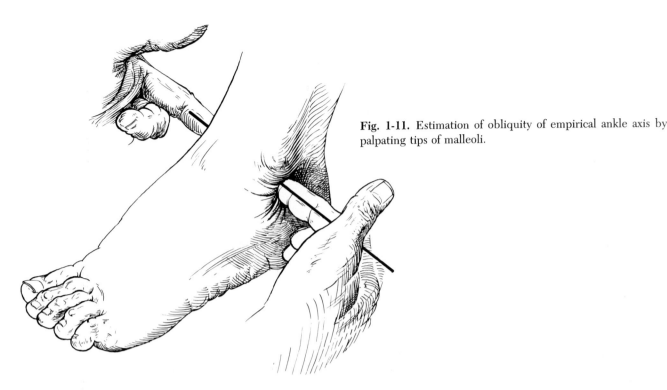

Fig. 1-11. Estimation of obliquity of empirical ankle axis by palpating tips of malleoli.

leg, it is not widely appreciated that the ankle axis is also directed laterally and downward as seen in the coronal plane. Inman (1976), in anthropometric studies, found that in the coronal plane the axis of the ankle may deviate 88° to 100° from the vertical axis of the leg (Fig. 1-10, *A*). Since the axis of the ankle passes just distal to the tip of each malleolus, the examiner should be able to obtain a reasonably accurate estimate of the position of the empirical axis by placing the ends of his index fingers at the most distal bony tips of the malleoli (Fig. 1-10, *B* and 1-11).

A horizontal axis that remains normal to the vertical axis of the leg can affect only the amount of toeing out or toeing in of the foot; no rotatory influence can be imposed in a transverse plane on either the foot or the leg during flexion and extension of the ankle. However, since the ankle joint axis is an obliquely oriented axis, it allows horizontal rotations to occur in the foot or the leg with movements of the ankle.

These rotations are clearly depicted in Figs. 1-12 and 1-13. With the foot free and the leg fixed, the oblique ankle joint axis causes the foot to deviate outward on dorsiflexion and inward on plantar flexion. The projection of the foot onto the transverse plane, as shown by the shadows in the sketches, reveals the extent of this external and internal rotation of the foot (Fig. 1-12). The amount of this rotation will vary with the obliquity of the ankle axis and the amount of dorsiflexion and plantar flexion.

With the foot fixed on the ground during midstance,

the body passing over the foot produces dorsiflexion of the foot relative to the leg (Fig. 1-13). The oblique ankle axis then imposes an internal rotation on the leg (Levens et al., 1948). Again, the degree of internal rotation of the leg on the foot will depend on the amount of dorsiflexion and the obliquity of the ankle axis. As the heel rises in preparaton for lift-off, the ankle is plantar flexed. This in turn reverses the horizontal rotation, causing the leg to rotate externally.

When the horizontal rotations of the leg are studied independently, the foregoing sequence of events can be seen to be precisely what occurs in human locomotion. The lower part of the leg rotates internally during the first third and externally during the last two thirds of stance. The average amount of this rotation is 19°, within a range of 13° to 25° (Levens et al., 1948). The recording of torques imposed on a force plate substantiates these rotations. Magnitudes vary from individual to individual but range from 7 to 8 newton-meters (Cunningham, 1950).

In summary, the oblique ankle axis produces the following series of events: from the instant of heel contact to the time the foot is flat, plantar flexion occurs and the foot appears to toe in. The more oblique the axis, the more apparent will be the toeing in. During midstance, the foot is fixed on the ground; relative dorsiflexion, with resulting internal rotation of the leg, occurs as the leg passes over the foot. As the heel rises, plantar flexion takes place and causes external rotation of the leg.

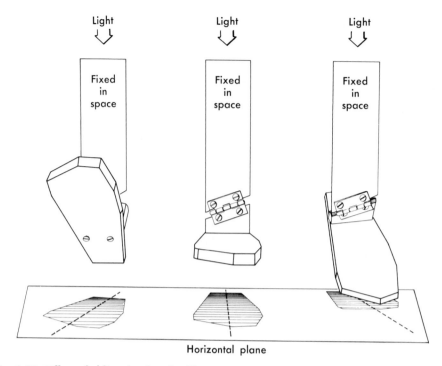

Fig. 1-12. Effect of obliquely placed ankle axis on rotation of foot in horizontal plane during plantar flexion and dorsiflexion, with foot free. Displacement is reflected in shadows of foot.

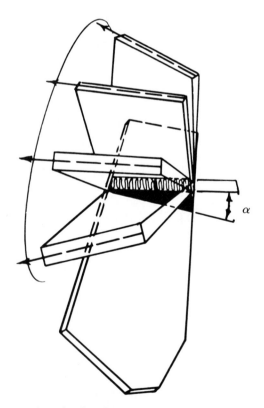

Fig. 1-13. Foot fixed to floor. Plantar flexion and dorsiflexion of ankle produce horizontal rotation of leg because of obliquity of ankle axis.

Rotations of the leg and movements of the foot caused by an oblique ankle axis, when observed independently, are seen to be qualitatively and temporarily in agreement. However, when the magnitudes of the various displacements are studied, irreconcilable disparities are evident. In normal locomotion ankle motion ranges from 20° to 36°, with an average of 24° (Berry, 1952; Ryker, 1952). The obliquity of the ankle axis ranges from 88° to 100° with an average of 93° from the vertical (Inman, 1979). Even in the most oblique axis and movement of the ankle through the maximum range of 36°, only 11° of rotation of the leg around a vertical axis will occur. This is less than the average amount of horizontal rotation of the leg as measured independently in normal walking. The average obliquity of the ankle, together with the average amount of dorsiflexion and plantar flexion, would yield values for the horizontal rotation of the leg that were much smaller than the degree of horizontal rotation of the leg that actually occurs while the foot remains stationary on the floor and is carrying the superincumbent body weight.

Subtalar joint

It is necessary to examine other articulations in the foot that could, in cooperation with the ankle, allow the leg to undergo the additional amount of internal and external rotation. The mechanism that appears to be

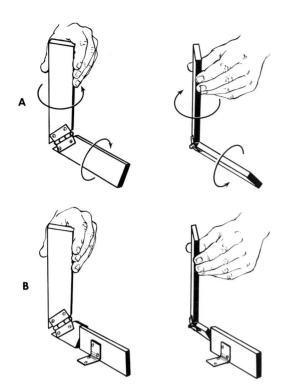

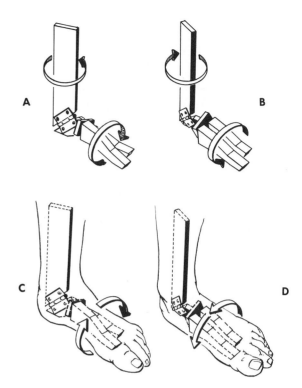

Fig. 1-14. Simple mechanism demonstrating functional relationships. **A,** Action of mitered hinge. **B,** Addition of pivot between two segments of mechanism.

Fig. 1-15. Distal portion of horizontal member replaced by two structures. **A** and **B,** Mechanical analog of principal components of foot. **C** and **D,** Mechanical components inserted into foot and leg.

admirably designed for this very function is the subtalar joint.

The subtalar joint is a single-axis joint that acts like a mitered hinge connecting the talus and the calcaneus. The direction of its axis is backward, downward, and lateral (Close and Inman, 1953; Manter, 1941). Individual variations are extensive and imply variations in the behavior of this joint during locomotion. Furthermore, the subtalar joint appears to be a determinative joint of the foot influencing the performance of the more distal articulations and modifying the forces imposed on the skeletal and soft tissues. Therefore we must understand the anatomic and functional aspects of this joint.

Based on the anatomic fact that the subtalar joint moves around a single inclined axis and functions essentially like a hinge connecting the talus and the calcaneus, the functional relationships that result from such a mechanical arrangement are easily illustrated. Fig. 1-14, *A,* shows two boards jointed by a hinge. If the axis of the hinge is at 45°, a simple torque converter has been created. Rotation of the vertical member causes equal rotation of the horizontal member. Changing the angle of the hinge will alter this one-to-one relationship. A more horizontally placed hinge will cause a greater rotation of the horizontal member for each degree of rotation of the vertical member; the reverse

holds true if the hinge is placed more vertically. In Fig. 1-14, *B,* to prevent the entire horizontal segment from participating in the rotatory displacement, the horizontal member has been divided into a short proximal and a long distal segment with a pivot in between. Thus the distal segment remains stationary while only the short segment adjacent to the hinge rotates.

To approach more closely the true anatomic situation of the human foot, in Fig. 1-15, *A* and *B,* the distal portion of the horizontal member has been replaced by two structures. The medial represents the three medial rays of the foot that articulate through the cuneiforms to the talus; the lateral represents the two lateral rays that articulate through the cuboid to the calcaneus. In Fig. 1-15, *C* and *D,* the entire mechanism has been placed into the leg and foot to demonstrate the mechanical linkages resulting in specific movements in the leg and foot. External rotation of the leg causes inversion of the heel, elevation of the medial side of the foot, and depression of the lateral side. Internal rotation of the leg produces the opposite effect on the foot.

Interestingly, in persons with flat feet the axis of the subtalar joint is more horizontal than in persons with "normal" feet; therefore the same amount of rotation of the leg imposes a greater supinatory and pronatory effect on the foot. This may partially explain why some individuals with asymptomatic and flexible pes planus break down their shoes and frequently prefer to go without shoes, which they find restrictive. Furthermore, people with asymptomatic flat feet usually show a greater range of subtalar motion than do persons with "normal" feet. The reverse holds true for people with pes cavus; in them, one is often surprised at the generalized rigidity of the foot and the limited motion in the subtalar joint. According to Wright et al. (1964) the range of motion in the subtalar joint during walking is approximately 6° for a normal foot and 12° for a flat foot. It is also interesting to note that the phasic activity of the intrinsic muscles of the foot seems to correlate fairly closely with the degree of subtalar joint rotation. It is noted that in a normal person the intrinsic muscles become active at about 30% of the walking cycle, whereas in an individual with flatfoot they become active during the first 15% of the walking cycle.

Transverse tarsal articulation

The calcaneocuboid and the talonavicular articulations together are often considered to make up the transverse tarsal articulation. Each possesses some independent motion and has been subjected to intensive study (Elftman, 1960). However, from a functional standpoint they perform together. In most textbooks of anatomy, movement is described as if the foot did not bear the weight of the body. The following statement is illustrative: Movement in the transverse tarsal articulation "consists of a sort of rotation by means of which the foot may be slightly flexed or extended, the sole being at the same time carried medially (inverted) or laterally (everted)."*

Actually, the importance of the transverse tarsal articulation lies not in its axes of motion while non-weight-bearing but in how it behaves during the stance phase of motion when the foot is required to support the body weight. Some specific changes occur in the amount of motion sustained by the transverse tarsal articulation with the forefoot fixed and the heel everted or inverted. Everting the heel produces relative pronation of the foot; varying amounts of flexion and extension in the sagittal plane, adduction and abduction in the transverse plane, and rotation between the forefoot and the heel now occur. The examiner gets the impression that the midfoot has become "unlocked" and that maximum motion is possible in the transverse tarsal articulation. However, if the forefoot is held firmly in one hand, something happens in the transverse tarsal artic-

---

*Goss, C.M., editor: Gray's anatomy, ed. 28, Philadelphia, 1970, Lea & Febiger, p. 368.

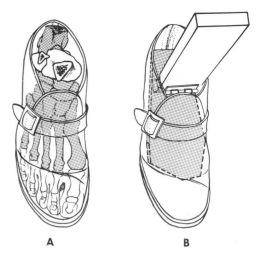

Fig. 1-16. Diagrammatic illustration of location of oblique metatarsophalangeal crease. **A,** Skeletal foot in shoe. **B,** Wooden mechanism in shoe.

ulation to make it appear "locked." The previously elicited motions all become suppressed and the midfoot becomes rigid (Fig. 1-7).

The mechanisms that might produce this dramatic change from flexibility to rigidity in the midfoot have not been adequately studied. Elftman (1960) has described one such mechanism, but others may exist that are as yet unidentified. In any case, inversion of the heel in the normal foot promptly occurs as weight is transferred from heel to forefoot when a person rises on his toes. As previously mentioned, such inversion of the heel causes the midfoot to convert from a mobile structure to a rigid lever. The reorientation of the skeletal components is the result of the function of the plantar aponeurosis, activity in the intrinsic and extrinsic muscles of the foot, the ligamentous structures, and the rotation imparted to the foot by the leg.

Metatarsophalangeal break

After wearing a new pair of shoes for a while, one notices the appearance of an oblique crease in the area overlying the metatarsophalangeal articulation (Fig. 1-16). Its obliquity is, of course, a result of the unequal forward extension of the metatarsals. The head of the second metatarsal is the most distal head; that of the fifth metatarsal is the most proximal. Although the first metatarsal is usually shorter than the second (because the first metatarsal head is slightly elevated and is supported by the two sesamoids), it often functionally approximates the length of the second.

When the heel is elevated during standing or at the time of lift-off, the weight of the body is normally shared by all the metatarsal heads. To achieve this fair division of the body weight among the metatarsals, the

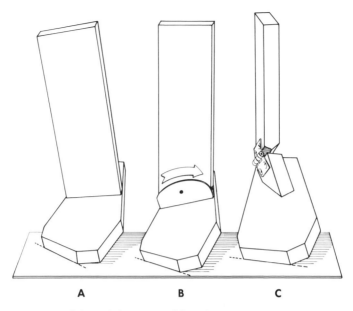

Fig. 1-17. Supination and lateral deviation of foot during raising of heel caused by oblique metatarsophalangeal break. **A,** Wooden mechanism without articulaton. If no articulation were present, leg would also deviate laterally. **B,** Wooden mechanism with articulation. Leg remains vertical; hence some type of articulaton must exist beween foot and leg. **C,** Articulation similar to that of subtalar joint. Fortunately, in addition to its other complex functions, subtalar joint also functions to permit leg to remain vertical.

foot must supinate slightly and deviate laterally. The oblique crease in the shoe gives evidence that these motions occur with every step. It has been demonstrated that the angle between the metatarsophalangeal break and the long axis of the foot may vary from 50° to 70° (Isman and Inman, 1969). Obviously, the more oblique the metatarsophalangeal break the more the foot must supinate and deviate laterally.

If the leg and foot acted as a single rigid member without ankle, subtalar, or transverse tarsal articulations, the metatarsophalangeal break would cause lateral inclination and external rotation of the leg (Fig. 1-17, A). However, to permit the leg to remain in a vertical plane during walking, an articulation must be provided between leg and foot (Fig. 1-17, B). Such an articulation is supplied by the subtalar joint (Fig. 1-17, C). Because of its anatomic arrangement, it is ideally suited to permit the foot to respond to the supinatory forces exerted by the oblique metatarsophalangeal break and still allow the leg to remain in a vertical plane.

All the essential mechanisms discussed in this chapter are pictorially summarized in Fig. 1-18. The two lower photographs were taken with the subject standing on a barograph; they reveal the distribution of pressure between the foot and the weight-bearing surface. (A barograph records reflected light through a transparent plastic platform; the intensity of the light is roughly proportionate to the pressure the foot imposes on the plate.)

In Fig. 1-18, A, the subject was asked to stand with muscles relaxed. Note that the leg is moderately rotated internally and the heel is slightly everted (in valgus position). The body weight is placed on the heel, the outer side of the foot, and the metatarsal heads.

In Fig. 1-18, B, the subject was asked to rise on his toes. Note that the leg is now externally rotated, the heel is inverted (in varus position), and the longitudinal arch is elevated. The weight is concentrated on the metatarsal heads and is equally shared by the metatarsal heads and the toes.

Even though such movements cannot be illustrated pictorially, it is easy to imagine the contraction of the intrinsic and extrinsic muscles that is necessary to stabilize the foot and ankle as the subject transfers the body weight to the forefoot and raises the heel. It should also be recalled that dorsiflexion of the toes tightens the plantar aponeurosis and assists in the inversion of the heel. The supinatory twist activates the "locking" mechanism in the foot, thus converting a flexible foot (Fig. 1-18, A) into a rigid lever (Fig. 1-18, B), an action that is necessary at lift-off.

Weight distribution on the plantar aspect of the foot

The distribution of weight on the plantar aspect of the foot has been demonstrated in many ways. The

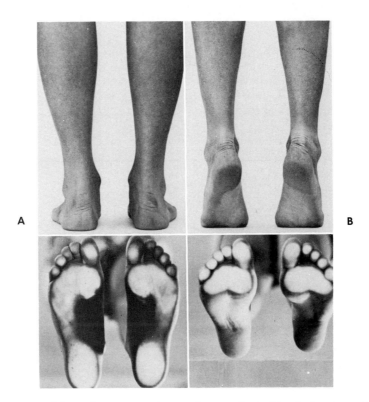

Fig. 1-18. Feet and legs of person standing on barograph. **A,** Weight bearing with muscles relaxed. **B,** Rising on toes.

work of Elftman (1934) using a barograph gives a good visual impression about the distribution of weight on the plantar aspect of the foot during a normal step (Fig. 1-19). Using a force plate gives us data regarding the location of the center of pressure on the plantar aspect of the foot. This type of data gives an average of the various pressures on the bottom of the foot as opposed to the barograph, which gives us a better picture of the overall distribution of weight bearing on the plantar aspect of the foot. Using newer techniques, Clark (1980) has graphically demonstrated the distribution of forces on the plantar aspect of the foot in such a way that one obtains a more quantitative visual concept of the weight distribution on the plantar aspect of the foot (Fig. 1-20).

MECHANICS OF RUNNING

In these times, with increased attention being given to athletics and to running in particular, it is essential for the physician to have a basic knowledge of the mechanics that occur during running. The same basic mechanisms that have been described thus far, insofar as the biomechanics of the foot and ankle are concerned, are not significantly altered during running. The same stabilization mechanism within the foot occurs during running as during walking. The major differences observed during running are that the gait cycle

is altered considerably, the amount of force generated—as measured by force-plate data—is markedly increased, the range of motion of the joints of the lower extremities is increased, and the phasic activity of the muscles of the lower extremities is altered. The changes that occur in the gait cycle are illustrated in Fig. 1-21. During walking one foot is always in contact with the ground; as the speed of gait increases, a float phase is incorporated into the gait cycle, during which time both feet are off the ground. There is also no longer a period of double limb support. It is noted that as the speed of gait continues to increase, the time the foot spends on the ground, both in real time and in percentage of cycle, decreases considerably.

The forces involved during running are considerable, as previously demonstrated in Fig. 1-4. The displacement of the center of gravity increases as the speed of gait increases, and the forces generated are in large part related to this. The main function of the body at the time of initial ground contact is that of absorption of these forces. This is carried out by increasing the range of motion at the ankle, knee, and hip joints. As the speed of gait further increases, the degree of motion in these joints also increases to help absorb the added impact.

Along with this increase in the range of motion and in the forces generated during running, the muscle

Hindfoot alignment

When a subtalar joint is fused, the transverse rotation that occurs in the lower extremity will be partially absorbed in the ankle joint, since it can no longer pass through the subtalar joint into the foot. The varus or valgus tilt of the subtalar joint will affect the position of the forefoot, so accurate alignment is essential. If the subtalar joint is placed into too much varus tilt, the forefoot will be rotated into supination, and the weight-bearing line of the extremity will then pass laterally to the calcaneus and fifth metatarsal. This results in increased stress on the lateral collateral ligament structure and abnormal weight bearing along the lateral aspect of the foot. This position also holds the forefoot in a semirigid position so that the patient either has to vault over it or place the foot in external rotation to roll over the medial aspect.

The position of choice is a valgus tilt of about 5° in the subtalar joint, since this permits satisfactory stability of the ankle joint, and the weight-bearing line of the body will pass medially to the calcaneus, and therefore no stress will be placed on the lateral collateral ligament structure. This position results in slight pronation of the forefoot, which permits an even distribution of weight on the plantar aspect of the foot. The slight valgus position also allows the forefoot to remain flexible, so that the body can easily pass over it.

Midfoot alignment

When surgical stabilization of the transverse tarsal joint or one of its components (talonavicular or calcaneocuboid) is carried out, motion in the entire joint system is eliminated. Motion of the subtalar joint directly affects the stability of the foot through its control of the transverse tarsal joint. When the subtalar joint is in valgus position in response to internal rotation of the lower extremity, the transverse tarsal joint is unlocked and the forefoot is flexible. Conversely, when the subtalar joint is inverted in response to external rotation of the lower extremity, the transverse tarsal joint is locked and the forefoot is fairly rigid. Because of the role the transverse tarsal joint plays in controlling the forefoot, it is essential that the foot be placed in a plantigrade position when the joints are stabilized. If the foot is placed into too much supination, the medial border of the foot is elevated and undue stress is placed on the lateral aspect of the foot. It also creates a rigid forefoot. The position of choice is neutral rotation or slight pronation, which ensures a flexible plantigrade foot.

When a triple arthrodesis is carried out, the position of choice is 5° of valgus for the subtalar joint and neutral rotation of the transverse tarsal joint. It should be emphasized, however, that it is better to err on the side of too much valgus and pronation to keep the weight-bearing line medial to the calcaneus, since that produces a flexible plantigrade foot. When carrying out a plantar arthrodesis the same basic principles apply.

Surgical stabilization of the intertarsal and tarsometatarsal joints can be carried out with minimum loss of function or increased stress on the other joints in the foot. The intertarsal joints that are distal to the transverse tarsal joint and proximal to the metatarsophalangeal joints have little or no motion between them.

Forefoot principles

Removal of the base of the proximal phalanx of the great toe results in instability of the medial longitudinal arch due to disruption of the plantar aponeurosis and the windlass mechanism. This results in decreased weight bearing of the first metatarsal head, which results in weight being transferred to the lesser metatarsal heads. If the base of the proximal phalanx of one of the lesser toes is removed, a similar problem of instability will occur but to a much lesser degree, particularly moving laterally across the foot. Conversely, resection of the metatarsal head, except in severe disease states such as rheumatoid arthritis, results in a similar problem because the windlass mechanism is destroyed as a result of the relative shortening of the ray. This will again cause increased stress and callus formation beneath the adjacent metatarsal head, which is subjected to increased weight bearing.

When carrying out an arthrodesis of the first metatarsophalangeal joint for such conditions as hallux rigidus, recurrent hallux valgus, or degenerative arthritis, the alignment of the arthrodesis site is critical. The metatarsophalangeal joint should be placed into approximately 10° to 15° of valgus and 15° to 25° of dorsiflexion in relation to the first metatarsal shaft. The degree of dorsiflexion is dependent to a certain extent on the heel height of the shoe that the patient desires to wear. An arthrodesis of the first metatarsophalangeal joint has a minimum effect on the patient's gait. The arthrodesis places an increased stress on the interphalangeal joint of the hallux. This increased stress may result in degenerative changes over a period of time, but these rarely become symptomatic. From a theoretical standoint increased stress is placed on the first metatarsocuneiform joint following arthrodesis of the metatarsophalangeal joint, but it is unusual to see any form of degenerative change occur.

An isolated arthrodesis of the interphalangeal joint of the great toe does not seem to have any significant effect on the biomechanics of gait. An arthrodesis of the proximal and distal interphalangeal joints of the lesser toes also does not seem to change the gait biomechanics.

Resection of a single sesamoid for a pathologic con-

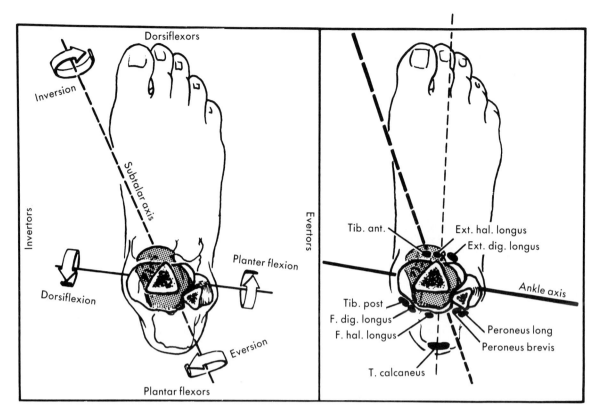

Fig. 1-26. Left-hand diagram demonstrates rotation that occurs about subtalar and ankle axes. Right-hand drawing demonstrates relationship of various muscles about subtalar and ankle axes. (From Mann, R.A.: Biomechanics of the foot. In American Academy of Orthopaedic Surgeons: Atlas of orthotics, St. Louis, 1975, The C.V. Mosby Co.)

dition such as a fracture, avascular necrosis, or intractable plantar keratosis may be done with relative impunity. If, however, one sesamoid has already been removed, the second sesamoid should not be removed because of risk of a cock-up deformity of the metatarsophalangeal joint. This occurs because the intrinsic muscle insertion into the proximal phalanx of the great toe encompasses the sesamoids, and when the sesamoid is removed, this insertion is impaired to a varying degree. If adequate intrinsic function is not present, then flexion of the proximal phalanx cannot be brought about, and the cock-up deformity results.

Tendon transfers

When evaluating a patient for muscle weakness or loss about the foot and ankle, the diagram in Fig. 1-26 can be most useful. It demonstrates the motion that occurs around each joint axis and the location of the muscles in relation to the axes. By considering the muscles in relation to the axes, it is possible to carefully note which muscles are functioning and thereby figure out which muscles might be transferred to rebalance the foot and ankle. Generally speaking, if inadequate

strength is present to balance the foot adequately, it is important to establish adequate plantar flexion function over that of dorsiflexion; an equinus gait is not as disabling as a calcaneal-type gait. One should also keep in mind that it is much more difficult to retrain a muscle that has been a stance phase muscle to become a swing phase muscle than retraining a swing phase muscle to become a stance phase muscle. Therefore, if possible, an in phase muscle transfer will produce a more satisfactory result, since no phase conversion is necessary.

BIOMECHANICS OF THE LIGAMENTS OF THE ANKLE JOINT

The configuration and alignment of the ligamentous structures of the ankle are such that they permit free movement of the ankle and subtalar joints to occur simultaneously. Since the configuration of the trochlear surface of the talus is curved in such a manner to produce a cone-shaped articulation whose apex is directed medially, the single fan-shaped deltoid ligament is adequate to provide stability to the medial side of the ankle joint (Fig. 1-27). On the lateral aspect of the ankle joint, however, where there is a larger area to be cov-

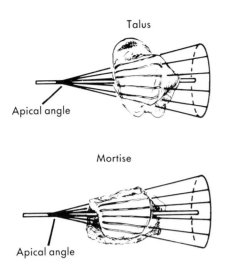

Talus

Apical angle

Mortise

Apical angle

Fig. 1-27. Curvature of trochlear surface of talus creates cone whose apex is based medially. From this configuration one can observe that deltoid ligament is well suited to function along medial side of ankle joint, whereas laterally, where more rotation is occurring, three separate ligaments are necessary. (From Inman, V.T.: The joints of the ankle, Baltimore, 1976, The Williams & Wilkins Co.)

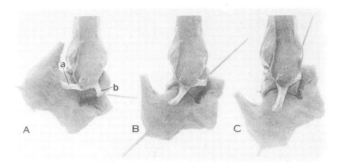

Fig. 1-28. Calcaneal fibular ligament (*a*) and anterior talofibular ligament (*b*) are shown. **A,** In plantar flexion anterior talofibular ligament is in line with fibula and is providing most of support to lateral aspect of ankle joint. **B,** In neutral position of ankle joint both anterior talofibular and calcaneofibular ligaments provide support to joint. Relationship of calcaneofibular ligament to subtalar joint axis, which is depicted in the background, is noted. Note that this ligament and axis are parallel to each other. **C,** In dorsiflexion calcaneofibular ligament is in line with fibula and provides support to lateral aspect of ankle joint. (From Inman, V.T.: The joints of the ankle, Baltimore, 1976, The Williams & Wilkins Co.)

ered by a ligamentous structure, the ligament is divided into three bands. These ligaments are the anterior talofibular and posterior talofibular ligaments and the calcaneofibular ligament. The relationship of these ligaments to each other and to the axes of the subtalar and ankle joints must always be considered carefully when these joints are examined or ligamentous surgery is contemplated.

Fig. 1-28 demonstrates the anterior talofibular and calcaneofibular ligaments in relation to the subtalar joint axis. It is noted that the calcaneofibular ligament is parallel to the subtalar joint axis in the sagittal plane. As the ankle joint is dorsiflexed and planter flexed, this relationship between the calcaneofibular ligament and the subtalar joint axis does not change. It should be further noted that the calcaneofibular ligament crosses both the ankle and subtalar joint. This ligament is constructed to permit motion to occur in both of these joints simultaneously. It is important to appreciate that when the ankle joint is in neutral position the calcaneofibular ligament is angulated posteriorly, but as the ankle joint is brought into more dorsiflexion, the calcaneofibular ligament is then brought into line with the fibula, thereby becoming a true collateral ligament. Conversely, as the ankle joint is brought into plantar flexion, the calcaneofibular ligament becomes horizontal in relation to the ground. In this position it provides little or no stability insofar as resisting inversion stress. The anterior talofibular ligament on the other hand is brought into line with the fibula when the ankle

joint is plantar flexed, thereby acting as a collateral ligament. When the ankle joint is brought up into dorsiflexion, the anterior talofibular ligament becomes sufficiently horizontal so that it does not function as a collateral ligament. It can thus be appreciated that, depending on the position of the ankle joint, either the calcaneofibular or the anterior talofibular ligament will be a true collateral ligament with regard to providing stability to the lateral side of the ankle joint.

The relationship between these two ligaments has been quantified and is presented in Fig. 1-29. This demonstrates the relationship of the angle produced by the calcaneofibular and the anterior talofibular ligaments to one another. The average angle in the sagittal plane is approximately 105°, although there is considerable variation from 70° to 140°. The significance of this is important because from a clinical standpoint it probably explains why some individuals have laxity of their collateral ligaments. If we assume that when the ankle is in full dorsiflexion the calcaneofibular ligament is providing most of the stability and in full plantar flexion the anterior talofibular ligament is providing stability, then as we pass from dorsiflexion to plantar flexion and back there will be a certain period of time in which neither ligament is truly functioning as a collateral ligament. If we assume an average angle of approximately 105° between these ligaments, then generally speaking an area in which an insufficient lateral collateral ligament is present is unusual, whereas if we have a range of 130° to 140° angulation between these two ligaments,

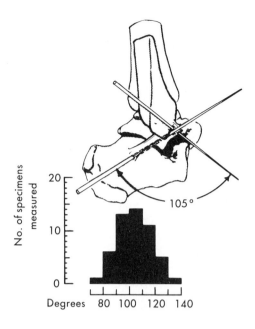

Fig. 1-29. Averge angle between calcaneofibular and talofibular ligaments in sagittal plane is shown. Although average angle is 105°, there is considerable variation from 70° to 140°. (From Inman, V.T.: The joints of the ankle, Baltimore, 1976, The Williams & Wilkins Co.)

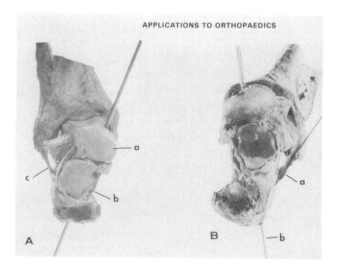

Fig. 1-30. A, Anterior view of the transverse tarsal joint. Head of talus (*A*). Head of calcaneus (*B*). Calcaneofibular ligament (*C*). Rod passing through head of talus and exiting on lateral aspect of calcaneus demonstrates axis of subtalar joint. **B,** Same specimen is viewed from below. Kirschner wire has now been placed through fibers of calcaneofibular ligament (*a*). Note direction of ligament extending from malleolus to lateral side of calcaneus. (From Inman, V.T.: The joints of the ankle, Baltimore, 1976, The Williams & Wilkins Co.)

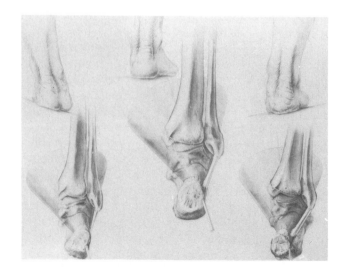

Fig. 1-31. Functional arrangement of calcaneofibular ligament. This drawing represents concept that explains mechanism in which free motion is permitted in the subtalar joint without restriction by calcaneofibular ligament. Imaginary cone has been drawn around axis of subtalar joint. Calcaneofibular ligament is shown converging from its fibular attachment to calcaneus. Since the ligament lies on surface of cone whose apex is point of intersection of functional extensions of ligament and axis of subtalar joint, motion of calcaneus under talus is allowed without undue restriction from ligament, which is merely displaced over surface of cone. (From Inman, V.T.: The joints of the ankle, Baltimore, 1976, The Williams & Wilkins Co.)

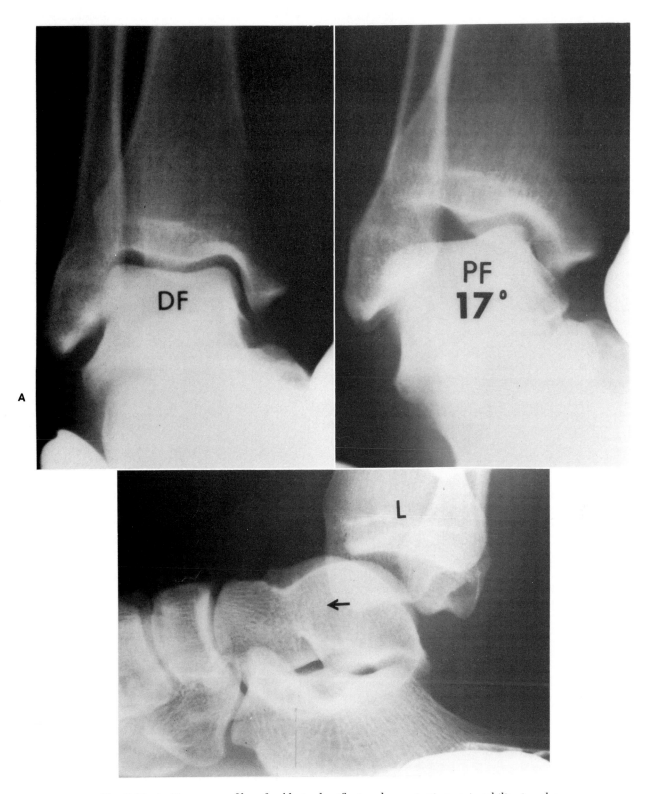

Fig. 1-32. A, Stress x-ray film of ankle in dorsiflexion demonstrating no instability in calcaneofibular ligament. Same ankle stressed in plantar flexion demonstrates loss of stability caused by disruption of anterior talofibular ligament. Note anterior subluxation that is present when this ligament is torn.   *Continued.*

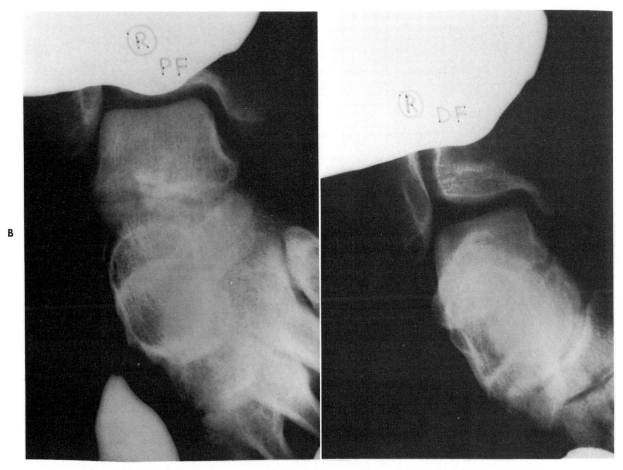

Fig. 1-32, cont'd. B, Stress x-ray film of ankle in plantar flexion demonstrating no ligamentous instability. Same ankle stressed in dorsiflexion demonstrates laxity of calcaneofibular ligament. **C,** Stress x-ray film of ankle joint in dorsiflexion, plantar flexion, and anteriorly all demonstrate evidence of ligamentous disruption. This indicates complete tear of lateral collateral ligament structure.

then there is a significant interval while the ankle is passing from dorsiflexion to plantar flexion and back in which neither ligament is functioning as a collateral ligament, and this may be the reason that some individuals might be susceptible to chronic ankle sprains. Some patients who are thought to have ligamentous laxity may in reality possess this anatomic configuration of their lateral collateral ligaments.

The other factor that needs to be considered is the relationship of the calcaneofibular ligament to subtalar joint motion. Motion in the subtalar joint occurs about an axis that deviates from medial to lateral as it passes from dorsal to a plantarward direction. Fig. 1-30 demonstrates the position of the subtalar joint axis in relation to a cadaver specimen. If a probe is now placed along the calcaneofibular ligament, it is noted that a V- or cone-shaped arc has been created. It is this cone-shaped arc of motion that permits the calcaneofibular

ligament to move in such a way to prevent restriction of subtalar joint or ankle joint motion (Fig. 1-31). This relationship of the calcaneofibular ligament to the ankle and subtalar joint axes is critical when contemplating ligamentous reconstruction, since any ligament reconstruction that fails to take this normal anatomic configuration into consideration will result in a situation in which motion in one or both of these joints will be restricted.

From a clinical standpoint when one is evaluating the stability of the lateral collateral ligament structure, the ankle joint should be tested in dorsiflexion to demonstrate the competency of the calcaneofibular ligament and in plantar flexion to test the competency of the anterior talofibular ligament. If both ligaments are completely disrupted, then there will be no stability in either position. Furthermore, to test for stability of the anterior talofibular ligament an anterior drawer sign

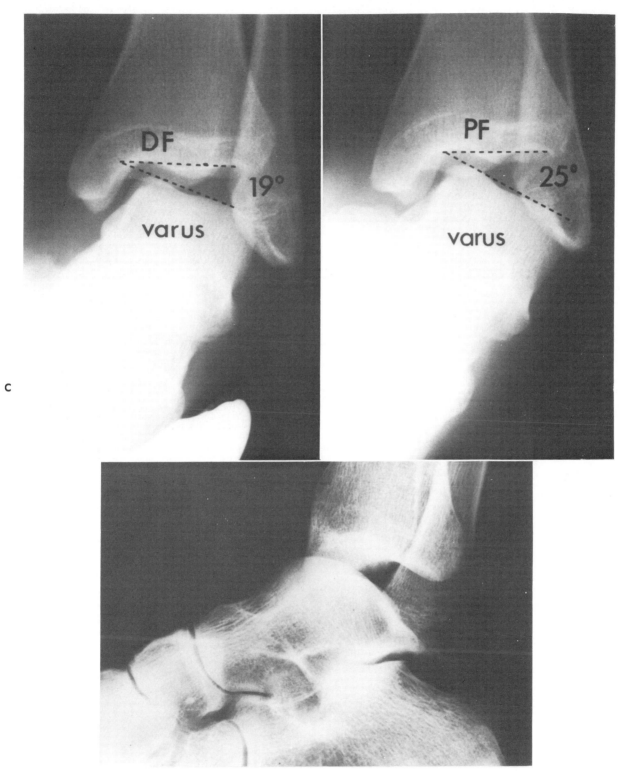

Fig. 1-32, cont'd. For legend see opposite page.

should be carried out, which is performed with the ankle joint in neutral position, at which time the anterior talofibular ligament should be in a position to resist anterior displacement of the talus from the ankle mortise (Fig. 1-32).

REFERENCES

Abbott, B.C., Bigland, B., and Ritchie, J.M.: The physiological cost of negative work, J. Physiol. (Lond.) **117:**380, 1952.

Asmussen, E.: Positive and negative muscular work, Acta Physiol. Scand. **28:**364, 1953.

Banister, E.W., and Brown, S.R.: The relative energy requirements of physical activity. In Falls, H.B., editor: Exercise physiology, New York, 1968, Academic Press, Inc.

Berry, F.R., Jr.: Angle variation patterns of normal hip, knee and ankle in different operations, Univ. Calif. Prosthet. Devices Res. Rep., Ser. 11, issue 21, February 1952.

Bresler, B., and Berry, F.R.: Energy and power in the leg during normal level walking, Univ. Calif. Prosthet. Devices Res. Rep., Ser. 11, issue 15, May 1951.

Clarke, T.E.: The pressure distribution under the foot during barefoot walking, doctoral dissertation, University Park, Pa., 1980, Pennsylvania State University.

Close, J.R., and Inman, V.T.: The action of the ankle joint, Univ. Calif. Prosthet. Devices Res. Rep., Ser. 11, issue 22, April 1952.

Close, J.R., and Inman, V.T.: The action of the subtalar joint, Univ. Calif. Prosthet. Devices Res. Rep. Ser. 11, issue 24, May 1953.

Cunningham, D.M.: Components of floor reactions during walking, Univ. Calif. Devices Res. Rep. Ser. 11, issue 14, November 1950.

Elftman, H.: The transverse tarsal joint and its control, Clin. Orthop. **16:**41, 1960.

Elftman, H.: A cinematic study of the distribution of pressure in the human foot, Anat. Rec. **59:**481, 1934.

Hicks, J.H.: The mechanics of the foot. II. The plantar aponeurosis and the arch. J. Anat. **88:**25, 1954.

Inman, V.T.: The joints of the ankle, Baltimore, 1976, Williams & Wilkins.

Isman, R.E., and Inman, V.T.: Anthropometric studies of the human foot and ankle, Bull. Prosthet. Res. **10-11:**97, 1969.

Levens, A.S., Inman, V.T., and Blosser, J.A.: Transverse rotation of the segments of the lower extremity in locomotion, J. Bone Joint Surg. **30A:**859, 1948.

Mann, R., and Inman, V.T.: Phasic activity of intrinsic muscles of the foot, J. Bone Joint Surg. **46A:**469, 1964.

Manter, J.T.: Movements of the subtalar and transverse tarsal joints, Anat. Rec. **80:**397, 1941.

Popova, T.: Quoted in Issledovaniia po biodinamike lokomotsii. Chapter 3, Vol. 1. Biodinamika khod'by normal'nogo vzroslogo muzhchiny (edited by N.A. Bernstein), Moscow, 1935, Idat. Vsesoiuz. Instit. Eksper. Med.

Ralston, H.J.: Energy-speed relation and optimal speed during level walking, Int. Z. Angew. Physiol. **17:**277, 1958.

Ryker, N.J., Jr.: Glass walkway studies of normal subjects during normal walking, Univ. Calif. Prosthet. Device. Res. Rep. Ser. 11, issue 20, January 1952.

Saunders, J.B.C.M., Inman, V.T., and Eberhart, H.D.: The major determinants in normal and pathological gait, J. Bone Joint Surg. **35A:**543, 1953.

Scott, E.: Personal communication.

Wright, D.G., Desai, M.E., and Henderson, B.S.: Action of the subtalar and ankle-joint complex during the stance phase of walking, J. Bone Joint Surg. **46A:**361, 1964.

2

Principles of examination of the foot and ankle

ROGER A. MANN

Fortunately the foot, ankle, and leg are parts of the body that are readily accessible to adequate physical examination. Usually a specific diagnosis can be reached by obtaining a careful history, by conducting a proper physical examination, and by using the indicated ancillary laboratory procedures. The techniques of examination available to the practitioner to gather information concerning the foot and to make proper diagnoses vary with the age of the patient. In examining the preambulatory infant the practitioner must rely on inspection, palpation, and manipulation. In examining the toddler, inspection, palpation, and manipulation may be supplemented with observations on the emerging patterns of locomotion. However, one should be aware that this period is a time of experimentation for the child, whose behavioral patterns are constantly changing. Since they may be based on transitory findings, definitive surgical procedures at this stage of a child's development should be undertaken with caution. Only in the older child and in the adult can all the anatomic features and the functional behavior of the various components be realistically evaluated.

NEONATE AND PREAMBULATORY INFANT— CONGENITAL ABNORMALITIES

Gross abnormalities of the lower limbs of children are easily recognized at birth or shortly thereafter. These congenital abnormalities present themselves in many different forms. During the past decade several attempts have been made to name and classify congenital limb defects based on the site and extent of the skeletal abnormality. Universal acceptance and use of such a system of classification with its standardized nomenclature would do much to improve communication and expedite the development of therapeutic principles. Currently the various types of limb deficiencies are reasonably well classified under the general heading of dysmelia, with the subdivisions of ectromelia, phocomelia, and amelia. Other abnormalities of the lower limb are still classified under specific descriptive names.

In a book of this nature, it is impossible to be encyclopedic. Therefore I am providing the reader with an extensive bibliography at the end of the present chapter as a vehicle for obtaining information of a more detailed nature than is here offered or for acquiring knowledge about deformities that occur infrequently. The following list attempts to be all-inclusive but should serve only as a reminder to the examiner. If more extensive discussions are available in chapters that follow, the chapter containing such a discussion is indicated; if the subject is covered minimally or not at all, the reader is referred to the bibliography.

Dysmelia. Under this heading are found all limb deficiencies, including congenital absence of skeletal parts and aplasia. See Bibliography and Chapter 22.

Dimelia. For supernumerary bones and skeletal elements see Chapter 22.

Anterior or posterior bowing of tibia. See Bibliography.

Length of leg discrepancies. See Bibliography.

Hemihypertrophy and local gigantism. See Bibliography and Chapter 22.

Calcaneovalgus foot. See Bibliography and Chapters 14 and 22.

Clubfoot. See Chapter 22.

Congenital metatarsus varus. See Chapter 22.

Congenital hammertoes. See Chapter 22.

Flatfoot. See Chapters 10 and 22.

The appearance of low arches in neonates and infants is primarily caused by the presence of fat deposits in the soles of the feet. However, it is mandatory during an examination to manipulate the feet gently to check the motion of the major articulations. There are two general categories of flatfoot—mobile and rigid—and the examiner should discern which type of flatfoot he is observing.

Mobile flatfoot. Mobile flatfoot is a condition in which there is a wide range of motion in the hindfoot and midfoot. The important factor to determine is whether there is a short Achilles tendon that may impose abnormal forces on the foot when the child begins to walk.

Rigid flatfoot. In the presence of rigid flatfoot, passive inversion of the heel and pronation of the forefoot will not produce elevation of the longitudinal arch, which is the case in the normal foot. Rigid flatfoot occurs in two conditions that should be recognized early: tarsal coalition and congenital vertical talus (see Chapter 22).

THE TODDLER

As the child begins to walk, it becomes possible to examine the behavior of all segments of the lower extremity and to observe the effects of weight bearing on them.

The degree of toeing in or toeing out should be observed. The position of the foot during stance is determined by (1) the degree of anteversion or retroversion of the neck of the femur (see Bibliography), (2) tibial or malleolar torsion (see Bibliography), (3) the mobility of the major joints, and (4) the musculature.

The degree of anteversion or retroversion of the neck of the femur should be checked. This position can be clinically determined by noting the amount of passive internal and external rotation that is possible in the extended leg. Also, as the child walks, the position and degree of horizontal motion of the patellas should be observed. To facilitate observation of the patella as the child walks, it is helpful to place a dot on the middle of each patella. As the child walks toward the examiner, the rotation of these dots to the plane of progression and to one another can be readily observed.

Tibial or malleolar torsion is still a controversial subject among clinicians; the measurements reported by many investigators vary widely. However, it is clear that when the child sits on the edge of the examining table with the knees flexed and the patellas and feet facing forward the plane of the long axes of the feet should not deviate markedly from the sagittal plane.

To obtain a fairly reproducible measurement of the degree of femoral rotation and tibial torsion and the relationship of the foot to the femur, the following examination technique may be used. The child is placed in a prone position on the examining table with the knee flexed to 90°. The internal and external rotation of the hip is recorded, the relationship of the malleoli to the long axis of the tibia is noted, and then the degree of rotation of the long axis of the foot to the long axis of the femur is recorded. In this manner a reproducible set of measurements is obtained, and the relationship between the degree of hip motion, tibial torsion, and long axis of the foot is established.

The degree of pronation of the foot while the child walks or stands barefoot is readily observed by the examiner. By encouraging the child to rise on tippy-toes or to walk on tiptoe and then on heels, the examiner is quickly able to determine the mobility of the major joints and the adequacy of the musculature.

A rough check of the musculature can often be made by tickling the feet and observing the various displacements of the feet and toes. Possible shortening of the Achilles tendon should be investigated.

OLDER CHILD AND ADULT

To prevent overlooking pertinent findings, every examiner should follow a rigorous routine. The particular routine adopted will vary depending on personal preference and arrangement of office facilities. However, it appears appropriate to emphasize that no matter what procedure he adopts, the examiner must consider the foot and ankle from three different points of view.

First, the foot and ankle should be seen as parts of the entire body. Since their examination may reveal the presence of systemic disease, evidence of circulatory, metabolic, and cutaneous abnormalities should be sought.

Second, the foot and ankle should be considered as important constituents of the locomotor system. They play reciprocal roles with the suprapedal segments, and abnormal function of any part of the locomotor apparatus is reflected in adaptive changes in the remaining parts. Therefore it is essential for the examiner to observe the patient walking over an appreciable distance to do the following:

1. Detect obvious abnormalities of locomotion. (For example, unequal step length or limp must be investigated.)
2. Perceive asymmetric behavior of the two sides of the body. (For example, asymmetric arm swing denotes unequal horizontal rotation of the components of the torso.)
3. Observe the position of the patellas, which are indicators of the degree of horizontal rotation of the leg in the horizontal plane.
4. Observe the degree of toeing in or out. (Toeing in or out that is relatively constant during the walk

cycle indicates the degree of malleolar torsion; toeing in or out occurring only during the interval between heel strike and foot flat indicates the degree of obliquity of the ankle axis.)

5. Observe the amount of pronation of the foot during the first half of stance-phase walking.

6. Note the amount of heel inversion and supination of the foot during lift-off, together with presence or absence of rotatory slippage of the forefoot on the floor. (These motions indicate the amount of movement in the subtalar joint at that moment.)

7. Observe the position of the foot in relation to the floor at the time of heel strike. (Normally the heel strikes the ground first, after which rapid plantar flexion occurs. If this sequence does not occur, further investigation is indicated. The time of heel rise should also be carefully noted, occurring normally at 34% of the walking cycle just after the swinging leg has passed the stance foot. Early heel rise may be indicative of tightness of the gastrocsoleus muscle complex. A delay in heel rise can indicate weakness in the same muscle group.)

It must be stressed that one sees only what one is looking for. If the implications of the preceding statements are not readily apparent, it is suggested that the reader review Chapter 1 at this time.

Third, the human foot and ankle should be viewed as relatively recent evolutionary acquisitions; thus they are subject to considerable individual anatomic and functional variation. It is regrettable that in most of the anatomic and orthopedic literature, only average values for the positions of axes of the major articulations and for ranges of motion about these axes are given (see Chapter 1). It so happens that an average individual is difficult to find, particularly among patients seeking help in the practitioner's office. The examiner should be aware of these variations and should also be cognizant of their functional implications. Only with such knowledge and insight will he be able to determine the proper therapeutic procedure to use and to evaluate realistically his success or failure with that procedure.

Sequence of examination

When examining the foot and ankle, the examiner should follow as closely as possible the procedural sequence taught in courses in introductory physical diagnosis. After taking an adequate history, the examiner first *inspects*, then *palpates*, and finally (in an orthopedic examination) *manipulates*. This sequence must be modified and repeated several times as the patient performs tasks with and without shoes, while walking, standing, and sitting on the edge of the examining table.

The following outline for the examination of the foot

and ankle has proved adequate in my experience; to increase its value, annotations have been inserted to elucidate the significance of some findings and to explain the use of special diagnostic procedures. Even if one does not wish to adopt the routine as presented here, it may prove useful as a checklist.

The patient is generally dressed in customary street clothes. It is usually convenient at that time for the examiner to observe the patient walking at various speeds, with shoes on, hands empty, and arms hanging freely at the sides. The following observations should be made.

Type of limp, if present. A pathologic condition of the lower extremity may produce a limp that is characteristic of the particular disorder. A patient with a painful hip, for example, will throw himself over the painful side during walking.

Symmetry of arm swing. As a rule, the shoulders rotate 180° out of phase with the pelvis; this is a passive response to pelvic rotation. If there are no abnormalities in the spine or upper extremities, rotation of the shoulders is reflected in equal and symmetric arm swing. If the arm swing is asymmetric, horizontal rotation of the pelvis is also asymmetric. Since such asymmetric pelvis rotation may be the result of abnormality in any of the components of the lower extremity, it is mandatory that the practitioner take extra care in examining not only the foot and ankle, but the knees and hips as well.

Degree of toe-in or toe-out. At toe-off the leg has achieved its maximal external rotation and the foot toes out slightly. During swing phase the entire leg and foot rotate internally. The average amount of rotation is about 15° but varies greatly among individuals. It may be almost imperceptible (3°) or considerable (30°) (Levens et al., 1948). At the time of heel strike the long axis of the foot has approached, to a varying degree, the plane of progression. The degree of parallelism between the long axis of the foot and the plane of progression at this point is subject to considerable individual variation. However, the transition from heel strike to foot flat, which occurs rapidly, should be carefully observed. Some individuals will show an increase in toe-in during the very short period of plantar flexion of the ankle, indicating a greater degree of obliquity of the ankle axis (Chapter 1).

Amount of pronation of foot during early stance phase. Normally the foot will pronate as it is loaded with the body weight during the first half of stance phase. The amount of pronation is subject to extreme individual variation. The important factor, however, is whether the foot remains pronated during the period of heel rise and lift-off. In the normally functioning foot, as the heel rises, an almost instantaneous inversion of the heel occurs. If the heel fails to invert at this time, the examiner should check the strength of the intrinsic and extrinsic muscles of the foot and the ranges of motion in the articulations of the hindfoot and midfoot.

Nature of heel strike and heel rise. The foot should contact the ground heel first, after which it rapidly plantar flexes so that it is flat on the ground by 7% of the walking cycle. In pathologic conditions the patient may contact the ground with the foot flat or possibly on his toes. The time when the heel begins to rise off the ground is at approximately 35% of the walking cycle, i.e., when the swinging leg is passing by the stance leg. If heel rise occurs too early in the walking cycle, tightness in the gastrocsoleus musculature is most likely the cause. If the heel-rise time is delayed significantly, this can be caused by weakness of the calf musculature.

Rotatory slippage of shoe on floor at lift-off. Except on slippery surfaces, the shoe does not visibly rotate externally or slip on the floor at the time of lift-off. Failure of the ankle and subtalar joints to permit adequate external rotation of the leg during this phase of walking may result in direct transmission of the rotatory forces to the interface between the sole of the shoe and the walking surface, with resultant rotatory slippage of the shoe on the floor. On noting slippage, the examiner should look for possible muscular imbalance and should check the obliquity of the ankle axis and the range of motion in the subtalar joint.

Type of shoe and height of heel. Since the type of shoe worn and its heel height affect the way a person walks, they must be noted. When wearing high heels, for example, women show less ankle-joint motion than when wearing flat heels, and in tennis shoes, show little difference from men in gait.

While the patient is disrobing, it is convenient for the examiner to inspect the shoes and note the following:

1. Path of wear from heel to toe
2. Presence of supportive devices or corrections in the shoes (Arch supports, Thomas heels, sole wedges, or metal tabs indicate previous difficulties.)
3. Obliquity of the angle of the crease in the toe of the shoe (The angle varies from person to person; the greater the obliquity of the crease in the shoe to its long axis, the greater the amount of subtalar motion that is required to distribute the body weight evenly over the metatarsal heads.)
4. Impression the forefoot has made on the insole of the shoe, which often gives important information about the patient's symptoms
5. Presence or absence of circular wear on the sole of the shoe (Such wear indicates rotatory slippage of the foot on the floor during lift-off from suppressed subtalar motion.)

6. The location of the wear pattern on the bottom of the shoe to ascertain whether it is too big or too small (The shape of the shoe, i.e., narrow pointed shoe or broad toe box, and the overall shape of the foot when the patient is weight bearing should be carefully observed.)

The patient, now barefoot, is requested to walk. The same sequence of observation is repeated. Any gross abnormalities that were obscured by stockings and shoes can now be seen.

For the convenience of the examiner who is seated, the patient is next requested to stand on a raised platform or lift, distributing his weight equally on the two feet. The examiner makes a preliminary evaluation of the patient's posture and a cursory inspection of the lower extremities from both front and back, taking note of the following.

Presence of pelvic tilt. To estimate pelvic tilt from the front, the examiner places his index fingers on either the anterior superior iliac spines or the iliac crests; from the back, he observes the gluteal creases. An anatomic or functional shortening of one leg can readily be seen if the shortening is greater than one-quarter inch. Inspection of the popliteal creases will reveal whether major shortening is in the thigh or in the leg.

Gross abnormalities of components of lower extremity. These abnormalities include differences in circumferences of the thigh and calves, excessive deviations in skeletal alignment, and the degree of pes planus or pes cavus.

There appear to be at least two general categories of pes planus. In one category the longitudinal arch is depressed, without the complicating factors of everted heel, abducted forefoot, or longitudinal rotation of the metatarsals and phalanges (Fig. 2-1). This type of flatfoot is seen typically in individuals with a plantar-flexed talus (Fig. 2-2). In the other category the foot appears to have fallen inward like the tilting of a half-hemisphere; the heel is everted, the outer border of the foot shows angulation at the midfoot, and the forefoot is abducted. There may also be varying degrees of rotation of the metatarsals and phalanges around their long axes (Fig. 2-3). In the first category the Achilles tendon remains relatively straight; in the second the Achilles tendon deviates laterally when the patient bears weight on the relaxed foot. The pathologic implications of these two types of flatfoot are different.

Movements occurring when patient rises on toes. When the patient is asked to rise onto his toes, if the foot is functioning normally, the heel will promptly invert, the longitudinal arch will rise, and the leg will rotate externally. Failure of these movements to occur may indicate a weak foot or a specific pathologic process.

Since inversion of the heel is achieved through

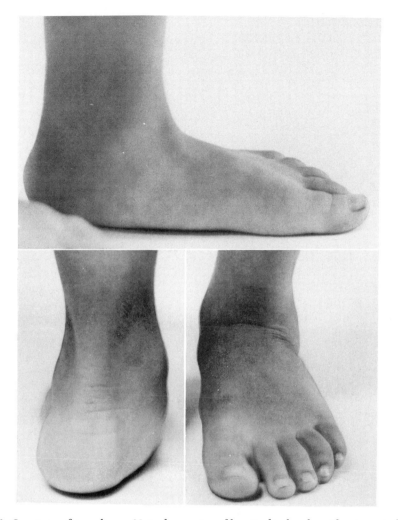

Fig. 2-1. One type of pes planus. Note depression of longitudinal arch, without everted heel, abducted forefoot, or longitudinal rotation of metatarsals and phalanges.

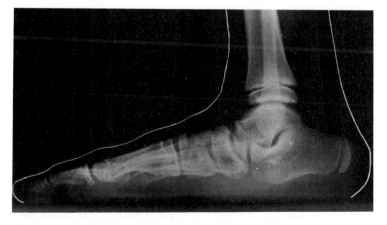

Fig. 2-2. Weight-bearing radiograph of foot of a youth. Note flatfoot and plantar-flexed talus.

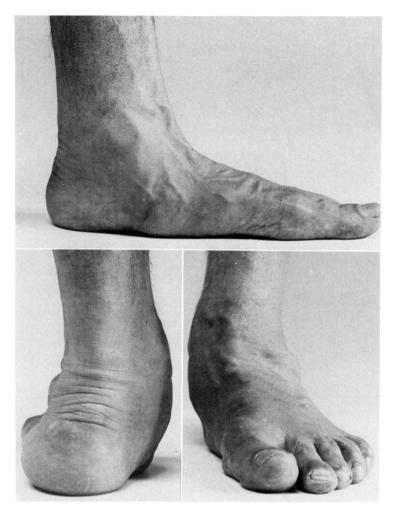

Fig. 2-3. Another type of pes planus. Foot appears to have fallen inward like a half-hemisphere.

proper performance of the subtalar and transverse tarsal articulations, failure to invert the heel should immediately focus the examiner's attention on possible malfunction of these structures. Conditions that may limit activity in these joints are muscular weakness, rupture or weakness of the tibialis posterior, arthritic changes in the subtalar joint, and such skeletal abnormalities as vertical talus and tarsal coalition.

Windlass action. Normally dorsiflexion of the toes increases the tension of the plantar aponeurosis, which causes the longitudinal arch to rise (Fig. 2-4, *A* and *B*). Failure of the longitudinal arch to rise suggests the presence or prolonged pes planus with attendant abnormal stretching and elongation of the plantar aponeurosis (Fig. 2-4, *C* and *D*).

Stability of subtalar joint. The weight-bearing line of the body normally falls medial to the axis of the subtalar joint; therefore, when the patient stands on one foot with muscles relaxed, the foot pronates. Because of the linkage between the foot and the leg provided by the subtalar articulation, when the examiner rotates the leg externally, the heel will invert and the weight-bearing line will move laterally. This position creates a metastable state, which in the normal foot extends over a moderate range of longitudinal rotation of the leg (10° to 15°). When the examiner exerts minimal external rotatory force on the leg with his hand, the patient's full body weight can be transmitted through the hindfoot to the floor. However, in some patients this metastable state cannot be achieved even if the examiner applies maximal external rotatory force to the leg. In others the metastable state is so tenuous that if the examiner exerts a few degrees of internal or external rotatory force on the leg the foot will promptly pronate or supinate.

The patient is next instructed to sit on the examining table with legs and feet hanging over the side. A more detailed examination is now possible.

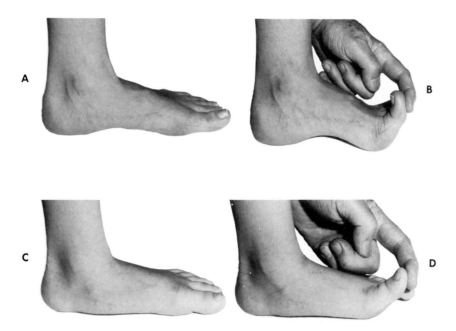

Fig. 2-4. A, "Normal" weight-bearing foot. **B,** Dorsiflexion of great toe causes elevation of the arch because of windlass action of aponeurosis. **C,** Flat weight-bearing foot. **D,** Dorsiflexion of great toe does not cause arch to rise.

Surface of foot, ankle, and leg. Any vascular abnormalities such as varicosities, areas of telangiectasia, and edema should be noted. The dorsalis pedis and posterior tibial pulses should be palpated. The speed of capillary filling after compression of the nail bed should be checked. The skin over joints is normally cooler than the skin over muscular areas of the extremity; inflammatory processes in or around deep structures cause increased temperature of the overlying skin. The examiner, by gently passing his hand over the extremity, can frequently localize "hot spots" that should alert him to investigate the underlying components. The distribution of hair on the foot should be carefully noted. The skin on the plantar aspect of the foot and about the toes is carefully inspected for callus formation, which often indicates abnormal pressure on the foot.

Skeletal structures (general appraisal). Gross skeletal deformities are readily discernible and can hardly be overlooked even by the most inexperienced examiner. Difficulties in making a diagnosis are more likely to arise in patients whose feet, on casual inspection, appear to be relatively normal.

Ranges of motion

After a sequential examination has been described in some detail, it is appropriate to discuss techniques of eliciting other pertinent information.

The passive ranges of motion of all the major articulations of the foot should be rapidly checked for limitation of motion, painful movement, and crepitus. These symptoms may occur separately or in any combination.

The ankle joint should be moved through its full range of motion. Although the ankle is essentially a single-axis joint, its axis is skewed to both the transverse and the coronal planes of the body passing downward and backward from the medial to the lateral side. A reasonably accurate estimate of the location of the ankle axis can be obtained by placing the tips of the index fingers just below the most distal projections of the two malleoli (Fig. 2-5). Depending on the degree of obliquity of the axis, dorsiflexion and plantar flexion produce medial and lateral deviation of the foot. If the examiner has noted previously that the patient tended to toe in during the interval between heel strike and flat foot, an oblique axis of the ankle as projected on the coronal plane of the body is to be expected. Since an oblique axis of the ankle will assist in absorbing the horizontal rotation of the leg, its range of motion is related to the range of motion in the subtalar joint. Thus range of subtalar motion should also be estimated.

The amount of motion in the subtalar joint varies; however, Isman and Inman (1969) found that in a series of feet in cadaver specimens a minimum of 20° and a maximum of 60° of motion were present. The simplest method of determining the degree of subtalar motion is to apply rotatory force on the calcaneus while permitting the rest of the foot to move passively. When rotatory force is applied to the forefoot, abnormally large

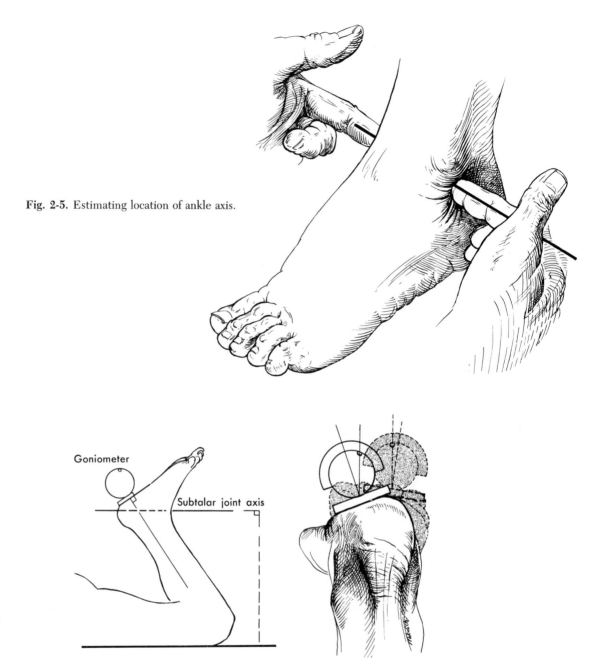

Fig. 2-5. Estimating location of ankle axis.

Goniometer

Subtalar joint axis

Fig. 2-6. Spherical goniometer attached to calcaneus to measure degree of subtalar motion.

displacements may be obtained through movements of the articulations in the midfoot that are additive to subtalar motion. By far the most accurate method of determining the degree of subtalar motion is to place the patient prone and flex his knee to approximately 135°. The axis of the subtalar joint now lies close to the horizontal plane. The examiner then passively inverts and everts the heel while measuring the extent of motion by attaching a gravity goniometer or level to the calcaneus with a metal spring clip (Fig. 2-6). Lack of subtalar motion should alert the examiner to the possibility of an arthritic process in the subtalar joint, of peroneal

spastic flatfoot, or of an anatomic abnormality such as tarsal coalition.

Normally there is no lateral play of the talus in the mortise even when the foot is in full plantar flexion. Any lateral displacement that can be imposed on the talus in its mortise by the examiner is indicative of abnormal widening of the mortise. Frequently the talus can be displaced forward and backward a millimeter or so in the mortise, but this is a normal finding.

Occasionally a degree of lateral talar tilt can be demonstrated in the normal ankle joint in the following manner: The examiner places the ankle in full plantar

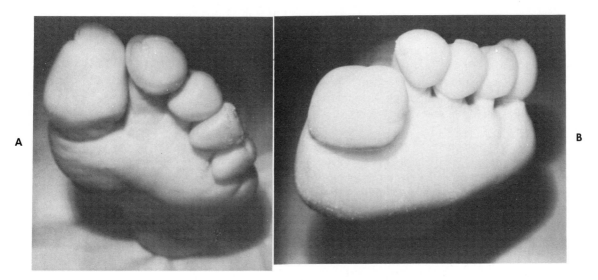

Fig. 2-7. A, Forefoot varus. **B,** Forefoot valgus.

flexion, thus displacing the trochlea anteriorly. He forcibly inverts the foot while placing his thumb just in front of the lateral malleolus and pressing against the anterior portion of the trochlea. He can then feel a slight medial rocking of the talus. Excessive talar tilt should alert the examiner to suspect injury to the lateral ligaments. The range of motion of the transverse tarsal, metatarsophalangeal, and interphalangeal joints should be observed for pain, joint stiffness, and deformities.

Relationship of forefoot to hindfoot

After the range of motion of the foot has been determined, the relationship of the hindfoot to the forefoot should be ascertained. This is an important measurement, since it may be the underlying cause of the patient's clinical problem. Determination of the relationship of the hindfoot to the forefoot may be carried out with the patient sitting on the examining table with the knees flexed at 90° or with the patient prone on the examining table, again with the knee flexed to 90° and the foot in the air. I prefer to carry out this examination with the patient sitting in front of me with the legs dangling. The hindfoot is grasped and placed into its neutral position, i.e., the calcaneus is in line with the long axis of the leg. When examining the right foot, the heel is grasped with the examiner's right hand, and the area of the fifth metatarsal head is grasped with the left hand. The examiner's right thumb is now placed over the talonavicular joint, and this joint is manipualted until the examiner feels that the head of the talus is covered by the navicular. This movement is brought about by the examiner's left hand moving the forefoot in relation to the hindfoot. Once neutral position has been achieved, the relationship of the forefoot as projected by a plane parallel to the metatarsals is related to a plane perpendicular to the long axis of the calcaneus. Based on this measurement, the forefoot will be in one of three positions in relation to the hindfoot: neutral, in which the plane of the metatarsals and the plane of the calcaneus are perpendicular to one another; forefoot varus, in which the plane of the metatarsals is supinated or internally rotated in relation to the plane of the calcaneus; or forefoot valgus, in which the plane of the metatarsal is pronated or externally rotated in relation to the plane of the calcaneus. This measurement should be carried out two or three times to be sure that an error is not made (Fig. 2-7).

The importance of this measurement is that by relating the position of the forefoot to the hindfoot, various types of clinical problems may be explained. Generally speaking, the forefoot and hindfoot planes are almost perpendicular to one another, although a moderate degree of variability in this measurement that is of no clinical significance can occur. An example of a clinical problem that might be detected by such an examination might be in a patient who has a problem with recurrent ankle sprains. Examination of the subtalar joint may demonstrate a lack of eversion past the midline, and, when the forefoot measurement is made, a valgus or pronation deformity is present so that the medial border of the foot is in a more plantar-flexed position than the lateral border. In such an individual, as the foot strikes the ground, the calcaneus does not have the ability to evert because of the structural alignment of the subtalar joint; when the forefoot strikes the ground, the medial border strikes before the lateral border, imparting an inversion twist to the hindfoot. In such a case, the ankle is being forced into an inverted position because of the anatomic alignment of the foot. If a condition such as this is not appreciated, treatment may be directed toward the chronically sprained lateral collateral ligament structure when indeed a postural problem of the foot is present. The most severe example of this condition, although associated with muscle weakness, is a patient with Charcot-Marie-Tooth disease who lacks eversion of the hindfoot and has marked plantar flexion of the medial border of the foot. The opposite would be with the hindfoot in a neutral position and the forefoot in marked varus position. In this case when the foot assumes a plantigrade position, the calcaneus, to compensate for it, must rotate into an everted position; this may in turn, if the degree of the deformity is severe, cause pain along the medial side of the foot or ankle. This occurs most frequently in persons involved in an active running program. If following a subtalar or triple arthrodesis the forefoot is placed anatomically into too much varus or valgus, an uncompensated condition exists in that, since the hindfoot is rigid, no accommodation is possible to place the forefoot into a plantigrade position. This may result in an abnormal wear pattern on the forefoot, often giving rise to a painful callosity as a result of localized pressure.

Ligamentous and muscular structures

The attachments of the collateral ligaments of the ankle should be palpated for tenderness. The deltoid, anterior talofibular, and calcaneofibular ligaments are readily palpable. The posterior talofibular ligament is too deeply situated to be felt. When examining the lateral collateral ligaments, it should be recalled that the anterior talofibular ligament should be tested with the foot in a plantar-flexed position. In this position, inversion of the hindfoot will demonstrate laxity in the anterior talofibular ligament, if such is present. When the foot is placed into dorsiflexion, the calcaneofibular ligament is placed on stretch, and with an inversion stress, laxity of this ligament may be detected. The anterior drawer sign is carried out with the ankle held at a right angle and the calcaneus pulled anteriorly and slightly internally while the examiner's other hand is holding the distal tibia and palpating the junction of the lateral aspect of the talus in relation to the anterior aspect of the fibula. Forward movement of more than 3 to 4 mm is an indication of laxity in the anterior talofibular ligament. The ligament structure on the involved side

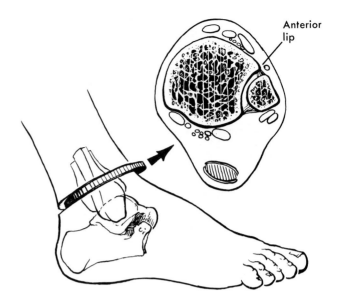

Fig. 2-8. Cross-section of leg just proximal to ankle joint showing fibula nestled in its groove in tibia. Note prominent anterior lip. (Adapted from Eycleshymer, A.C., and Schoemaker, D.M.: A cross-section anatomy, New York, 1970, Appleton-Century-Crofts.)

should always be compared to the opposite side to determine whether indeed a difference in the ligamentous structure exists. A variation of the anterior drawer sign that may be useful is to note how much internal rotation seems to occur when the lateral aspect of the foot is grasped with one hand and the other hand is placed on the distal tibia while palpating the articulation between the lateral articular surface of the talus and the anterior aspect of the distal fibula. This is carried out with the ankle in neutral position. Pulling forward on the forefoot while internally rotating will at times demonstrate a rotatory laxity as a result of an injury to the anterior talofibular ligament.

Injuries to the distal fibular syndesmosis are too frequently overlooked by orthopedists, although patients with such injuries may suffer pain when walking, jumping, and running. The construction of this articulation is such that the fibula is nestled into a groove on the lateral side of the tibia (Fig. 2-8). The anterior lip of the tibial groove is prominent, whereas the posterior lip is less pronounced. When attempting to displace the fibula anteriorly in an uninjured ankle, the examiner cannot elicit movement; but he frequently can feel movement, even in a normal ankle, when he attempts to displace the fibula posteriorly. In patients who have sustained injuries to the ligamentous structures supporting the syndesmosis, rarely can the examiner initiate an increase in anterior displacement of the fibula; only occasionally does the attempt produce an increase

McElvenny, R.T.: Congenital pseudo-arthrosis of the tibia, Q. Bull. Northwest. Univ. Med. Sch. **23**:413, 1949.

McFarland, B.: Birth fracture of the tibia, Br. J. Surg. **27**:706, 1940.

McFarland, B.: Pseudarthrosis of the tibia in childhood, J. Bone Joint Surg. **33B**:36, 1951.

Middleton, D.S.: Studies on prenatal lesions of striated muscle as a cause of congenital deformity, Edinburgh Med. J. **41**:401, 1934.

Milgram, J.E.: Impaling (telescoping) operation for pseudarthrosis of long bones in childhood, Bull. Hosp. Joint Dis. **17**:152, 1956.

Moore, B.H.: Some orthopaedic relationships of neurofibromatosis, J. Bone Joint Surg. **29**:199, 1941.

Moore, J.R.: Delayed autogenous bone graft in the treatment of congenital pseudarthrosis, J. Bone Joint Surg. **31A**:23, 1949.

Moore, J.R.: Congenital pseudarthrosis of the tibia. In American Academy of Orthopaedic Surgeons, Instructional Course Lectures, vol. 14, Ann Arbor, 1957, J.W. Edwards.

Nicoll, E.A.: Infantile pseudoarthrosis of the tibia, J. Bone Joint Surg. **51B**:589, 1969.

Purvis, G.D., and Holder, J.E.: Dual bone graft for congenital pseudarthrosis of the tibia: variations of technic, South. Med. J. **53**:926, 1960.

Sofield, H.A., and Millar, E.A.: Fragmentation, realignment and intramedullary rod fixation of deformities of the long bones in children: a ten-year appraisal, J. Bone Joint Surg. **41A**:1371, 1959.

Williams, E.R.: Two congenital deformities of the tibia: congenital angulation and congenital pseudarthrosis, Br. J. Radiol. **16**:371, 1943.

Wilson, P.D.: A simple method of two-stage transplantation of the fibula for use in cases of complicated and congenital pseudarthrosis of the tibia, J. Bone Joint Surg. **23**:639, 1941.

Congenital vertical talus

Axer, A.: Into-talus transposition of tendons for correction of paralytic valgus foot after poliomyelitis in children, J. Bone Joint Surg. **42A**:1119, 1960.

Clark, M.S., Dambrosia, R.D., and Ferguson, A.B., Jr.: Congenital vertical talus, J. Bone Joint Surg. **59A**:861, 1977.

Dickson, J.W.: Congenital vertical talus, J. Bone Joint Surg. **44B**:229, 1962.

Eyre-Brook, A.L.: Congenital vertical talus, J. Bone Joint Surg. **49B**:618, 1967.

Grice, D.S.: The role of subtalar fusion in the treatment of valgus deformities of the feet. In American Academy of Orthopaedic Surgeons, Instructional Course Lectures, vol. 16, St. Louis, 1959, The C.V. Mosby Co.

Hark, F.W.: Rocker-foot due to congenital subluxation of the talus, J. Bone Joint Surg. **32A**:344, 1950.

Harrold, A.J.: Congenital vertical talus in infancy, J. Bone Joint Surg. **49B**:634, 1967.

Herndon, C.H., and Heyman, C.H.: Problems in the recognition and treatment of congenital convex pes valgus, J. Bone Joint Surg. **45A**:413, 1963.

Heyman, C.H.: The diagnosis and treatment of congenital convex pes valgus or vertical talus. In American Academy of Orthopaedic Surgeons, Instructional Course Lectures, vol. 16, St. Louis, 1959, The C.V. Mosby Co.

Hughes, J.R.: On congenital vertical talus, J. Bone Joint Surg. **39B**:580, 1957.

Lamy, L., and Weissman, L.: Congenital convex pes valgus, J. Bone Joint Surg. **21**:79, 1939.

Lloyd-Roberts, G.C., and Spence, A.J.: Congenital vertical talus, J. Bone Joint Surg. **40B**:33, 1958.

Mead, N.C., and Nast, G.: Vertical talus (congenital talonavicular dislocation), Clin. Orthop. **21**:198, 1961.

Osmond-Clarke, H.: Congenital vertical talus, J. Bone Joint Surg. **38B**:334, 1956.

Outland, T., and Sherk, H.H.: Congenital vertical talus, Clin. Orthop. **16**:214, 1960.

Silk, F.F., and Wainwright, D.: The recognition and treatment of congenital flat foot in infancy, J. Bone Joint Surg. **49B**:628, 1967.

Steindler, A.: Orthopedic operations, Springfield, Ill. 1940, Charles C Thomas, Publisher.

Stone, K.H.: Congenital vertical talus: a new operation, Proc. R. Soc. Med. **56**:12, 1963.

Thompson, J.E.M.: Treatment of congenital flatfoot, J. Bone Joint Surg. **28**:787, 1946.

Townes, P.L., DeHart, G.K., Hecht, F., and Manning, J.A.: Trisomy 13-15 in a male infant, J. Pediatr. **60**:528, 1962.

Uchida, I.A., Lewis, A.J., Bowman, J.M., and Wang, H.C.: A case of double trisomy: trisomy no. 18 and triplo-X, J. Pediatr. **60**:498, 1962.

Wainwright, D.: The recognition and care of congenital flat foot, Proc. R. Soc. Med. **57**:357, 1964.

White, J.W.: Congenital flatfoot: a new surgical approach, J. Bone Joint Surg. **22**:547, 1940.

Whitman, A.: Astragalectomy and backward displacement of the foot: an investigation of its practical results, J. Bone Joint Surg. **4**:266, 1922.

Hemihypertrophy and gigantism

Barsky, A.J.: Macrodactyly, J. Bone Joint Surg. **49A**:1255, 1967.

Ben-Bassat, M., Casper, J., Kaplan, I., and Laron, Z.: Congenital macrodactyly, J. Bone Joint Surg. **44B**:359, 1966.

Bryan, R.S., Lipscomb, P.R., and Chatterton, C.C.: Orthopedic aspects of congenital hypertrophy, Am. J. Surg. **96**:654, 1958.

Charters, A.D.: Local gigantism, J. Bone Joint Surg. **39B**:542, 1957.

Dennyson, W.D., Bear, J.N., and Bhoola, K.D.: Macrodactyly in the foot, J. Bone Joint Surg. **59B**:355, 1977.

Goidanich, I.F., and Campanacci, M.: Vascular hamartomata and infantile angioectatic osteohyperplasia of the extremities: a study of ninety-four cases, J. Bone Joint Surg. **44A**:815, 1962.

Hutchinson, W.J., and Burdeaux, B.D., Jr.: The influence of stasis on bone growth, Surg. Gynecol. Obstet. **99**:413, 1954.

Peabody, C.W.: Hemihypertrophy and hemiatrophy: congenital total unilateral somatic asymmetry, J. Bone Joint Surg. **18**:466, 1936.

Pease, C.N.: Local stimulation of growth of long bones, J. Bone Joint Surg. **34A**:1, 1952.

Peremans, G.: An unusual case of congenital asymmetry of the pelvis and of the lower extremities, J. Bone Joint Surg. **5**:331, 1923.

Sabanas, A.O., and Chatterton, C.C.: Crossed congenital hemihypertrophy, J. Bone Joint Surg. **37A**:871, 1955.

Strobino, L.J., French, G.O., and Colonna, P.C.: The effect of increasing tensions on the growth of epiphyseal bone, Surg. Gynecol. Obstet. **95**:694, 1952.

Thomas, H.B.: Partial gigantism: overgrowth and asymmetry of bones and skeletal muscle, Am. J. Surg. **32**:108, 1936.

Thorne, F.L., Posch, J.L., and Mladick, R.A.: Megalodactyly, Plast. Reconstr. Surg. **41**:232, 1968.

Trueta, J.: The influence of the blood supply in controlling bone growth, Bull. Hosp. Joint Dis. **14**:147, 1953.

Ward, J., and Lerner, H.L.: A review of the subject of congenital hemihypertrophy and a complete case report, J. Pediatr. **31**:403, 1947.

Inequality of length of leg

Abbott, L.C.: The operative lengthening of the tibia and fibula, J. Bone Joint Surg. **9**:128, 1927.

Aitken, A.P.: Overgrowth of the femoral shaft following fracture in children, Am. J. Surg. **49**:147, 1940.

Anderson, M.S., Green, W.T., and Messner, M.B.: Growth and predictions of growth in the lower extremities, J. Bone Joint Surg. **45A**:1, 1963.

Arkin, A.M., and Katz, J.F.: The effects of pressure on epiphyseal growth, J. Bone Joint Surg. **38A:**1057, 1956.

Barfod, B., and Christensen, J.: Fractures of the femoral shaft in children with special reference to subsequent overgrowth, Acta Chir. Scand. **116:**235, 1959.

Barr, J.: Growth and inequality of leg length in poliomyelitis, N. Engl. J. Med. **238:**737, 1948.

Barr, J.S., Lingley, J.R., and Gall, E.A.: The effect of roentgen irradiation on epiphyseal growth. I. Experimental studies on the albino rat. Am. J. Roentgenol. Radium. Ther. **49:**104, 1943.

Barr, J.S., Stinchfield, A.J., and Reidy, J.A.: Sympathetic ganglionectomy and limb length in poliomyelitis, J. Bone Joint Surg. **32A:**793, 1950.

Bell, J.S., and Thompson, W.A.L.: Modified spot scanography, Am. J. Roentgenol. Radium Ther. **63:**915, 1950.

Bisgard, J.D.: Longitudinal bone growth: the influence of sympathetic deinnervation, Ann. Surg. **97:**374, 1933.

Bisgard, J.D., and Bisgard, M.E.: Longitudinal growth of long bones, Arch. Surg. **31:**568, 1935.

Blount, W.P.: Unequal leg length in children, Surg. Clin. North Am. **38:**1107, 1958.

Blount, W.P.: Unequal leg length. In American Academy of Orthopaedic Surgeons, Instructional Course Lectures, vol. 17, St. Louis, 1960, The C.V. Mosby Co.

Blount, W.P., and Clarke, G.R.: Control of bone growth by epiphyseal stapling: a preliminary report, J. Bone Joint Surg. **31A:**464, 1949.

Blount, W.P., and Zeier, F.: Control of bone length, J.A.M.A. **148:**451, 1952.

Bohlman, H.R.: Experiments with foreign materials in the region of the epiphyseal cartilage plate of growing bones to increase their longitudinal growth, J. Bone Joint Surg. **11:**365, 1929.

Bost, F.C., and Larsen, L.J.: Experiences with lengthening of the femur over an intramedullary rod, J. Bone Joint Surg. **38A:**567, 1956.

Brockway, A., Craig, W.A., and Cockrell, B.R., Jr.: End-result of sixty-two stapling operations, J. Bone Joint Surg. **36A:**1063, 1954.

Brodin, H.: Longitudinal bone growth, the nutrition of the epiphyseal cartilages and the local blood supply, Acta Orthop. Scand. (supp.) **20:**1, 1955.

Brookes, M.: Femoral growth after occlusion of the principal nutrient canal in day-old rabbits, J. Bone Joint Surg. **39B:**563, 1957.

Cameron, B.M.: A technique for femoral-shaft shortening: a preliminary report, J. Bone Joint Surg. **39A:**1309, 1957.

Carpenter, E.B., and Dalton, J.B.: A critical evaluation of a method of epiphyseal stimulation, J. Bone Joint Surg. **38A:**1089, 1956.

Coleman, S.S., and Noonan, T.D.: Anderson's method of tibial-lengthening by percutaneous osteotomy and gradual distraction: experience with thirty-one cases, J. Bone Joint Surg. **49A:**263, 1967.

Compere, E.L., and Adams, C.O.: Studies of longitudinal growth of long bones. I. The influence of trauma to the diaphysis, J. Bone Joint Surg. **19:**922, 1937.

Dalton, J.B., Jr., and Carpenter, E.B.: Clinical experiences with epiphyseal stapling, South. Med. J. **47:**544, 1954.

David, V.C.: Shortening and compensatory overgrowth following fractures of the femur in children, Arch. Surg. **9:**438, 1924.

Doyle, J.R., and Smart, B.W.: Stimulation of bone growth by short-wave diathermy, J. Bone Joint Surg. **45A:**15, 1963.

Duthie, R.B.: The significance of growth in orthopaedic surgery, Clin. Orthop. **14:**7, 1959.

Ferguson, A.B.: Surgical stimulation of bone growth by a new procedure: preliminary report. JAMA **100:**26, 1933.

Ferguson, A.B.: Growth as a factor in relation to deformity and disease. In American Academy of Orthopaedic Surgeons, Instructional Course Lectures, vol. 9, Ann Arbor, 1952, J.W. Edwards.

Ford, L.T., and Key, J.A.: A study of experimental trauma to the distal femoral epiphysis in rabbits, J. Bone Joint Surg. **38A:**84, 1956.

Gardner, E.: The development and growth of bones and joints. In American Academy of Orthopeadic Surgeons, Instructional Course Lectures, vol. 13, Ann Arbor, 1956, J.W. Edwards.

Gatewood and Mullen, B.P.: Experimental observations on the growth of long bones, Arch. Surg. **15:**215, 1927.

Geiser, M., and Trueta, J.: Muscle action, bone rarefaction and bone formation: an experimental study, J. Bone Joint Surg. **40B:**282, 1958.

Gelbke, H.: The influence of pressure and tension on growing bones in experiments with animals, J. Bone Joint Surg. **33A:**947, 1951.

Gill, G.G., and Abbott, L.C.: Practical method of predicting the growth of the femur and tibia in the child, Arch. Surg. **45:**286, 1942.

Goetz, R.H., Du Toit, J.G., and Swart, B.H.: Vascular changes in poliomyelitis and the effect of sympathectomy on bone growth, Acta Med. Scand. (suppl.) **306:**56, 1955.

Goff, C.W.: Growth determinations. In American Academy of Orthopaedic Surgeons, Instructional Course Lectures, vol. 8, Ann Arbor, 1951, J.W. Edwards.

Goff, C.W.: Surgical care of unequal extremities: measuring and predicting growth. In American Academy of Orthopaedic Surgeons, Instructional Course Lectures, vol. 16, St. Louis, 1959, The C.V. Mosby Co.

Goff, C.W.: Surgical treatment of unequal extremities, Springfield, Ill., 1960, Charles C Thomas, Publisher.

Green, W.T.: Discussion following prediction of unequal growth of the lower extremities in anterior poliomyelitis, J. Bone Joint Surg. **31A:**485, 1949.

Green, W.T., and Anderson, M.: Experiences with epiphyseal arrest in correcting discrepancies in length of the lower extremities in infantile paralysis, J. Bone Joint Surg. **29:**659, 1947.

Green, W.T., and Anderson, M.: Discrepancy in length of the lower extremities. In Americn Academy of Orthopaedic Surgeons, Instructional Course Lectures, vol. 8, Ann Arbor, 1951, J.W. Edwards.

Green, W.T., and Anderson, M.: The problem of unequal leg length, Pediatr. Clin. North Am. **2:**1137, 1955.

Green, W.T., and Anderson, M.: Epiphyseal arrest for the correction of discrepancies in length of the lower extremities, J. Bone Joint Surg. **39A:**853, 1957.

Green, W.T., and Anderson, M.: Skeletal age and control of bone growth. In American Academy of Orthopaedic Surgeons, Instructional Course Lectures, vol. 17, St. Louis, 1960, The C.V. Mosby Co.

Green, W.T., Wyatt, G.M., and Anderson, M.S.: Orthoroentgenography as a method of measuring the bones of lower extremities, J. Bone Joint Surg. **28:**60, 1946.

Gruelich, W.W., and Pyle, S.I.: Radiographic atlas of skeletal development of the hand and wrist, Stanford, Calif., 1950, Stanford University Press.

Greville, N.R., and Ivins, J.C.: Fractures of the femur in children: an analysis of their effect on the subsequent length of both bones of the lower limb, Am. J. Surg. **93:**376, 1957.

Greville, N.R., and Janes, J.M.: An experimental study of overgrowth after fractures, Surg. Gynecol. Obstet. **105:**711, 1957.

Gross, R.H.: An evaluation of tibial lengthening procedures, J. Bone Joint Surg. **53A:**693, 1971.

Gullickson, G., Jr., Olson, M., and Koettke, F.J.: The effect of paralysis of one lower extremity on bone growth, Arch. Phys. Med. Rehabil. **31:**392, 1950.

Haas, S.L.: The relation of the blood supply to the longitudinal growth of bone, Am. J. Orthop. Surg. **15:**157, 1917.

Haas, S.L.: Interstitial growth in growing long bones, Arch. Surg. **12**:887, 1926.

Haas, S.L.: Retardation of bone growth by a wire loop, J. Bone Joint Surg. **27**:25, 1945.

Haas, S.L.: Femoral shortening in subtrochanteric region combined with angulation at site of resection, Am. J. Surg. **80**:461, 1950.

Haas, S.L.: Restriction of bone growth by pins through the epiphyseal cartilaginous plate, J. Bone Joint Surg. **32A**:338, 1950.

Haas, S.L.: Stimulation of bone growth, Am. J. Surg. **95**:125, 1958.

Harris, H.A.: The growth of the long bones in childhood (with special reference to certain bony striations of the metaphysis and to the role of vitamins), Arch. Intern. Med. **38**:785, 1926.

Harris, H.A.: Lines of arrested growth in the long bones in childhood: the correlation of histological and radiographic appearances in clinical and experimental conditions, Br. J. Radiol. **4**:561, 1931.

Harris, H.A.: Bone growth in health and disease, London, 1933, Oxford University Press.

Harris, R.I., and McDonald, J.L.: The effect of lumbar sympathectomy upon the growth of legs paralyzed by anterior poliomyelitis, J. Bone Joint Surg. **18**:35, 1936.

Hayes, J.T., and Brody, G.L.: Cystic lymphangiectasis of bone, J. Bone Joint Surg. **43A**:107, 1961.

Herndon, C.H., and Spencer, G.E.: An experimental attempt to stimulate linear growth of long bones in rabbits, J. Bone Joint Surg. **35A**:758, 1953.

Hiertonn, T.: Arteriovenous anastomoses and acceleration of bone growth, Acta Orthop. Scand. **26**:322, 1956.

Hutchinson, W.J., and Burdeaux, B.D.: The influence of stasis on bone growth, Surg. Gynecol. Obstet. **99**:413, 1954.

James, C.C.M., and Lassman, L.P.: Spinal dysraphism: the diagnosis and treatment of progressive lesions in spina bifida occulta, J. Bone Joint Surg. **44B**:828, 1962.

Janes, J.M., and Musgrove, J.E.: Effect of arteriovenous fistula on growth of bone: an experimental study, Surg. Clin. North Am. **30**:1191, 1950.

Kruger, L.M., and Talbott, R.D.: Amputation and prosthesis as definitive treatment in congenital absence of the fibula, J. Bone Joint Surg. **43A**:625, 1961.

Maresh, M.M.: Linear growth of long bones of extremities from infancy through adolescence, Am. J. Dis. Child. **89**:725, 1955.

Marino-Zuco, C.: Treatment of length discrepancy of the lower limbs, J. Bone Joint Surg. **38B**:934, 1956.

Moore, B.H.: A critical appraisal of the leg lengthening operation, Am. J. Surg. **52**:415, 1941.

Morgan, J.D., and Somerville, E.W.: Normal and abnormal growth at the upper end of the femur, J. Bone Joint Surg. **42B**:264, 1960.

Neer, C.S., II, and Cadman, E.F.: Treatment of fractures of the femoral shaft in children, JAMA **163**:634, 1957.

Park, E.A., and Richter, C.P.: Transverse lines in bone: mechanism of their development, Johns Hopkins Med. J. **93**:234, 1953.

Pearse, H.E., and Morton, J.J.: The stimulation of bone growth by venous stasis, J. Bone Joint Surg. **12**:97, 1930.

Pease, C.N.: Local stimulation of growth of long bones: a preliminary report, J. Bone Joint Surg. **34A**:1, 1952.

Phemister, D.B.: Operative arrestment of longitudinal growth of bones in the treatment of deformities, J. Bone Joint Surg. **15**:1, 1933.

Ratliff, A.H.C.: The short leg in poliomyelitis, J. Bone Joint Surg. **41B**:56, 1959.

Reidy, J.A., Lingley, J.R., Gall, E.A., and Barr, J.S.: The effect of roentgen irradiation on epiphyseal growth. II. Experimental studies upon the dog, J. Bone Joint Surg. **29**:853, 1947.

Rezaian, S.M.: Tibial lengthening using a new extension device: report of thirty-two cases, J. Bone Joint Surg. **58A**:239, 1976.

Richards, V., and Stofer, R.: The stimulation of bone growth by internal heating, Surgery **46**:84, 1959.

Ring, P.A.: Shortening and paralysis in poliomyelitis, Lancet, **2**:980, 1957.

Ring, P.A.: Experimental bone lengthening by epiphyseal distraction, Br. J. Surg. **46**:169, 1958.

Ring, P.A.: Congenital short femur: simple femoral hypoplasia, J. Bone Joint Surg. **41B**:73, 1959.

Ring, P.A.: The influence of the nervous system upon the growth of bones, J. Bone Joint Surg. **43B**:121, 1961.

Ring, P.A., and Less, J.: The effect of heat upon the growth of bone, J. Pathol. **75**:405, 1958.

Schneider, M.: Experimental epiphyseal arrest by intraosseous injection of papain, J. Bone Joint Surg. **45A**:25, 1963.

Siffert, R.: The effect of staples and longitudinal wires on epiphyseal growth, J. Bone Joint Surg. **38A**:1077, 1956.

Siffert, R.S.: The effect of juxta-epiphyseal pyogenic infection on epiphyseal growth, Clin. Orthop. **10**:131, 1957.

Sofield, H.A., Blair, S.J., and Millar, E.A.: Leg-lengthening, J. Bone Joint Surg. **40A**:311, 1958.

Sofield, H.A., and Millar, E.A.: Fragmentation, realignment and intramedullary rod fixation of deformities of the long bones in children, J. Bone Joint Surg. **41A**:1371, 1959.

Stewart, S.F.: Effect of sympathectomy on the leg length in cortical rigidity, J. Bone Joint Surg. **19**:222, 1937.

Stinchfield, A.J., Reidy, J.A., and Barr, J.S.: Prediction of unequal growth of the lower extremities in anterior poliomyelitis, J. Bone Joint Surg. **31A**:478, 1949.

Straub, L.R., Thompson, T.C., and Wilson, P.D.: The results of epiphysiodesis and femoral shortening in relation to equilization of limb length, J. Bone Joint Surg. **27**:255, 1945.

Strobino, L.J., Colonna, P.C., Brodey, R.D., and Leinbach, T.: The effect of compression on the growth of epiphyseal bone, Surg. Gynecol. Obstet **103**:85, 1956.

Strobino, L.J., French, G.O., and Colonna, P.C.: The effect of epiphyseal bone, Surg. Gynecol. Obstet. **95**:694, 1952.

Thompson, T.C., Straub, L.R., and Arnold, W.D.: Congenital absence of the fibula, J. Bone Joint Surg. **39A**:1229, 1957.

Thompson, T.C., Straub, L.R., and Campbell, R.D.: An evaluation of femoral shortening with intramedullary nailing, J. Bone Joint Surg. **36A**:43, 1954.

Truesdell, E.D.: Inequality of the lower extremities following fracture of the shaft of the femur in children, Ann. Surg. **74**:498, 1921.

Trueta, J.: Stimulation of bone growth by redistribution of the intraosseous circulation, J. Bone Joint Surg. **33B**:476, 1951.

Trueta, J.: The influence of the blood supply in controlling bone growth, Bull. Hosp. Joint Dis. **14**:147, 1953.

Trueta, J., and Amato, V.P.: The vascular contribution to osteogenesis, J. Bone Joint Surg. **42B**:571, 1960.

Tupman, G.S.: Treatment of inequality of the lower limbs, J. Bone Joint Surg. **42B**:489, 1960.

Tupman, G.S.: A study of bone growth in normal children and its relationship to skeletal maturation, J. Bone Joint Surg. **44B**:42, 1962.

White, J.W.: A simplified method for tibial lengthening, J. Bone Joint Surg. **12**:90, 1930.

White, J.W.: Femoral shortening for equilization of leg length, J. Bone Joint Surg. **17**:597, 1935.

White, J.W.: A practical graphic method of recording leg length discrepancies, South. Med. J. **33**:946, 1940.

White, J.W.: A method of subtrochanteric limb shortening, J. Bone Joint Surg. **31A**:86, 1949.

White, J.W.: Leg-length discrepancies. In American Academy of Orthopaedic Surgeons, Instructional Course Lectures, vol. 6, Ann Arbor, 1949, J.W. Edwards.

White, J.W., and Stubbins, S.G.: Growth arrest for equalizing leg lengths, JAMA, **126**:1146, 1944.

White, J.W., and Warner, W.P.: Experiences with metaphyseal arrests, South. Med. J. 31:41, 1938.

Wilson, C.L., and Percy, E.C.: Experimental studies on epiphyseal stimulation, J. Bone Joint Surg. 38A:1096, 1956.

Wise, C.S., Castlemann, B., and Watkins, A.L.: Effect of diathermy (short wave and microwave) on bone growth in the albino rat, J. Bone Joint Surg. 31A:487, 1949.

Wu, Y.K., and Miltner, L.J.: A procedure for stimulation of longitudinal growth of bone, J. Bone Joint Surg. 19:909, 1937.

Tarsal coalitions

Anderson, R.J.: The presence of an astralagoscaphoid bone in man, J. Anat. 14:452, 1880.

Austin, F.H.: Symphalangism and related fusions of tarsal bones, Radiology 56:882, 1951.

Badgley, C.E.: Coalition of the calcaneus and the navicular, Arch. Surg. 15:75, 1927.

Bersani, F.A., and Samilson, R.L.: Massive familial tarsal synotosis, J. Bone Joint Surg. 39A:1187, 1957.

Boyd, H.B.: Congenital talonavicular synostosis, J. Bone Joint Surg. 26:682, 1944.

Bullitt, J.B.: Variations of the bones of the foot: fusion of the talus and navicular, bilateral and congenital, Am. J. Roentgenol. Radium Ther. 20:548, 1928.

Conway, J.J., and Cowell, H.R.: Tarsal coalition: clinical significance and roentgenographic demonstration, Radiology 92:799, 1969.

Cowell, H.R.: Talo-calcaneal coalition and new causes of peroneal spastic flat foot, Clin. Orthop. 85:16, 1972.

Harris, B.J.: Anomalous structures in the developing human foot (abstr.), Anat. Rec. 121:399, 1955.

Harris, R.I.: Rigid valgus foot due to talonaccaneal bridge, J. Bone Joint Surg. 37A:169, 1955.

Harris, R.I.: Peroneal spastic flatfoot. In American Academy of Orthopaedic Surgeons, Instructional Course Lectures, vol. 15, Ann Arbor, 1958, J.W. Edwards.

Harris, R.I.. Follow-up notes on articles previously published in this journal, J. Bone Joint Surg. 47A:1657, 1965.

Harris, R.I., and Beath, T.: Etiology of peroneal spastic flat foot, J. Bone Joint Surg. 30B:624, 1948.

Harris, R.I., and Beath, T.: John Hunter's specimen of talocalcaneal bridge, J. Bone Joint Surg. 32B:203, 1950.

Hodgson, F.G.: Talonavicular synostosis, South. Med. J. 39:940, 1946.

Holl, M.: Beiträge zur chirurgischen Osteologie des Fusses, Arch. Klin. Chir. 25:211, 1880.

Illievitz, A.B.: Congenital malformations of the feet: report of a case of congenital fusion of the scaphoid with the astragalus, and complete absence of one toe, Am. J. Surg. 4:550, 1928.

Jack, E.A.: Bone anomalies of the tarsus on relation to "peroneal spastic flat foot," J. Bone Joint Surg. 36B:530, 1954.

Kendrick, J.I.: Treatment of calcaneonavicular bar, JAMA 172:1242, 1960.

Lapidus, P.W.: Congenital fusion of the bones of the foot: with a report of a case of congenital astragaloscaphoid fusion, J. Bone Joint Surg. 14:888, 1932.

Lapidus, P.W.: Bilateral congenital talonavicular fusion: report of a case, J. Bone Joint Surg. 20:775, 1938.

Lapidus, P.W.: Spastic flat-foot, J. Bone Joint Surg. 28:126, 1946.

Mahaffey, H.W.: Bilateral congenital calcaneocuboid synostosis: a case report, J. Bone Joint Surg. 27:164, 1945.

Nievergelt, K.: Positiver Vaterschaftsnachweis auf Grund erblicher Missbildungen der Extremitäten, Arch. Julius Klaus-Stiftg. Vererbungsforschg. 19:157, 1944.

O'Donoghue, D.H., and Sell, L.S.: Congenital talonavicular synostosis: a case report of a rare anomaly, J. Bone Joint Surg. 25:925, 1943.

Outland, T., and Murphy, I.D.: Relation of tarsal anomalies to spastic and rigid flatfeet, Clin. Orthop. 1:217, 1953.

Outland, T., and Murphy, I.D.: The pathomechanics of peroneal spatic flat foot, Clin. Orthop. 16:64, 1960.

Pearlman, H.S., Edkin, R.E., and Warren, R.F.: Familial tarsal and carpal synostosis with radial-head subluxation (Nievergelt's syndrome), J. Bone Joint Surg. 46A:585, 1964.

Pfitzner, W.: Ein Beitrag zur Kenntniss der sekundären Geschlectsunterschiede beim Menschen, Morphol. Arb. 7:473, 1897.

Schreiber, R.R.: Talonavicular synostosis, J. Bone Joint Surg. 45A:170, 1963.

Seddon, H.J.: Calcaneo-scaphoid coalition, Proc. R. Soc. Med. 26:419, 1933.

Shands, A.R., Jr., and Wentz, I.J.: Congenital anomalies, accessory bones and osteochondritis in the feet of 850 children, Surg. Clin. North Am. 33:1643, 1953.

Simmons, E.H.: Tibialis spastic varus foot with tarsal coalition, J. Bone Joint Surg. 47B:533, 1965.

Slomann: On coalition calcaneo-navicularis, J. Orthop. Surg. 3:586, 1921.

Vaughan, W.H., and Segal, G.: Tarsal coalition, with special reference to roentgenographic interpretation, Radiology 60:855, 1953.

Wagoner, G.W.: A case of bilateral congenital fusion of the calcanei and cuboids, J. Bone Joint Surg. 10:220, 1928.

Waugh, W.: Partial cubo-navicular coalition as a cause of peroneal spastic flat foot, J. Bone Joint Surg. 39B:520, 1957.

Webster, F.S., and Romerts, W.M.: Tarsal anomalies and peroneal spastic flatfoot, JAMA 146:1099, 1951.

Weitzner, I.: Congenital talonavicular synostosis associated with its hereditary multiple ankylosing arthropathies, Am. J. Roentgenol. Radium Ther. 51:185, 1946.

Wray, J.B., and Herndon, C.N.: Hereditary transmission of congenital coalition of the calcaneus to the navicular, J. Bone Joint Surg. 45A:365, 1963.

Torsional deformities of lower extremities

Appleton, A.B.: Postural deformities and bone growth, Lancet 1:451, 1934.

Arkin, A.M., and Katz, J.F.: Effects of pressure on epiphyseal growth, J. Bone Joint Surg. 38A:1056, 1956.

Backman, S.: The proximal end of the femur: investigations with special reference to the etiology of femoral neck fractures, Acta Radiol. (supp.) 146:1, 1957.

Badgley, C.E.: Correlation of clinical and anatomical facts leading to a conception of the etiology of congenital hip dysplasias, J. Bone Joint Surg. 25:503, 1943.

Badgley, C.E.: Etiology of congenital dislocation of the hip, J. Bone Joint Surg. 31A:341, 1949.

Baker, L.D., and Hill, L.M.: Foot alignment in the cerebral palsy patient, J. Bone Joint Surg. 46A:1, 1964.

Bergmann, G.A.: Die Bedeutung der Innendrehung der Unterschenkel für die Entwicklung des Senk-Knickfusses mit der Angabe einer Messmethode von Messergebnissen, Acta Orthop. 96:177, 1962.

Billing, L.: Roentgen examination of the proximal femur end in children and adolescents, Acta Radiol. (suppl.) 110:1, 1954.

Blount, W.P.: Bow leg, Wis. Med. J. 40:484, 1941.

Blumel, J., Eggers, G.W.N., and Evans, E.B.: Eight cases of hereditary bilateral medial tibial torsion in four generations, J. Bone Joint Surg. 39A:1198, 1957.

Böhm, M.: The embryologic origin of club-foot, J. Bone Joint Surg. 11:229, 1929.

Böhm, M.: Infantile deformities of the knee and hip, J. Bone Joint Surg. 15:574, 1933.

Browne, D.: Congenital deformities of mechanical origin, Proc. R. Soc. Med. 29:1409, 1936.

Chapple, C.C., and Davidson, D.T.: A study of the relationship between fetal position and certain congenital deformities, J. Pediatr. **18**:483, 1941.

Crane, L.: Femoral torsion and its relation to toeing-in and toeing-out, J. Bone Joint Surg. **41A**:421, 1959.

Doyle, M.R.: Sleeping habits of infants, Phys. Ther. Rev. **25**:74, 1945.

Dunlap, K., Shands, A.R., Hollister, L.C., Gahl, J.S., and Streit, H.A.: A new method for determination of torsion of the femur, J. Bone Joint Surg. **35A**:289, 1953.

Dunn, D.M.: Anteversion of the neck of the femur, J. Bone Joint Surg. **34B**:181, 1952.

Durham, H.A.: Anteversion of the femoral neck to the normal femur and its relation to congenital dislocation of the hip, JAMA **65**:223, 1915.

Elftman, H.: Torsion of the lower extremity, Am. J. Phys. Anthropol. **3**:255, 1945.

Fitzhugh, M.L.: Faulty alignment of the feet and legs in infancy and childhood, Phys. Ther. Rev. **21**:239, 1941.

Garden, R.S.: The structure and function of the proximal end of the femur, J. Bone Joint Surg. **43B**:576, 1961.

Geist, E.S.: An operation for the after treatment of some cases of congenital club-foot, J. Bone Joint Surg. **6**:50, 1924.

Howorth, M.B.: A textbook of orthopedics, Philadelphia, 1952, W.B. Saunders Co.

Hutter, C.G., and Scott, W.: Tibial torsion, J. Bone Joint Surg. **31A**:511, 1949.

Irwin, C.E.: The iliotibial band: its role in producing deformity in poliomyelitis, J. Bone Joint Surg. **31A**:141, 1949.

Kaplin, E.B.: The iliotibial tract: clinical and morphological significance, J. Bone Joint Surg. **40A**:817, 1958.

Khermosh, O., Lior, G., and Weissman, S.L.: Tibial torsion in children, Clin. Orthop. **79**:25, 1971.

Kingsley, P.C., and Olmstead, K.L.: A study to determine the angle of anteversion of the neck and of the femur, J. Bone Joint Surg. **30A**:745, 1948.

Kite, J.H.: Torsion of the lower extremities in small children, J. Bone Joint Surg. **36A**:511, 1954.

Kite, J.H.: Torsion of the legs in small children, Med. Assoc. Georgia **43**:1035, 1954.

Kite, J.H.: Torsional deformities of the lower extremities, West Va. Med. J. **57**:92, 1961.

Knight, R.A.: Developmental deformities of the lower extremities, J. Bone Joint Surg. **36A**:521, 1954.

Lanz, Wachsmuth: Praktische Anatomie, Berlin, 1938, Springer-Verlag.

LeDamany, P.: La torsion du tibia, normale, pathologique, expérimentale, J. Anat. Physiol. **45**:598, 1909.

Lowman, C.L.: Rotation deformities, Boston Med. Surg. J. **21**:581, 1919.

Lowman, C.L.: The sitting position in relation to pelvic stress, Phys. Ther. Rev. **21**:30, 1941.

MacKenzie, I.G., Seddon, H.J., and Trevor, D.: Congenital dislocation of the hip, J. Bone Joint Surg. **42B**:689, 1960.

Majestro, T.C., and Frost, H.M.: Spastic internal femoral torsion, Clin. Orthop. **79**:44, 1971.

Milch, H.: Subtrochanteric osteotomy, Clin. Orthop. **22**:145, 1962.

Morgan, J.D., and Somerville, E.W.: Normal and abnormal growth at the upper end of the femur, J. Bone Joint Surg. **42B**:264, 1960.

Nachlas, I.W.: Medial torsion of the leg, Arch. Surg. **28**:909, 1934.

Nachlas, I.W.: Common defects of the lower extremity in infants, South. Med. J. **41**:302, 1948.

O'Donoghue, D.H.: Controlled rotation osteotomy of the tibia, South. Med. J. **33**:1145, 1940.

Rabinowitz, M.S.: Congenital curvature of the tibia, Bull. Hosp. Joint Dis. **12**:63, 1951.

Rosen, H., and Sandick, H.: The measurement of tibiofibular torsion, J. Bone Joint Surg. **37A**:847, 1955.

Sell, L.S.: Tibial torsion accompanying congenital clubfoot, J. Bone Joint Surg. **23**:561, 1941.

Statham, L., and Murray, M.P.: Early walking patterns of normal children, Clin. Orthop. **79**:8, 1971.

Sterling, R.I.: "Derotation" of the tibia, Br. Med. J. **1**:581, 1936.

Sutherland, D.H., Schottstaedt, E.R., Larsen, L.S., Ashley, R.K., Callander, J.N., and James, P.M.: Clinical and electromyographic study of seven spastic children with internal rotation gait, J. Bone Joint Surg. **51A**:1070, 1969.

Swanson, A.B., Green, P.W., and Allis, H.D.: Rotational deformities of the lower extremity in children and their clinical significance, Clin. Orthop. **27**:157, 1963.

Thelander, H.E., and Fitzhugh, M.L.: Posture habits in infancy affecting foot and leg alignments, J. Pediatr. **21**:306, 1942.

Yount, C.C.: The role of tensor fasciae femoris in certain deformities of the lower extremities, J. Bone Joint Surg. **8**:171, 1926.

3

Radiographic examination of the normal foot

IGOR Z. DROBOCKY

Standard radiographic film examination of the foot still offers the best overall detail for the rapid analysis of foot morphology. The standard radiographic projections of the foot are the best means by which the numerous variations of normal can be examined fully. Special projections, together with the standard projections, are usually all that is necessary for full evaluation of the precise interrelationships of the individual digits and other small bones of the foot. Numerous technologic advances have occurred in radiology over the past 5 years, and a number of these modalities have been found useful in the examination of the foot. Computed tomography (CT scanning), xeroradiography, digital subtraction angiography, bone detail subtraction techniques, and nuclear magnetic resonance (NMR) scanning have all found application in the routine and specialized examination of the foot. The application of some of these newer modalities in the examination of the foot will be discussed at the end of this chapter.

STANDARD RADIOGRAPHIC PROJECTIONS

Standard radiographic projections of the foot can be either weight-bearing or passive views. If the biomechanics of the foot are to be evaluated, the weight-bearing views in anteroposterior (AP; dorsoplantar) and lateral projections (Figs. 3-1 and 3-2) are chosen. For completeness the recumbent oblique projections can be added. For an analysis of function, standing lateral views centered at the first metatarsophalangeal joint and standing AP views of the talotarsal joints with various degrees of flexion of the foot are used. If only the structural anatomy of the foot is to be evaluated, the recumbent or non-weight-supporting views are suffi-cient, easier, and quicker to perform—i.e., the standard AP, lateral, and oblique views (Figs. 3-3 to 3-6).

SPECIAL RADIOGRAPHIC PROJECTIONS

It may be necessary to evaluate certain areas of interest in the foot. For these, special projections are used. The most common regions of interest are the *individual digits*. To visualize the digits adequately, the examiner must direct his attention to the variable length and direction of the digits. The position of the AP projection is standard, but the lateral projection must be adapted to the requirements of the patient; usually modified oblique projections are necessary. The *middle* and *distal phalanges* can sometimes best be demonstrated with placement of a dental film between the individual digits, extending to the midproximal phalanx; and with flexion of the adjacent toes, the particular area can be seen (Fig. 3-7).

Regardless of the area of interest to be examined, at least two projections at right angles to each other must be obtained.

1. Attention to the *great toe* is given by dorsoplantar (AP) and lateral projections. The AP view is standard, but the lateral projection is usually a modification of the true lateral. To obtain the most satisfactory projection of the great toe, from the base of the metatarsal bone to the distal aspect, the technician should place the foot with the great toe and medial aspect of the leg in contact with the table and the heel raised on a sandbag so the film will be in contact with the foot. In this position the plantar aspect of the foot is obliquely forward relative to the film (Fig. 3-8), and an unobscured lateral view of the great toe is obtained. The AP view of the great toe is the basic dorsoplantar projection.

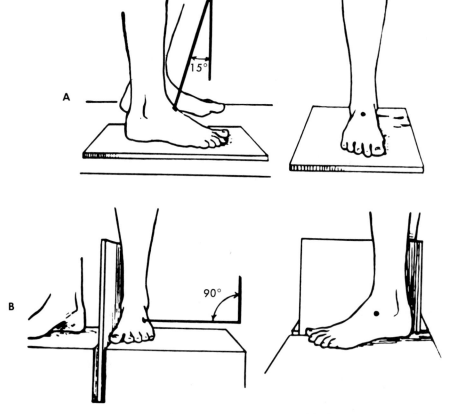

Fig. 3-1. Standard positioning for projections of foot in weight bearing. **A,** Weight-bearing anteroposterior view. **B,** Weight-bearing lateral view. (From Meschan, I.: Semin. Roentgenol. **5:**327, 1970. By permission of Grune & Stratton, Inc.)

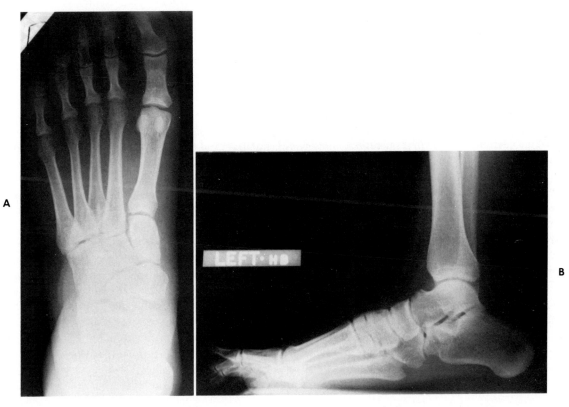

Fig. 3-2. Standard projections of foot in weight bearing. **A,** Weight-bearing anteroposterior view. **B,** Weight-bearing lateral view.

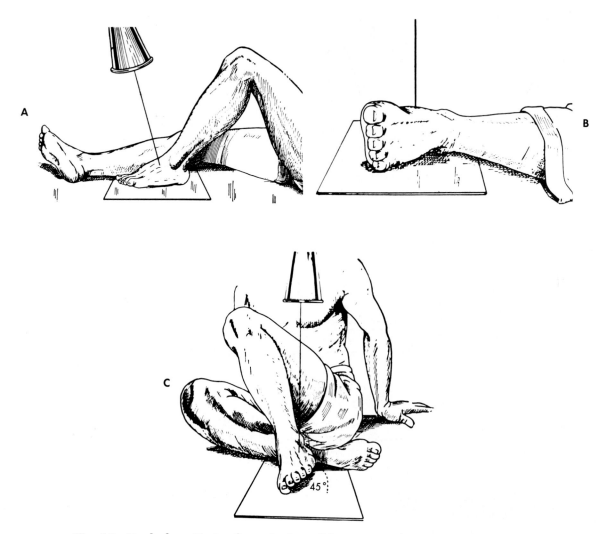

Fig. 3-3. Standard positioning for projections of foot in recumbency. **A,** Anteroposterior view. **B,** Lateral view. **C,** Oblique view. (From Meschan, I.: An atlas of anatomy basic to radiology, vol. 1, Philadelphia, 1975, W.B. Saunders Co.)

2. Special projections of the *first metatarsophalangeal sesamoid bones* are sometimes necessary. These are usually gained well enough in the standard AP and lateral views, but an axial projection of this area is sometimes diagnostic (Fig 3-9, *A* and *B*). There is a choice of two particularly suitable axial projections. The first is with the patient sitting and the film held firmly against the instep. Flexion at the joint is aided by a tightened bandage passed around the digit of the great toe (Fig. 3-9, *A* and *B*). The second is with the limb in a 15° oblique angle and the great toe pulled foreward. The film is placed horizontally for vertical tube projection (Fig. 3-9, *C*).

3. To examine the *os calcis* adequately, the physician must employ AP, lateral, oblique, and axial projections. The AP, lateral, and oblique projections are standard, but the axial views may be a number of variations. The axial projection generally employed is centered on the plantar aspect between both heels with the tube angled 40° from the vertical and the patient supine with ankles flexed and film placed under the heels (Fig. 3-10). A variation of this is to place the patient prone, ankle extended, with the tube angled 60° from the vertical and the film placed perpendicular to the table against the plantar aspect of the foot. These same projections can be used with the patient laterally positioned when necessary to maintain the position without discomfort. When this is done, attention must be given to maintaining the limbs in horizontal alignment by the use of pads and by making the exposure with the tube in a horizontal projection.

Another method of obtaining the axial projection of

Text continued on p. 59.

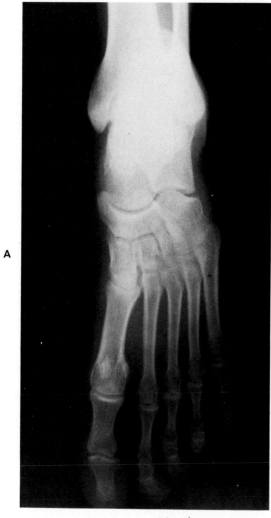

A

Fig. 3-4. A, Standard anteroposterior view of foot. **B,** Line drawing for anatomic points of interest.

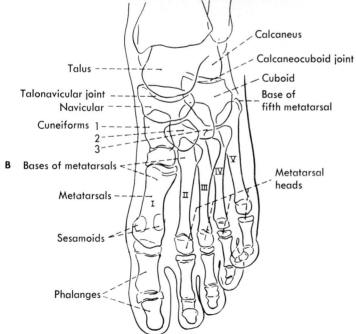

B

Talus

Talonavicular joint

Navicular

Cuneiforms 1
2
3

Bases of metatarsals

Metatarsals

Sesamoids

Phalanges

Calcaneus

Calcaneocuboid joint

Cuboid

Base of
fifth metatarsal

Metatarsal
heads

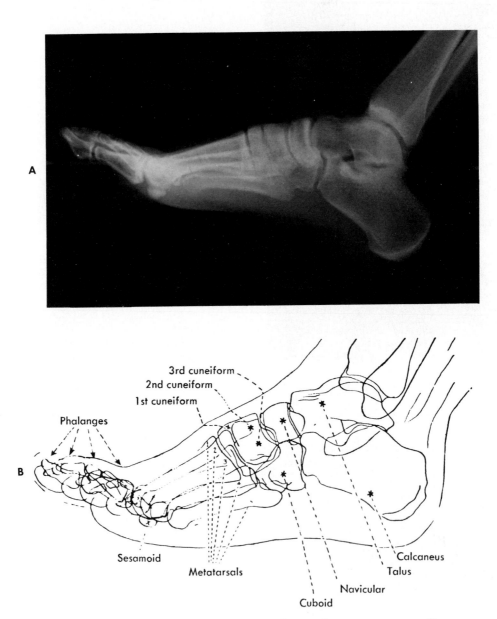

Fig. 3-5. **A,** Standard lateral view of foot. **B,** Line drawing for anatomic points of interest.

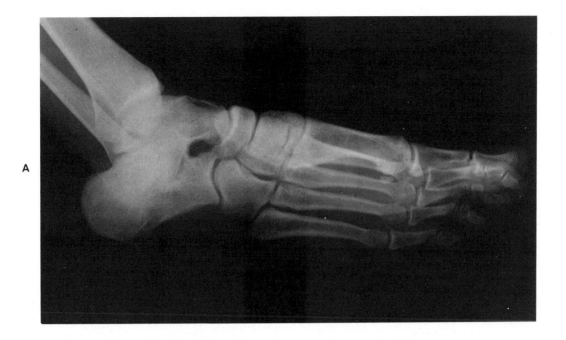

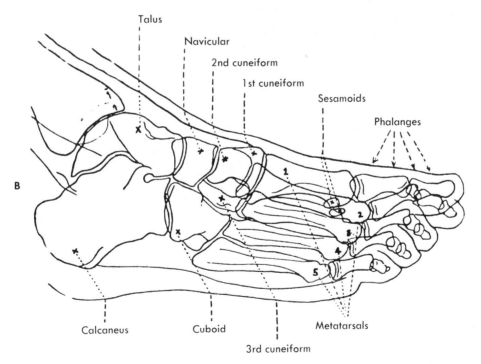

Fig. 3-6. **A**, Standard oblique view of foot. **B**, Line drawing for anatomic points of interest.

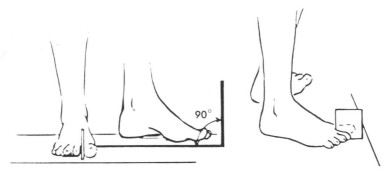

Fig. 3-7. Special projection for individual digits of foot. Here for great toe. (From Meschan, I.: Semin. Roentgenol. **5:**327, 1970. By permission of Grune & Stratton, Inc.)

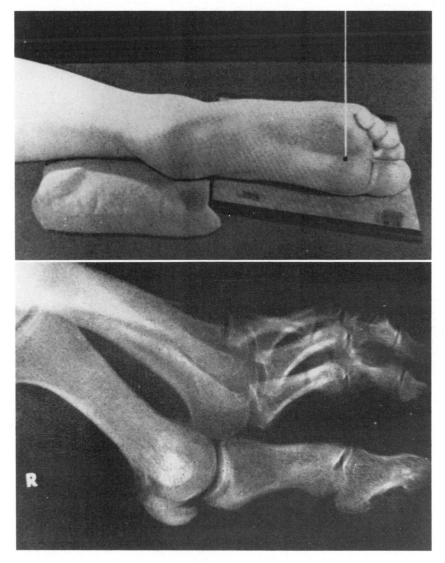

Fig. 3-8. Special projection for great toe in lateral projection. Entire toe from base to distal aspect. (From Clarke, K.C.: Positioning in radiography, ed. 9, London, 1973, Ilford, Ltd.)

4

Hallux valgus and complications of hallux valgus

ROGER A. MANN and MICHAEL J. COUGHLIN

Hallux valgus and treatment

The metatarsophalangeal joint is the most complex joint in the forefoot because of the sesamoid mechanism (Fig. 4-1). It is composed of relatively large bones with powerful intrinsic muscles that insert into the base of the proximal phalanx. Since no muscles insert into the metatarsal head, it is vulnerable to extrinsic factors. It is also influenced by the extrinsic muscles: the extensor and flexor hallucis longus, the tibialis anterior, and the peroneus longus. Furthermore, the metatarsophalangeal joint plays a major role in the transmission of body weight during locomotion, and if there is abnormal stress placed on the joint it may become deformed. Static deformities such as hallux valgus, hallux rigidus, and degenerative arthritis have a tendency to affect this joint and may require surgical intervention.

NOMENCLATURE

The term *bunion* is derived from the Latin word *bunio*, meaning "turnip," and this has led to some confusing misapplications in regard to disorders of the first metatarsophalangeal joint. The term *bunion* has been used to denote any enlargement or deformity of the metatarsophalangeal joint, including such diverse diagnoses as an enlarged bursa, a ganglion, hallux valgus, hallux rigidus, and proliferative changes secondary to arthritis at the metatarsophalangeal joint. The term *hal-*

lux valgus was introduced by Carl Hueter (1871) and has come to define a static subluxation of the first metatarsophalangeal joint with lateral deviation of the great toe and medial deviation of the first metatarsal. It is occasionally accompanied by rotation or pronation of the great toe in severe cases. Other characteristics of the deformity include displacement of the sesamoids, which lie within the tendons of the flexor hallucis brevis (caused by the medial deviation of the first metatarsal); plantar displacement of the abductor hallucis tendon; and lateral bow-stringing of the flexor hallucis longus and extensor hallucis longus tendons.

The hallux valgus deformity thus comprises a common but complex forefoot deformity and may not only encompass deformities of the metatarsophalangeal articulation but also be associated with significant pathophysiologic changes in the soft tissue–supporting structures, the sesamoid mechanism, and the metatarsocuneiform articulation. It may also be involved with abnormal foot mechanics such as a contracted Achilles tendon, severe pes planus, or a more generalized neuromuscular problem such as cerebral palsy.

ETIOLOGY

Hallux valgus occurs almost exclusively in people who wear shoes; however, it does occasionally occur in the unshod. The notion of footwear being the principal contributor in the development of hallux valgus was substantiated by the study of Lam Sim-Fook and Hodgson (1958), in which 33 percent of shod individuals had some degree of hallux valgus as compared to 1.9% of

The authors would like to thank Craig Schonhardt, who drew some of the illustrations in this chapter.

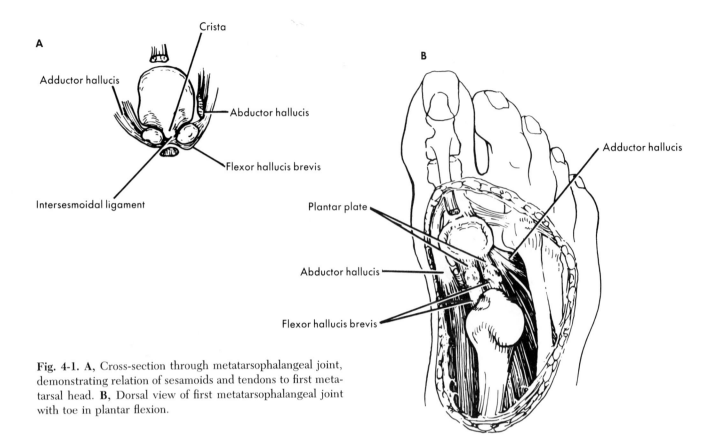

Fig. 4-1. A, Cross-section through metatarsophalangeal joint, demonstrating relation of sesamoids and tendons to first metatarsal head. **B,** Dorsal view of first metatarsophalangeal joint with toe in plantar flexion.

the unshod. Hallux valgus deformity in the Japanese was extremely rare until the 1970s because of the nature of their traditional footwear—the clog. It was not until the manufacture of leather shoes greatly exceeded the manufacture of clogs that the hallux valgus deformity began occurring in the Japanese (Kato and Watanabe, 1981). Conversely, physicians in France referred to hallux valgus as early as the eighteenth century, whereas before that time the common footwear was a Greco-Roman style flat-soled thong. Studies by MacLennan (1966) in New Guinea, Wells (1931) in South African natives, Barnicot (1955) in West Africa, Engle and Morton (1931) in the Belgian Congo, and James (1939) in the Solomon Islands all seemed to find some element of metatarsus primus varus and an occasional hallux valgus deformity that was asymptomatic in the indigenous population. One might conclude from these studies that an asymptomatic hallux valgus deformity in an unshod person might be attributed to hereditary causes. More commonly in shoe-wearing populations, however, the painful bunion is an acquired deformity.

Although the shoe appears to be the essential extrinsic factor in the causation of hallux valgus, the fact remains that there are many individuals who wear fashionable footwear who do not develop this deformity. Therefore there must be some intrinsic predisposing factors that make some feet more vulnerable to the effect of footwear and likewise cause some unshod feet to exhibit a tendency toward the development of hallux valgus. Rare cases of congenital and juvenile hallux valgus may also be explained by these predisposing factors. That modern footwear is the principal contributor to the development of hallux valgus appears certain (Fig. 4-2). Although several studies have provided statistical data showing some predilection of the female population for the development of hallux valgus, this may be merely a reflection of poorer footwear. Wilkins (1941) in his study of feet with reference to schoolchildren reported a predilection of 2:1 in females in the general population. Hewitt, et al. (1953), and Marwil and Brantingham (1943), in investigating male and female military recruits, found predilection of approximately 3:1 in the female population. Creer (1938) and Hardy and Clapham (1951), in reporting statistics from their surgical practices, reported this ratio to be approximately 15:1. Certainly shoes that are worn by women are generally speaking less physiologic than those worn by men, and shoes of any type are prone to lead to hallux valgus in susceptible individuals.

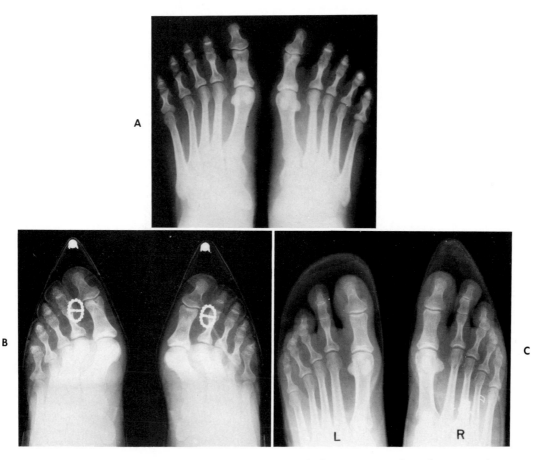

Fig. 4-2. **A,** Normal feet of young woman during weight bearing. **B,** In shoes during weight bearing. She is developing hallux valgus. **C,** Effects of different types of shoes. Left shoe permits freedom of forefoot function; right shoe restricts function of four lesser toes.

Intrinsic causes

Hereditary. Although hallux valgus deformities will commonly occur unilaterally or in patients with no familial history, there are instances in which hallux valgus deformities will show definite hereditary characteristics. Juvenile hallux valgus deformities are more noted for their familial tendency. Johnson (1956), in investigating the inheritance of hallux valgus, felt that in some cases it was transmitted as an autosomal dominant trait with incomplete penetrance.

Pes Planus. The tendency for the pronated foot to develop a hallux valgus deformity has been noted by many authors (Anderson, 1929; Craigmile, 1953; Ewald, 1912; Galland and Jordan, 1938; Hiss, 1931; Joplin, 1950; Jordan and Brodsky, 1951; Mayo, 1920; Rogers and Joplin, 1947; Schede, 1927; Silver, 1923; Stein, 1938; and Verbrugge, 1933). Hohmann (1925) was the most definitive, asserting that hallux valgus is always combined with pes planus and that pes planus is always a causative factor in hallux valgus. The role played by pronation of the foot in the pathophysiology

of hallux valgus is readily depicted in any normal foot, as noted in Figs. 4-3 to 4-7.

In Fig. 4-3, a pendulum has been glued to the nail of the great toe. As the foot is pronated, the rotation of the first ray around its longitudinal axis is clearly seen. In Fig. 4-4, a skeletal model has been photographed. Note that with longitudinal rotation of the first metatarsal head, the fibular sesamoid becomes visible on the lateral side of the first metatarsal head. In Fig. 4-5 a dorsal plantar weight-bearing radiograph is shown of the same foot as in Fig. 4-3. Note that in the pronated position the sesamoids appear to have been displaced laterally. The fibular sesamoid is now visible in the interval between the first and second metatarsals, as would be anticipated from the skeletal model in Fig. 4-4. That this appearance is caused solely by the longitudinal rotation of the first metatarsal and not by an actual lateral displacement is revealed in tangential radiographs of the foot, in which the sesamoids can be seen to remain in a normal relationship to their facets located on the plantar surface of the metatarsal head (Fig. 4-6).

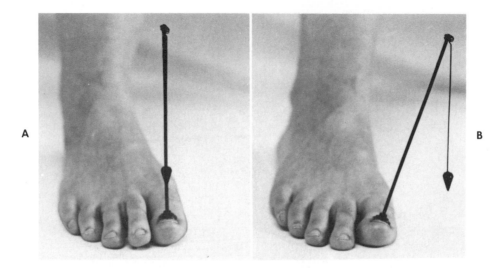

Fig. 4-3. Longitudinal rotation of first ray. **A,** Supination. **B,** Pronation. Pendulum is glued to nail of great toe.

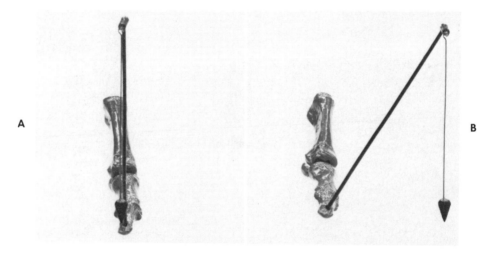

Fig. 4-4. Skeletal model of demonstration in Fig. 4-3. **A,** Supination; **B,** pronation.

In Fig. 4-7, the distribution of weight bearing through the sole of the foot is demonstrated by the barograph. Note that in the pronated foot the area of weight bearing transmitted through the great toe has been displaced medially and a degree of hallux valgus has been created.

Pronation of the foot imposes a longitudinal rotation of the first ray (metatarsal and phalanges), which places the axis of the metatarsophalangeal joint in an oblique plane relative to the floor. In this position the foot appears to be less able to withstand the deforming pressures exerted on it, either by shoes or by weight-bearing. Unfortunately, there are no data available on the relationship between the degree of pes planus and the degree of hallux valgus in the small percentage of unshod individuals who develop the condition. Fur-

thermore, authors who have noted a relationship between pes planus and hallux valgus in shod individuals have presented no quantitative data.

In children who have severe pes planus secondary to a neuromuscular disorder such as poliomyelitis or cerebral palsy there is a much higher incidence of hallux valgus deformity, because these children exert pressure along the medial border of the foot during the stance and lift-off phase of walking, thereby forcing the great toe laterally or into valgus. This, in effect, stretches the medial capsular structures and produces a severe, rapidly occurring hallux valgus deformity.

Therefore in a limited number of patients pronation of the foot may be a predisposing factor to hallux valgus because the medial capsular structures offer limited resistance to the strong deforming forces.

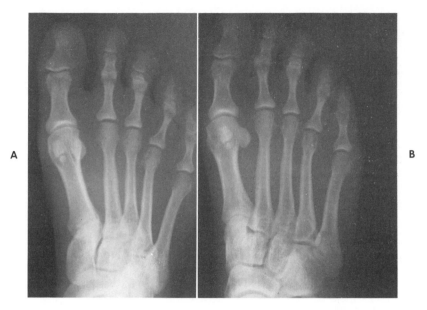

Fig. 4-5. Foot in Fig. 4-3 during weight bearing. **A,** Supination. **B,** Pronation. Note apparent lateral displacement of sesamoids.

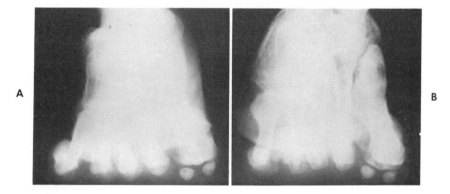

Fig. 4-6. Tangential views of sesamoids during weight bearing. **A,** Supination. **B,** Pronation. Degree of longitudinal rotation of metatarsal is clearly demonstrated by position of sesamoids, which still retain normal relationship to their facets beneath metatarsal head.

Metatarsus primus varus. The simultaneous occurrence of hallux valgus and metatarsus varus has been frequently noted in the literature. Hardy and Clapham (1951) reported a correlation between the degree of hallux valgus and the size of the intermetatarsal angle (coefficient of 0.71). Of all the variables considered in their studies, the highest correlation was between metatarsus primus varus and hallux valgus. The question of cause and effect between medial deviation of the first metatarsal and valgus of the toe will continue to be debated, but it is sufficient to say that they present a combined deformity to a greater or lesser extent in practically all deformities. Truslow (1925) proposed the term *metatarsus primus varus* for a congenital anomaly

that, if present, "inevitably resulted in hallux valgus" when the individual was forced to wear shoes. Studies by Hardy and Clapham (1951) and Craigmile (1953) seem to indicate that metatarsus primus varus is secondary to the hallux valgus deformity. Obviously there is a close relationship between the degree of metatarsus primus varus and hallux valgus, and this must be considered in any corrective surgery. Metatarsus primus varus may predispose a foot at risk, and poor footwear may enhance the development of the hallux valgus deformity.

It is our impression that metatarsus primus varus is more frequently associated with the juvenile form of hallux valgus than the adult, and it is probably a strong

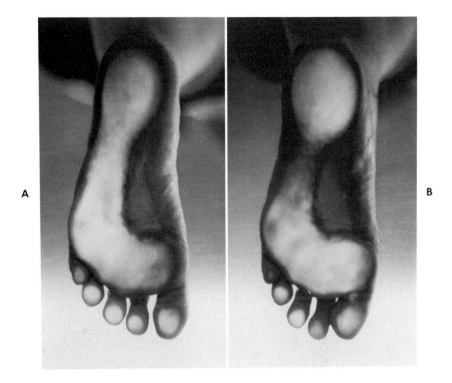

Fig. 4-7. Barographic view during weight bearing. **A,** Supination. **B,** Pronation. Note that pressure area of great toe has moved medially and has produced mild hallux valgus.

predisposing factor, whereas in adults it is probably more often a secondary change.

Metatarsus primus varus may be associated with an adducted forefoot as well. This is congenital in origin and may present as a fixed juvenile bunion.

First metatarsal length. Based on minimal supporting data, both a short first metatarsal (Harris and Beath, 1949; Morton, 1935) and a long first metatarsal (Haines and McDougall, 1954; Mayo, 1908, 1920; and Simon, 1918) have been proposed as essential factors in the develoment of hallux valgus. It appears that the relationship between metatarsal length and the development of hallux valgus is fortuitous and there is no direct etiologic factor.

Miscellaneous factors

Amputation of the second toe will often result in a hallux valgus deformity (Fig. 4-8). This is probably caused by loss of the support afforded by the second toe. A mild form of hallux valgus may be seen after resection of the second metatarsal head.

Cystic degeneration of the medial capsule of the first metatarsophalangeal joint resulting in ganglion formation may sufficiently attenuate the capsule to permit development of a hallux valgus deformity in a foot that might otherwise have only a slight predisposition toward it (Fig. 4-9).

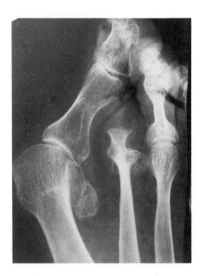

Fig. 4-8. Severe hallux valgus following amputation of second toe.

Contracture of the Achilles tendon secondary to any cause that results in restriction of normal ankle dorsiflexion may produce a gait pattern in which the individual slightly externally rotates the foot and/or has a tendency to roll off the medial border of the foot. This repetitive stress against the hallux may lead to a hallux valgus deformity. This is frequently seen in patients

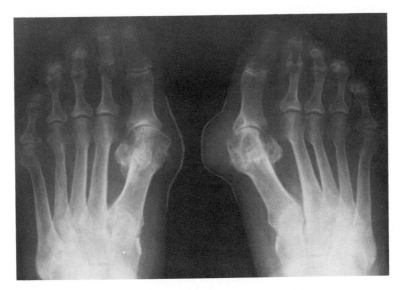

Fig. 4-9. Moderately advanced hallux valgus associated with large ganglionic cyst.

who have neuromuscular disorders, such as cerebral palsy or poliomyelitis, or who have had a stroke, but, may also occur on an idiopathic basis.

Joint hyperelasticity, often presenting as a heritable trait, not infrequently is associated with hallux valgus. Ehlers-Danlos syndrome is the most severe form of hyperelasticity, and most patients with hyperelastic joints do not have this clinical syndrome.

ANATOMIC CONSIDERATIONS OF HALLUX VALGUS

The specialized articulation of the metatarsophalangeal joint of the great toe differs from that of the lesser toes in that it has a sesamoid mechanism. The head of the first metatarsal is rounded and cartilage covered and articulates with the somewhat smaller, concave, elliptically shaped base of the proximal phalanx. From the medial and lateral metatarsal epicondyles originates a fan-shaped ligamentous band, which constitutes the collateral ligaments of the metatarsophalangeal joint (Fig. 4-10). These ligaments interdigitate with the ligaments of the medial and lateral sesamoid. The strong collateral ligaments run distally and plantarward to the base of the proximal phalanx, while the sesamoid ligaments fan out plantarward to the margins of the sesamoid and the plantar plate. The two tendons of the flexor hallucis brevis, the abductor and adductor hallucis, the plantar aponeurosis, and the joint capsule condense on the plantar aspect of the metatarsophalangeal joint to form the plantar plate (Fig. 4-10, *B*). Located on the plantar surface of the metatarsal head are two longitudinal cartilage-covered grooves, which are separated by a rounded ridge (the crista). A sesamoid bone

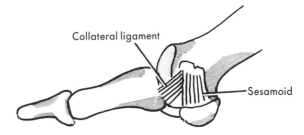

Fig. 4-10. Collateral ligament structure around first metatarsal head.

is contained in each tendon of the flexor hallucis brevis that articulates by means of cartilage-covered convex facets on its superior surface with those corresponding longitudinal grooves on the inferior surface of the first metatarsal head. Distally the two sesamoids are attached by the fibrous plantar plate to the base of the proximal phalanx; thus the sesamoid complex is attached to the base of the proximal phalanx rather than to the metatarsal head. The sesamoids are connected by the intersesamoidal ligament, and this recess conforms to the crista on the plantar surface of the metatarsal head.

The tendons and muscles that move the great toe may be arranged around the metatarsophalangeal joint in four groups. The long and short extensor tendons pass dorsally, and the extensor hallucis longus is anchored medially and laterally by the hood ligament (Fig. 4-11). The extensor hallucis brevis inserts beneath the hood ligament into the dorsal aspect of the base of the proximal phalanx. The long and short flexor tendons pass on the plantar surface, the tendon of the flexor hallucis longus coursing through a centrally located ten-

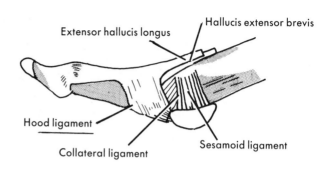

Fig. 4-11. Collateral ligament structure and extensor mechanism about first metatarsophalangeal joint.

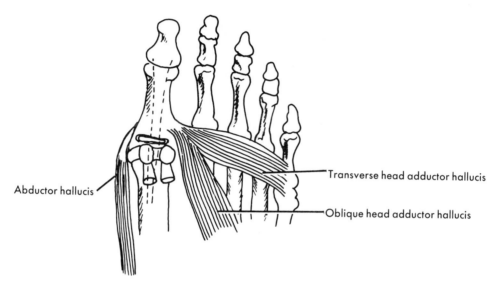

Fig. 4-12. Normal anatomic configuration of first metatarsophalangeal joint, demonstrating stabilizing effect of abductor and adductor hallucis muscles.

don sheath on the plantar aspect of the sesamoid complex. It is firmly anchored within this tunnel to the sesamoid complex. The tendons of the abductor and adductor hallucis pass medially and laterally, respectively, but much nearer the plantar surface than the dorsal surface, so that the dorsomedial and dorsolateral aspects of the joint capsule are covered only by the hood ligaments that maintain the alignment of the extensor hallucis longus tendon.

The abductor hallucis, in addition to its action in maintaining the alignment of the hallux, also has a splinting effect on the first metatarsal head (Fig. 4-12). Acting in a line parallel to this bone and using the head of the first metatarsal as a fulcrum, the abductor hallucis pushes the first metatarsal toward the second metatarsal. The adductor hallucis, arising from the lesser metatarsal shafts, is made up of two segments, the transverse and oblique heads, which insert on the plantar lateral aspect of the base of the proximal phalanx and also blend with the plantar plate and the sesamoid complex. The adductor hallucis balances the abductor forces of the abductor hallucis.

The base of the first metatarsal has a mildly sinusoidal articular surface that articulates with the distal articular surface of the first cuneiform. The joint has a slight medioplantar inclination. The mediolateral dimension is approximately one half the length of the dorsoplantar dimension. The joint is stabilized by capsular ligaments and is bordered laterally by the proximal aspect of the second metatarsal, which extends more cephalad and offers a stabilizing lateral buttress to the first metatarsocuneiform articulation. Occasionally a facet may be present between the proximal first and second metatarsals (Fig. 4-13). The orientation of the metatarsocuneiform joint may determine the amount of metatarsus primus varus, while the shape of the articulation may affect the metatarsal mobility. Normal dorsoplantar motion is believed to be 10° to 15°, while 5° of mediolateral motion is believed to be normal.

A medial inclination of up to 8° at the metatarsocuneiform joint is normal. Increased obliquity at this joint may increase the degree of the metatarsus primus varus.

The tarsometatarsal articulation is quite stable in the

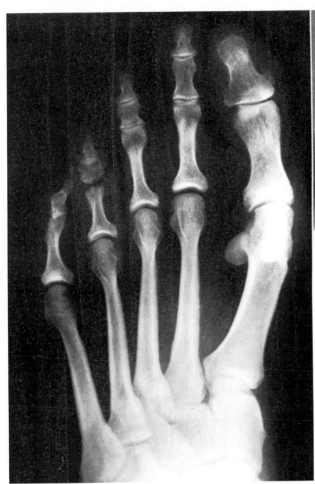

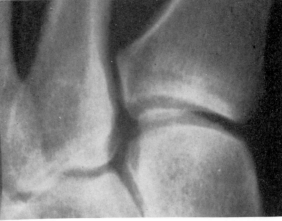

Fig. 4-13. Radiograph demonstrating first metatarsal being maintained in varus position by facet on its plantar lateral aspect.

Fig. 4-14. Stability of tarsometatarsal articulation is maintained by interlocking of central metatarsals.

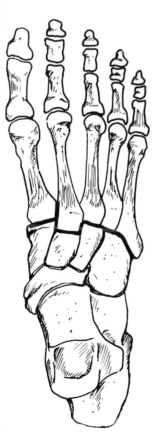

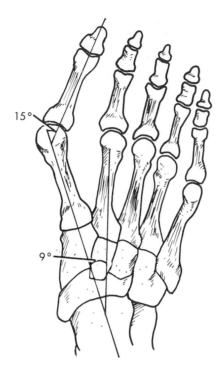

Fig. 4-15. Normal first metatarsophalangeal joint angle should be less than 15°. Intermetatarsal angle should be less than 9°.

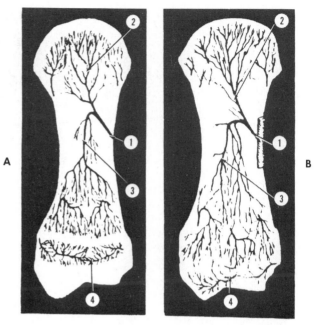

Fig. 4-16. Blood supply to first metatarsal bone. **A,** In adolescent aged 12 to 13 years. Nutrient artery *(1)* divides into short distal *(2)* and long proximal *(3)* branches. Distal branch anastomoses with distal metaphyseal and capital vessels. Proximal branch is stronger and is directed proximally toward epiphysis, which in turn is supplied by arterial branches entering from its medial and lateral side; *(4)* epiphyseal vessels. **B,** In adult: *(1)* nutrient artery; *(2)* distal division branch of nutrient artery; *(3)* proximal division branch of nutrient artery anastomosing with *(4)* epiphyseal vessels. (From Anseroff, N.J.: Die Arterien des Skelets der Hand und des Fusses des Mensche, Z Anat. Entwicklungs, **106:**204, 1937.) (From Sarrafian, S.K.: Anatomy of the foot and ankle, Philadelphia, 1983, J.B. Lippincott Co.)

central portion because of the interlocking of the central metatarsals and cuneiforms (Fig. 4-14). This is not necessarily the case for the first and fifth metatarsals, where stability is determined not only by the inherent stability of the tarsometatarsal articulation but also by the surrounding capsular structures. Therefore in some situations where there is ligamentous laxity, the first metatarsal may deviate medially and the fifth metatarsal laterally in the development of a splayfoot deformity.

Normal values of first metatarsophalangeal joint and intermetatarsal angulation

In evaluating a large group of normal patients, as well as patients with hallux valgus deformities, Hardy and Clapham (1952) determined that a metatarsophalangeal angle of greater than 15° was abnormal and an intermetatarsal angle of greater than 9° was abnormal (Fig. 4-15). Piggott (1960), in evaluating 100 adolescent patients, found a variation in the orientation of the articular surface of the metatarsophalangeal joint. He concluded, however, that a normal metatarsal head is tilted in a slightly lateral direction and that this accounts for the normal valgus alignment of the great toe.

Blood supply to the metatarsal head

The blood supply to the first metatarsal passes through the nutrient artery, which traverses the lateral cortex of the midshaft of the metatarsal in a distal direction. The vessel divides within the medullary canal, sending branches both distally and proximally. Whereas the blood supply through the nutrient artery demonstrates little variation, the blood supply to the metatarsal head and that to the base of the metatarsal demonstrate great variability. Distally there is a network of vessels that penetrates the head and neck of the metatarsal, but, as mentioned previously, a great deal of individual variation occurs. Proximally the blood supply is centered around the area of the old epiphyseal plate region and seems to demonstrate a more uniform pattern (Fig. 4-16).

PATHOPHYSIOLOGY OF HALLUX VALGUS

The dynamics of the hallux valgus deformity can be best understood by first examining the articulation where the deformity occurs, i.e., the metatarsophalangeal and metatarsocuneiform joints.

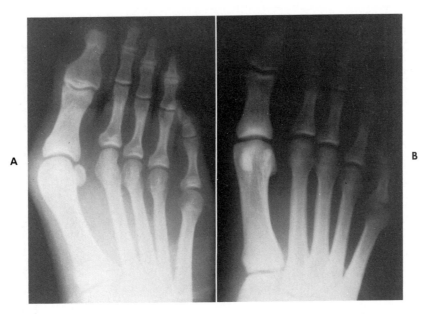

Fig. 4-17. A, Round metatarsal head. This type of articulation tends to predispose patient to hallux valgus deformity. **B,** Flat type of metatarsal head. This type resists hallux valgus deformity.

A flattened metatarsophalangeal articulation is a very stable joint that will resist deforming forces, while the rounded head will be more prone to the development of a hallux valgus deformity (Fig. 4-17). Congruity of the articulation is another factor that must be considered. In a congruous relationship, the base of the proximal phalanx articulates with the central region of the metatarsal articular surface. In an incongruous articulation, the base of the proximal phalanx may be slightly deviated or subluxed laterally so that the metatarsal head is slightly uncovered (Fig 4-18). The congruity of the joint is determined by measuring the orientation of the articular surface of the proximal phalanx and the metatarsal head. Piggott (1960) found that a congruous articulation was a very stable joint and not specifically inclined toward a hallux valgus deformity, while an incongruous articulation was at significant risk for later metatarsophalangeal decompensation.

The orientation of the first metatarsocuneiform joint may determine the stability of the joint. A horizontal setting tends to resist an increase in the intermetatarsal angle, while an oblique setting is a less stable articulation (Fig. 4-19). A greater curvature or rounding of the metatarsocuneiform joint may enhance the mobility of the metatarsocuneiform joint and hence the tendency of the metatarsal to deviate medially.

Anatomic variations in the shape and stability of these joint surfaces may predispose the forefoot to deformity by extrinsic pressure of various types of footwear or abnormal foot mechanics, such as a contracted Achilles tendon.

The presence of a lateral facet, exostosis, or an accessory bone between the base of the first and second metatarsals will resist any attempt to decrease the intermetatarsal angle. In the face of a hallux valgus deformity, failure to address this rigid articulation may result in a failure of the operative procedure (Fig 4-20).

The intrinsic musculature, which under normal circumstances stabilizes the first metatarsophalangeal joint, plays a key role in the development and progression of the hallux valgus deformity once it begins (Fig. 4-21). As the hallux valgus progresses, the phalanx is displaced laterally and may be pronated on the head of the first metatarsal. The adductor hallucis tendon, besides being a relatively fixed structure that inserts into the plantar lateral aspect of the base of the proximal phalanx, also anchors the sesamoids along with the transverse metatarsal ligament so that they cannot drift medially with the metatarsal head (Fig. 4-22). As the hallux valgus deformity progresses, the great toe is forced laterally by extrinsic deforming forces. As the medial joint capsule becomes attenuated, the hallux migrates into valgus, and the first metatarsal is pushed into a medial or varus position. The only structure that affords medial stability to the metatarsophalangeal joint is the medial ligamentous complex. With increasing angulation at the metatarsophalangeal joint, sesamoid subluxation occurs as the head of the first metatarsal progressively moves off the sesamoid mechanism (Fig. 4-23). The sesamoid mechanism retains its anatomic relationship to the second metatarsal. As this displacement occurs, the intersesamoid ridge is eroded, so that

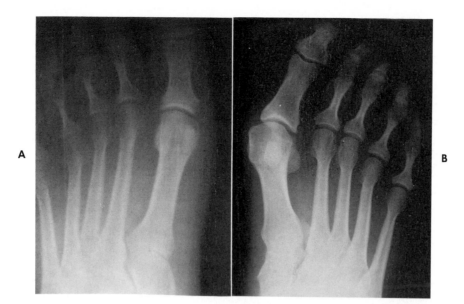

Fig. 4-18. A, Radiograph demonstrating congruent joint surface. Base of proximal phalanx is centered over metatarsal head. **B,** Lateral tilt to metatarsal head creates incongruous relationship, which predisposes to hallux valgus deformity.

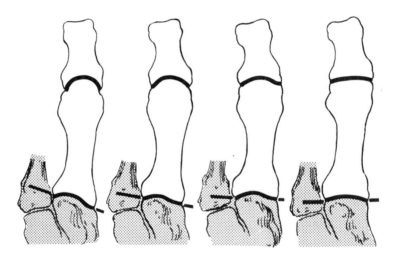

Fig. 4-19. Variations in shape of first metatarsal head and angle of articulation of first metatarsal cuneiform joint of right foot. These may contribute to or resist deformity of first metatarsophalangeal joint. Round metatarsal head predisposes to hallux valgus, as does oblique first metatarsocuneiform joint.

there remains no further bony resistance to this migration. Although the term *sesamoid subluxation* is frequently used, technically speaking the sesamoids retain their anatomic relationship to the second metatarsal because they are anchored by the transverse metatarsal ligament and adductor hallucis. In a severe hallux valgus deformity, the lateral sesamoid may come to be located in a position on the lateral aspect of the metatarsal head and may come to lie vertically above the medial sesamoid (associated with severe pronation of the hallux), with the medial sesamoid articulating with the lateral aspect of the first metatarsal (Fig. 4-24). Sesamoid views confirm the progressive displacement of the metatarsal head off the sesamoids. As the metatarsal head migrates medially, the medial joint capsule is further attenuated, and the abductor hallucis is pulled into a plantar position beneath the metatarsal head, further rotating the proximal phalanx into pronation. The base

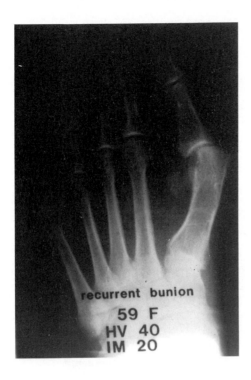

Fig. 4-20. Recurrent hallux valgus caused by failure to correct metatarsus primus varus.

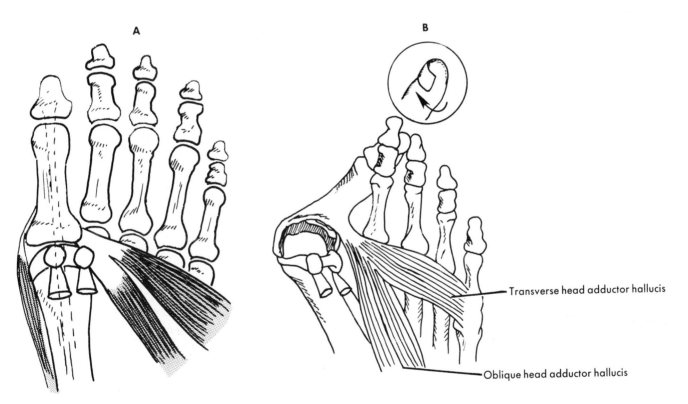

Fig. 4-21. Pathologic anatomy of hallux valgus. **A,** Normal anatomic configuration of first metatarsophalangeal joint. **B,** Hallux valgus with distortion of anatomic structures around first metatarsophalangeal joint. Inset demonstrates pronation of great toe.

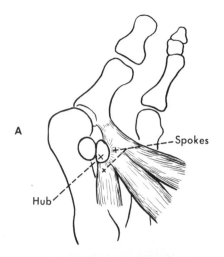

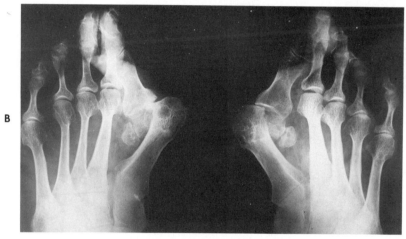

Fig. 4-22. **A,** Proximal phalanx and sesamoids are anchored by conjoint tendon consisting of adductor hallucis and fibular portion of flexor hallucis brevis. **B,** As first metatarsal head drifts medialward, it slides off sesamoids, which become displaced into first interspace, and proximal phalanx is pulled into valgus.

of the proximal phalanx remains firmly anchored to the adductor hallucis and the sesamoids, so that as the metatarsal head drifts medially the base of the proximal phalanx is not only anchored laterally but also is forced to rotate along its longitudinal axis, with the pivot point being the insertion of the adductor tendon (Fig. 4-25). This is the mechanism of pronation of the great toe. Pronation is frequently observed with hallux valgus deformities of 35° or greater (Mann and Coughlin, 1980).

Because of abnormal rotation, calluses may develop along the medial aspect of the interphalangeal joint as well as underneath the second metatarsal head. This is caused by increased weight bearing, which results from the loss of stability at the first metatarsophalangeal joint.

In a marked hallux valgus deformity the extensor hallucis longus tendon displaces, and the medial hood lig-

ament and capsule become stretched. The extensor hallucis longus tendon displaces laterally with the hallux. Therefore when the extensor tendon contracts it not only extends the toe but also adducts it. The abductor hallucis tendon, by migrating plantarward, loses any remaining abductor power. The flexor hallucis longus tendon retains its relationship to the sesamoids and, with the "migration of the sesamoids," also becomes a dynamic deforming force.

If the medial drift of the metatarsal continues unabated, in time there will be subluxation or frank dislocation of the metatarsophalangeal joint with the fibular and sometimes the tibial sesamoid becoming displaced into the first intermetatarsal space. The flexor hallucis longus tendon is displaced with the sesamoids and becomes a plantar-deforming force, while the extensor hallucis longus tends to drift laterally with the hallux, becoming a dorsal-deforming force. Together these

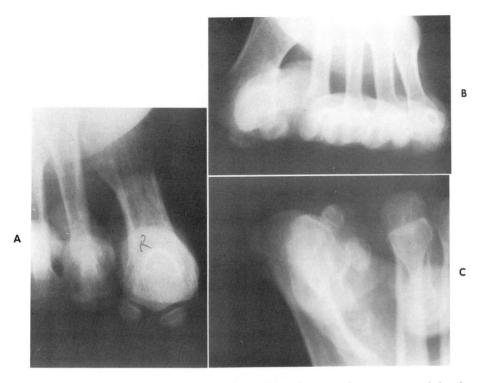

Fig. 4-23. Radiograph demonstrating relationship of sesamoids to metatarsal head. **A,** Normal position. **B,** Moderate hallux valgus. **C,** Severe hallux valgus.

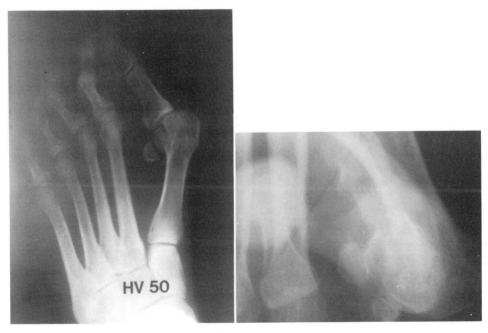

Fig. 4-24. Radiograph of severe hallux valgus deformity, demonstrating subluxation of metatarsal head off of sesamoids so that fibular sesamoid is in first interspace.

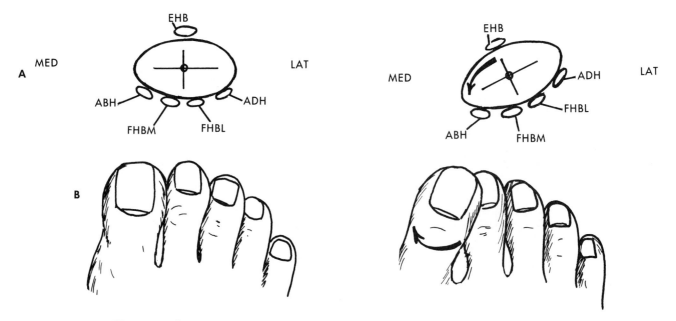

Fig. 4-25. Schematic representation of tendons about first metatarsal head. **A,** Normal articulation in balanced state. **B,** Relationship of tendons in patient with hallux valgus deformity. *EHB,* extensor hallucis brevis; *ABH,* abductor hallucis; *ADH,* adductor hallucis; *FHBM,* flexor hallucis brevis medial head; *FHBL,* flexor hallucis brevis lateral head.

structures become secondarily contracted in long-standing, severe deformities.

In early cases of hallux valgus there appears to be minimal bony outgrowth on the medial aspect of the first metatarsal head. This prominence is accounted for by the displacement of the proximal phalanx in a lateral direction, uncovering the medial aspect of the metatarsal head. Even in a severe hallux valgus deformity the medial aspect of the metatarsal head itself may not hypertrophy more than 1 to 2 mm, but at other times it may hypertrophy 3 to 5 mm. Some patients, however, demonstrate little deformity but have a large medial prominence (Fig. 4-26). At times inflammatory bursitis and thickening of the bursa overlying the metatarsal head may accentuate the medial eminence.

The ligament of the medial sesamoid and the medial collateral ligament overlying the metatarsophalangeal joint may be thickened over the medial eminence; however, this ligamentous complex at other times becomes thin and soft, and occasionally it is completely attenuated because of chronic inflammation when an adventitious bursa overlies this eminence. Where complete erosion of the capsule has occurred, postsurgical recurrence is more commonly noted. Enlargement of the adventitious bursa over the first metatarsal head can be severe and at times may break down, forming a chronic draining sinus.

The splayed appearance of the forefoot in advanced hallux valgus, we believe, occurs primarily because the first metatarsal is no longer contained by the base of the proximal phalanx, into which all intrinsic muscles are inserted. The phalanx and the sesamoids remain fixed by the adductor and the transverse metatarsal ligament, while the first metatarsal drifts medially. The middle metatarsals do not splay because of the stable articulation at their tarsometatarsal joints. However, the fifth metatarsal may drift in a lateral direction as well.

The medial deviation of the first metatarsal, giving rise to the so-called metatarsus primus varus, may be brought about by the lateral deviation of the proximal phalanx pushing against the first metatarsal head, which will result in medial deviation of the first metatarsal. Generally speaking, this usually occurs in patients with some ligamentous laxity. Conversely, the medial deviation of the first metatarsal may be the anatomic alignment for the particular patient, and as such is a rather fixed, rigid structure. In the former condition, the medial deviation of the metatarsal is secondary to its hypermobility and the pressure of the proximal phalanx against the first metatarsal head, whereas in the latter, the hallux valgus deformity was brought about by the fixed medial position of the first metatarsal and the resultant pressure against the proximal phalanx pushing it into a valgus position.

The lesser toes are often pushed laterally by the deviating hallux. This in turn may cause problems with

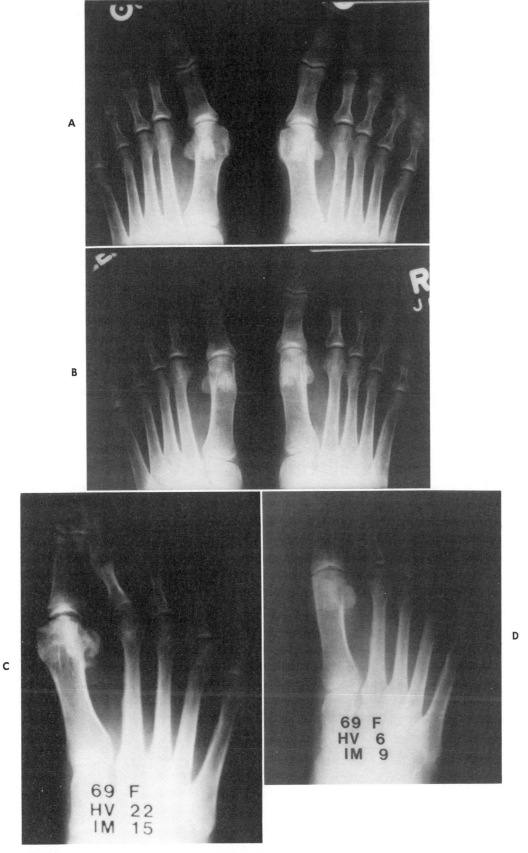

Fig. 4-37. A, Preoperative radiograph of moderate hallux valgus deformity. **B,** Postoperative radiograph following soft tissue procedure. Note improvement in alignment of first metatarsophalangeal joint as well as intermetatarsal angle. **C,** Preoperative radiograph of moderate hallux valgus deformity. **D,** Postoperative radiograph following soft tissue procedure.

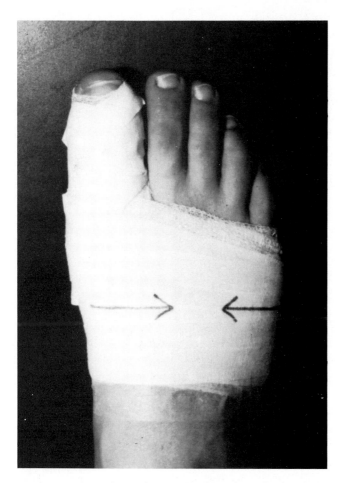

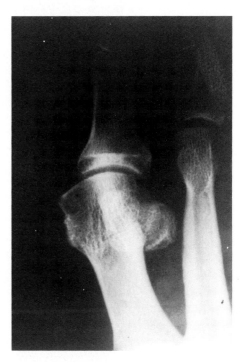

Fig. 4-39. Radiograph demonstrating hallux valgus deformity in patient with short first metatarsal. Further shortening of this metatarsal would only result in significant weight transfer to second metatarsal and probable significant metatarsalgia.

Fig. 4-38. Postoperative dressing consists of 2-inch Kling bandage and ½-inch adhesive tape. Essential part of dressing is firm binding of metatarsal heads together, as demonstrated by arrows, and proper positioning of first metatarsophalangeal jont to be maintained by dressing.

modification of the McBride procedure. Using the DuVries modification of the McBride procedure, a review of 200 of our cases demonstrated a 4% incidence of severe hallux varus deformity. In this group the hallux varus averaged 15°. Another group, comprising 7% of our patients, had a mild hallux varus deformity, averaging 4° of varus. Although the mild degree of varus was evident on x-ray film, none of these patients had any clinical symptoms. The patients with the severe degree of hallux varus were symptomatic and required further treatment.

In an effort to further diminish the possibility of developing a hallux varus deformity, we have modified the DuVries modification of the McBride procedure and presented it as a soft-tissue procedure. The alteration in the procedure was designed to leave the fibular sesamoid in place but to carefully release the transverse metatarsal ligament from it, which permits the sesamoids to be reduced beneath the metatarsal head.

Through this modification we have been able to reduce the incidence of postoperative varus deformities to about 2% incidence of mild hallux varus (averaging 3°) and no patients with a severe deformity. In the previous review of our patients, most of the hallux varus deformities occurred in patients with severely deformed feet (that is, with a hallux valgus deformity of greater than 40°) and it was believed that the hallux varus was probably caused by attempting to correct too much deformity of the metatasophalangeal joint without using a metatarsal osteotomy. At present, with the use of a metatarsal osteotomy and the retention of the lateral sesamoid, we believe that hallux varus will rarely be a significant complication.

For a further discussion of hallux varus, see p. 126.

Proximal first metatarsal osteotomy

Use of a metatarsal osteotomy to correct a hallux valgus deformity has been advocated in the distal metatarsal by Austin et al. (1968), Hawkins et al. (1945), Hohmann (1921, 1925), and Reverdin (1881); in the metatarsal shaft by Ludloff (1918); an opening wedge proximal osteotomy by Bonney and MacNab (1952); and a closing wedge proximal osteotomy by Balacescu (1903). Many others have advocated various forms of osteotomies for correction of hallux valgus deformity.

Our indication for the use of a metatarsal osteotomy in the treatment of a hallux valgus deformity is when the first metatarsal cannot be reduced to the second when carrying out a soft tissue procedure. As a general rule this occurs if the angle of metatarsus primus varus is greater than 15°, although it must be emphasized that there are exceptions to this generalization.

One of the more common causes for recurrent hallux valgus postoperatively, particularly when only a soft tissue procedure is used, is the inadequate correction of either a significant metatarsus primus varus or the residual pronation of the great toe.

In most individuals, the second metatarsal is slightly longer than the first. In carrying out a metatarsal osteotomy it is important to maintain adequate length of the first metatarsal to prevent metatarsalgia from occurring beneath the second metatarsal because of weight transfer. With the surgeon bearing this thought in mind, the preoperative length of the metatarsal may determine in part the type of osteotomy employed. A short first metatarsal should not be further shortened by an osteotomy that sacrifices length of the metatarsal, and conversely an abnormally long first metatarsal should not be further lengthened by an opening wedge osteotomy (Fig. 4-39). In general, we prefer a crescentic osteotomy, which has a minimal effect on metatarsal length. It is carried out in a cancellous portion of the proximal first metatarsal, where rapid healing occurs because of the broad stable interface of the osteotomy site. The proximal osteotomy is employed in conjunction with the soft tissue repair described previously.

Technique

1. The skin incision is made over the dorsal aspect of the proximal portion of the first metatarsal and is approximately 2.5 cm in length (Fig. 4-32, *C*). The extensor hallucis longus tendon is usually swept laterally. The first metatarsocuneiform joint is identified, and the proximal portion of the first metatarsal is stripped of its soft tissue attachments.

2. A crescentic osteotomy is then created using a curved osteotomy* saw (Fig. 4-40, *B*). The osteotomy is carried out approximately 1 cm distal to the metatarsocuneiform joint, with the concave aspect of the osteotomy oriented proximally (Fig. 4-40, *C*). Care should be taken to orient the osteotomy in a dorsoplantar plane at about a right angle to the first metatarsal shaft.

3. After the osteotomy is completed, displacement of the metatarsal is carried out. As this is done, the head

---

*Produced by Stryker or Zimmer Corporation.

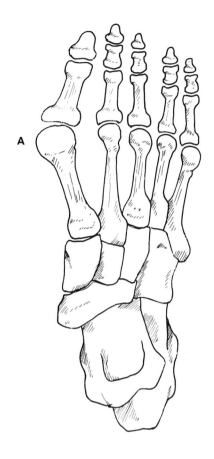

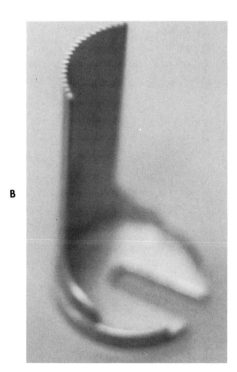

Fig. 4-40. Technique of proximal metatarsal osteotomy. **A,** Diagram of foot with hallux valgus deformity and uncorrectable metatarsus primus varus. **B,** Curved osteotomy saw blade.

Continued.

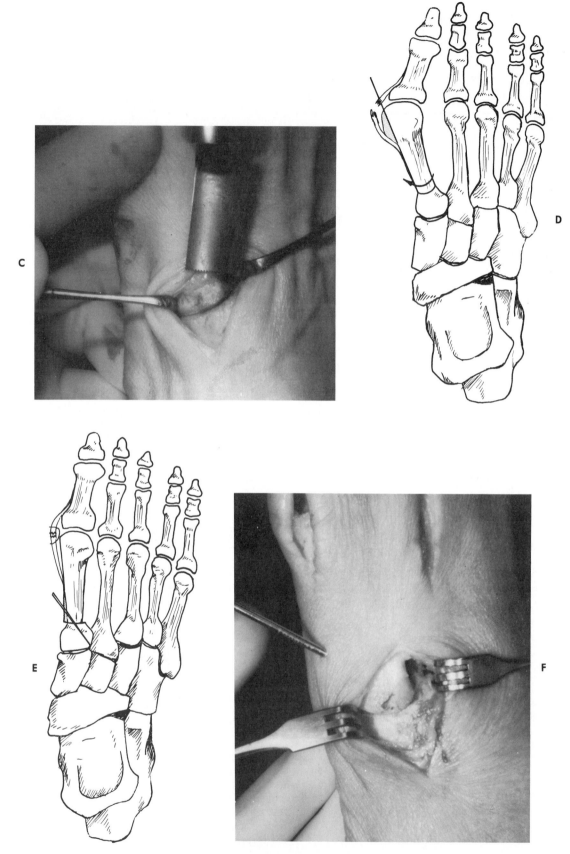

Fig. 4-40, cont'd. For legend see opposite page.

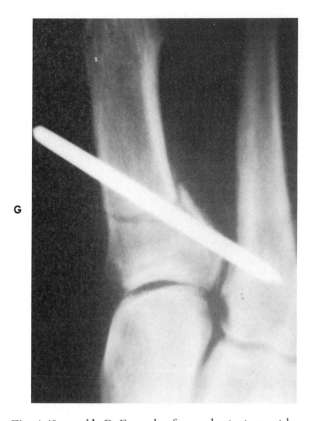

G

Fig. 4-40, cont'd. **C,** Example of curved osteotomy at base of metatarsal. Concavity is based proximally. **D,** Osteotomy site is displaced slightly medially as metatarsal head is displaced laterally. **E,** Diagram of displaced osteotomy with pin fixation. **F,** Demonstration of medial displacement of osteotomy site with pin fixation. **G,** Radiograph demonstrating the osteotomy site with pin fixation.

of the metatarsal moves laterally and the site of the osteotomy is displaced slightly medially. This displacement occurs within the curve of the osteotomy site and, generally speaking, the metatarsal is displaced medially approximately 2 mm. A displacement of more than this may give rise to too much correction distally.

4. The osteotomy site is stabilized at this point by using a small elevator, which is held in the osteotomy site to produce stability. A ⁵⁄₆₄-inch smooth Steinmann pin is then drilled across the osteotomy site from medial to lateral and embedded into the tarsal bones (Fig. 4-40, *E* to *G*). From a technical standpoint it is easier to predrill the medial cortex of the metatarsal through a short incision with a ¹⁄₁₆-inch drill bit. By predrilling the hole, a more accurate pin placement can usually be achieved. As a general rule, one pin is sufficient to stabilize the osteotomy site, but if necessary more pins may be used. The Steinmann pin is cut so that approximately 5 mm protrudes beyond the skin

margin. This facilitates easy removal of the pin in the office.

An alternative method of stabilizing the osteotomy site is to use one or two smooth Kirschner wires. These are cut off at the skin edge and driven beneath the skin with a nail punch. Occasionally, if the operating surgeon is not happy with the bony apposition of the osteotomy site, it may be augmented by bone graft excised from the medial eminence. Following the stabilization of the osteotomy site, the wound is approximated and a soft tissue dressing is applied.

Since the osteotomy is only used in conjunction with the soft tissue repair, the postoperative care is the same as that described for the soft tissue bunion repair. A cast is not used. Ambulation in the previously described dressing and shoe is permitted (see p. 92 and Fig. 4-38). The osteotomy site is usually stable by the fourth to sixth postoperative week, and at that time the pin is removed and the dressings continued as for the soft tissue procedure for the full 8-week period (Fig. 4-41).

When the osteotomy is used in conjunction with soft tissue bunion repair, the following sequence of steps should be followed:

1. Release of the structures on the lateral side of the first metatarsophalangeal joint
2. Medial capsular tissue preparation and medial eminence excision
3. Metatarsal osteotomy
4. Placement of sutures in the first web space between the first and second metatarsal heads, incorporating the adductor tendon
5. Fixation of the osteotomy site
6. Repair of the medial capsular structures
7. Sutures tied in the first web space

In our hands this osteotomy has been very successful. There have been no cases of a nonunion, nor has there been angulation dorsally or plantarward of the osteotomy site. Care must be taken when displacing the osteotomy that the metatarsal shaft is not moved too far laterally. The lateral displacement can be judged by carefully palpating the interval between the first and second metatarsal heads when the metatarsal site is being secured with the Steinmann pin. If a problem arises at the pin site before the healing of the osteotomy, the pin may be removed sooner than 4 to 6 weeks, and in some cases it has been removed as early as 2 weeks postoperatively. In these cases there has been no significant displacement of the osteotomy site. We believe that it is the firm dressing holding the metatarsal heads together that supports the oseotomy site.

Complications. Complications that may result following any metatarsal osteotomy include delayed union, nonunion, or malunion.

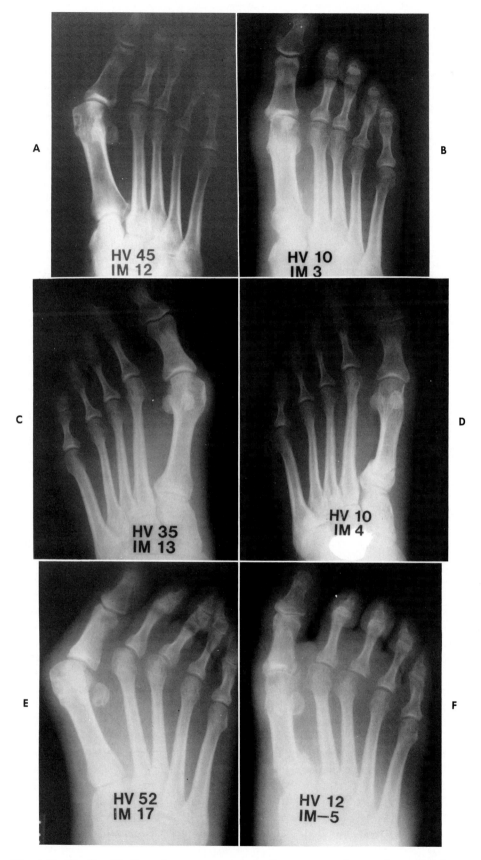

Fig. 4-41. Results of hallux valgus surgery using soft tissue procedure and metatarsal osteotomy. **A,** Preoperative radiograph. **B,** Postoperative radiograph. **C,** Preoperative radiograph. **D,** Postoperative radiograph. **E,** Properative radiograph. **F,** Postoperative radiograph.

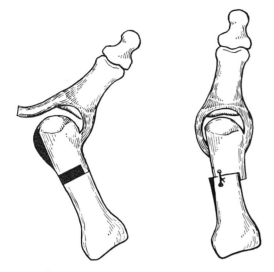

Fig. 4-42. Hawkins et al. (1945) step-cut osteotomy of first metatarsal shaft for hallux valgus.

Distal metatarsal osteotomy
Mitchell procedure

The Mitchell procedure was described by Hawkins et al. (1945). They described a double step-cut osteotomy through the neck of the first metatarsal. It is indicated for moderate hallux valgus deformities with an intermetatarsal angle of up to approximately 18° and, generally speaking for patients less than 50 years of age.

Technique

1. The skin incision is made over the dorsomedial aspect of the first metatarsophalangeal joint. The incision begins distally at the midportion of the proximal phalanx and is carried proximally about 6 cm. Care must be taken to protect the dorsal and plantar medial nerves.

2. A Y-shaped capsular incision is developed over the medial joint capsule. The apex of the distally based V-shaped flap is located approximately 0.5 cm proximal to the metatarsophalangeal joint.

3. A subperiosteal dissection is then carried out on the dorsal and medial aspect of the distal metatarsal, with care being taken not to devascularize the lateral aspect of the metatarsal head. The medial eminence is then excised in line with the medial metatarsal shaft. The surgeon must remember that the remaining blood supply to the metatarsal head traverses the lateral capsular attachments, and disruption of this may result in avascular necrosis of the metatarsal head.

4. A drill hole is placed 1 cm proximal to the metatarsophalangeal joint and is oriented in a dorsoplantar direction. This drill hole is oriented slightly toward the medial metatarsal cortex. A second drill hole, 1 cm

proximal to the first hole and located closer to the lateral aspect of the metatarsal shaft, is now drilled in a similar manner.

5. A double osteotomy is created (Fig. 4-42). The more proximal cut completely transects the metatarsal shaft in a transverse fashion, while a more distal cut is incomplete on the lateral border of the metatarsal shaft. Approximately 2 to 4 mm of bone is resected by this double osteotomy, depending on how much shortening is desired to decompress the contracted lateral structures. The width of the lateral spike remaining depends on the degree of the intermetatarsal angle. In a severe deformity the spike constitutes approximately one third of the metatarsal shaft, while in a more moderate deformity it comprises approximately one sixth of the metatarsal width.

6. If one of the osteotomies is oriented in a slightly plantar direction, the metatarsal head will rotate slightly plantarward with the correction, which will improve the weight bearing on the first metatarsal head, compensating, it is hoped, for the metatarsal shortening. The osteotomy is displaced so that the metatarsal head is shifted laterally until the lateral spike displaces over the proximal shaft.

7. The osteotomy site is stabilized with heavy suture material or wire passed through the prepared drill holes.

8. With the toe held in a slightly overcorrected position, the medial capsular tissues are reefed with interrupted 00 chromic sutures. The skin is closed in the usual manner (Fig. 4-43).

A soft dressing is applied, and the toe is protected with tongue blade splints, which maintain the toe in slight varus and slight plantar flexion. The dressing is removed 1 week postoperatively, and a slipper cast is applied. This is used for 6 to 8 weeks until the osteotomy site has healed.

Complications. Avascular necrosis was initially reported by Hawkins et al. (1945), and continues to be a noteworthy problem. Malunion resulting in incomplete correction of the metatarsus primus varus, dorsal or plantar angulation, hallux varus, significant shortening of the first metatarsal resulting in metatarsalgia, recurrence because of inadequate soft tissue release, and nonunion have been reported (Fig. 4-44).

Chevron osteotomy

The chevron osteotomy was described by Austin and Leventen (1968, 1981), Corless (1976), and Johnson et al. (1979). These authors believe the procedure is useful in adolescents and in adults up to the age of about 50 years who have a hallux valgus deformity of up to approximately 30° and an intermetatarsal angle of 15° or less, without evidence of pronation of the great toe. It

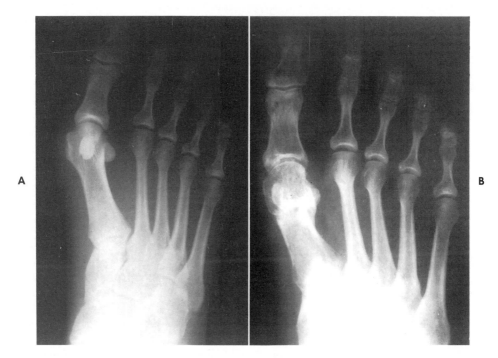

Fig. 4-43. Preoperative and postoperative radiographs following a Mitchell procedure. **A,** Preoperative. **B,** Postoperative. (Courtesy James J. Coughlin, M.D.)

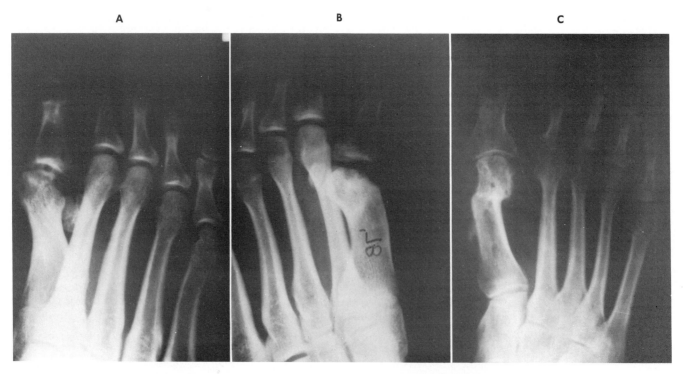

Fig. 4-44. Complications following Mitchell procedure. **A,** Dorsiflexion of distal fragment. **B,** Plantar flexion of distal fragment. **C,** Avascular changes within metatarsal head.

Fig. 4-45. Technique of chevron osteotomy. **A,** Location of chevron osteotomy within metatarsal head. **B,** Lateral displacement of osteotomy site and excision of medial eminence.

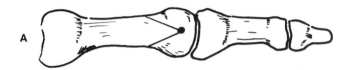

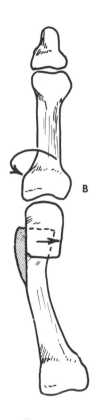

is imperative that an adequate range of motion and a congruous relationship of the metatarsophalangeal articulation are present. Hallux valgus deformities of greater than 30° to 35°, an intermetatarsal angle of greater than 15°, an incongruous metatarsophalangeal joint articulation, and excessive pronation of the great toe may be considered contraindications to the procedure.

Technique

1. The skin incision is made over the medial aspect of the metatarsophalangeal joint. It is started distally at the midportion of the proximal phalanx and carried proximally about 6 cm. The dissection is carried down to the joint capsule; and a dorsal and plantar flap is created, with care being taken to protect the cutaneous nerves.

2. A distally based U-shaped flap is created medially, thus exposing the prominent medial eminence.

3. The medial eminence is then resected with an osteotome oriented in or just medial to the sagittal sulcus. A rasp or rongeur is then used to smooth the edges.

4. The conjoint tendon and lateral capsular structures are not released, as this may place the first metatarsal head at significant risk for the development of avascular necrosis caused by disruption of its blood supply.

5. The chevron osteotomy is carried out with its base oriented proximally (Fig. 4-45). A ⅚₄-inch drill hole may be used to mark the apex of the osteotomy within the metatarsal head. The drill hole is placed at the center of the metatarsal head and oriented in a medial to lateral plane, parallel to the articular surface of the metatarsal. The biplane horizontal osteotomy is then carried out, using an oscillating saw with a very fine blade. The angle of the osteotomy approximates 60°. If the apex of the osteotomy is located in the center of the metatarsal head, the osteotomy site will be within the cancellous metaphyseal region, which will provide not only stability but a broad surface of bony contact for rapid healng. The most lateral aspect of the osteotomy must be completed with a thin osteotome if the power saw has not completed the osteotomy.

6. The metatarsal head is then displaced in a lateral direction a distance not to exceed one third of the width of the metatarsal shaft. If the toe still retains a valgus component, a small wedge of bone may be removed from the superior medial and inferior medial aspects of the proximal fragment. The osteotomy is carefully impacted on itself.

7. The osteotomy site may be stabilized with a Kirschner wire if the surgeon feels this is necessary. Although the osteotomy is quite stable in a dorsoplantar direction, medial displacement of the osteotomy may allow some recurrence of the deformity.

8. The medial capsular flap is then secured to the proximal metatarsal with 00 chromic sutures fixed into the periosteum or small drill holes in the cortex of the proximal metatarsal fragment. The toe is held in a corrected position during this portion of the repair.

9. A compression dressing is used postoperatively, followed by a short-leg walking cast for approximately 3 weeks. The Kirschner wire, if used, may be removed when healing has occurred, at approximately 4 to 6 weeks. After the short-leg case is removed, a soft compression dressing and a bunion shoe are used for ambulation (Fig. 4-46).

Complications. Malunion of the osteotomy site caused by postoperative migration (Wagner, 1981), avascular necrosis of the metatarsal head (Mann, 1982)

A   B

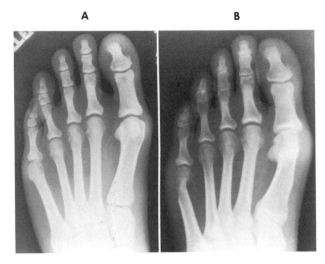

Fig. 4-46. Results of chevron osteotomy. **A,** Preoperative radiograph. **B,** Postoperative radiograph. (Courtesy, Kenneth Johnson, M.D.)

A   B

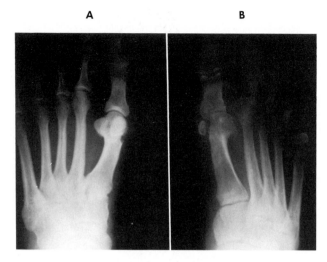

Fig. 4-47. Possible complications following chevron osteotomy. **A,** Excessive shortening. **B,** Too much lateral displacement resulting in hallux varus (see Fig. 4-64).

excessive shortening secondary to bone resorption, and hallux varus has been observed (Fig. 4-47). Recurrence caused by the use of the procedure for severe hallux valgus deformities with metatarsus primus varus of greater than 20° and pronation of the great toe may be a complication of this procedure.

Resection arthroplasty—Keller procedure

The procedure first described by Davies-Colley (1887) was popularized by Keller (1904, 1912). Its purpose was to decompress the metatarsophalangeal joint by resection of one third to one half of the proximal phalanx, thereby relaxing the contracted lateral structures. Although the Keller procedure was probably the most widely used bunion procedure in the past, with the development of other surgical techniques, along with the critical clinical evaluation of the results of the Keller procedure, we believe that this procedure should be used in patients who will place minimal demands on the foot. We do not believe that the Keller procedure should be the bunion procedure of choice for active individuals, since there are other techniques available that will give a far more functional result. The Keller procedure is indicated in an older person in whom extensive surgery is contraindicated or in whom hallux rigidus is not amenable to treatment by cheilectomy, arthrodesis, or Silastic joint interposition. It is also indicated as a salvage for failed bunion surgery or for the older person who has a severe hallux valgus deformity that has resulted in chronic skin breakdown and who is considered essentially a house-bound ambulator. Contraindications include a short first metatarsal, be-

cause of the possibility of the patient developing metatarsalgia beneath the second metatarsal.

Technique

1. The joint capsule is exposed through a dorsomedial incision, with care being taken to protect the dorsomedial nerve.

2. The metatarsophalangeal joint capsule and periosteum are dissected off the medial aspect of the proximal phalanx to create a rectangular flap that is based proximally on the metatarsal shaft.

3. Using an osteotome or an oscillating saw, the proximal phalanx is resected by osteotomizing it at the proximal flare of the metaphysis (Fig. 4-48). Up to one half of the proximal phalanx may be resected; however, excessive resecton may result in a cock-up deformity.

4. The medial eminence is then resected flush with the metatarsal shaft, and the remaining osteophytes on the metatarsal head are removed with the rongeur. If motion is still compromised, further bone may be removed from the dorsal aspect of the first metatarsal head to decompress the joint further to permit dorsiflexion.

5. Two or three drill holes are then made on the medial and plantar aspects of the diaphysis of the proximal phalanx.

6. The medial capsular structure and the plantar plate with the attached sesamoids and tendons of the flexor hallucis brevis are then fixed to the proximal phalanx to stabilize it. The attachment of the intrinsic muscles affords some plantar flexion strength, as well as stability to the hallux.

7. A ⁵⁄₆₄-inch Steinmann pin is driven distally through

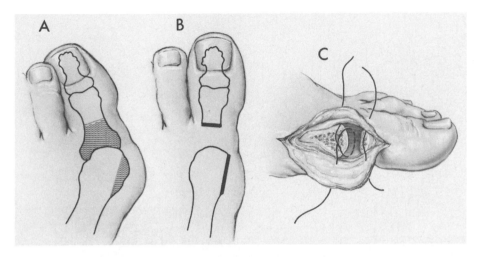

Fig. 4-48. Keller operation for correction of hallux valgus.

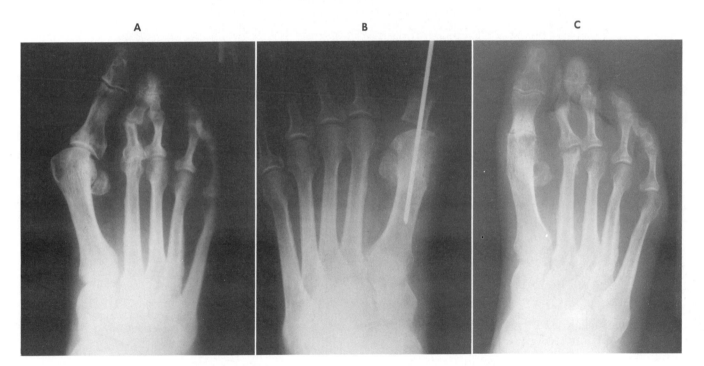

Fig. 4-49. Results following Keller procedure. **A,** Preoperative roentgenogram. **B,** Pin fixation of joint following surgery. **C,** Postoperative radiograph.

the intramedullary canal of the proximal phalanx, across the interphalangeal joint, and through the distal phalanx, exiting through the tip of the hallux. It is then driven in a retrograde fashion into the metatarsal head to stabilize the great toe and create a 5 mm space. The pin is bent at the tip of the toe to prevent proximal migration, and the capsular structures are then repaired.

8. A soft compression dressing is used postoperatively, and ambulation is permitted in a bunion shoe.

At 3 weeks the pin is removed and motion is commenced. Dressings may be discontinued 6 weeks after surgery (Fig. 4-49).

Complications. The major problem following the Keller procedure is occurrence of significant metatarsalgia beneath the second and possibly third metatarsal heads. This is caused by the decreased weight bearing by the first metatarsal, which results from the instability created by the resection of the proximal phalanx. Resection of more than half of the proximal phalanx

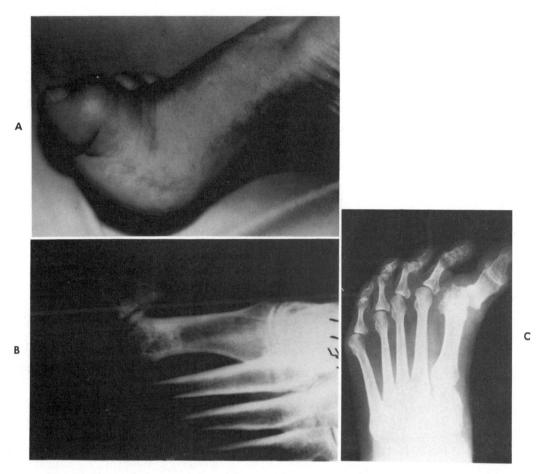

Fig. 4-50. Complications following Keller procedure. **A,** Cock-up deformity of metatarsophalangeal joint. **B,** Radiograph of cock-up deformity. **C,** Varus deformity.

may cause excessive shortening of the great toe. At times a cock-up deformity and recurrence of the hallux valgus result, caused by loss of stability (Fig. 4-50).

Proximal phalangeal osteotomy and soft tissue correction—Akin procedure

The Akin procedure was described by Akin in 1925. It involves an excision of the medial eminence, a lateral capsular release, and a closing wedge osteotomy in the proximal metaphysis of the proximal phalanx to correct hallux valgus.

The closing wedge osteotomy of the proximal phalanx may be indicated for hallux interphalangeus, a hallux valgus of up to 30° without significant metatarsus primus varus, a recurrent hallux valgus deformity in which the congruity of the joint precludes a soft tissue repair, or in conjunction with a proximal first metatarsal osteotomy as a means of correcting the metatarsus primus varus and the hallux valgus without significantly altering the congruity of the metatarsophalangeal joint. The Akin procedure maintains the congruity of the articular surface but does little to realign the metatarsal.

Technique

1. The joint capsule and base of the proximal phalanx are exposed through a medial skin incision that begins at the level of the interphalangeal joint and is carried proximal to the medial eminence. The dorsal and plantar digital nerves are carefully protected within the skin flaps.

2. The capsule is cut vertically, using a no. 11 blade, 2 to 3 mm proximal to the base of the proximal phalanx. A second, parallel cut is made more proximally, removing 3 to 5 mm of joint capsule. The amount of capsule excised depends on the size of the medial eminence to be excised.

3. The medial eminence is excised in line with or slightly medial to the sagittal sulcus. If the sagittal sulcus remains, a rongeur is used to remove any prominent lip.

4. The osteotomy of the phalanx is made with either a small oscillating saw or a needle-nosed rongeur. A small medially based wedge is removed, with the lateral cortex left intact. The osteotomy is carried out approximately 7 mm distal to the metatarsophalangeal

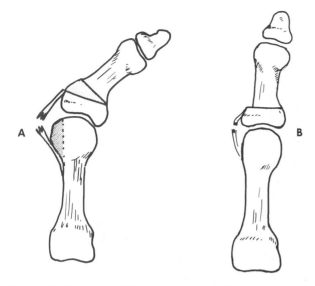

Fig. 4-51. Diagram of Akin procedure. **A,** Location of osteotomy in base of proximal phalanx. Shaded area on metatarsal head demonstrates excision of medial eminence. **B,** Closure of osteotomy site and plication of medial capsule.

joint and up to but not through the lateral cortex (Fig. 4-51).

5. The osteotomy site is then closed and fixed with an 0.045 Kirschner wire that exits through the tip of the toe. The wire is bent at the tip of the toe to prevent proximal migration. An alternative to using wire fixation is to make several drill holes on the medial side of the osteotomy site and pass suture material through it, close the osteotomy site down, and tie the sutures. If there is a slight pronation of the toe, it may be corrected by excising slightly more bone on the dorsomedial aspect of the osteotomy site.

6. The medial capsular defect is closed with interrupted 00 chromic suture (Fig. 4-52).

Although Akin advised a release of the lateral capsule and adductor tendon, this may devascularize the proximal fragment. If the hallux valgus deformity is of such a severe nature that a lateral release would be required, a more aggressive bunion procedure should probably be considered.

In cases in which there has been a recurrent hallux valgus deformity and an Akin procedure is being used to realign the great toe to keep the pressure off the second toe, the capsular portion of the procedure is not carried out but only the osteotomy is made in the base of the proximal phalanx.

A soft compression dressing holding the hallux slightly overcorrected is used postoperatively and changed weekly for 6 to 8 weeks while the patient is allowed to ambulate in a bunion shoe. If a pin is used, it is removed at approximately 4 to 6 weeks postoperatively.

Complications. Nonunion in this area is an extremely uncommon occurrence. However, a malunion in the form of undercorrection or overcorrection may occur. If the soft tissues are not supported adequately following the repair, a lateral subluxation of the metatarsophalangeal joint caused by lack of adequate capsular healing may occur. Avascular necrosis is a definite possibility if the proximal phalangeal fragment is devascularized through circumferential dissection (Fig. 4-53). Inadequate correction is the most significant complication with this procedure, and because it does not correct the metatarsus primus varus deformity for moderate and severe deformities, it must be used in conjunction with a procedure that addresses the increased intermetatarsal angle.

Metatarsophalangeal arthrodesis

Arthrodesis of the metatarsophalangeal joint of the great toe for treatment of hallux valgus deformity was described by Broca (1852) and Clutton (1894). DuVries (1965), McKeever (1952), and many others have advocated the use of an arthrodesis of the first metatarsophalangeal joint when this joint demonstrates degenerative arthritis. The rationale for this method of treatment is that the metatarsal length is preserved and the stability of the first ray is maintained. The indications for an arthrodesis, we believe, are rheumatoid arthritis of the metatarsophalangeal joints with an associated hallux valgus deformity, as a salvage procedure for a recurrent hallux valgus deformity or failed implant, some cases of hallux rigidus, degenerative arthritis following trauma, and hallux valgus secondary to loss of the second toe.

Concomitant degenerative arthritis of the interphalangeal joint as well as the insensate foot may be a contraindication.

Technique

1. Through a dorsal incision just medial to the extensor hallucis longus tendon, the metatarsophalangeal joint is exposed.

2. The joint capsule is dissected transversely, and care is taken to protect the dorsomedial cutaneous nerve and extensor tendon.

3. The tendons that insert into the base of the proximal phalanx and joint capsule are released along the skeletal plane.

4. The distal portion of the first metatarsal head is exposed and, with the use of a power saw or osteotome, is resected to create a flat surface that is angulated slightly dorsally and laterally.

5. The base of the proximal phalanx is likewise removed to obtain a position of the great toe that approximates 10° to 15° of valgus and about 15° of dorsiflexion in relation to the plantar aspect of the foot (Fig. 4-54).

In defining the position of the great toe for arthrod-

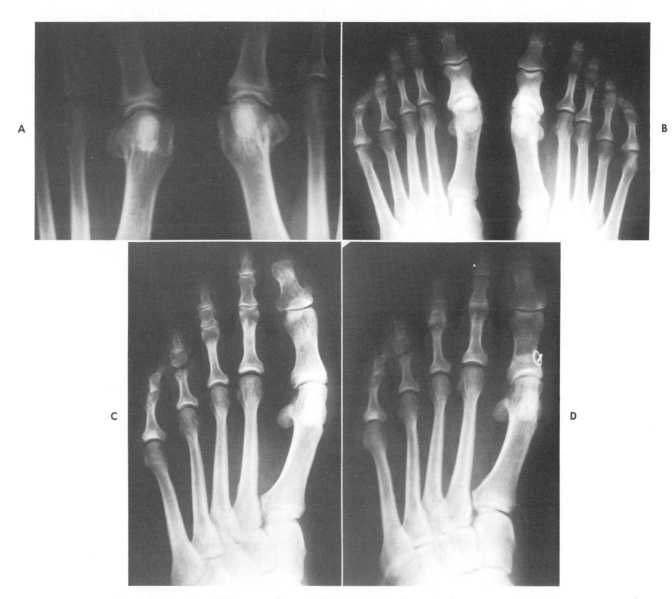

Fig. 4-52. Results of Akin procedure. **A,** Preoperative radiograph demonstrating an irregularly shaped metatarsal head. Such a metatarsal head will not permit correction by medial displacement, because an incongruent articular surface would result. **B,** Postoperative radiograph demonstrating satisfactory alignment with removal of medial eminence without affecting articular surface. **C,** Preoperative radiograph of mild recurrence of hallux valgus deformity. **D,** Correction of recurrence using Akin procedure.

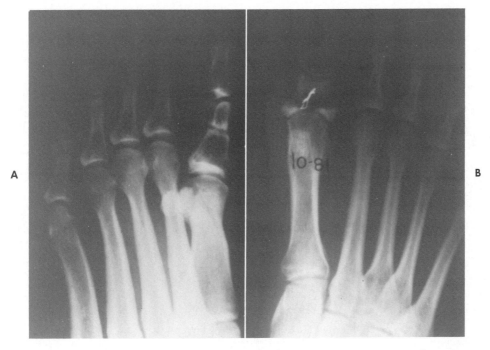

Fig. 4-53. Complications following Akin procedure. **A,** Delayed or nonunion of osteotomy site. **B,** Avascular necrosis.

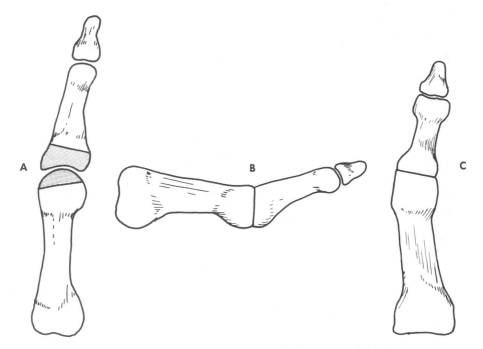

Fig. 4-54. Diagram of arthrodesis of metatarsophalangeal joint. **A,** Shaded area represents amount of bone surface that is usually removed when arthrodesis is carried out. **B,** Lateral view of metatarsophalangeal joint demonstrating that arthrodesis site should be placed in approximately 30° of dorsiflexion in relation to metatarsal shaft. **C,** Anteroposterior view of metatarsophalangeal joint demonstrating that there should be approximately 15° of valgus at the arthrodesis site.

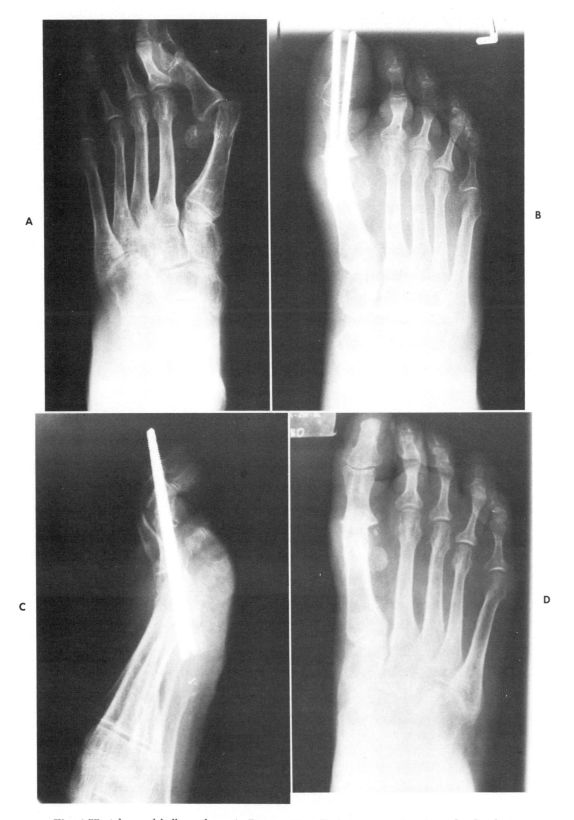

Fig. 4-55. Advanced hallux valgus. **A,** Preoperative. **B,** Anteroposterior view of arthrodesis of metatarsophalangeal joint using heavy threaded Steinmann pins. **C,** Lateral view. Note about 20° of dorsiflexion at metatarsophalangeal joint. **D,** Postoperative.

esis, the surgeon must remember that the first metatarsal is normally angled approximately 15° in a plantar direction. Therefore when one speaks of the angle of fusion it is in reference either to the ground or to the first metatarsophalangeal joint angle. The optimal position for men is approximately 30° of dorsiflexion (15° of dorsiflexion plus 15° of inclination of the first metatarsal). The optimal position for women, depending on heel height, is approximately 45° (30° of dorsiflexion and 15° of plantar inclination of the first metatarsal). If a woman does not desire to wear a high-heeled shoe, the angle of dorsiflexion would be correspondingly decreased. As McKeever (1952) stated, "It is the arthrodesis and its position that is important and not the method by which it is obtained." If the arthrodesis creates a long first ray in relation to the lesser toes, resection of a portion of the proximal phalanx primarily and the metatarsal head secondarily should be undertaken at the time of the arthrodesis.

6. After apposition of the prepared surfaces, care must be taken that no bony prominences are produced. The metatarsophalangeal joint is then stabilized with staples, a screw, crossed Kirschner wires, or axially threaded Steinmann pins.

7. We prefer the use of heavy threaded Steinmann pins measuring ⅛-inch and %4-inch. The Steinmann pins are placed using a power driver distally through the proximal phalanx to exit through the tip of the toe. They are then driven in a retrograde fashion across the arthrodesis site while the bone surfaces are firmly compressed by the surgeon.

8. The wound is closed in layers, and a compression dressing is applied. A new dressing is applied approximately 12 to 18 hours postoperatively. Using our method of fixation permits weight bearing in a postoperative wooden shoe the day following surgery (Fig. 4-55). Using other methods of fixation, if there is any question about stability, weight bearing is delayed until early healing has been demonstrated roentgenographically.

In our cases we have a fusion rate of 98% using this technique of fixation and early mobilization (Mann and Oates, 1981). In our experience, it usually takes between 10 and 14 weeks for the arthrodesis to take place.

Complications. Complications following an arthrodesis include nonunion, the incidence of which is reported in the literature as being from approximately 5% to 25%. Malposition of the arthrodesis site with excessive varus, valgus, dorsiflexion, or plantar flexion is occasionally a problem. Degenerative arthritis of the interphalangeal joint of the great toe has been reported in the literature as occurring in approximately 40% of patients.

Using our technique of placing the heavy threaded

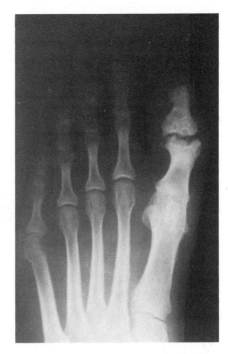

Fig. 4-56. Degenerative arthritis of interphalangeal joint following arthrodesis of metatarsophalangeal joint.

Steinmann pins across the interphalangeal joint we too have found an incidence of degenerative change of approximately 40% (Fig. 4-56). From a clinical standpoint, however, few patients who manifest degenerative changes within the interphalangeal joint have clinical symptoms. It is quite unusual to see a patient with degenerative arthritis of the interphalangeal joint who is significantly disabled. In a few cases in which both the metatarsophalangeal joint and the interphalangeal joint have become arthrodesed, the patients seemed to have little or no disability. Their main problem, however, is attempting to place their foot into a boot because of lack of mobility in the foot.

The degenerative changes in the interphalangeal joint appear to be related to the valgus position of the hallux. The less valgus that is present at the arthrodesis site, the greater is the possibility of the patient developing degenerative change at the interphalangeal joint.

ADOLESCENT OR JUVENILE HALLUX VALGUS

The problem of the adolescent patient with hallux valgus has not been specifically discussed in this chapter. In most cases of adolescent hallux valgus a metatarsus primus varus exists, so we consider the soft tissue procedure previously discussed along with a proximal metatarsal osteotomy to be the treatment of choice for this problem. It is important, however, when carrying out the osteotomy that it be made approximately 0.5 cm distal to the epiphyseal plate so that no growth abnormality can occur. As mentioned previously, however, we prefer to defer bunion surgery in the adolescent until skeletal maturity has been reached. Generally speaking, the results of bunion surgery in the adolescent patient do not seem to be as good as those which can be achieved in the adult. In treating the adolescent it is important to identify all of the predisposing factors that might be contributing to the hallux valgus deformity and correct them, if possible, before surgical repair.

HALLUX VALGUS ASSOCIATED WITH HYPERMOBILITY OF FIRST METATARSOCUNEIFORM JOINT

Occasionally a patient with hallux valgus deformity has marked hypermobility of the first metatarsocuneiform joint. This may be caused by either marked medial sloping of the articulation or ligamentous laxity. In either case, when carrying out a correction of the hallux valgus deformity in these patients the first metatarsocuneiform joint should be arthrodesed. Lapidus (1934) believed that the arthrodesis should include the first metatarsocuneiform joint as well as the tibial side of the base of the second metatarsal. We believe that just carrying out the first metatarsocuneiform arthrodesis is sufficient to produce a satisfactory result (Fig. 4-57). From a technical standpoint this procedure is somewhat difficult, because it is hard to achieve perfect alignment of the first metatarsocuneiform joint.

HALLUX VALGUS ASSOCIATED WITH SPASTICITY

At times patients with neuromuscular disorders, e.g., cerebral palsy or stroke, develop a hallux valgus deformity. The deformity is usually caused by the spasticity of the calf producing an equinus deformity at the ankle joint, and then, secondarily, these patients develop a severe hallux valgus because they tend to roll off the medial border of their foot. In these situations, unless the predisposing factor is corrected before the bunion surgery, recurrence is a distinct possibility. Generally speaking, an arthrodesis will probably produce a more satisfactory long-term result than any of the soft tissue procedures.

Complications of hallux valgus surgery

The basic goal of the repair of a hallux valgus deformity is to achieve a satisfactory correction of the deformity and foot function that is as normal as possible. To achieve this goal the patient needs to be carefully evaluated preoperatively and then informed as to what type of correction may be achieved. It is conceivable that following surgery the patient may not be able to return to as full a level of activity as he desires, and the patient should be made aware of the possible functional limitations.

As an example of functional limitations, a person with an arthrodesis of the first metatarsophalangeal joint

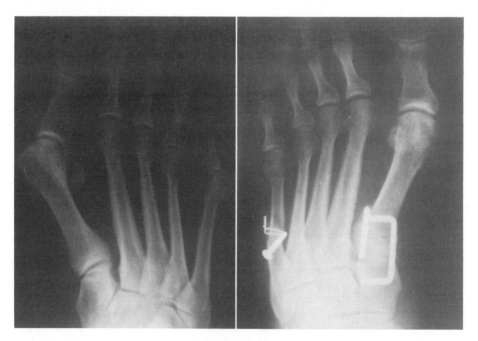

Fig. 4-57. Results following first metatarsocuneiform fusion along with soft tissue procedure at metatarsophalangeal joint.

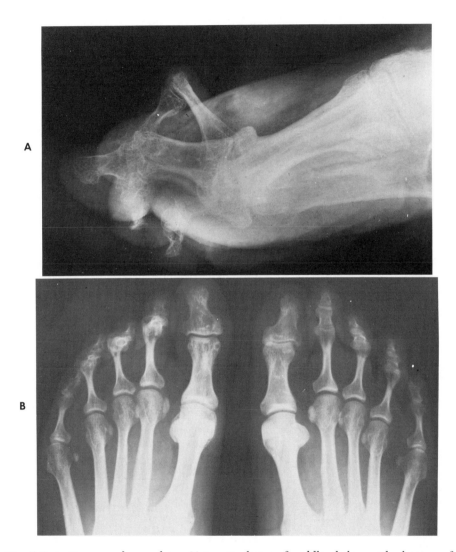

Fig. 5-7. **A,** Hammered second toe. Note articulation of middle phalanx with plantar surface of head of proximal phalanx. **B,** Right foot: hammered third and fourth toes. Second toe is normal. Left foot: hammered second, third, and fourth toes.

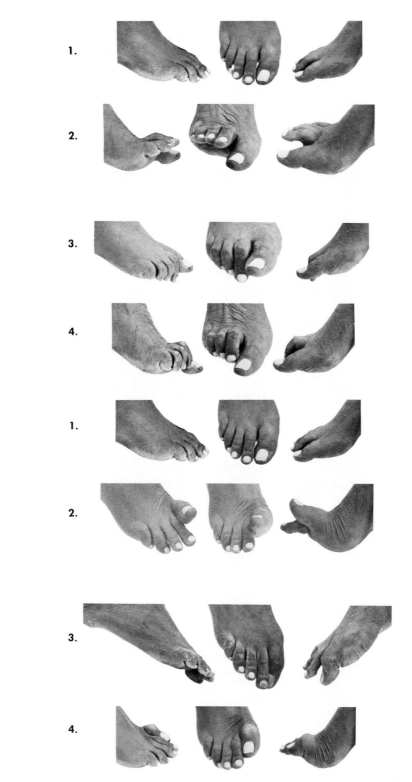

Fig. 5-8. **A,** Action of the muscles in clawtoe deformity. Fresh cadaver foot. **1,** At rest. **2,** Tension on extensor digitorum longus alone. Note extension of metatarsophalangeal joints and minimal extension of interphalangeal joints. **3,** Tension on flexor digitorum longus alone. Note that maximal flexion occurs in interphalangeal joints. **4,** Tension simultaneously on extensor digitorum longus and flexor digitorum longus. Note resulting deformities in all but great toe. **B,** Action of muscles in clawtoe deformity. Cadaver foot. **1,** At rest. **2,** Tension on the extensor hallucis longus alone. Note extension of metatarsophalangeal and interphalangeal joints. **3,** Tension on flexor hallucis longus alone. Note maximal flexion in interphalangeal joint. **4,** Simultaneous tension on extensor hallucis longus and flexor hallucis longus, with resulting hammertoe deformity.

strike the top of the shoe, and the metatarsal heads are forced into the plantar aspect of the foot. As the toes are drawn up into the metatarsal heads, the fat pad is pulled distally and the metatarsal heads become more prominent on the plantar aspect of the foot. This can result in painful plantar callosities that may ulcerate in severe cases, particularly if sensation of the foot is impaired.

Anatomy and pathophysiology

An understanding of the anatomy and pathophysiology is helpful in selecting a treatment regimen. The most common deformity is of course the hammertoe, and this will be used as the prototype for discussing the pathophysiology of all three anomalies.

The central dorsal structure of the toe is formed by the tendon of the extensor digitorum longus, which divides into three slips over the proximal phalanx; the middle slip inserts into the base of the middle phalanx, and the two lateral slips extend over the dorsolateral aspect of the middle phalanx and converge to form the terminal tendon, which inserts into the base of the distal phalanx (Fig. 5-9). The tendon is held in a central

position dorsally by a fibroaponeurotic sling that anchors the long extensor to the plantar aspect of the metatarsophalangeal joint and to the base of the proximal phalanx. Surprisingly, there is no dorsal insertion of the extensor digitorum longus to the proximal phalanx, the phalanx being virtually suspended by the extensor digitorum longus tendon and its extensor sling (Fig. 5-10). The main function of the extensor digitorum longus is to dorsiflex the proximal phalanx (Fig. 5-11). Only when the proximal phalanx is held in flexion or in a neutral position at the metatarsophalangeal joint can this tendon become an extensor of the proximal interphalangeal joint. This is an important concept because with a hammertoe deformity the long extensor tendon function may be neutralized by extension of the proximal phalanx.

The flexor digitorum longus tendon inserts into the distal phalanx and flexes the distal interphalangeal joint, whereas the flexor digitorum brevis inserts into the middle phalanx, flexing the proximal interphalangeal joint. There is no insertion into the proximal phalanx, so the flexor influence on the proximal phalanx is minimal. As a result of this, with the proximal phalanx in

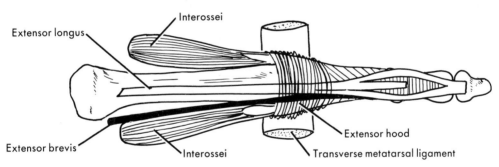

Fig. 5-9. Diagram of a dorsal view of extensor mechanism of toes. (Redrawn from Sarrafian, S.K., and Topouzian, L.K.: J. Bone Joint Surg. 51A:669, 1969.)

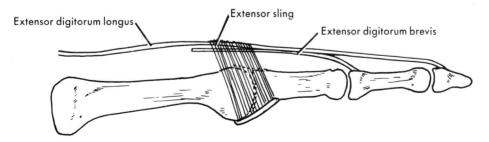

Fig. 5-10. Lateral view of extensor mechanism of lesser toe. Note that extensor digitorum longus inserts only into distal phalanx and secondarily suspends metatarsophalangeal joint through extensor sling mechanism. (Redrawn from Sarrafian, S.K.: Anatomy of the foot and ankle, Philadelphia, 1983, J.B. Lippincott Co.)

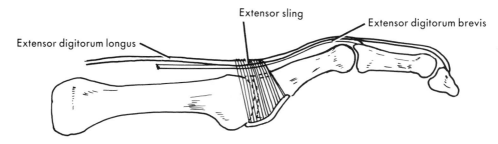

Fig. 5-11. Lateral view of extensor mechanism demonstrating main function of extensor digitorum longus, which is to dorsiflex proximal phalanx. (Redrawn from Sarrafian, S.K.: Anatomy of the foot and ankle, Philadelphia, 1983, J.B. Lippincott Co.)

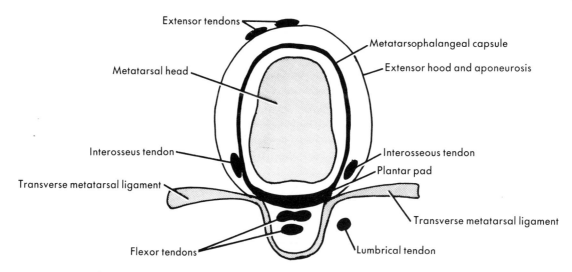

Fig. 5-12. Cross-section through metatarsal head of a lesser toe, demonstrating structures that pass through this region. Note that interossei tendons are dorsal to transverse metatarsal ligament, whereas lumbrical is plantar to it. (Redrawn from Sarrafian, S.K.: Anatomy of the foot and ankle, Philadelphia, 1983, J.B. Lippincott Co.)

an extended position, there are no major antagonists to the long and short flexors, and the toe buckles, resulting in hyperextension of the distal interphalangeal joint and flexion of the proximal interphalangeal joint. Over a long period of time, if this position becomes fixed, a hammertoe deformity occurs. Resistance to flexion at the metatarsophalangeal joint is maintained in the normal toe by the long extensor. The most important factor is probably the reactive force of the foot against the ground, pushing the metatarsophalangeal joints into extension.

The interossei tendons are located dorsal to the transverse metatarsal ligament, whereas the lumbrical is located plantar to this ligament (Fig. 5-12). Both tendons of the intrinsic muscles, however, pass plantar to the axis of motion of the metatarsophalangeal joint, flexing the metatarsophalangeal joint (Fig. 5-13), and pass

dorsal to the axis of the proximal interphalangeal joint and distal interphalangeal joint, extending these joints. The plantar and dorsal interossei have only a few fibers that reach the extensor sling and are therefore weak extensors of the interphalangeal joints. The lumbrical, with all of its fibers terminating in the extensor sling, is a stronger extensor of these joints. The interossei flex the proximal phalanx by their direct attachment to the base of the proximal phalanx, whereas the lumbrical achieves flexion by placing tension on the extensor sling (Fig. 5-14). It is obvious with marked dorsiflexion at the metatarsophalangeal joint that the lumbrical flexion power is quite limited by the fact that it is pulling at a 90° angle.

Probably the most significant stabilizing factor of the metatarsophalangeal joint is that the plantar aponeurosis and plantar capsule combine to form the plantar

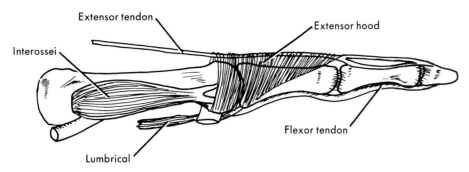

Fig. 5-13. Lateral view of a lesser toe demonstrating that both tendons of intrinsic muscles pass plantar to axis of motion of metatarsophalangeal joint, thereby flexing it. They pass dorsal to axis of motion of proximal and distal interphalangeal joints, thereby extending them. Lumbrical does not insert into bone but rather into extensor hood and as such is stronger extensor of interphalangeal joints. (Redrawn from Sarrafian, S.K.: Anatomy of the foot and ankle, Philadelphia, 1983, J.B. Lippincott Co.)

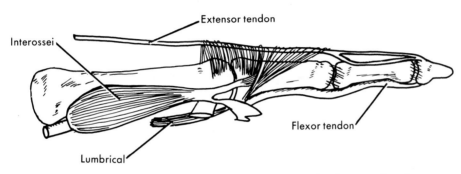

Fig. 5-14. Lateral aspect of lesser toe with portion of extensor hood removed to demonstrate insertion of interossei into base of proximal phalanx. This insertion permits interossei to plantar flex proximal phalanx on metatarsal head. (Redrawn from Sarrafian, S.K.: Anatomy of the foot and ankle, Philadelphia, 1983, J.B. Lippincott Co.)

pad. During the walking cycle varying degrees of dorsiflexion occur at the metatarsophalangeal joints. The static resistance of the plantar capsule combines with the dynamic force of the intrinsic flexors to pull the proximal phalanx back into a neutral position at the metatarsophalangeal joint (Fig. 5-15). It should be reiterated, however, that the major structure that resists dorsiflexion at the metatarsophalangeal joint is the plantar pad. With chronic hyperextension forces on the proximal phalanx, these plantar structures may become stretched and are rendered less efficient (Fig. 5-16).

The position of the proximal phalanx at the metatarsophalangeal jont is subject to the antagonistic actions of the strong extensor digitorum longus, through its sling mechanism, in opposition with the decidedly weaker intrinsics and the more static capsule and plantar aponeurosis complex. The position of the middle

and distal phalanges, on the other hand, are subject to the forces of the long and short flexors, which are opposed by the directly weaker intrinsics. At each of these joints an obvious "mismatch" can occur, and in each case the extrinsic muscle overpowers the intrinsic muscle (Fig. 5-17). The extensor digitorum longus will help to extend the interphalangeal joints, if the proximal phalanx is not hyperextended, and the flexor digitorum longus will help to flex the metatarsophalangeal joint, if the proximal phalanx is not hyperextended. The hyperextended proximal phalanx, then, is definitely the key to the production of most hammertoe deformities.

Hammertoes most commonly occur in older women. The elevated heel and small toe box of ladies' footwear, over a long period of time, is the major contributing factor maintaining the metatarsophalangeal joint in varying states of hyperextension. Furthermore, crowd-

Fig. 5-15. Diagram demonstrating plantar plate and capsule of metatarsophalangeal joint, which is sufficiently resilient to bring metatarsophalangeal joint back into neutral position after joint has been dorsiflexed at time of lift-off.

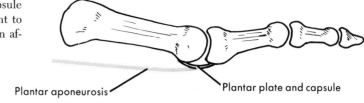

Plantar aponeurosis   Plantar plate and capsule

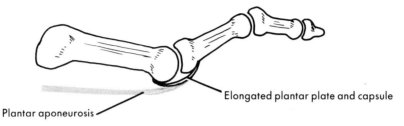

Elongated plantar plate and capsule

Plantar aponeurosis

Fig. 5-16. Diagram to illustrate effects of elongated plantar plate and capsule. As a result of certain disease states, this capsular structure is no longer sufficiently viable to restore joint to its normal position following lift-off.

Fig. 5-17. Diagram demonstrating relationship of intrinsic and extrinsic muscles about a lesser toe.

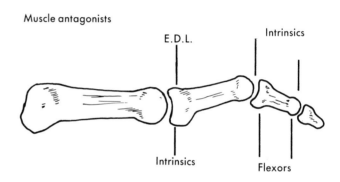

Muscle antagonists

E.D.L.   Intrinsics

Intrinsics   Flexors

ing of the toes in the forepart of the shoe may lead to a hallux valgus deformity with subsequent pressure on the second toe, forcing the proximal phalanx into dorsiflexion. Likewise, a relatively short toe box in a patient with a long second toe causes a buckling effect on the toe, with a concomitant hyperextension deformity at the metatarsophalangeal joint. With a chronic hyperextended position of the proximal phalanx being maintained throughout the entire walking cycle (by the wearing of high-heeled shoes), the plantar structures gradually become inefficient, and thus the proximal phalanx remains chronically dorsiflexed.

Therefore with chronic extension of the proximal phalanx, the extensor digitorum longus tendon loses its tenodesing effect on the interphalangeal joints, allowing the distal phalanges to migrate into flexion, and as the proximal phalanx extends, the intrinsic flexors are under greater tension, further increasing the flexion deformity at the interphalangeal joint. The only counteracting forces to this flexion deformity are the lumbricals and the interossei, which are easily overpowered by the long flexor tendons.

Treatment
Treatment of hammertoe

When evaluating a patient with a hammertoe deformity, which is often thought of as a relatively simple problem, certain factors need to be carefully considered to fully appreciate the nature of the deformity. These include the rigidity of the toe, the position of the metatarsophalangeal joint while standing, the overall tightness of the flexor digitorum longus tendon in the involved and adjacent toes, and whether or not there is sufficient space for the toe if it were to be placed back into its normal position.

A hammertoe may be a flexible, semiflexible, or rigid deformity. If the deformity is flexible, the toe may be passively corrected to neutral. At the other end of the spectrum, if it is a rigid deformity, there are joint contractures that preclude passive correction. The rigidity

5. Attention is directed to the dorsal aspect of the toe where a longitudinal incision is made over the proximal phalanx, centered over the extensor tendon. A hemostat is now passed from dorsal to plantar along the extensor hood to enter into the wound on the plantar aspect of the foot. Care is taken to stay along the extensor hood to avoid the neurovascular bundle.

6. A mosquito clamp is placed along the extensor hood into the plantar wound on each side of the toe, and the tails of the flexor digitorum longus tendon are brought up onto the medial and lateral aspects of the hood.

7. The toe is placed into approximately 20° plantar flexion at the metatarsophalangeal joint, and the flexor tendon is sutured to the extensor digitorum longus tendon approximately over the midportion of the proximal phalanx under a slight degree of tension.

8. The wounds are closed, and the patient is placed in a compression dressing and ambulates in a postoperative wooden shoe.

9. After 3 weeks of ambulation in a protected shoe, the patient is permitted to once again resume activities as tolerated.

This procedure will usually provide satisfactory correction not only of idiopathic flexible hammertoe, but also for patients with cerebral palsy or following cerebrovascular accident, compartment syndrome, and neuromuscular diseases such as Charcot-Marie-Tooth disease. It is important for the surgeon to remember that if a fixed contracture is present this procedure will not produce a satisfactory result.

The complications seen following this procedure have been few but include the following:

1. Occasionally swelling of varying degrees will persist for a short period of time.
2. Some transient numbness probably caused by contusion of the cutaneous nerves may occur, but this rarely persists.
3. Hyperextension of the distal interphalangeal joint has been noted in a few patients with severe spasticity. This may be a result of concomitant tightness of the flexor digitorum brevis.
4. Occasionally in the patient with dynamic hammertoes an element of clawing is also present. A release of the extensor digitorum longus tendon and dorsal capsulotomies of the metatarsophalangeal joint may be carried out at the same time as the flexor tendon transfer.

Treatment of the hammered fifth toe. The hammertoe deformity involving the fifth toe as an isolated entity is uncommon. When it is symptomatic and conservative measures have failed, it will respond well to a condylectomy, which is carried out through a longitudinal incision centered over the proximal interphalangeal joint.

The condyles are generously removed, and the skin is closed, following which a compression dressing is used. Following this procedure it is important to keep the toe taped adjacent to the fourth toe for approximately 6 weeks so that adequate scar tissue will form, thereby precluding any problem with a floppy toe.

Treatment of the mallet toe deformity

A mallet toe deformity is usually a fixed deformity, but occasionally in a young patient it may be flexible. The symptoms are caused by the tip of the toe striking the ground, which results in a callosity on the tip of the toe. This can be treated conservatively with a small felt pad placed beneath the toe to prevent the tip from striking the ground. The patient must be placed into a shoe with an adequate toe box to accommodate the toe with the felt pad beneath it.

Occasionally if the deformity is flexible, release of the flexor digitorum longus tendon percutaneously may be sufficient. If the deformity is fixed, which is usually the case, it may require surgical treatment. When surgical intervention is required, resection of the head of the middle phalanx and release of the flexor digitorum longus tendon result in a most satisfactory correction. The procedure is carried out as follows (Fig. 5-21).

1. An elliptic incision is made over the dorsal aspect of the distal interphalangeal joint and carried down through the extensor tendon and joint capsule. The distal portion of the ellipse should be sufficiently proximal to avoid injuring the nail matrix.

2. The collateral ligaments are cut on the medial and lateral sides of the distal interphalangeal joint, and the head of the middle phalanx is delivered into the wound. It is resected proximal to the condyles.

3. The plantar capsule is incised, and the flexor digitorum longus tendon is identified and cut under direct vision.

4. The toe is brought into satisfactory alignment without tension. If the toe cannot be completely corrected, more bone is resected from the middle phalanx.

5. A single suture of 3-0 silk incorporating two Telfa bolsters is inserted similarly to that carried out for the hammertoe repair. As the tension is applied to the suture, leverage is created to bring the toe into satisfactory alignment.

6. The suture and bolsters are removed in 1 week, and the toe is held in the corrected position with adhesive tape for 7 weeks to assure adequate soft tissue scarring.

The expected result following this procedure has been most satisfactory. The alignment of the toe remains good, and complications are rare. The few problems that have been observed are as follows:

1. Occasionally swelling will persist for several

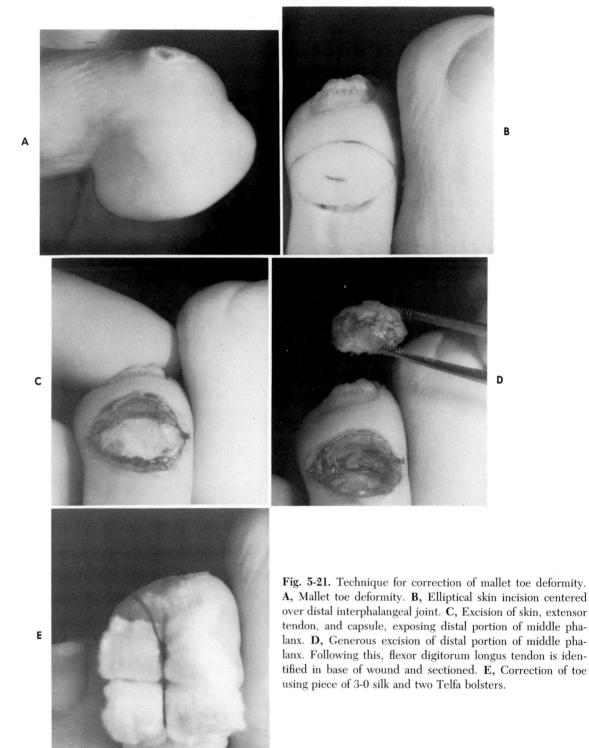

Fig. 5-21. Technique for correction of mallet toe deformity. **A,** Mallet toe deformity. **B,** Elliptical skin incision centered over distal interphalangeal joint. **C,** Excision of skin, extensor tendon, and capsule, exposing distal portion of middle phalanx. **D,** Generous excision of distal portion of middle phalanx. Following this, flexor digitorum longus tendon is identified in base of wound and sectioned. **E,** Correction of toe using piece of 3-0 silk and two Telfa bolsters.

in the proximal phalanx, and sutured to the lateral side of the fifth metatarsophalangeal joint in the region of the abductor digiti minimi. This procedure should be used for the recurrent or failed overlapping fifth toe deformity.

4. The toe is immobilized for 6 weeks, and the patient ambulates in a wooden shoe.

• • •

Problems involving the fifth toe, such as hard corns and soft corns, are discussed in Chapter 7.

REFERENCES

Barnicot, N.A., and Hardy, R.H.: The position of the hallux in West Africans, J. Anta. **89**:355, 1955.

Branch, H.E.: Pathological dislocation of the second toe, J. Bone Joint Surg. **19**:978, 1937.

Creer, W.S.: The feet of the industrial worker: clinical aspect—relation to footwear. Lancet **2**:1482, 1938.

Duchenne, G.B.: Physiology of motion (translated and edited by E.B. Kaplan), Philadelphia, 1949, J.B. Lippincott Co. (Original French edition, 1867.)

DuVries, H.L.: Dislocation of toe, JAMA **160**:728, 1956.

Engle, E.T., and Morton, D.J.: Notes on foot disorders among natives of the Belgian Congo, J. Bone Joint Surg. **13**:311, 1931.

Girdlestone, G.R.: Physiotherapy for hand and foot, J. Chartered Soc. Physiother. **32**:167, 1947.

Hewitt, D., Stewart, A.M., and Webb, J.W.: The prevalence of foot defects among wartime recruits, Br. Med. J. **2**:745, 1953.

Higgs, S.L.: Hammer-toe, Postgrad. Med. J. **6**:130, 1931.

James, C.S.: Footprints and feet of natives of the Soloman Islands, Lancet **2**:1390, 1939.

Lapidus, P.W.: Transplantation of the extensor tendon for correction of the overlapping fifth toe, J. Bone Joint Surg. **24**:555, 1942.

Marwil, T.B., and Brantingham, C.R.: Foot problems of women's reserve, Hosp. Corps Q. **16**:98, 1943.

Parrish, T.F.: Dynamic correction of claw toes, Orthop. Clin. North Am. **4**:97, 1973.

Ruiz-Mora, J.: Plastic correction of over-riding 5th toe, Orthopaedic Letters Club, vol. 6, 1954.

Sarrafian, S.K.: Anatomy of the foot and ankle, Philadelphia, 1983, J.B. Lippincott Co.

Taylor, R.G.: The treatment of claw toes by multiple transfers of flexor into extensor tendons, J. Bone Joint Surg. **33B**:539, 1951.

Wells, L.H.: The foot of the South African native, Am. J. Phys. Anthropol. **15**:185, 1931.

Wilson, J.N.: V-Y correction for varus deformity of the fifth toe, Br. J. Surg. **41**:133, 1953.

6

Arthritides

FRANCESCA M. THOMPSON and ROGER A. MANN

The foot is subject to disabling arthritides of multiple sites and variable causes (Gold, 1982; Guerra, 1982). The major categories are degenerative joint disease, or osteoarthritis; crystal-induced arthritis; the seronegative spondyloarthropathies; and rheumatoid arthritis.

DEGENERATIVE JOINT DISEASE
General concepts

Degenerative joint disease usually occurs in middle-aged and elderly persons, but it can also occur in younger individuals as the end stage of posttraumatic conditions or osteochondritis. Obesity, occupational stress, and excessive levels of physical activity have also been implicated as causes of degenerative joint disease in the foot. The most common sites of degenerative joint disease in the foot are the first metatarsophalangeal joint and the first metatarsocuneiform joint, but it can occur within any joint of the foot.

The cause of degenerative joint disease is still controversial, but biochemical changes occur within the articular cartilage along with proliferation of bone about the joint and subsequent distortion of the joint. As the degenerative process continues, structural changes occur in the joint that over time result in functional loss. This funcitonal loss in turn places stress on other areas of the foot, causing further pain because of the abnormal use of the foot. The foot is unique insofar as it is constantly under stress during gait; consequently, an abnormality within the foot that causes pain will cause the person to alter his gait pattern. This may result in further discomfort that may manifest itself in the other joints of the lower extremity and back.

The typical history given depends somewhat on the joint or joints involved. Generally, however, the symptoms are worse in the mornings until the person has had a chance to "loosen up," but symptoms are also aggravated by prolonged walking and standing. "Weatherache" is common.

A physical examination demonstrates that the affected joint is tender and may be warmer than usual. Motion of the joint often causes discomfort. Bony proliferation around the margin of the affected joint can be palpated and is frequently visible.

A radiographic examination demonstrates a decrease in the joint space, sclerotic joint margins, proliferative bone about the periphery of the joint, and subchondral cyst formation.

Conservative management

In general, conservative treatment should be provided initially. Antiinflammatory medicine can be given systemically and judiciously by local injections. This can be helpful if pain originates from local inflammation and synovitis.

The key to conservative management of degenerative joint disease is stress reduction. When indicated, patients should be encouraged to lose weight. Activity modification can reduce symptoms; joggers should be advised to bike or swim, and standing jobs should be modified to sedentary ones.

Properly fitted shoes should be prescribed, particularly to relieve friction over bony excrescences. Orthoses that will remove stress from the rigid and painful area may be useful (Chapter 21). In general, we have found that semiflexible orthoses disperse more stress than rigid orthoses when the degenerative joint disease occurs in the hindfoot or midfoot. Orthotic devices could include a molded leather ankle brace for ankle and midtarsal dysfunction or a rocker-bottom shoe to help take the stress off the proximal and distal joints of the foot. A rocker-bottom shoe causes a rolling motion, which in turn reduces stress on the foot. The more rigid

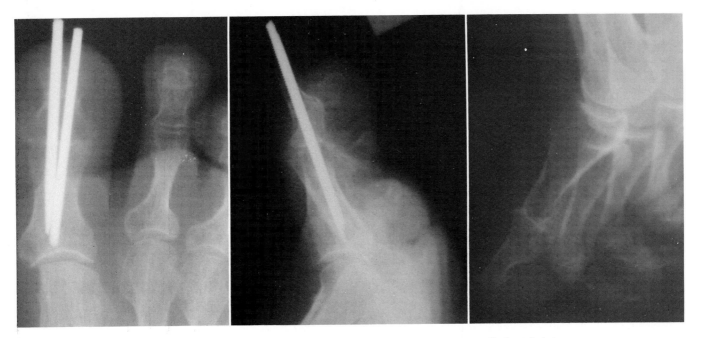

Fig. 6-1. Arthrodesis of interphalangeal joint of great toe using two small threaded Steinmann pins.

the sole is, the less the stress on the forefoot (Grundy et al., 1975).

SURGICAL TREATMENT OF DEGENERATIVE JOINT DISEASE OF THE FOOT

The primary indication for surgical intervention in degenerative joint disease is disabling pain in a patient without local or systemic contraindications to surgery. The major techniques available are arthrodesis, excisional arthroplasty, and occasionally osteotomy (Moberg, 1979). Implant arthroplasty in the foot has had generally disappointing results. We believe there is little reason to recommend implant arthroplasty because the stress concentrations in the foot are so high that there is a significant risk of implant failure over time. Postimplant salvage is compromised by the bone loss required by the implant technique.

Degenerative arthritis of interphalangeal joint

Degenerative arthritis of the interphalangeal joint of the great toe usually is the result of trauma. At times a claw-toe deformity, which is quite painful because of the prominence it creates is present with fibrous ankylosis of the interphalangeal joint.

If conservative management with a broad-toed, firm-soled shoe fails to bring about satisfactory relief, arthrodesis of the interphalangeal joint is indicated. This arthrodesis of the great toe is carried out through a dorsal approach, following which the joint surfaces are denuded and the arthrodesis site fixed with two small,

threaded Steinmann pins. We believe it is important to use two pins to prevent any possibility of toggling of the attempted arthrodesis site. These people can be treated postoperatively in a wooden shoe, and we do not believe they require cast immobilization (Fig. 6-1).

Degenerative arthritis of the lesser metatarsophalangeal joints, which usually results from trauma but occasionally is associated with Freiberg's infraction, is discussed on p. 191 and seen in Fig. 7-13. Degenerative arthritis of the interphalangeal joints of the lesser toes may be treated either with an excisional arthroplasty or by arthrodesis as described on p. 141 and seen in Fig. 5-18.

Hallux rigidus (hallux limitus)

Hallux rigidus, or hallux limitus, is second to hallux valgus in prevalence among disabling deformities of the great toe joint (Fig. 6-2). Indeed, it may be more disabling than hallux valgus because in hallux valgus the patient is distressed mainly by the inability to obtain shoes to accommodate the deformity. In hallux rigidus the patient cannot obtain relief even when not wearing shoes because dorsiflexion of the metatarsophalangeal joint of the great toe is severely limited and painful. The main complaint is the pain in the metatarsophalangeal joint of the great toe, which is well localized to the dorsal aspect of the joint. The degree of disability is directly related to the extent of the deformity and the limitation of dorsiflexion.

The pathologic anatomy of hallux rigidus demonstrates degenerative arthritis of the metatarsophalangeal

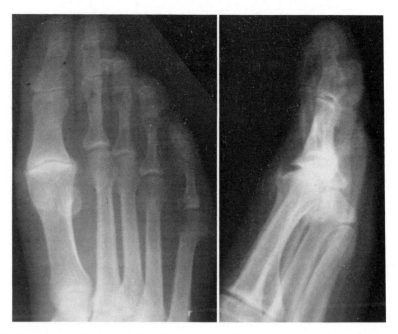

Fig. 6-2. Classic case of hallux rigidus. Note osseous changes on the dorsum of first metatarsal head, which block dorsiflexion.

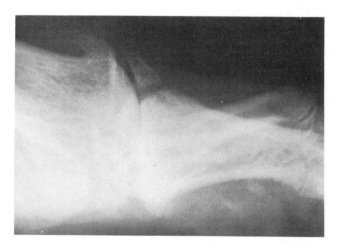

Fig. 6-3. Moderately severe hallux rigidus with large dorsal spur on base of the proximal phalanx. Note probable fracture line through base of large spur.

joint of the great toe. As a result the great toe is either fixed in plantar flexion or limited in dorsiflexion because of proliferation of bone around the articular surface of the head of the first metatarsal, particularly on the dorsal aspect. The bony proliferation usually does not involve the plantar surface of the metatarsal head. Not infrequently concomitant degenerative changes are noted about the base of the proximal phalanx (Fig. 6-3). In advanced cases the entire hallux is fixed in a plantar attitude, which forces the patient to walk on the outer border of the foot, thereby inverting the ankle and frequently producing secondary changes in the soft tissue and bones of the whole foot (Fig. 6-4).

Etiology. For convenience, hallux rigidus may be divided into three types: (1) congenital or juvenile, (2) acquired as a result of traumatic arthritis, and (3) acquired as a result of one of the general arthritides.

Congenital or juvenile. The congenital or juvenile type of hallux rigidus usually becomes manifest in the early teen-age years. It may or may not be associated with trauma to the first metatarsophalangeal joint. The main complaint is pain and swelling about the metatarsophalangeal joint that is aggravated by activities and at times only partially relieved by rest. The physical examination demonstrates some degree of synovial thickening about the metatarsophalangeal joint and marked restriction of motion, in particular dorsiflexion. Plantar flexion usually can be carried out without too much difficulty. The radiographic findings usually demonstrate an osteochondritic defect in the metatarsal head (Fig. 6-5).

The treatment in juvenile cases should be directed toward rest and immobilization. If the osteochondritic defect is large or appears to be loose, then excision of the defect may be of benefit, but unfortunately adequate dorsiflexion is usually not achieved. The procedure that may be beneficial to the adolescent patient is resection of a wedge of bone from the proximal portion of the proximal phalanx (Moberg, 1979). By removing a wedge of bone whose base is oriented dorsally, dorsi-

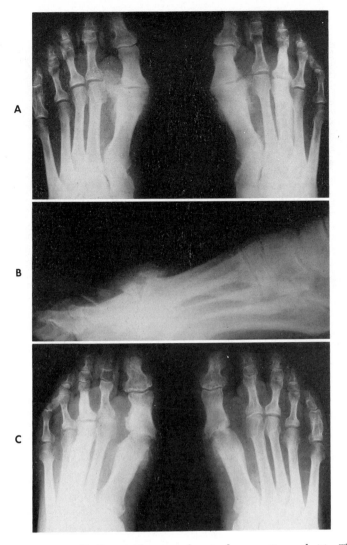

Fig. 6-4. A, Severe case of hallus rigidus secondary to degenerative arthritis. Third metatarsophalangeal joint on right side also shows degenerative changes. B, Note extensive new growth of bone on dorsum of first metatarsophalangeal joint. C, After correction by cheilectomy.

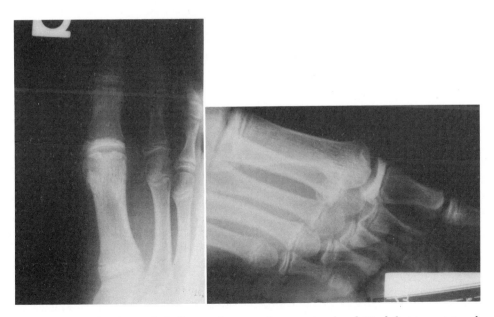

Fig. 6-5. Example of juvenile hallux rigidus secondary to osteochondritic defect in metatarsal head.

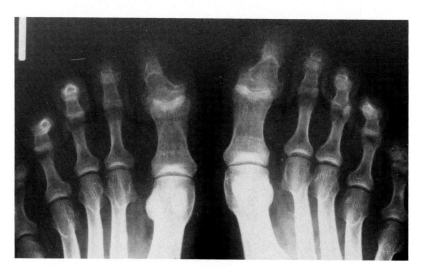

Fig. 6-6. Congenitally flat metatarsal heads of both feet.

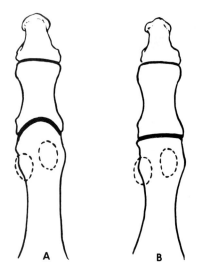

Fig. 6-7. Extreme variations in shape of first metatarsal head. **A,** Oval. Medial side of shoe will force hallux into valgus position, producing hallux valgus. **B,** Flat. Pressure of side of shoe cannot push hallux into valgus but will cause constant trauma to articular surface of base of proximal phalanx and to head of first metatarsal. Ultimately traumatic osteoarthritis will occur, resulting in hallux rigidus.

flexion of the proximal phalanx can be achieved, which may result in a less symptomatic first metatarsophalangeal joint. In the adolescent patient any type of prosthetic replacement is contraindicated.

Acquired. The acquired type of hallux rigidus is more common than the congenital type. It is essentially a traumatic osteoarthritis resulting from a combination of any of the following factors: (1) intraarticular fracture, (2) osteochondritis dissecans of the first metatarsal head, (3) repeated use of the great toe as a striking or anchor point, and (4) a congenitally flat head of the first metatarsal (Figs. 6-6 and 6-7, *B*).

The metatarsophalangeal joint of the hallux has a moderate ball-and-socket articulation, and the periarticular structures have normal resistance to external pressure. If abnormal stress is applied to the hallux by a short and/or a pointed-toe shoe, excessive pressure can be brought against the articular surface of the joint. If the joint has a ball-and-socket type of relationship (Fig. 6-7, *A*), a hallux valgus may result. Conversely, the flatter the articular surface of this joint (Fig. 6-7, *B*) and the more resistant the periarticular structures, the greater will be the pressure applied in an irregular manner; and this pressure may, over time, lead to traumatic osteoarthritis and to a hallux rigidus.

Acquired secondary to one of the general arthritides. Gout and psoriatic or rheumatoid arthritis are possible causes of hallux rigidus. In gout the great toe joint is often the only joint of the foot involved, whereas in rheumatoid and psoriatic arthritis other joints of the foot are also affected. Complete ankylosis of the joint may be consequent to infection after surgical correction for hallux valgus.

From a historical standpoint, other theories have been advanced as to the cause of hallux rigidus. Mau (1928) believed that an inefficient foot such as a pes valgus or a pes valgoplanus is the forerunner of hallux rigidus. Miller and Arendt (1940) expressed the opinion that hallux rigidus is related to a congenital proximal displacement of the sesamoid. Bingold and Collins (1950) stated it is a result of gait abnormality.

Treatment. Conservative treatment for hallux rigidus is directed toward alleviating the pain at the metatarsophalangeal joint of the great toe and can be accomplished by obtaining a shoe large enough to prevent excessive pressure against the enlarged joint. A stiff-soled shoe will help decrease motion at the metatarsophalangeal joint, thereby alleviating some discomfort (see Fig. 11-3). Alleviation can also be accomplished, particularly in adolescence, by placing the patient in a short leg cast, which extends out over the toes, to immobilize the joint for a 4-to-6-week period. Occasionally intraarticular injection of steroid will be of benefit. If conservative methods fail, surgical intervention may be indicated.

Treatment for congenital cases differs because the deformity varies. The faulty articular surface of the joint must be carefully evaluated in each case and an arthroplasty performed so a nearly normal ball-and-socket articular relation will be reestablished between the base of the proximal phalanx and the head of the first metatarsal.

Surgical treatment of hallux rigidus in adults is directed toward establishing a pain-free metatarsophalangeal joint and can be accomplished by arthrodesis of the first metatarsophalangeal joint, which eliminates the motion and hence the pain. Such a procedure has been advocated by Harrison and Harvey (1963) and by Moynihan (1967). To permit more dorsiflexion of the metatarsophalangeal joint, Kessel and Bonney (1958) and Moberg (1979) recommended a wedge osteotomy on the dorsum of the base of the proximal phalanx to bring the great toe out of its plantar-flexed position and into some dorsiflexion, thereby reducing the pressure against the joint during walking. Procedures to reestablish motion at the metatarsophalangeal joint usually do so at the expense of stability of the joint. The arthroplasty using a Silastic implant in the base of the proximal phalanx has been advocated for this condition. In our experience there have been as many poor results because of soft tissue reaction, joint stiffness, and loosening of the prosthesis as there have been satisfactory results with establishment of active dorsiflexion. We do not recommend the use of a prosthesis in any patient under the age of 50, since there are other procedures that will give a more satisfactory result, and the long-term results of prosthetic replacement thus far are not well established.

DuVries (1965) advocated a cheilectomy for the treatment of hallux rigidus. The procedure is applicable in essentially all acquired types of hallux rigidus and involves removal of the proliferative bone around the metatarsal head, thus allowing dorsiflexion to recur at the joint. With the return of dorsiflexion, the joint pain is effectively eliminated. The procedure has the advantage that if it happens to fail (which occurs in less than 10% of the patients), an arthrodesis or prosthetic replacement can still be easily effected at the metatarsophalangeal joint.

The surgical technique of cheilectomy is as follows.

1. Make a longitudinal incision immediately over the first metatarsophalangeal joint on either side of the extensor hallucis longus, extending it from the middle of the proximal phalanx to a point about the middle of the shaft of the first metatarsal.

2. Retract the skin and extensor hallucis longus.

3. Incise the joint capsule longitudinally and free it from the proliferative bone to which it is usually attached, retract the margins, carry out a complete synovectomy, and remove any excessively thick capsular material.

4. Deliver the head of the first metatarsal dorsally. Plantar flexion of the great toe at this stage aids delivery (Figs. 6-8, A and 6-9, A).

5. Observation of the articular surface of the first metatarsal head will demonstrate the outline of the original articular cartilage. Using this as the starting point, remove proliferative bone on the dorsum and sides of the metatarsal head. The bone is often granite-like in consistency. Include some of the normal bone of the head to form an accentuated rounded dorsal surface but never a pointed surface (Figs. 6-8, B, and 6-9, B).

6. Smooth the surface with a rasp. Be sure 60° to 80° of extension has been achieved. If the base of the proximal phalanx is also exostotic, remove excess bone and smooth (Fig. 6-8, C and D).

7. Instill 1 ml of steroid into the joint space to help inhibit formation of extensive scar tissue in the capsule.

8. Suture the capsule if possible with fine chromic; close the skin as usual. Apply a compression bandage for 12 to 18 hours.

9. Institute gentle motion of the great toe joint on the third or fourth postoperative day, to be increased in vigor and extent daily for 3 months, to prevent formation of adhesions in the periarticular structures. The patient can usually be ambulatory by the first postoperative day in a wooden shoe worn for 2 weeks.

The results following a cheilectomy have been most satisfactory as a whole. Although at surgery 60° to 80° of dorsiflexion is achieved, postoperatively the patient will usually retain about one half of this motion. This, however, is a sufficient degree of motion to make walking and other activities quite comfortable. The patient often notes some aching feeling in the joint after prolonged standing or activities, but rarely is the degree of discomfort sufficient to preclude any activity on the part of the patient. The majority of patients have been able to resume their previous athletic endeavors such as jogging, tennis, and golf with little or no disability. The fact that the large amount of proliferative bone has been removed makes wearing shoes much simpler for the patient. It is uncommon that following a cheilectomy the patient will require a revision of the metatarsophalan-

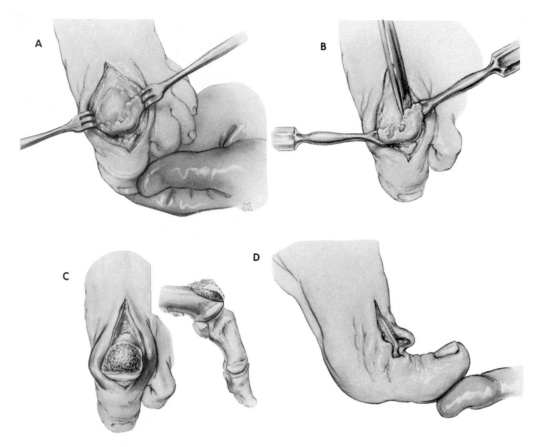

Fig. 6-8. Dorsal delivery of head of first metatarsal. **A,** Exposure of head with hallux plantar flexed, showing proliferated bony change. **B,** Removal of excess bone with osteotome. **C,** Smoothing and rounding raw bone surface. **D,** Dorsiflexion of hallux in normal excursion.

geal joint to either a fusion or possibly a prosthetic replacement.

Based on the results of this procedure in our hands, we believe that a cheilectomy is the treatment of choice for hallux rigidus.

Degenerative arthritis of metatarsocuneiform joints

Degenerative arthritis of the first metatarsocuneiform joint is usually the result of trauma. It often is the result of a Lisfranc fracture-dislocation. Degenerative arthritis, however, also occurs spontaneously. In either case it is an extremely disabling condition as it becomes more advanced because of the stress placed on this portion of the arch while standing. Several sequelae may result from degenerative changes at the metatarsocuneiform joint, namely, a moderate degree of bony proliferation that results in discomfort while wearing shoes and a progressive flatfoot deformity resulting from the collapse of the metatarsocuneiform joints. The foot may swing out into a moderate degree of abduction and lose the longitudinal arch. When dealing with the patient who has what appears to be degenerative arthritis of the

metatarsocuneiform joints but cannot recall a history of trauma, one should always be cognizant of this representing a Charcot foot, possibly as a result of diabetes.

The conservative management of this problem is the use of a rigid orthosis that will provide the longitudinal arch sufficient support so that the patient is more comfortable. If this is added to a rocker-bottom shoe, it may significantly improve the function of the foot, particularly in the early stages. Unfortunately, as degenerative arthritis of the metatarsocuneiform joints progresses and in particular if there is progressive loss of the longitudinal arch and abduction of the forefoot, surgical intervention is indicated.

Surgery consists of carrying out an arthrodesis of the first metatarsocuneiform joint and any other metatarsocuneiform joints that may be involved with degenerative changes. In patients who have developed flatfoot with abduction of the forefoot it is important to attempt to reestablish the normal alignment of the foot at the time of the surgery. This is done by bringing the first metatarsal joint into normal alignment with the remainder of the foot by adducting it slightly and usually

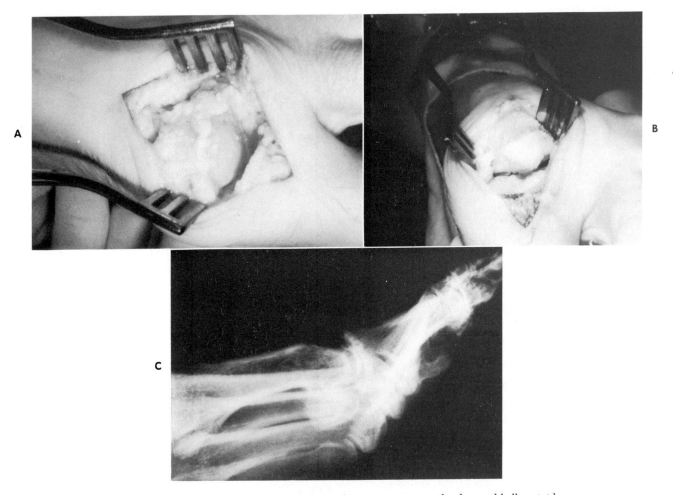

Fig. 6-9. A, Dorsal view of metatarsophalangeal joint in patient with advanced hallux rigidus. Note marked proliferative bone around metatarsal head as well as at base of proximal phalanx. **B,** View of metatarsal head following excision of proliferative bone. **C,** Radiograph demonstrating first metatarsophalangeal joint following excision of proliferative bone. Note marked amount of dorsal bone that has been removed. This is essential to permit return of dorsiflexion.

by plantar flexing it to help reestablish the longitudinal arch. The arthrodesis site requires internal fixation, which can be in the form of staples, compression screw, or Steinmann pins.

Technique for carrying out first metatarsocuneiform fusion

1. A medial longitudinal incision is made slightly above the medial midline and centered over the metatarsocuneiform joint. This is carried down through subcutaneous tissue and fat to expose the periosteum.

2. The joint capsule is opened, and the proliferative bone is removed, particularly along the dorsal aspect.

3. Using a power saw or osteotome, the articular surfaces are removed, and if necessary, the first metatarsocuneiform joint is brought into slight abduction and plantar flexion to realign the forefoot.

4. The arthrodesis site is then fixed with either staples or screws.

5. Following the initial compression dressing, the patient's leg is placed in a short leg walking cast until healing is complete at about 2 months.

If multiple metatarsocuneiform joints are to be fused, the second incision is made on the dorsal aspect of the foot centered over the second metatarsal, or if the second and third metatarsocuneiform joints are undergoing arthrodesis, the second incision is made between them.

It has been our experience that a single metatarsocuneiform joint fusion will often give the patient a most satisfactory result, but when it is carried out at multiple joints because of an old Lisfranc fracture-dislocation, although a solid union may occur, the foot often remains sufficiently symptomatic that the patient is not able to

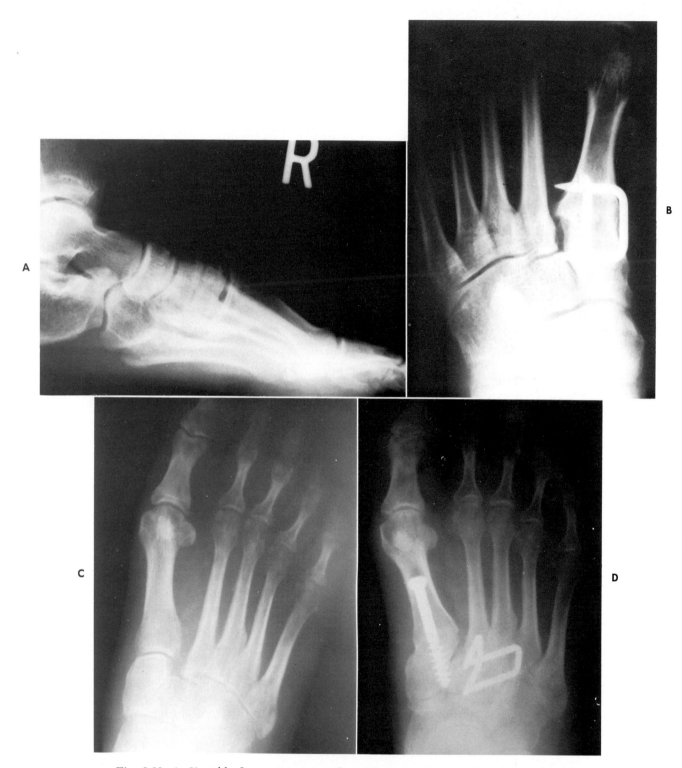

Fig. 6-10. A, Unstable first metatarsocuneiform joint secondary to old trauma with early degenerative changes. **B,** Postoperative arthrodesis of first metatarsophalangeal joint using staple fixation. **C,** Degenerative arthritis of metatarsocuneiform articulation secondary to an old Lisfranc fracture-dislocation. **D,** Postoperative arthrodesis of metatarsocuneiform joints.

return to his preinjury level of activities. Most workers would have difficulty standing on their feet for a full 8-hour day following multiple metatarsocuneiform fusions (Fig. 6-10).

Degenerative arthritis of talonavicular joint

Degenerative arthritis of the talonavicular joint usually is the result of trauma to the foot, although it may occur spontaneously or in association with rheumatoid arthritis. As the degenerative process progresses, there may be increasing loss of the longitudinal arch, particularly in patients with rheumatoid arthritis. Most patients who have degenerative arthritis of the talonavicular joint either following trauma or spontaneously do not show the loss of the longitudinal arch to the degree that is seen in patients with rheumatoid arthritis. The loss of the longitudinal arch in rheumatoid arthritis probably is caused by the involvement of the ligamentous structure about the talonavicular joint, which is not affected in patients with degenerative arthritis.

The conservative management of degenerative arthritis of the talonavicular joint is the use of some type of an arch-support device. This may take the form of a firm, well-padded longitudinal arch support, a University of California Biomechanics Laboratory (UCBL) type of insert, or a polypropylene ankle-foot orthosis to prevent motion in the forefoot but still allow ankle joint motion. If these measures fail to give the patient adequate relief, arthrodesis of the talonavicular joint is the treatment of choice.

For patients in whom the degenerative changes only involve the talonavicular joint, we believe that an isolated fusion of this joint would produce a satisfactory result. Since the subtalar joint complex depends on mo-

tion in the subtalar joint for proper function, arthrodesis of this joint will essentially eliminate all subtalar joint and transverse tarsal joint motions. If there is any question regarding degenerative changes in the calcaneocuboid or subtalar joints, either a double arthrodesis—in the talonavicular and calcaneocuboid joint—or a triple arthrodesis would then be the treatment of choice.

Arthrodesis of the talonavicular joint should be carried out through a dorsomedial or medial approach to the joint, following which the joint undergoes arthrodesis either by denuding the joint surfaces and fixing them with a staple or screw or by an inlaid bone graft. Following the surgery, the patient's foot is immobilized in a nonwalking cast for 4 to 6 weeks, after which a walking cast should be used for another 4 to 6 weeks (Fig. 6-11).

There may be evidence of avascular necrosis of the navicular bone at times, either following trauma or, more frequently, on a spontaneous basis. This should be observed for carefully, and if it is present, the possibility of obtaining a solid fusion may be jeopardized. In cases such as this it may be necessary to extend the fusion from the talus into the cuneiform bones.

CRYSTAL-INDUCED ARTHRITIS

Two types of crystal deposits cause arthritis: gout results from sodium urate cystals that are strongly negatively birefringent and sharply needle shaped when viewed under a polarized microscope, and pseudogout results from calcium pyrophosphate dihydrate crystals that are weakly positively birefringent under polarized light and variably shaped.

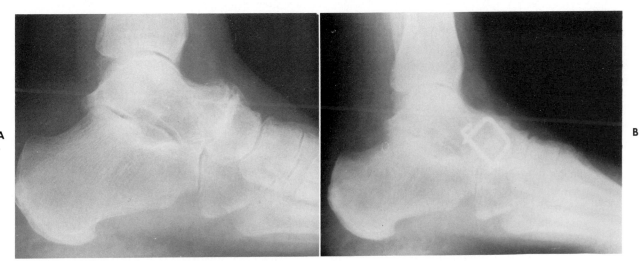

Fig. 6-11. A, Degenerative arthritis of talonavicular joint on spontaneous basis. **B,** After arthrodesis of talonavicular joint using staple fixation.

Calcium pyrophosphate dihydrate deposition disease

Calcium pyrophosphate dihydrate (CPPD) deposition disease, also known as chondrocalcinosis or pseudogout, is believed to cause symptoms when crystals are shed into a joint, leading to phagocytosis and chemotactic enzyme release by leukocytes, which results in a painful inflammatory response. Although fine curvilinear calcifications are sometimes seen at metatarsophalangeal joints, this does not usually cause a destructive arthropathy at these articulations. The talonavicular and subtalar joints are more often implicated and in the end stage resemble advanced degenerative joint disease.

Treatment. For acute synovitis, systemic antiinflammatory medications are recommended. When joint destruction is advanced, surgical approaches used in degenerative joint disease are indicated.

Gouty arthritis

Gout has been known since antiquity and is caused by an alteration in purine metabolism so that sodium urate crystals precipitate into synovial fluid, causing an inflammatory reaction, which is the acute stage, or are deposited into tophi, which is the chronic stage, that cause periarticular destruction.

Gout occurs more frequently in men than in women and exhibits a definite inheritance pattern. Approximately 50% to 75% of initial attacks involve the great toe. About 90% of patients with gout experience one or more acute attacks in the toes during their lifetime (Stanbury et al., 1972). Gout can also manifest as an acute periarthritis of the great toe joint, which is often referred to as gouty bursitis or podagra.

The onset of an acute gouty arthritis attack is sudden; the great toe joint becomes swollen and excruciatingly painful. The overlying skin is hyperesthetic. The attack is self-limiting but tends to recur at intervals. Gout can also occur in the plantar fascia as a plantar fasciitis, tenosynovitis, or occasionally in any of the joints of the foot. Acute attacks often occur after the stress of a surgical procedure. The patient with postoperative pain in the foot should be evaluated for possible gout. When an acute attack occurs, it can last from several days to weeks.

Although the diagnosis is best made by the identification of sodium urate crystals aspirated from the acutely involved joint and examined under polarized light, the diagnosis can be inferred on the basis of the clinical examination, the serum uric acid level, or the response to a trial of treatment with colchicine. Once the diagnosis is established and the acute stage has resolved, allopurinol can be used to prevent further attacks and the formation of tophi. The patient should have the regular supervision of an internist or rheumatologist.

Chronic gouty arthritis with its tophaceous deposits is rare today probably because of the excellent medical management of most patients who have gouty arthritis; however, 10% of patients with untreated gout develop chronic tophaceous deposits in the soft tissues followed by invasion and destruction of joints and bones (Fig. 6-12). Patients with primary gout who have serum urate levels of 9 mg/100 ml or less usually do not develop tophi, even if left untreated. When the serum urate level exceeds 11 mg/100 ml, tophaceous deposits are inevitable and, unless preventive measures are taken, are likely to occur within a few years of the initial acute attack.

Radiographic findings of patients with joint involvement vary from no detectable abnormality to severe destruction of the joints of the foot. There is a characteristic periarticular erosion just proximal to the joint, often on both the tibial and fibular aspects of the first metatarsal head (Fig. 6-13). A feature that distinguishes gouty arthritis from other arthritides is the presence of destructive lesions in bones remote from the articular surface. Miskew (1980) described gouty invasion of the talus resulting in aseptic necrosis requiring ankle arthrodesis but sparing the subtalar articulation. Many of the lesions are expansile with overhanging margins of periosteal new bone at the limits of a tophus with secondary calcifications within the tophi or degenerative tissues (Martel, 1968). There may be tophaceous deposits below the deep fascia that can encircle and invade tendons, but the nerves and blood vessels are spared, although they are surrounded by the tophaceous material. Areas of cartilage are also often spared, resulting in some preservation of joint space, which is a feature that distinguishes gouty arthritis from rheumatoid arthritis.

Treatment. The acute attack is treated symptomatically with elevation and rest of the foot. The sooner colchicine or other antiinflammatory medication is administered at therapeutic levels after the onset of an attack, the sooner the pain will diminish.

In patients with chronic tophaceous gout removal of the tophaceous material by curetting usually prevents the return of deforming overgrowth (Woughter, 1959). Kurtz (1965) has emphasized that (1) amputation is rarely indicated, (2) for draining sinuses over tophi, local currettement removing as much of the deposit as possible followed by application of wet dressings will promote healing, and (3) if the skin sloughs and a surgical wound exude urates, treatment with wet dressings and antibiotics usually results in healing with surprisingly little scarring (see Fig. 6-12, *B*).

Medical treatment of chronic tophaceous gout can result in rapid dissolution of tophi with failure of bony ingrowth into former erosions; the phalanges and meta-

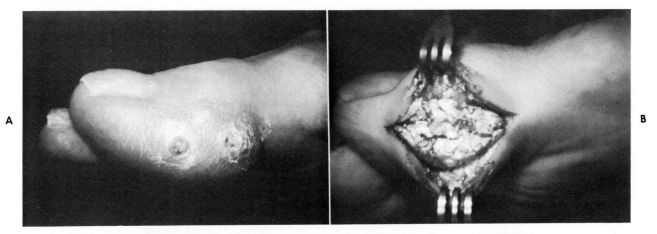

Fig. 6-12. **A,** Gouty ulcerations along medial side of great toe. **B,** Surgical debridgement of gouty deposits.

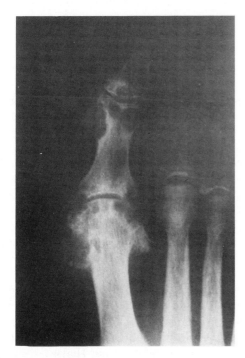

Fig. 6-13. Radiograph of first metatarsophalangeal joint in patient with gouty arthritis. Note characteristic periarticular erosion.

tarsals were markedly and rapidly shortened by such treatment as described by Gottlieb (1977).

SERONEGATIVE SPONDYLOARTHROPATHIES

The three seronegative spondylarthropathies, ankylosing spondylitis, psoriatic arthritis, and Reiter's syndrome, have radiologic features and clinical manifestations that differentiate them from rheumatoid arthritis. The key radiologic differences are (1) the absence of generalized osteoporosis; (2) the presence of adventitious calcification, or "whiskering," about the joints in association with erosive changes; and (3) intraarticular ankylosis, which is rarely seen in rheumatoid arthritis of the foot except in the tarsus (Resnick, 1979). Clinically, rheumatoid arthritis does not present with painful heel syndrome; a review of 222 cases of patients with rheumatoid arthritis showed no Achilles tendinitis and rare plantar fasciitis, whereas 20% of 150 patients with seronegative spondyloarthritis had plantar fasciitis, Achilles tendinitis, or both (Gerster, 1980).

Ankylosing spondylitis

Ankylosing sponylitis has overwhelming involvement in the axial skeleton so that foot and ankle manifestations seem relatively insignificant. However, enthesopathy, or pathologic process, involving the attachments of tendons and ligaments to the calcaneus occurs in ankylosing spondylitis in a way identical to that appearing in Reiter's syndrome and psoriatic arthritis. Metatarsophalangeal joints are afflicted in a way similar to that seen in rheumatoid arthritis but with less intense synovitis, smaller erosions, and more periosteal new bone formation, which results in bony ankylosis or joint capsule ossification (Ball, 1971). Subchondral sclerosis is more apparent than osteoporosis and is a differentiating feature from rheumatoid arthritis. Grossly, however, the toes become dorsiflexed and have a lateral drift that is similar to the forefoot deformity of rheumatoid arthritis.

Psoriatic arthritis

Patients with psoriasis have a greater incidence of arthritis than the population in general. The arthritis antedates, often by years, the skin lesions in 10% to 15% of patients so that the diagnosis is suggested by the type

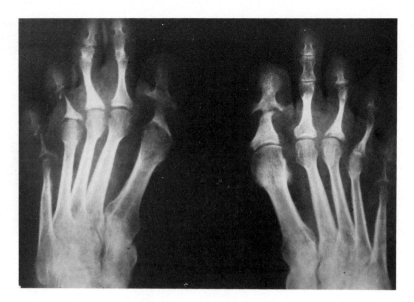

Fig. 6-14. Psoriatic arthritis; extensive destruction of some proximal phalanges.

of arthritis that manifests. Often there is symmetric involvement of both hands and feet. There is a striking involvement of the distal interphalangeal joints and psoriatic changes in the adjacent nails. Dorsal tuft resorption can be seen with soft tissue atrophy. Arthritis mutilans causes destruction of the proximal phalanges wherein the bone atrophies to needle points (Fig. 6-14), producing the "cup and saucer" appearance of the destroyed joint. Heel pain syndrome is indistinguishable from that seen in Reiter's syndrome, but otherwise many of the cases resemble rheumatoid arthritis clinically, and the details of management are similar to those for rheumatoid arthritis.

Reiter's syndrome

First described in the early 1800s, the triad of conjunctivitis, urethritis, and asymmetric arthritis in men following dysentery has been termed Reiter's syndrome by common consent since 1916. The cause is not understood, but the association with enteritides suggests an infectious origin, and the high incidence (up to 96%) of HLA-B27 positivity in Reiter's syndrome suggests an immunologic predisposition in afflicted individuals (Ford, 1979). The lower extremities are usually involved, particularly the knees, feet, and ankles. Chand (1980) found that one half of the patients with Reiter's syndrome had foot and ankle involvement, half of which was bilateral. Another joint, most often the knee, was involved in two thirds of these patients. Because the arthritis commonly appears some time after the infectious process, which can be a minimally symptomatic genitourinary infection, Reiter's syndrome should be suspected when a male patient has several lower extremity complaints, especially if one is heel pain syndrome.

The painful area usually has tenderness and swelling without erythema. "Sausage toes" are common. The metatarsophalangeal joints and posterior calcaneus are also frequently affected, while the midtarsal area, metatarsal shafts, and subtalar area are relatively spared. When the ankle is involved, an effusion is common and is sometimes associated with erosions that could be confused radiographically with osteochondritis dissecans of the talus.

There can be no radiographic findings at all in up to one third of the cases. Sometimes only soft tissue swelling is apparent on radiographic examinations early in the appearance of the syndrome. However, persistent heel pain as a result of Reiter's syndrome characteristically evolves fluffy calcifications at the insertions of the plantar fascia and the Achilles tendon and small irregular erosions around heel spurs. The interphalangeal and metatarsophalangeal joints can demonstrate small intraarticular and extraarticular erosions. Occasionally there is demineralization of the proximal interphalangeal joints, but otherwise osteoporosis is not notable. Rarely is there severe joint destruction with bony ankylosis.

Treatment. Surgery is usually not required in Reiter's syndrome. Heel spur surgery was assayed in a few of Gerster's patients (1980) and was deemed worthless or worse. For end stage, "burned-out" joint destruction, procedures similar to those used for rheumatoid arthritis can be used.

Most researchers agree that Reiter's syndrome is a self-limited disease that requires supportive management in the acute or subacute phase. The time course varies from a few weeks to more than 1 year but most patients undergo spontaneous remission within a few months. Antiinflammatory medication may relieve symptoms. Heel pads and felt metatarsal supports in rocker-bottom, crepe-soled shoes may decrease mechanical stress on the afflicted areas while the disease is symptomatic.

RHEUMATOID ARTHRITIS

Rheumatoid arthritis is a systemic disease that primarily affects the synovial tissues in a symmetric pattern, but extraarticular disease is common as a result of vasculitis. The cause of rheumatoid arthritis is not understood but is thought to be an aberration of the immune-response system in individuals who may be genetically predisposed by having the HLA-DRW4 cell surface marker; the inflammatory response is instigated by interactions between antigens, antibodies, complement, and immune complexes formed by the rheumatoid factor (IgM antibody directed against IgG) and the antigens of rheumatoid arthritis (Spiegel, 1982). Women are affected three times as often as men; as many as 2% to 3% of the population over 55 years of age may develop rheumatoid arthritis.

Diagnosis

A diagnosis of rheumatoid arthritis is based on clinical, laboratory, and radiographic findings. Although the disease commonly begins insidiously, an acute onset is not by any means rare. Radiographic studies and laboratory tests give little diagnostic help during the acute phase, although an elevated erythrocyte sedimentation rate is suspicious and should be measured serially. Generally the diagnosis must be tentative for several weeks until the disease has progressed and its true nature becomes apparent. A test for rheumatoid factor is frequently positive, although a negative result does not in any way preclude the diagnosis.

Rheumatoid arthritis begins in the feet in approximately 17% of reported cases. The forefoot is more commonly involved than the hindfoot. The condition may begin asymmetrically, but with progression to a subacute or chronic arthritis, symmetric involvement usually occurs. Swelling is chiefly intraarticular with effusion, but periarticular soft tissue swelling is often present; initially there is tenderness accompanied by erythema over the involved joint. Involvement of the proximal interphalangeal and metatarsophalangeal joints is particularly suggestive. A radiographic examination may reveal only soft tissue swelling and juxtaarticular osteoporosis early in the course of the disease.

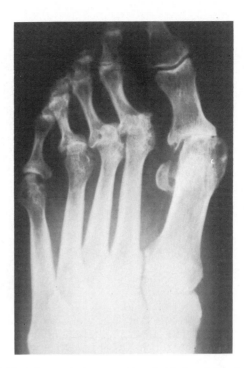

Fig. 6-15. Advanced rheumatoid arthritis involving forefoot. Note marked deformity of metatarsophalangeal joints.

Clinical course

The natural history of rheumatoid arthritis in the foot is one of inexorably progressive deformity associated with pain and disability. Vainio (1956) reported 89% of 955 adult patients with rheumatoid arthritis had foot problems. Spiegel (1982) found that synovitis was the hallmark of the first 3 years of the disease (65%) with only 6% having moderate to severe deformity of any metatarsophalangeal joint, whereas patients with more than 10 years of disease duration had less incidence of synovitis (18%) but more than 40% had moderate to severe deformities of the metatarsalphalangeal joints. Hallux valgus occurs in more than 60% of the patients when mild (15° to 35°) deformities are included.

Rheumatoid foot problems are dynamic because the mechanical stress of walking is superimposed on gradual joint destruction brought about by the chronic synovitis. In the forefoot, soft tissue support of the first metatarsophalangeal joint is destroyed by the disease process, which results in the hallux deviating into severe valgus (Fig. 6-15), but it may become displaced dorsally or into varus. This severe hallux valgus deformity decreases the weight-bearing capacity of the joint, and increased stress is placed on the lesser toes. The lesser toes frequently drift with the hallux and become subluxed or frankly dislocated because of loss of intrinsic soft tissue support brought about by the synovitis and capsular distention of the metatarsophalangeal

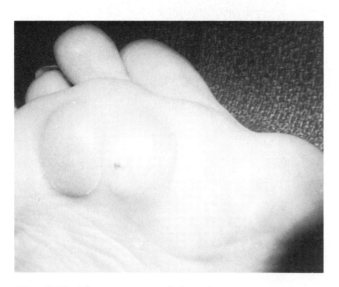

Fig. 6-16. Plantar aspect of foot demonstrating changes caused by fixed plantar flexion of metatarsal heads secondary to dislocation of metatarsophalangeal joints.

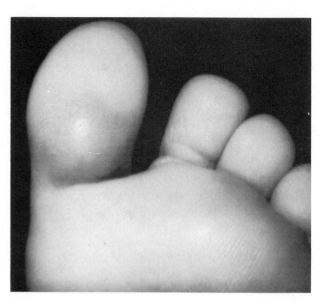

Fig. 6-17. Large rheumatoid nodule beneath great toe.

joint. Finally the plantar fat pad is pulled distally by the dorsal soft tissue contractures of the lesser toes. The metatarsal heads are fixed in a plantar-flexed position, and diffuse intractable plantar keratoses develop over bony prominences (Fig. 6-16). Dorsal callosities develop over interphalangeal joints because of shoe pressure, and terminal callosities form on the tips of the toes as a result of the direct pressure of their flexed position.

The great toe can develop additional deformities after long-standing disease. Jacoby (1976) described hallux tortus, a pronation deformity greater than 20° of the great toe associated with severe hallux valgus, which causes pain at the site of a callus over the medial aspect of the interphalangeal joint that assumes the weight-bearing load. More than 40% of rheumatoid great toes had interphalangeal hyperextension; half of these demonstrated chisel toe, a combination of pressure of the nail plate against the toe box of the shoe with nail dystrophy and concomitant plantar callosity or nodule formation under the crease of the interphalangeal joint (Fig. 6-17).

The midfoot can be involved with chronic synovitis and eventual loss of joint space with initially fibrous and ultimately bony ankylosis. Osteoporosis is common and thought to be part of the systemic disease, but erosions are rare in the midfoot. Loss of the longitudinal arch is often seen on weight-bearing lateral radiographs, and the naviculocuneiform joint frequently sags at this articulation (Vainio, 1956).

Hindfoot involvement in rheumatoid arthritis is slowly progressive in about one third of patients with rheumatoid foot problems. Subtalar synovitis with subsequent relaxation of hindfoot ligamentous support results in hindfoot valgus deformities associated with flatfoot that progresses from a flexible deformity to a rigid one. However, a stiff equinovarus deformity can develop in a patient with rheumatoid arthritis and subtalar involvement, particularly one who has had prolonged bed rest with splinting inadequate to preserve a plantigrade foot (Heywood, 1983).

The ankle is the least involved joint of the major weight-bearing joints in rheumatoid arthritis (Wagner, 1982). When it is affected, however, the subtalar and midtarsal joints are often involved as well, so that tibiopedal motion is drastically reduced (Fig. 6-18).

Rheumatoid arthritis can be divided into four stages (Fig. 6-19).

1. In the first stage there is no bony deformity, and no surgery is indicated.
2. In the second stage there is early involvement without fixed deformity. Radiographs show minimal erosive changes. Synovectomy as a prophylactic and therapeutic measure may be employed if there has been unremitting synovitis despite adequate nonsurgical measures for a period of not less than 6 months and if the patient has had the disease for not less than 1 year. The ankle and metatarsophalangeal and interphalangeal joints lend themselves to synovectomy. Vainio (1979) found that performing metatarsophalangeal synovectomies early in the course of the disease reduced

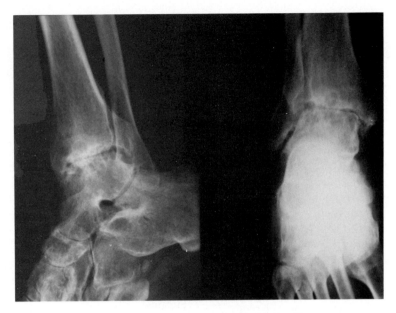

Fig. 6-18. Rheumatoid arthritis of tarsus and ankle joints.

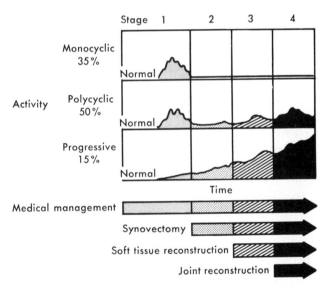

Fig. 6-19. Clinical course of rheumatoid arthritis.

the rate of interdigital neuroma excision in patients with rheumatoid arthritis from 4.5 to 0.6 operations per year.

3. At the third stage of involvement soft tissue deformity has occurred, but there have been no significant erosive changes. Under these circumstances, synovectomy, tendon transfer, repair and release, and a capsulotomy are indicated.

4. In the fourth stage deformity and articular destruction have occurred, and reconstructive surgical procedures such as arthroplasty or arthrodesis are required.

Conservative treatment

An appreciation of the clinical course just outlined is essential to the proper planning of a treatment program. Treatment is directed toward (1) relief of pain, (2) prevention of deformity, (3) correction of deformity, (4) restoration of function, and (5) preservation of function. Medical management should be continued throughout all stages of the disease and may be the only treatment necessary during the early phases. Treatment should include antiinflammatory medication and orthopaedic appliances.

Drug therapy. Agents that reduce inflammation and relieve pain are recommended. Salicylates are prescribed as the first line of defense and may be the only drug needed, although other nonsteroidal antiinflammatory medications can be used. Remissive agents such as gold, antimalarial medication, and D-penicillamine and immunosuppressive agents are often prescribed by rheumatologists to arrest the disease before joint destruction occurs. Systemic steroid therapy is less favored by rheumatologists because of the well-known side effects that are deleterious. Steroid injections into the ankle and subtalar joints are occasionally beneficial, but restraint should be exercised.

Physical therapy. Bardwick (1982) reports that physical modalities are of limited usefulness in treating the pain of rheumatoid arthritis, but some patients benefit by thermal modalities such as cold baths for acute inflammatory pain, moist heat or warmth (104° F) (40° C) for subacute chronic pain, or contrast bathing. However, cold should not be used in patients with Raynaud's phenomenon or cryoglobulinemia. Heat must be used with caution in those patients with vasculitis. Diathermy is no longer considered to be a useful modality of physical medicine; ultrasound may provide temporary relief of heel pain syndrome.

Heel cord stretching of a gentle passive nature that is not painful should be practiced daily by patients with rheumatoid arthritis and ankle and subtalar joint involvement. Maintaining a full range of motion of all the metarsophalangeal and interphalangeal joints of the rheumatoid foot can be accomplished by active or passive means. The patient should range each joint once a day to maintain motion; more frequent joint manipulation may be required to regain motion lost during an acute attack. Picking up marbles with the toes or wrinkling a towel are active exercises that can be easily performed. If pain prevents this, passive manipulation of the forefoot joints can be performed by the patient or a family member.

Orthotic devices. Metatarsalgia can be relieved in the early phase by using felt metatarsal arch supports fixed to the shoe just proximal to the metatarsal heads. When the metatarsal heads become more prominent, the addition of a Spenco liner with a felt pad glued to it can offer additional protection. Crepe or rubber-soled, rocker-bottom shoes decrease the stress on the metatarsal area. As the toes become hammered, it may be necessary to accommodate them in an extra-depth shoe into which a customized orthosis of Plastizote may be used to accommodate plantar lesions such as large intractable keratoses and synovial cysts (Glass et al., 1982). Because rheumatoid forefoot deformities are dynamic and Plastizote is a deformable substance, new orthotic devices need to be constructed every 6 to 8 months. This may seem expensive and time-consuming, but when a patient can be maintained as an employed person or a community ambulator, the effort seems worthwhile.

Patients with tarsal pain but no fixed deformity can be maintained in a functional position with a UCBL insert (see Fig. 11-10). This orthosis also relieves pain in the plantar area. The orthosis may be used as long as necessary, depending on the activity of the disease process, and should be removed at least once (and preferably several times) a day for the patient to carry out active and passive range of motion exercises.

Ambulatory aids such as canes and crutches can provide significant reduction in weight bearing of the afflicted lower extremity, but the upper extremity involvement so typical of rheumatoid arthritis often precludes this option. Special cane hand-grips and platform crutches are useful when there is hand and wrist disease, but shoulder affliction is not spared by these modifications.

Bracing may be required when foot and ankle pain and disability are refractory to other methods of treatment or when the deformity has become fixed. A molded leather ankle brace with metal stays can be worn inside a shoe to provide support and pain relief to the tarsal and ankle region. A lightweight polypropylene ankle-foot orthosis can also provide similar relief. When weight bearing and motion at the ankle and subtalar region are very painful, weight bearing can be transferred proximally by means of a below-the-knee bearing brace (BKBB) or a patellar tendon–bearing brace (PTB). The BKBB uses double-upright steel bars and a leather calf corset that is laced; free ankle motion can be retained. The PTB is molded of plastic and can be worn in a regular shoe. The use of a solid ankle cushion heel (SACH) and a rocker-bottom shoe will increase tibiopedal motion and thus facilitate a more normal heel-toe gait.

Surgical treatment

Although medical management should continue throughout the progression of the disease, surgical procedures are indicated in the later phases.

Forefoot deformity. The typical forefoot deformities are hallux valgus, subluxation or dislocation of the metatarsophalangeal joints, and flexion of the interphalangeal joints of the lesser toes. There is a loss of effectiveness of the plantar fat pad that results in painful plantar calluses under the metatarsal head. When conservative treatment fails, surgical treatment must be directed toward reestablishing the alignment of the metatarsal bones and phalanges, restoring adequate padding on the plantar surface of the foot, and correcting the deformed position of the interphalangeal joints.

Resectional arthroplasty of the first metatarsal joint has been recommended for generations in reconstructing the severely deformed forefoot found in patients with rheumatoid arthritis (Amuso et al., 1971; Barton, 1973; Benson et al., 1971; Clayton, 1960, 1963; Fowler, 1959; Hoffman, 1912, Kates et al., 1967; Lipscomb et al., 1972; Marmor, 1975; Peterson, 1968; Schwartzmann, 1964; Scranton, 1980). There have been suggestions that relief by excisional arthroplasty is short-lived, and Silastic implant arthroplasty of the first ray has been recommended as a modern alternative (Cracchiolo, 1980, 1981). However, Silastic implants are frought with potential problems, as has been noted by Shereff and Jahss (1980) and Gordon and Bullough (1982). Some have advocated amputation of all the toes (Flint and Sweetnam, 1960). DuVries (1959) has long maintained that the rheumatoid foot requires the stabilization offered by arthrodesis of the first metatarsophalangeal joint to best preserve its function. Others also prefer arthrodesis of the first metatarsophalangeal joint (Fitzgerald, 1969; Henry and Waugh, 1975; Mann and Coughlin, 1979; Mann and Oates, 1980; Mann and Thompson, 1984; Moynihan, 1967; Raymakers and Waugh, 1971; Watson, 1974).

Henry and Waugh (1975) have shown that the hallux maintains a weight-bearing role after arthrodesis but not after Keller arthroplasty, and they believed this accounted for their improved results obtained with arthrodesis. In 1974 Watson reported a long-term follow-up of forefoot arthroplasties, stating that the chief aim of the operation was pain relief. In the long-term study he concluded that arthrodesis of the metatarsophalangeal joint of the great toe resulted in the highest proportion of painless feet. After a Keller procedure, he observed that the natural valgus position of the flail great toe was not supported by the abnormal lesser toes. Consequently, during the take-off phase of gait the great toe and lateral toes were displaced dorsally and laterally. As the toes migrated laterally and dorsally, the brunt of the patient's weight was shifted onto the metatarsal ends, causing calluses to develop once again at the distal ends of the remaining metatarsal shafts. When the first metatarsophalangeal joint was fused, it prevented the great toe from pushing the lesser toes laterally.

We prefer arthrodesis to other methods of surgical management of the rheumatoid forefoot. The results of reconstruction of the rheumatoid forefoot by arthrodesis of the first metatarsophalangeal joint were reviewed (Mann and Thompson, 1984). Follow-up averaged 4.1 years and ranged between 2 and 7¼ years. There were 18 feet in 11 women operated on; 12 feet underwent total forefoot reconstruction consisting of arthrodesis of the first metatarsophalangeal joint and excision of all lesser metatarsophalangeal joints; 6 feet underwent subtotal forefoot reconstruction that included arthrodesis of the first metatarsophalangeal joints in all cases. Results were classified as excellent in 14, good in 2, and fair in 2. There were no poor results. All but 1 achieved fusion for a fusion rate of 95%; the fibrous ankylosis was painless and had satisfactory function. Interphalangeal degenerative joint disease is a radiographic but not a clinical sequela. Arthrodesis of the first metatarsophalangeal joint provides stability that permanently corrects deformity, permits ordinary shoe wear, and, in combination with excisional arthroplsty of involved lesser metatarsophalangeal joints, relieves disabling pain in the rheumatoid forefoot. The arthrodesed first metatarsophalangeal joint in the patient with rheumatoid arthritis provides stability to the first ray, and because of the rigidity of the metatarsophalangeal joint, minimum stress is placed on the lesser metatarsophalangeal joints. This results in permitting the fat pad to remain well positioned beneath the lesser metatarsal heads, resulting in a painless foot with little likelihood of the need for further surgical intervention.

If only one or two metatarsophalangeal joints are affected, the entire forefoot usually does not have to reconstructed. If the great toe is affected, an arthrodesis of the first metatarsophalangeal joint is performed. If only one or two metatarsophalangeal joints are involved, an arthroplasty is performed only on those joints. If the entire forefoot is involved except for the fifth metatarsophalangeal joint, which is frequently seen, it is important, however, to also do an arthroplasty of the fifth metatarsophalangeal joint or the fifth toe will drift underneath the fourth toe because of loss of stability of the adjacent metatarsophalangeal joint.

Method of surgical reconstruction of rheumatoid forefoot

1. Expose the capsule and perform a thorough synovectomy through a longitudinal dorsal incision over the first metatarsophalangeal joint.

2. Resect the distal portion of the metatarsal head with a sagittal saw to create a flat surface of cancellous bone angled slightly dorsally and laterally.

3. Resect the base of the proximal phalanx perpendicular to its shaft. The bone cuts should provide bone-to-bone contact with the resulting position of the hallux being 15° to 20° of valgus and 10° to 15° of dorsiflexion measured from the floor, or 25° to 30° of dorsiflexion measured from the metatarsal. Before fixing the hallux, the lesser toe procedures should be performed so that the overall length of the hallux can be shortened to the appropriate length if necessary.

4. Approach the lesser toes through dorsal longitudinal incisions, one between the second and third metatarsal heads and the other between the fourth and fifth metatarsal heads. Identify the base of each proximal phalanx and divest it of its soft tissue attachments. Resect one third to one half of the proximal phalanx.

5. Continue the dissection on the dorsum of the distal metatarsal neck and head to release the contracted soft tissues and relocate them plantarward. This will allow the plantar fat pad to slide proximally. Decide how much of the metatarsal head to resect. When the contracture is severe, it is usually necessary to resect the entire head and bevel the neck to reduce its plantar protrusion. Generally speaking, the second metatarsal is resected back to the level of the end of the first metatarsal, and then each subsequent lateral metatarsal is shortened approximately 2 to 3 mm more. If only one or possibly two metatarsophalangeal joints are involved, resect the base of the proximal phalanx and remove only as much metatarsal head as is necessary to permit easy reduction of the joint. Avoid a single dominant metatarsal prominence.

6. Recheck the length of the first ray against the lesser toes, and if necessary, resect more length from

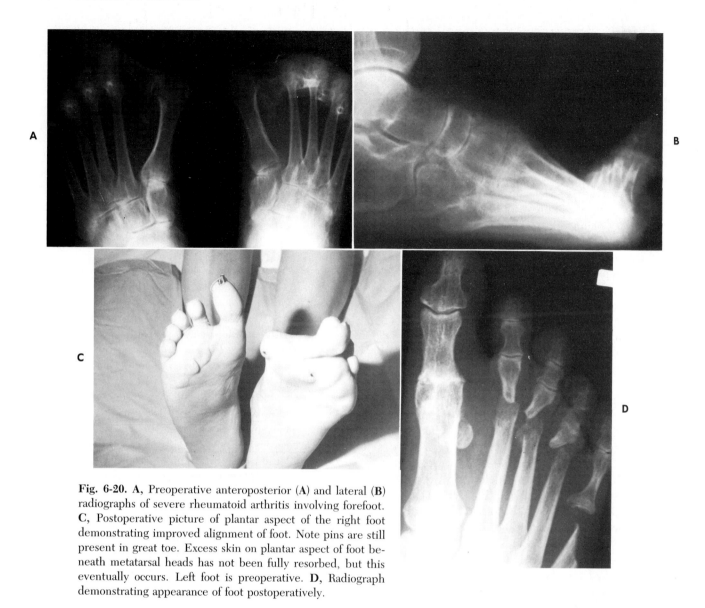

Fig. 6-20. A, Preoperative anteroposterior (**A**) and lateral (**B**) radiographs of severe rheumatoid arthritis involving forefoot. **C,** Postoperative picture of plantar aspect of the right foot demonstrating improved alignment of foot. Note pins are still present in great toe. Excess skin on plantar aspect of foot beneath metatarsal heads has not been fully resorbed, but this eventually occurs. Left foot is preoperative. **D,** Radiograph demonstrating appearance of foot postoperatively.

the base of the phalanx. The amount of bone resected from the first ray should leave the great toe no more than 3 to 4 mm longer than the lateral rays.

7. To stabilize the fusion site use two heavy (%4 inch and ⅛ inch) double-ended threaded Steinmann pins. Place them retrograde with power equipment out the end of the hallux, and then advance them retrograde across the arthrodesis site and into the metatarsal shaft. Be sure the hallux is in proper rotation before the second pin is advanced. Drill slowly so the threads in the soft rheumatoid bone are not stripped. Amputate the pins ¼ inch from the tip of the big toe.

8. The deformity of the proximal interphalangeal joint, which is usually a fixed hammer toe, is corrected by "crunching" the joint with digital pressure. The bone is usually soft enough to completely straighten the

toe and can be maintained in that position with either a pin or adhesive tape.

9. Close one layer of soft tissue under the extensor hallucis longus tendon, then close all the skin incisions, and apply a well padded compression dressing before releasing the tourniquet.

10. Change the dressing to a firm, soft dressing after 18 to 24 hours. In our experience fixation is adequate to allow weight bearing in a wooden shoe immediately.

11. Change the firm, soft dressing every 7 to 10 days for 6 weeks. The soft tissue dressing should be applied to bring the lesser toes over toward the great toe and hold them in a slightly plantar-flexed position. This is accomplished by wrapping the 2-inch Kling bandage counterclockwise as one sits in front of the right foot and clockwise as one sits in front of the left foot.

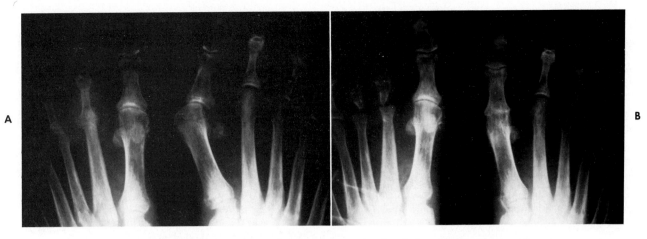

Fig. 6-21. A, Preoperative radiograph demonstrating localized rheumatoid changes. On one foot, only first metatarsophalangeal joint was involved, and in the other foot, second and third metatarsophalangeal joints were involved. **B,** Postoperative radiograph demonstrating arthrodesis of first metatarsophalangeal joint. Resectional arthroplasty of second and third metatarsophalangeal joints produced satisfactory alignment. In patients who have localized involvement, it is not necessary to repair entire foot but merely to correct involved joints.

If desired, the lesser toes may be pinned for 3 weeks to hold them in correct alignment. After 6 weeks, when the dressings are removed, the patient is allowed to shower or bathe even with the pins still in place in the hallux but is still required to wear the wooden shoe. Fusion usually occurs in 3 months but it can take up to 5 months in rare cases. During the postoperative period do not allow the patient to walk without the wooden shoe, even around the house.

The pins are removed in the office using a digital block at the base of the hallux and a Craig pin remover. The patient can then resume ordinary shoe wear (Figs. 6-20 and 6-21).

Hindfoot and ankle deformity. When rheumatoid arthritis primarily affects the talonavicular joint and has not yet involved the subtalar joint, a talonavicular arthrodesis may relieve pain and correct deformity. This can only be done while the foot is still passively correctable, before it reaches the stage of a fixed valgus deformity. Elboar et al. (1976) have described 35 talonavicular arthrodeses in 31 patients with rheumatoid arthritis. In more than 85% of their cases there was complete relief of pain and improvement in ambulatory status. They believe this relatively simple talonavicular fusion arrested the natural course of the disease and eliminated the need for more elaborate corrective surgery.

Rheumatoid arthritis involvement of the hindfoot usually is more clinically apparent as an affliction of the subtalar joint. The ankle joint is frequently spared. If significant involvement of the subtalar joint has failed to respond to nonsurgical measures (e.g., an orthosis, short leg brace, or both) and if the ankle joint is only minimally involved, a subtalar arthrodesis or triple arthrodesis is indicated. The problem that arises at times with a patient with rheumatoid arthritis and severe valgus of the hindfoot is that the forefoot has also become distorted and rigid. When examining this type of patient, once the hindfoot is brought into satisfactory alignment in relation to the tibia from a severe valgus deformity, the forefoot often remains in a markedly supinated position. In this type of patient a triple arthrodesis needs to be carried out to produce a plantigrade foot. If only the hindfoot is corrected, the forefoot will remain in a supinated and nonplantigrade position, making walking extremely difficult. At times it is difficult to achieve a satisfactory position of the severely distorted rheumatoid foot, and the overall correction may not be optimal. If only a severe valgus deformity exists along with a rather supple forefoot, so that the treating physician believes that only a subtalar joint fusion is reqired to produce a plantigrade foot, then usually a bone graft will be necessary to fill in the space created within the subtalar joint when the calcaneus is brought out of its severe valgus position to one of approximately 5° of valgus. If one does not bone graft the subtalar joint in such a case, the initial deformity may recur in the postoperative period. In our hands the results of hindfoot surgery in the patient with rheumatoid arthritis have been most satisfactory, and it is highly recommended when the deformity of the foot no longer permits comfortable plantigrade gait.

The technique for subtalar arthrodesis and for triple arthrodesis is found on pp. 294-296.

Wagner (1982) reports that ankle fusion is rarely required in patients with rheumatoid arthritis, and of all ankle fusions performed only 2% to 10% of the fusions in the literature were performed for patients with collagen diseases. He noted that the indications for ankle fusion were identical to those for total ankle arthroplasty but noted that no ankle arthroplasties had been performed in a 2-year period, during which 100 total hip or knee arthroplasties were performed. Most follow-up studies of total ankle replacement arthroplasties have shown that although it is technically feasible and achieves early good results, these are not maintained over time (Samuelson et al., 1982; Thomas, 1983). The technique for ankle arthrodesis is described on pp. 285-288.

For hindfoot disease that causes an ankylosed foot with equinovarus deformity and limited tarsal motion, Heywood (1983) has found supramalleolar osteotomy to be useful in correcting varus deformity permanently, although equinus did recur if ankle dorsiflexion was not maintained.

For rheumatoid involvement of the subtalar and the ankle joints Adam and Ranawat (1976) have reported on six patients who underwent pantalar arthrodesis. In each case a solid fusion resulted, and the authors expressed satisfaction with their results.

REFERENCES

Gold, R.H., and Bassett, L.W.: Radiologic evaluation of the arthritic foot, Foot Ankle 2:332, 1982.
Guerra, J., and Resnick, D.: Arthritides affecting the foot: radiographic-pathological correlation, Foot Ankle 2:325, 1982.

Degenerative joint disease

Grundy, M., Tosh, P.A., McLeish, R.D., and Smidt, L.: An investigation of the centers of pressure under the foot while walking, J. Bone Joint Surg. 57B:98, 1975.

Hallux rigidus

Bingold, A.C., and Collins, D.H.: Hallux rigidus, J. Bone Joint Surg. 32B:214, 1950.
DuVries, H.L.: Surgery of the foot, ed. 2, St. Louis, 1965, The C.V. Mosby Co.
Harrison, M.H., and Harvey, F.J.: Arthrodesis of the first metatarsophalangeal joint for hallux valgus and rigidus, J. Bone Joint Surg. 45A:471, 1963.
Kessel, L., and Bonney, G.: Hallux rigidus in the adolescent, J. Bone Joint Surg. 40B:668, 1958.
Mau, C.: Das Krankheitsbild des Hallux rigidus, Munch. Med. Wochenschr. 75:1193, 1928.
Moberg, E.: A simple operation for hallux rigidus, Clin. Orthop. 142:55, 1979.
Miller, L.F., and Arendt, J.: Deformity of first metatarsal head due to faulty foot mechanics, J. Bone Joint Surg. 22:349, 1940.
Moynihan, F.J.: Arthrodesis of the metatarsophalangeal joint of the great toe, J. Bone Joint Surg. 49B:544, 1967.

Crystal-induced arthritis

Gottlieb, N.L., and Gray, R.G.: Allopurinol: associated hand and foot deformities in chronic tophaceous gout, JAMA 238:1663, 1977.
Kurtz, J.F.: Surgery of tophaceous gout in the lower extremity, Surg. Clin. North Am. 45:217, 1965.
Martel, W.: The overhanging margin of bone: a roentgenologic manifestation of gout, Radiology 91:755, 1968.
Miskew, D.B.W., and Goldflies, M.L.: Atraumatic avascular necrosis of the talus associated with hyperuricemia, Clin. Orthop. 148:156, 1980.
Stanbury, J.B., Wyngaarden, J.B., and Fredrickson, D.S., editors: The metabolic basis of inherited disease, ed. 3, New York, 1972, McGraw-Hill, Inc.
Woughter, H.W.: Surgery of tophaceous gout: a case report. J. Bone Joint Surg. 41A:116, 1959.

Seronegative spondyloarthropathies

Ball, J.: Enthesopathy of rheumatoid and ankylosing spondylitis, Ann. Rheum. Dis. 30:213, 1971.
Chand, Y., and Johnson, K.A.: Foot and ankle manifestations of Reiter's syndrome, Foot Ankle, 1:167, 1980.
Ford, D.K.: The clinical spectrum of Reiter's syndrome and similar postenteric arthropathies, Clin. Orthop. 143:59, 1979.
Gerster, J.C.: Plantar fasciitis and Achilles tendinitis among 150 cases of seronegative spondarthritis, Rheum. Rehab. 19:218, 1980.
Resnick, D.: Radiology of seronegative spondyloarthopathies, Clin. Orthop. 143:38, 1979.

Rheumatoid arthritis

Adam, W., and Ranawat, C.: Arthrodesis of the hindfoot in rheumatoid arthritis, Orthop. Clin. North Am. 7:827, 1976.
Amuso, S.J., Wissinger, H.A., Margolis, H.M., Eisenbeis, C.H., Jr., and Stolzer, B.L.: Metatarsal head resection in the treatment of rheumatoid arthritis, Clin. Orthop. 74:94, 1971.
Bardwick, P.A., and Swezey, R.L.: Physical modalities for treating the foot affected by connective tissue disease, Foot Ankle 3:41, 1982.
Barton, N.J.: Arthroplasty of the forefoot in rheumatoid arthritis, J. Bone Joint Surg. 55B:126, 1973.
Benson, G.M., and Johnson, E.W., Jr.: Management of the foot in rheumatoid arthritis, Orthop. Clin. North Am. 2:733, 1971.
Clayton, M.L.: Surgery of the forefoot in rheumatoid arthritis, Clin. Orthop. 16:136, 1960.
Clayton, M.L.: Surgery of the lower extremity in rheumatoid arthritis, J. Bone Joint Surg. 45A:1517, 1963.
Cracchiolo, A. III: Results of implant arthroplasty in the arthritic forefoot, Orthop. Trans. 4:150, 1980.
Cracchiolo, A. III: Implant arthroplasty of all metatarsophalangeal (MTP) joints of the rheumatoid forefoot, Orthop. Trans. 5:454, 1981.
DuVries, H.L.: Surgery of the foot, ed. 1, St. Louis, 1959, The C.V. Mosby Co.
Elboar, J.E., Thomas, W., Weinfeld, M., and Potter, T.: Talonavicular arthrodesis for rheumatoid arthritis of the hindfoot, Orthop. Clin. North Am. 7:821, 1976.
Fitzgerald, J.A.W.: A review of long-term results of arthrodesis of the first metatarsophalangeal joint, J. Bone Joint Surg. 51B:488, 1969.
Flint, M., and Sweetnam, R.: Amputation of all toes: a review of forty-seven amputations, J. Bone Joint Surg. 42B:90, 1960.
Fowler, A.W.: A method of forefoot reconstruction, J. Bone Joint Surg. 41B:507, 1959.
Glass, M.K., Karno, M.L., Sella, E.J., and Zeleznik, R.: An office-based orthotic system in treatment of the arthritic foot, Foot Ankle 3:37, 1982.

Gordon, M., and Bullough, P.G.: Synovial and osseous inflammation in failed silicone-rubber prostheses: a report of six cases, J. Bone Joint Surg. **64A**:574, 1982.

Henry, A.P.J., and Waugh, W.: The use of footprints in assessing the results of operations for hallux valgus: a comparison of Keller's operation and arthrodesis, J. Bone Joint Surg. **57B**:478, 1975.

Heywood, A.W.B.: Supramalleolar osteotomy in the management of the rheumatoid hindfoot, Clin. Orthop. **177**:76, 1983.

Hoffman, P.: An operation for severe grades of contracted or clawed toes, Am. J. Orthop. Surg. **9**:441, 1912.

Jacoby, R.K., Vidigal, E., Kirkup, J., and Dixon, A.S.J.: The great toe as a clinical problem in rheumatoid arthritis, Rheum. and Rehab. **15**:143, 1976.

Kates, A., Kessel, L., and Kay, A.: Arthroplasty of the forefoot, J. Bone Joint Surg. **49B**:552, 1967.

Lipscomb, P.R., Benson, G.M., and Sones, D.A.: Resection of proximal phalanges and metatarsal condyles for deformity of the forefoot due to rheumatoid arthritis, Clin. Orthop. **82**:24, 1972.

Mann, R.A., and Coughlin, M.J.: The rheumatoid forefoot: a review of the literature and method of treatment, Orthop. Rev. **8**:105, 1979.

Mann, R.A., and Oates, J.C.: Arthrodesis of the first metatarsophalangeal joint, Foot Ankle, **1**:159, 1980.

Mann, R.A. and Thompson, F.M.: Arthrodesis of the first metatarsophalangeal joint for hallux valgus in rheumatoid arthritis, J. Bone Joint Surg. **66A**:687, 1984.

Marmor, L.: Resection of the forefoot in rheumatoid arthritis, Clin. Orthop. **108**:223, 1975.

Moynihan, F.J.: Arthrodesis of the metatarsophalangeal joint of the great toe, J. Bone Joint Surg. **49B**:544, 1967.

Peterson, L.F.A.: Surgery for rheumatoid arthritis: timing and technique: the lower extremity, J. Bone Joint Surg. **50A**:559, 1968.

Raymakers, R. and Waugh, W.: The treatment of metatarsalgia with hallux valgus, J. Bone Joint Surg. **53B**:684, 1971.

Samuelson, K.M., Freeman, M.A.R., and Tuke, M.A.: Development and evolution of the ICLH ankle replacement, Foot Ankle **3**:32, 1982.

Schwartzmann, J.R.: The surgical management of foot deformities in rheumatoid arthritis, Clin. Orthop. **36**:86, 1964.

Scranton, P.I.: Metatarsalgia: diagnosis and treatment, J. Bone Joint Surg. **62A**:723, 1980.

Shereff, M., and Jahss, M.: Complications of silastic implant arthroplasty in the hallux, Foot Ankle **1**:95, 1980.

Spiegel, T.M., and Spiegel, J.S.: Rheumatoid arthritis in the foot and ankle: diagnosis, pathology, and treatment: the relationship between foot and ankle deformity and disease duration in 50 patients, Foot Ankle **2**:318, 1982.

Thomas, W.: Total ankle arthroplasty: experience at Birmingham Women's Hospital. Presented at American Academy of Orthopaedic Surgeons Course on Ankle and Foot, New Orleans, April 1983.

Vainio, K.: The rheumatoid foot: a clinical study with pathologic and rheumatologic comments, Ann. Chir. Gynaecol. Suppl. **45**:1, 1956.

Vainio, K.: Morton's metatarsalgia in rheumatoid arthritis, Clin. Orthop. **142**:85, 1979.

Wagner, F.W.: Ankle fusion for degenerative arthritis secondary to the collagen diseases, Foot Ankle, **3**:24, 1982.

Watson, M.S.: A long-term follow-up of forefoot arthoplasty, J. Bone Joint Surg. **56B**:527, 1974.

7

Keratotic disorders of the plantar skin

ROGER A. MANN

Disorders of the skin to which the foot is particularly susceptible are either (1) callosities, caused by friction and pressure over a bony prominence, which are by far the most common lesions of the foot; or (2) intrinsic diseases of the skin itself, which are covered in Chapter 18 and in texts on dermatology. Friction or pressure may result in hard or soft corns, calluses, keratoses, suppurating sinuses, or ulcers. Keloids and hypertrophic scars are usually secondary to the healing of lacerations, burns, or surgical wounds. Some intrinsic diseases of the skin are verrucae, dermatoses (especially tinea infections), epidermal cysts, and the rare diastasis of the fifth toe known as ainhum.

The various types of solitary lesions appearing on the plantar surface of the foot are (1) common diffuse calluses; (2) small, deep-seated, circumscribed, nucleated calluses—seed corns; (3) solitary or multiple verrucae plantaris; (4) circumscribed ulcerating areas; (5) epidermal cysts; and (6) intractable plantar keratoses. These conditions are frequently not specifically diagnosed and are often treated as though they were verrucae plantaris.

EXCRESCENCES CAUSED PRIMARILY BY FRICTION, PRESSURE, OR FAULTY WEIGHT-BEARING

Corns and calluses are common disorders of mechanical cause. They are essentially localized keratoses caused by intermittent pressure from without and solid resistance from within; the outside pressure is produced by the shoe, and it is resisted from within by the bones. Therefore one rarely sees corns or calluses over the shafts of long bones. They occur either on the con-

dyles of the epiphyses of long bones or on the prominent projections of short bones.

A hard corn (heloma durum) will form primarily on the exposed surfaces of the toes. The fibular side of the fifth toe is by far the most common site of the hard corn; occasionally it will develop on the fibular side of the fifth metatarsal head. A soft corn (heloma molle) forms over a condyle of the phalanx between the toes. A callus (tyloma) may form over or under any bony prominence of the foot but commonly forms on the plantar surface of the foot and heel. The terms *heloma* and *tyloma* are somewhat misleading because they imply that the lesion is neoplastic, whereas the lesion is actually a reactive proliferation of the epidermal layer secondary to pressure. The findings of an extensive study of corns by Bonavilla (1968) support this hypothesis.

Corns (heloma, clavus)

A corn is an accumulation of horny layers of epidermis over a bony prominence.

Etiology. The bones of the foot have numerous projections, especially over the condyles of the heads and bases of the metatarsals and phalanges. The shoe presses on these prominent condylar processes, and the soft tissues over the prominence bear the brunt of the pressure and friction exerted on the foot by the shoe. Nature attempts to protect the irritated part by accumulating horny epithelium, but the accumulation so elevates the prominence that the pressure of the shoe on the underlying live tissues is increased. At times, if the localized area of pressure is too great, the skin will break down rather than form a callus. This usually oc-

180

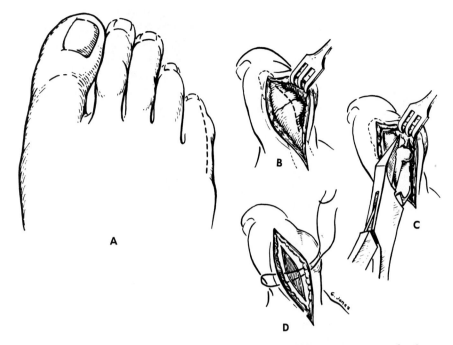

Fig. 7-1. DuVries' technique for condylectomy of corn on fifth toe. **A,** Longitudinal incision over dorsolateral aspect of fifth toe. **B,** Skin and capsule retracted. **C,** Fibular condyles of phalanges amputated. **D,** Skin and capsule closed by mattress sutures.

curs if the pressure is applied rapidly rather than over a long period of time. The patient with an insensitive foot is not aware of the pressure and often will develop ulcerations over bony prominences rather than hyperkeratotic changes. Again, this occurs because of the severity of the pressure against the bony prominence. Occasionally if the callosity becomes too thick, a cleavage plane between the callus and the normal skin will occur, which may become secondarily infected.

General treatment. Palliative measures, such as reducing the horny accumulation, changing the patient's footwear to a broad-toed, soft-soled shoe with a larger toe box, and padding of the area to relieve the pressure, give relief in most cases, especially if the site of the corn is a non-weight-bearing area. In many cases the patients can be taught to care for the callus themselves by using a pumice stone after bathing. Callosities on the weight-bearing surface may require an orthosis (see Chapter 22). An intractable callus over a non-weight-bearing area will respond to excision of the condylar prominence immediately underlying the lesion (Billig, 1956; Rutledge and Green, 1957). Callosities on the weight-bearing areas, which usually occur under a metatarsal head, may be caused by an abnormal alignment of the metatarsal heads or may be the result of the deforming restriction of the forefoot by an improper shoe. This will be discussed in detail later in this chapter under Intractable Plantar Keratoses.

Corn on the lateral side of the fifth toe. Corns on the lateral side of the fifth toe are common, because the fifth toe receives the maximal pressure of the curve of the outer border of the forepart of standard shoes. Ordinarily the head of the proximal phalanx of the fifth toe is the most prominent surface at that point, which is why the corn is nearly always over the fibular condyle of the head of the proximal phalanx.

Operative treatment. The following procedure for condylectomy of the phalanx under a corn on the fibular side of the fifth toe usually involves the head of the proximal phalanx, but may also involve the lateral condyle of the middle phalanx (Fig. 7-1).

1. After digital block, the skin incision is made longitudinally over the dorsal aspect of the small toe just medial to the corn, extending from the middle phalanx to the base of the proximal phalanx. The corn itself should not be excised because the scar would be exposed to further friction. Moreover, callous tissue tends to be somewhat devitalized, and therefore healing might be delayed.

2. The incision is deepened to the bone, through the subcutaneous tissue and extensor tendon.

3. The knife is now inserted into the proximal interphalangeal joint, and the collateral ligaments are cut to expose the condyles of the proximal phalanx.

4. If the condyle is particularly prominent it should be excised, leaving the remainder of the joint intact. If

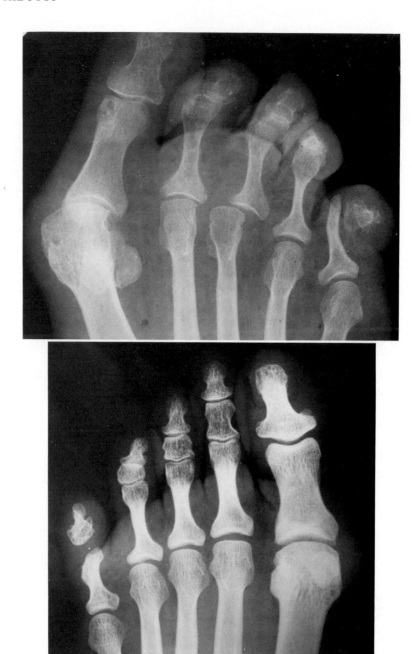

Fig. 7-2. Flail toes produced by phalangectomy.

both the distal portion of the proximal phalanx and the lateral aspect of the middle phalanx are involved, the lateral aspect of the middle phalanx should likewise be excised. If, however, the lesion is caused by a large bulbous condyle at the head of the proximal phalanx, the distal portion of the phalanx should be excised.

5. The edges are smoothed with a rongeur, and the skin is closed in a single layer with mattress sutures.

6. Postoperatively the patient is treated with a compression dressing for several days, after which a small dressing is placed on the toe. Care is taken to keep the toe taped down to the fourth toe for 6 weeks to prevent excessive floppiness of the toe.

Postoperatively these patients may ambulate either in a postoperative wooden shoe or in a sandal that does not place pressure over the operated area.

The expected result following this procedure is most satisfactory. In about 2% of patients there tends to be a persistence of the keratotic lesion despite the relief of the bony prominence beneath it. In these cases frequent trimmings usually result in eventual reduction of the keratotic lesion to a minimally symptomatic state.

vision is extremely important, since the etiology is different and the correct diagnosis is imperative for proper treatment of the lesion.

The *small discrete* plantar keratotic lesion is caused by the sharp condylar process present under the metatarsal head (Fig. 7-12). The condylar projection on the fibular side is always the larger of the two (Fig. 7-7). The condition becomes symptomatic for various reasons. The metatarsal may be slightly plantar flexed, which will cause the condyle to be pushed into the plantar skin and thereby produce a keratotic lesion; the condition may follow a fractured metatarsal that has healed in a slightly plantar-flexed position; or the condition may be caused by a tight shoe. In the last condition the buckling of the toes would force the metatarsal heads into the plantar aspect of the foot, causing the keratotic lesion (Fig. 7-6).

Regardless of the etiology of the small punctate lesion, conservative treatment should be initially undertaken. The conservative treatment consists of trimming of the keratotic lesion and placing the patient in a proper soft-soled shoe with adequate padding to relieve the pressure on the keratotic area.

DuVries' arthroplasty. The surgical treatment of choice for the localized keratotic lesion is a condylectomy as described by DuVries (1953) and modified (1965) to include an arthroplasty. A long term follow-up of the procedure has been reported by Mann and DuVries (1973).

The technique for the arthoplasty is as follows:

1. Make a hockey stick–shaped incision, starting in the web space, and carry it down over the metatarsal head and distal third of the metatarsal shaft (Fig. 7-13, A).

2. Identify the transverse metatarsal ligament on the medial and lateral sides of the involved metatarsal head and cut the transverse metatarsal ligament.

3. Make an incision next to the extensor tendon through the dorsal capsule to expose the metatarsophalangeal joint.

4. Cut the collateral ligament and plantar flex the involved toe with the thumb of the left hand while applying pressure against the metatarsal shaft with the index finger of the same hand (Fig. 7-13, B and C).

5. Remove about 2 mm of the distal portion of the metatarsal head (Fig. 7-13, D).

6. Remove at least half the plantar condyle with an osteotome, angulating the osteotome slightly toward the fibular side (Fig. 7-13, E).

7. Round off the metatarsal head with a rasp or rongeur, irrigate, and reduce the metatarsophalangeal joint. Close the skin in a routine manner (Fig. 7-13, F).

8. Apply a compression dressing for 12 to 18 hours postoperatively, following which the patient can walk in

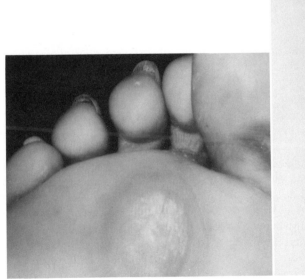
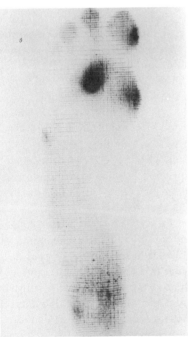

Fig. 7-14. A, Diffuse intractable plantar keratosis beneath second metatarsal head. **B,** Harris mat print of patient with diffuse intractable plantar keratosis beneath second metatarsal head. Heavy smudge indicates increased localized weight bearing.

a supportive dressing and wooden shoe for 3 weeks.

This type of arthroplasty will produce a satisfactory result 85% of the time. In approximately 5% of cases, the lesion will not be helped by the surgical procedure; and in about 10% a transfer lesion will result. Following an arthroplasty of the metatarsophalangeal joint of a lesser toe, roughly 25% of the motion of the metatarsophalangeal joint is lost; but I do not believe the loss is of any real clinical significance.

• • •

The *large diffuse* plantar keratosis, which is an intractable lesion, is caused by an elongated or plantar flexed metatarsal (Fig. 7-14). It usually occurs under the second metatarsal but occasionally develops under the third and rarely under the fourth or fifth metatarsal unless caused by old trauma. The plantar lesion is diffuse, generally measuring 1 to 1.5 cm across, and does not have a small keratotic core as is found in the lesion caused by prominence of the plantar metatarsal condyle.

Metatarsal osteotomy. If the diffuse lesion persists after adequate conservative treatment, surgical intervention is indicated. The procedure of choice is a metatarsal osteotomy based on the concept of Giannestras (1954).

The technique for the osteotomy is as follows.

1. Make dorsal incision over the affected metatarsal, taking care to avoid the superficial nerves as the metatarsal is exposed. Expose the metatarsal shaft subperiosteally.

2. Make two small nicks on the metatarsal shaft a measured distance from one another so that a precise amount of shortening can be carried out.

3. Make long oblique osteotomy in the anteroposterior plane through the metatarsal shaft.

4. The amount of shortening of the metatarsal will have been predetermined from the preoperative radiograph. It is usually 4 to 8 mm.

5. Shorten the metatarsal a specific distance using the marks made on it previously. Place a drill hole through the midportion of the osteotomy site, and fix the site with a piece of 22-gauge wire.

6. Tighten the wire sufficiently that the osteotomy site is well fixed and the metatarsal is in anatomic alignment and neither plantar flexed nor dorsiflexed distally.

7. Close the wound in a routine manner, and apply a compression dressing for 12 to 18 hours. A snug dressing is then applied, and the patient ambulates in a wooden shoe until the osteotomy site is healed. Healing time is approximately 6 weeks (Fig. 7-15).

The results of this procedure for the diffuse keratotic lesion have been most satisfactory. The satisfactory results approach 90% to 95%. A transfer lesion has been observed in about 5% of cases, but this rarely requires further surgical treatment. At times there is delayed healing, but only one case of nonunion has been observed, and this was not symptomatic.

If a symptomatic transfer lesion does occur following this procedure, I believe it should be treated by a basilar closing wedge metatarsal osteotomy to relieve the pressure underneath the transfer lesion. In these cases the dorsal wedge should only be about 2 mm in width.

• • •

There are other procedures described for treatment of intractable plantar keratoses that involve a proximal or distal osteotomy of the metatarsal shaft. Most of these are dorsal wedge osteotomies that allow the metatarsal to rise. The osteotomy at the base of the metatarsal, I believe, has a place in the treatment of intractable plantar keratoses, although I personally do not use the procedure frequently. The osteotomy at the neck of the metatarsal to allow the metatarsal head to angulate dorsally causes, in my opinion, too much scarring and loss of motion about the metatarsophalangeal joint to be used in lieu of the previously mentioned, more successful procedure.

I have seen a number of cases in which a high-speed burr has been used to produce a distal metatarsal osteotomy. Unfortunately, this procedure seems to be associated with a rather high incidence of nonunion, a great deal of scarring, and loss of motion about the metatarsophalangeal joint. Whether this is caused by bone particles that are left behind or the possible bone necrosis brought about by the heat of the burr is difficult to state. Generally speaking, I believe that this is an ill-advised procedure (Fig. 7-16).

I believe that in most cases only one metatarsal should be shortened at a single procedure, although on rare occasions I have shortened two metatarsals on the same foot simultaneously. More than two metatarsals should never be shortened at a single procedure on the same foot.

There are other procedures reported in the literature for treatment of intractable plantar keratoses. I previously have mentioned the procedures I believe to be most successful. Excision of a metatarsal head for the treatment of an intractable plantar keratosis is mentioned just to condemn it. This procedure will only lead to more difficulty, secondary transfer lesions, and shortening of the involved toe (Fig. 7-17).

At times the intractable keratosis has been misdiagnosed as a verruca plantaris, and the keratotic lesion has been treated by various modalities that produce severe dense scarring on the plantar aspect of the foot. When there is a dense scar on the plantar aspect of the foot under a metatarsal head, none of the aforemen-

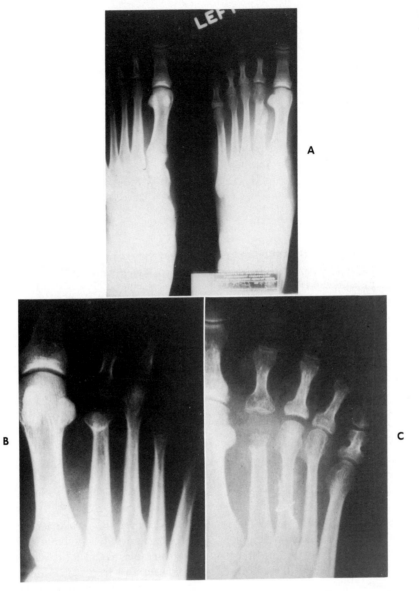

Fig. 7-15. Results following metatarsal shortening. **A,** Preoperative and postoperative radiographs demonstrating shortening of second metatarsal to improve weight bearing pattern of first three metatarsals. **B,** Preoperative radiograph demonstrating long third metatarsal after second metatarsal had been removed for treatment of intractable plantar keratosis. **C,** Postoperative appearance after shortening of third metatarsal to improve weight-bearing pattern of metatarsal heads.

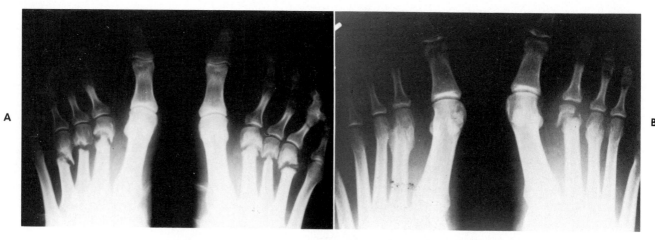

Fig. 7-16. A, Nonunion of metatarsal necks secondary to use of high-speed burr to produce osteotomy. **B,** Left hand radiograph demonstrates abundance of bone formation following osteotomy of second metatarsal neck that was produced by high-speed burr. Right hand radiograph demonstrates nonunion of second metatarsal neck as the result of use of high-speed burr.

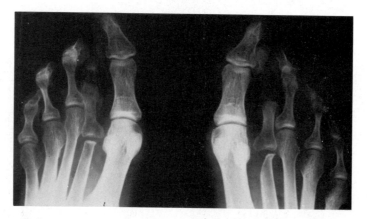

Fig. 7-17. Feet of a 42-year-old man who complained of disability from previous surgical procedures.

tioned procedures is successful in relieving the keratotic lesion. In such cases consideration should be given to excising the lesion at the same time the metatarsal procedure is done. The skin margins are then sutured so they are not under tension. These patients treated with excision of the plantar skin should be kept non-weight-bearing for a total of 6 weeks to allow the plantar skin to heal with minimal scar formation.

Scars on plantar aspect of foot

Although plantar incisions for excision of a neuroma or a procedure on the metatarsal head have been advocated in the literature, I believe they should be avoided if possible. Although most plantar incisions will heal in a benign fashion, if the patient forms a hypertrophic scar it may lead to an unsolvable problem. Most

foot surgery can be carried out through a dorsal approach, and I strongly advise this if possible. The fibular sesamoid can also be removed through a dorsal incision in the first web space, which I believe to be preferable to the plantar approach.

If a plantar incision is used, it is imperative that the incision be placed between the metatarsal heads to avoid a scar directly beneath a metatarsal.

Fig. 7-18 demonstrates a hypertrophic scar that resulted from a plantar approach to remove a fibular sesamoid.

Tailor's bunion (bunionette)

The term *tailor's bunion* is applied to any enlargement of the fibular side of the fifth metatarsophalangeal joint. In time past, tailors would sit with their legs

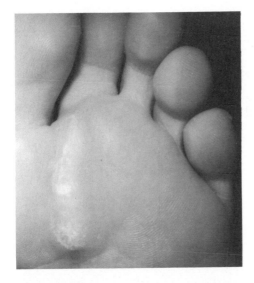

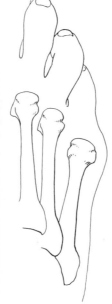

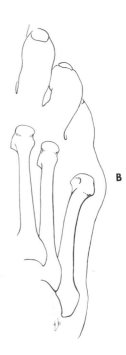

Fig. 7-18. Hypertrophic scar following plantar incision.

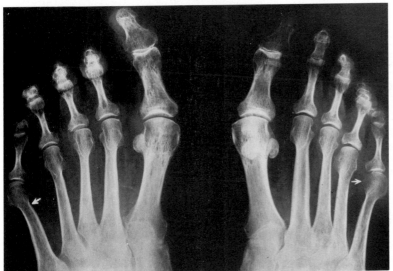

Fig. 7-19. Tailor's bunion. **A,** Two types of bone variation in same person: Left, Lateral deviation at neck of fifth metatarsal. Right, wide fifth metatarsal head. **B,** Schematic drawing: left, wide head; right, lateral deviation of head.

crossed as they sewed clothes by hand, thereby placing abnormal pressure on the fifth metatarsal head, which often caused painful symptoms.

The enlargement may be the result of one or a combination of three conditions: (1) hypertrophy of the soft tissue overlying the fifth metatarsophalangeal joint, (2) a congenitally wide dumbbell-shaped fifth metatarsal head or (3) lateral deviation of the fifth metatarsal shaft and head (Fig. 7-19).

Etiology. As a result of the prominence of the metatarsal head, regardless of the etiology, increased pressure results over the fifth metatarsophalangeal joint because of the wearing of tight shoes. In response to the

pressure over a period of time, a thickened bursa results, which becomes progressively more symptomatic. Once this bursa becomes too large, even placing the foot in a broad-toed shoe will not adequately correct the problem.

Occasionally, besides lateral deviation of the metatarsal head, some plantar deviation is present. In these cases, along with a developing bursa over the fibular side of the joint, there is an intractable plantar keratosis beneath the metatarsal head.

Symptoms. The overlying bursa becomes painful, swollen, and tender. The symptoms are usually aggravated by wearing any shoe that places pressure on the

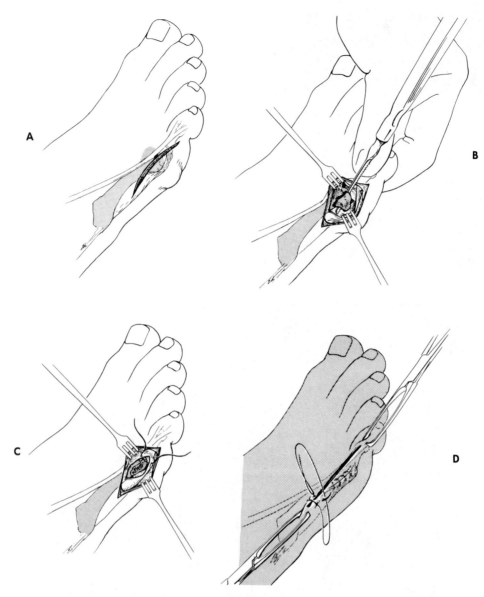

Fig. 7-20. DuVries' technique of correction of tailor's bunion (congenitally wide type). **A,** Semielliptical incision over dorsum of fifth metatarsophalangeal joint. **B,** Skin, capsule, and tendon of abductor digiti minimi retracted. Fibular condyle of fifth metatarsal head is excised with nasal saw or osteotome. **C,** Capsule and tendon of abductor digiti minimi sutured. **D,** Skin closed.

area and alleviated by going barefoot or cutting out this area of the shoe.

In patients with plantar flexion of the metatarsal shaft and head, an intractable plantar keratosis develops accompanied by subsequent pain and disability.

Treatment. In mild and moderate cases treatment with a broad-toed shoe and sometimes padding will help alleviate the symptoms. In protracted cases, however, operative correction is indicated. In the patient who has a congenitally wide fifth metatarsal head, the recommended surgical procedure is as follows.

1. Make a longitudinal incision over the dorsolateral aspect of the fifth metatarsophalangeal joint, extending it proximally from the middle of the proximal phalanx to the juncture of the middle and distal thirds of the fifth metatarsal. The dorsal cutaneous nerve to the fifth toe should then be identified (Fig. 7-20, *A*).

2. Retract the skin, subcutaneous tissue, and dorsal cutaneous nerve to expose the joint capsule.

3. Incise the joint capsule longitudinally just dorsal to the insertion of the abductor digiti minimi tendon.

4. Denude the fibular border of its capsule. At this

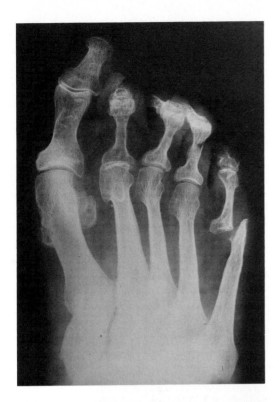

Fig. 7-21. Result of failure to suture capsule and tendon of abductor digiti minimi and excessive removal of head of fifth metatarsal.

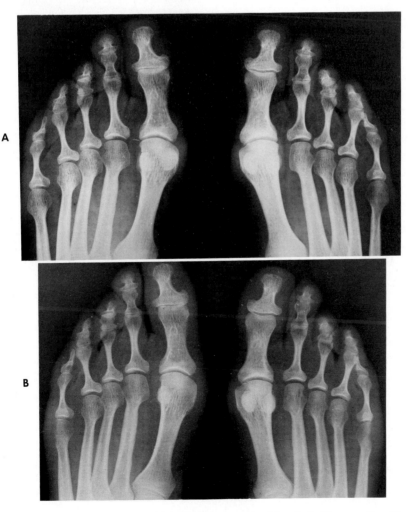

Fig. 7-22. Tailor's bunion caused by wide fifth metatarsal head. **A,** Preoperative; **B,** postoperative.

point the dorsal capsular flap may be retracted dorsally and the abductor digiti minimi retracted plantarward to expose the fibular condyle of the metatarsal head.

5. Excise the fibular condylar process longitudinally by means of an osteotome. The sharp edges should be rounded off with a rasp or rongeur (Fig. 7-20, *B*). Do not excise the adventitious bursa unless excessively thickened. If the bursa is greatly enlarged and needs to be excised, be sure to identify the dorsal cutaneous nerve to the small toe to prevent cutting it when the bursa is removed.

6. Repair the capsule by suturing the dorsal capsule to the abductor digiti minimi (Fig. 7-20, *C* and *D*). Failure to do this may result in dislocation of the fifth metatarsophalangeal joint (Fig. 7–21). Fig. 7-22 shows the end result of the operation.

When there is a mild intractable plantar keratosis, excision of the plantar condyle is indicated at the time the fibular condyle is removed.

If, however, there is a large diffuse intractable plantar keratosis beneath the fifth metatarsal head, and radiographs demonstrate lateral and plantar deviation of the fifth metatarsal shaft, the treatment of choice is an osteotomy of the fifth metatarsal. This is carried out on an oblique plane so as to allow the metatarsal head to move both dorsally and medially. This type of osteotomy is carried out as follows.

1. Make the skin incision over the lateral aspect of the fifth metatarsal shaft for a distance of approximately 5 cm. Deepen it through subcutaneous tissue and fat, taking great care not to interrupt twigs of the sural nerve. The nerve should be located just dorsal to the skin incision.

2. Expose the fifth metatarsal subperiosteally by stripping off the abductor digiti minimi muscle.

3. With a sagittal saw, make an oblique osteotomy that passes from plantar-lateral and proceeds in a dorsomedial direction.

4. Displace the osteotomy site dorsally and medially. Fix the site with either a small fragment screw or a wire loop.

5. The foot is immobilized in a compression dressing, and the patient ambulated in a wooden shoe. Healing usually occurs in 8 weeks.

This procedure has yielded satisfactory results relieving the intractable plantar keratoses as well as of the lateral prominence caused by the condyle. Union of the osteotomy site has occurred in all but one case. With the use of the small fragment screw, good bony fixation can be obtained (Fig. 7-22).

REFERENCES

Billig, H. E., Jr.: Condylectomy for metatarsalgia: indications and results, J. Int. Coll. Surgeons **25**:220, 1956.

Bonavilla, E. J.: Histopathology of the heloma durum: some significant features and their implications, J. Am. Podiatry Assoc. **58**:423, 1968.

DuVries, H. L.: New approach to the treatment of intractable verruca plantaris (plantar wart), J.A.M.A. **152**:1202, 1953.

DuVries, H. L.: Surgery of the foot, ed. 2, St. Louis, 1965, The C.V. Mosby Co.

Giannestras, N. J.: Shortening of the metatarsal shaft for the correction of plantar keratosis, Clin. Orthop. **4**:225, 1954.

Mann, R. A., and DuVries, H. L.: Intractable plantar keratosis, Orthop. Clin. North Am. **41**:67, 1973.

Rutledge, B. A., and Green, A. L.: Surgical treatment of plantar corns, U.S. Armed Services Med. J. **8**:219, 1957.

8

Diseases of the nerves of the foot

ROGER A. MANN

Diagnosis and treatment of diseases of the peripheral nerves about the foot at times may be quite straightforward but at other times present a most complex clinical problem. In this section the interdigital plantar neuroma, tarsal tunnel syndrome, reflex sympathetic dystrophy, and peripheral nerve entrapments about the foot will be discussed.

INTERDIGITAL PLANTAR NEUROMA

The history of the interdigital neuroma has been a long and colorful one. This description provided by Kelikian (1965) presents a detailed chronology of the condition. The history will only be briefly summarized at this time. The condition was first described by the Queen's Surgeon-chiropodist, Louis Durlacher (1845). He described a "form of neuralgic affection" involving "the plantar nerve between the third and fourth metatarsal bones." Morton (1876) related the problem to the fourth metatarsophalangeal joint and suspected a neuroma or some type of hypertrophy of the digital branches of the lateral plantar nerve. Mason (1877) related a case with pain about the second metatarsophalangeal joint and suspected involvement of a digital branch of the medial plantar nerve. It was Hoadley (1893) who actually explored the digital nerves under the painful area, "found a small neuroma," and excised it, claiming he obtained a "prompt and perfect cure." Tubby (1912) reported observing on two occasions that the plantar digital nerves were congested and thickened. Betts (1940) stated, "Morton's metatarsalgia is a neuritis of the fourth digital nerve," and McElvenny (1943) stated that it was caused by a tumor involving the lateralmost branch of the medial plantar nerve.

Pathology

There are differing opinions regarding the underlying pathologic process observed in the neuroma specimens in patients diagnosed as having an interdigital neuroma. This is probably caused by the fact that the pathologic material that has been acquired represents different stages in the development of the condition. According to Lassman (1979), normal endoneural structures are frequently found in the proximal end of the resected nerve, with most of the pathologic changes noted in the region of the bifurcation of the digital nerve. From a quantitative standpoint, he noted a decrease in the amount of the thick myelinated fibers and a decrease in the diameter in individual nerve fibers resulting from attenuation of their myelin sheaths. Alterations of the interdigital arteries could not be correlated with the alterations found in the nerves themselves. Although hyalinization of vessel walls has been observed in patients with interdigital neuroma, it has also been observed in control material in patients without interdigital neuroma. In a study of 133 cases with a clinical diagnosis of Morton's syndrome, light and electron microscopic investigations revealed that in the early stages of the disease the histologic findings are dominated by the following alterations of the nerves, independent of alterations of their interdigital vessels:

1. Sclerosis and edema of the endoneurium
2. Thickening and hyalinization of the walls of the endoneural vessels, caused by multiple layers of basement membranes
3. Thickening of the perineurium
4. Deposition of an amorphous eosinophilic material built up by filaments of tubular structures
5. Demyelinization and degeneration of the nerve fi-

Fig. 8-1. Plantar nerves of right foot.

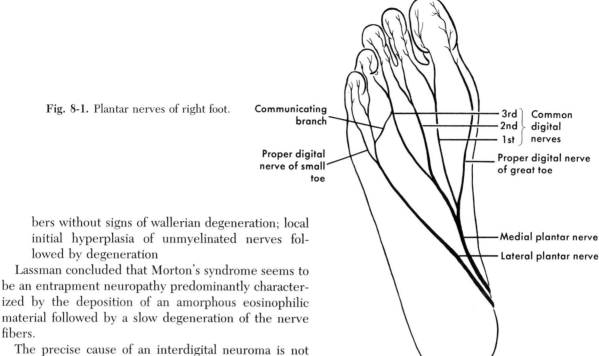

Communicating branch

Proper digital nerve of small toe

3rd 2nd 1st } Common digital nerves

Proper digital nerve of great toe

Medial plantar nerve

Lateral plantar nerve

bers without signs of wallerian degeneration; local initial hyperplasia of unmyelinated nerves followed by degeneration

Lassman concluded that Morton's syndrome seems to be an entrapment neuropathy predominantly characterized by the deposition of an amorphous eosinophilic material followed by a slow degeneration of the nerve fibers.

The precise cause of an interdigital neuroma is not known. There are many possible causes that either singly or together may indeed be the origin. These may be divided into anatomic factors, traumatic causes, and extrinsic pressure.

From an anatomic standpoint the medial plantar nerve has four digital branches. The most medial branch is the proper digital nerve to the medial aspect of the great toe. The next three branches are named the first, second, and third common digital nerves and are distributed to both the medial and lateral aspects of the first, second, and third interspaces, respectively. The lateral plantar nerve divides into a superficial branch (which splits into a proper digital nerve to the lateral side of the small toe) and a common digital nerve to the fourth interspace. The common digital nerve frequently leads to a communicating branch that passes to the third digital branch of the medial plantar nerve in the third interspace. It has been speculated that since the common digital nerve to the third interspace consists of branches from the medial and lateral plantar nerves, the common digital nerve has increased thickness and therefore is more subject to trauma and possible neuroma formation (Fig. 8-1). The mobility of the third and fourth metatarsals has also been implicated in that the three medial metatarsals are rather fixed at their metatarsocuneiform joints and the fourth and fifth metatarsals are fixed to the cuboid. This anatomic fact results in an increased mobility in the third web space compared with other web spaces, and possibly as a result of the upward and downward movement across the nerve in this area it may traumatize the nerve. The in-

timate association of the nerve with the flexor digitorum brevis has also been implicated (Wagner, 1980) in that contraction of the flexor digitorum brevis may put pressure on the lateral plantar nerve (pulling it proximally) and as the toes are dorsiflexed a stretching of the nerve will occur as it passes beneath the transmetatarsal ligament. These anatomic speculations are interesting, but in our series of interdigital neuromas (Mann and Reynolds, 1983) we have found just about as many neuromas in the second interspace as in the third, which would possibly negate some of the etiologic reasons stated previously.

Trauma to the plantar aspect of the foot, both in chronic form brought on by wearing tight, high-heeled shoes with thin soles and in the acute form as by falling from a height or stepping onto a sharp object, may also produce neuritic symptoms.

Extrinsic pressure on the nerve, either resulting from a benign tumor or from the metatarsal heads, has also been implicated. Since the nerve is below the transverse metatarsal ligament, any thickening arising from the metatarsophalangeal joint, such as a synovial cyst or a ganglion, may cause impingement against the common digital nerve that could result in neuritic symptoms (Fig. 8-2). I have also seen a lipoma in the web space that applied pressure to the common digital

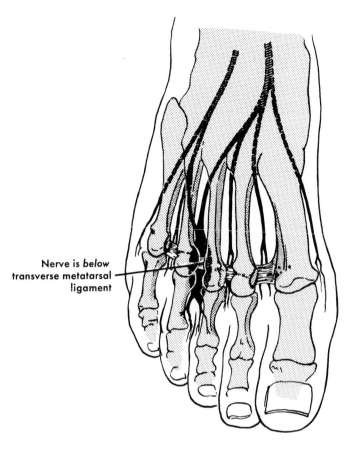

Nerve is *below* transverse metatarsal ligament

Fig. 8-2. Schematic view of third branch of medial plantar nerve. Note that it courses plantarward, under transverse metatarsal ligament.

nerve and thereby caused neuritic symptoms. When the metatarsal heads are squeezed together by the medial or lateral subluxation of one of the metatarsophalangeal joints to force the two metatarsal heads together, neuritic symptoms probably secondary to impingement from the metatarsal heads may result (Fig. 8-3). The possibility that an interdigital neuroma is caused by a nerve entrapment was speculated by Gauthier (1979). It was his belief that during terminal stance phase when the toes are in sharp dorsiflexion, the nerve is drawn against the transverse metatarsal ligament, thereby giving rise to the neuritic complaints.

Symptom complex

In a critical analysis of 56 of our patients with 76 neuromas that were excised, there were 53 women and 3 men (Mann and Reynolds, 1983). This represents a greater female-to-male ratio than observed by Bradley et al. (1976), who reported a ratio of about 4:1. The average age of the patient in our series was 55 years, with a range of 29 to 81 years. The condition is generally unilateral, but bilateral neuromas are seen approximately 15% of the time. Two neuromas occurring simultaneously in the same foot is very rare in my experience. Although most of the literature states that the neuroma usually involves the third interspace, in

our study there was an equal number of neuromas in the second and third interspaces. Neuromas of the first and fourth interspaces are exceedingly rare.

The most common symptoms of an interdigital neuroma is pain localized to the plantar aspect of the foot between the metatarsal heads. The pain is aggravated by activities and relieved by resting the foot, particularly rubbing it with the shoe off. At times a patient notes no symptoms when walking barefoot on a soft surface but develops pain promptly when putting on a tight-fitting shoe, particularly with a high heel. The pain tends to be fairly well localized to the plantar aspect of the foot but occasionally radiates toward the tip of the toe of the involved interspace. Occasionally the pain is noted to radiate toward the dorsum of the foot or more proximally into the plantar aspect of the foot.

The pain is usually characterized as burning in nature but without a sharp component to it. Occasionally the patient notes that there is something moving around in the plantar aspect of the foot that periodically gets "caught" and causes an acute, sharp pain. This is probably a result of the nerve being trapped beneath the metatarsal head, following which the patient steps on it.

The following is a list of the preoperative symptoms

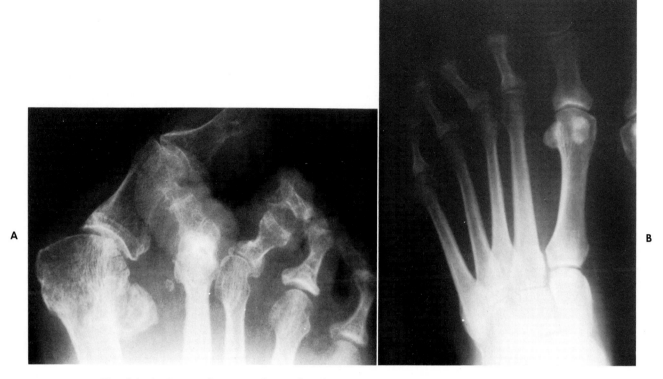

Fig. 8-3. A, Severe deviation of second and third toes close down second intermetatarsal space, putting pressure on underlying digital nerve. **B,** Similar problem but less severe deformity.

by percent in patients with interdigital neuroma in our series:

Plantar pain increased by walking	91%
Relief of pain by resting	89%
Plantar pain	77%
Relief of pain by removing shoe	70%
Pain radiating into toes	62%
Burning pain	54%
Aching or sharp pain	40%
Numbness of toes or foot	40%
Pain radiating up foot or leg	34%
Cramping sensation	34%

Diagnosis

Palpation of the plantar aspect of the involved interspace often causes a sharp, stabbing pain similar to that occurring when the patient bears weight on the foot. The involved nerve can be palpated in about one-third of the patients. When palpated, a mass may be felt beneath the examiner's fingers and can actually be rolled back and forth. If the examiner then sequeezes the mass against the metatarsal head, the patient experiences a moderate amount of discomfort and usually notes that the pain beneath the examiner's fingers radiates out toward the toes of the involved interspace. Care must always be taken to carefully examine the metatarsophalangeal joint on each side of the involved interspace to be sure that some type of pathology of the joint is not mimicking that of interdigital neuroma.

The diagnosis of a neuroma is therefore based on the history and physical examination, since neither radiographs nor laboratory data are helpful.

The preoperative physical findings noted in analysis of our patients was as follows:

Plantar tenderness	95%
Radiation of pain into toes	46%
Palpable mass	12%
Numbness	3%
Widening of the interspace	3%

In considering the differential diagnosis of an interdigital neuroma, the possibility of a tarsal tunnel syndrome, some problem involving the metatarsophalangeal joint (i.e., synovitis of the joint, degeneration of the plantar pad, or subluxation or dislocation of the joint), or lumbar disc disease should always be considered.

Treatment

Conservative management of the patient with the interdigital neuroma begins with obtaining a broad shoe with a soft sole and low heel. This allows the foot to be spread out, relieving some of the pressure between the metatarsal heads and, it is hoped taking some of the stress off the interdigital nerves. A soft metatarsal support just proximal to the metatarsal head region also helps to spread out the metatarsal heads, relieving pressure on the nerve. At times the use of a metatarsal bar or a molded leather arch support may be helpful.

Local injection of the interspace with local anesthetic may be useful as a diagnostic tool, particularly if there is tenderness in two interspaces of the same foot. The injection of one interspace may give the examiner a clue as to which nerve is the most symptomatic. The use of steroids may occasionally be helpful, but care must be taken to avoid injecting the joint capsule of the adjacent metatarsophalangeal joints, which might result in deterioration of the capsule and a subsequent divergent toe.

Most of the patients will respond fairly well to conservative management in that they obtain some relief of their clinical symptoms, but the physical findings of localized plantar pain rarely change. The majority of the patients usually remain sufficiently symptomatic so that in time approximately 70% to 80% elect to have excision of the neuroma.

Generally speaking, I believe it important to reevaluate the patient with an interdigital neuroma on several occasions to be sure that the area of pain can be well localized to a single interspace.

If the patient does not respond to conservative management and desires excision of the nerve, a satisfactory result can usually be obtained.

In Europe excision of the neuroma is often carried out through a plantar approach, as described by Betts (1940) and Nissen (1948). In the United States the approach is usually through the dorsum of the foot, as described by McElvenny (1943) and McKeever (1952). The dorsal approach has as its main advantage the prevention of scar formation on the plantar surface of the foot. Although, generally speaking, a plantar approach is safe, if placed in such a way that it does not pass directly under the metatarsal head, occasionally a painful scar will result, or hypertrophic skin will develop about the scar, making it painful. The treatment of the painful plantar scar is extremely difficult. The dorsal approach does not present any obstacle to observing the nerve in the intermetatarsal space.

Surgical technique

1. Under tourniquet control, make an incision on the dorsal aspect of the foot starting in the web space between the involved toes. Carry the incision proximally about 1 inch to the level of the metatarsal head. It is important to keep the incision directly in the web space because deviation to either side may result in cutting one of the fine dorsal digital nerves, which could cause a painful neuroma within the scar.

2. Carry the incision down directly between the metatarsal heads. Place a Weitlander between the metatarsal heads to spread them apart. This will put the transverse metatarsal ligament under tension.

3. Using a neurologic freer, dissect out the common digital nerve and identify the transverse metatarsal ligament. Carefully transect the transverse metatarsal ligament, being careful not to cut the underlying structures. Once this has been accomplished, the nerve can be readily freed from the surrounding vessels and fat.

4. The common digital nerve is now lying free in the base of the wound. Grasp it with the forceps, pull distally, and cut it as proximally as possible. It should be cut just proximal to the level of the metatarsal head. This having been accomplished, the nerve is then easily dissected distally and cut just past the bifurcation into its terminal branches. Dorsiflex the ankle to pull the stump more proximally into the foot.

5. Suture only the skin and apply a compression bandage for 18 to 24 hours. After this time the compression bandage is released and another firm dressing is applied. Ambulation is then begun in a wooden shoe.

6. The foot is kept wrapped with a firm dressing for 3 weeks following the procedure.

Results. Few papers have appeared in the literature discussing the clinical results of excision of a neuroma. In an analysis of our patients following excision of an interdigital neuroma, 71% were essentially asymptomatic, 9% were significantly improved, 6% were marginally improved, and 14% considered the operation a failure. The patients in the latter two groups were carefully reexamined, and no other local pathology involving the metatarsophalangeal joints or surrounding tissue could be identified that would account for their lack of a better clinical response. Until this careful study was carried out, I believed that the results of an excision of a neuroma were better. With these results in mind, however, it is important to be sure the patient is aware of the fact that excision of a neuroma may not always result in complete relief.

The further evaluation of the patients following the excision of the neuroma demonstrated the following postoperative findings:

Local plantar pain	65%
Numbness in the interspace	68%
An area of plantar numbness adjacent to the interspace	51%

The comparison of patients who had neuromas excised from the second interspace with those who had them excised from the third interspace did not show any difference in clinical response.

RECURRENT NEUROMA

Months to years following excision of an interdigital neuroma a certain group of patients will develop recurrent symptoms. These patients at times will feel the recurrent symptoms are even more severe than before their surgery. The physical findings in this group of patients usually demonstrate a well-localized area of tenderness, usually beneath a metatarsal head or just adjacent to it, which when percussed demonstrates a positive Tinel sign, and the patient notes pain radiating out toward the tip of the toes of the involved interspace.

Patients with a recurrent neuroma should be treated in a manner similar to the patient with a virgin neuroma, namely, by placing them into a broad-toed, soft-soled shoe with a soft metatarsal support. If these conservative measures fail and symptoms persist, reexploration of the interspace may be indicated. At times I have found the use of a transcutaneous nerve stimulator useful in helping to "break up" the patient's pain pattern.

When considering reexploring an interspace, the foot should be carefully examined to attempt to accurately localize the neuroma, which (as I mentioned previously) is often adjacent to a metatarsal head. By carefully localizing the area of the neuroma preoperatively, finding the neuroma during surgery—and at times it can be embedded in rather dense scar tissue—can be made much easier. The reexploration of the interspace is carried out as in the original exploration. Once again the transverse metatarsal ligament is cut (it always reforms), and the underlying tissue is carefully and gently explored using a neurologic freer. It is important to start as far proximally as possible in as normal appearing tissue as possible to facilitate exposure of the common digital nerve. Once the nerve is identified, the neuroma is freed from its adhesions and transected at a more proximal level. Postoperatively the patient wears a wooden shoe for a period of 3 weeks.

Analysis of 11 recurrent neuromas in 7 patients demonstrated that 81% of the patients were essentially asymptomatic, 9% considered their improvement marginal, and 9% considered the procedure a failure.

REFLEX SYMPATHETIC DYSTROPHY (CAUSALGIA)

Reflex sympathetic dystrophy is a clinical entity in which the patient after major or minor trauma or surgery develops a symptom complex consisting of burning pain, swelling, and motor dysfunction that can be extremely disabling. The condition has been called Sudek atrophy and causalgia, but reflex sympathetic dystrophy is the preferred term.

Reflex sympathetic dystrophy has been divided into several categories by Lankford and Thompson (1977). In their clinical classification, trauma to a purely sensory nerve is "minor causalgia"; when caused by a non-nerve injury, "minor traumatic dystrophy"; when caused by more severe trauma, "major traumatic dystrophy"; and when caused by trauma to a major mixed nerve, "major causalgia."

Insofar as the foot is concerned, a minor causalgia or minor traumatic dystrophy is usually seen after foot surgery, lacerations of the foot, minor trauma such as a twisting injury to the foot and ankle, or fracture of a metatarsal bone. Major traumatic dystrophy is seen after a severe injury or crush injury to the lower extremity; major causalgia can be seen after trauma to the sciatic nerve or its terminal trunks—common peroneal and posterior tibial nerves.

Etiology

The cause of reflex sympathetic dystrophy is poorly understood, although the condition is generally thought to be a result of an abnormal autonomic response to trauma.

In their review Lankford and Thompson (1977) pointed out that three factors must be present at the same time for reflex sympathetic dystrophy to occur: a painful lesion resulting from trauma (either major or minor), a diathesis or susceptibility of the patient, and an abnormal autonomic reflex.

Symptoms

Symptoms vary somewhat depending on the type of reflex sympathetic dystrophy the patient may manifest.

Minor causalgia, affecting a purely sensory nerve, will involve only the foot. The patient describes the pain as burning and experiences marked dysethesias. The pain usually follows the course of a sensory nerve.

Minor traumatic dystrophy is the most common type seen and usually involves the toes, often following a crush injury to the toes. The patient manifests fairly well localized pain, mild to moderate generalized edema of the affected foot and ankle, some motor dysfunction, and vasomotor changes indicated by cool moist skin.

Major traumatic dystrophy follows a more extensive injury to the foot and ankle. The symptoms are similar to those seen in minor traumatic dystrophy although the changes may be more extensive and marked demineralization of the bone is noted radiographically.

Major causalgia, which follows an injury to a major mixed nerve—namely, the sciatic, posterior tibial, or common peroneal—is not common, but the symptoms may be extremely severe and disabling. The patient manifests an intense burning pain generally following the sensory distribution of the nerve but that cannot be well localized. The clinical findings are again the marked sensitivity of the extremity to any type of touch, increased vasomotor response in the form of cool moist skin, and marked motor dysfunction.

Treatment

The most critical factor in the treatment of reflex sympathetic dystrophy is early recognition of the problem. This is particularly important in the minor causalgic and minor traumatic forms of the condition. In these two entities the problem may be thwarted early in its clinical course before more severe changes occur.

Initial treatment should be directed toward vigorous physical therapy in the form of range-of-motion exercises and using the extremity, whirlpool exercises, and control of the edema by an elastic stocking. Approximately 90% of these patients respond favorably when such treatment is started early.

Once the condition has become more severe, it is much more difficult to treat. In the more chronic cases there may be permanent changes in the soft tissues and joints. In the later stages treatment consists of lumbar sympathetic blocks (preferably by an anesthesiologist), which will interrupt the abnormal sympathetic reflex. These can be repeated on three or four occasions to provide complete relief. If after successful sympathetic block the symptoms continue to recur, a sympathectomy may be considered.

In the treatment of major traumatic dystrophy or major causalgia, it may be necessary to do a neurolysis of the involved nerve and the other treatment modalities mentioned.

TARSAL TUNNEL SYNDROME

The tarsal tunnel syndrome is caused by pressure exerted on the posterior tibial nerve or one of its terminal branches as it passes beneath the flexor retinaculum at the level of the ankle or more distally as it divides into its terminal branches—medial plantar nerve, lateral plantar nerve, and medial calcaneal branch (Fig. 8-4). The condition is analogous to the carpal tunnel syndrome in the wrist and was first described by Keck (1962) and later in the same year by Lam.

The diagnosis of a tarsal tunnel syndrome, I believe, should be based on three criteria: the nature of the pain as described by the patient, a positive Tinel sign over the tarsal tunnel region, and a positive electrodiagnostic study indicating some abnormality in the function of the posterior tibial nerve or its terminal branches.

Etiology

In approximately 50% of the patients with tarsal tunnel syndrome, a specific cause can be identified. This might include a previous severe ankle sprain, crush injury, fracture of the distal tibia, fracture or dislocation of the ankle, or fracture of the calcaneus.

There are certain local causes that may result in a tarsal tunnel syndrome, and these include the following:

1. A ganglion of one of the tendon sheaths passing adjacent to the tarsal canal or one of the terminal branches of the posterior tibial nerve
2. A lipoma within the tarsal canal exerting pressure against the posterior tibial nerve
3. An exostosis or a fracture fragment from the distal tibia or tarsal bones

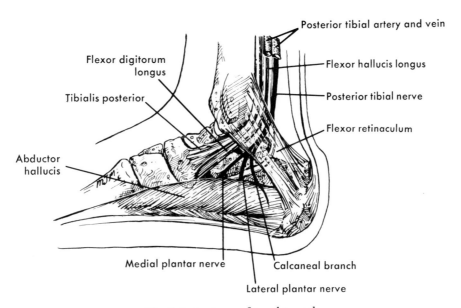

Fig. 8-4. Anatomy of tarsal tunnel.

4. A tarsal coalition involving a medial talocalcaneal bar that protrudes into the inferior aspect of the tarsal canal
5. An enlarged venous plexus surrounding the posterior tibial nerve within the tarsal canal
6. Severe pronation of the hindfoot that may produce a stretching of the posterior tibial nerve

Symptoms

Whereas the patient with an interdigital neuroma is usually able to localize the area of maximum tenderness, the patient with the tarsal tunnel syndrome usually complains of a more diffuse type of pain on the plantar aspect of the foot. This pain is characterized as burning or tingling in nature and, generally speaking, is aggravated by the patient's activity and usually diminished by rest. Some patients note that the pain is worse when they are in bed at night and that it actually is relieved by getting up and moving around. The burning, tingling, numb feeling cannot be well localized but on occasions will follow one of the terminal branches of the posterior tibial nerve. About one third of the patients will note some proximal radiation of pain along the medial aspect of the leg to the midcalf region. If the pain passes much more proximal to this, I believe that another diagnosis should be considered.

Physical findings

The examination of the patient will demonstrate a positive Tinel sign over the tarsal tunnel area, which is located behind the medial malleolus. It is important to percuss the entire course of the posterior tibial nerve and its terminal branches, looking for a positive Tinel sign, since this will help localize the area of the pathologic condition. The percussion of the nerve will cause localized discomfort and pain radiating out along the distribution of the medial or lateral plantar nerve. The neurologic examination may be confusing in that although the patient complains of pain and numbness, clinically it is unusual to demonstrate actual numbness or loss of two-point discrimination. Weakness of the intrinsic muscles has been a very infrequent finding in my experience.

Although a tarsal tunnel syndrome may be caused by severe valgus of the hindfoot, I have not been able to reproduce the patient's symptoms by holding the foot into a marked valgus position.

In the patient who has a local cause for the tarsal tunnel syndrome, such as a ganglion, lipoma, or exostosis, the diagnosis is easily made, since the area of the nerve overlying the lesion will be extremely sensitive when percussed. If the lesion causing the tarsal tunnel syndrome occurs distal to the tarsal canal along one of the tendon sheaths, the diagnosis can be easily made when the nerve in this area is percussed.

Electrodiagnostic studies

The diagnosis of a tarsal tunnel syndrome is confirmed by obtaining electrodiagnostic studies of the posterior tibial nerve and its branches.

The conduction velocity of the posterior tibial nerve before the tarsal tunnel will help to rule out an abnormality of the posterior tibial nerve before it enters the area of the tarsal canal, such as a peripheral neuritis. The terminal latency of the medial plantar nerve to the abductor hallucis and of the lateral plantar nerve to the abductor digiti quinti should be obtained. The terminal latency of the medial plantar nerve to the abductor hallucis should be less than 6.2 msec and of the lateral plantar nerve to the abductor digiti quinti should be less than 7 msec. If the difference in the terminal latency to the abductor hallucis and abductor digiti quinti is greater than 1 msec, it may indicate the presence of tarsal tunnel syndrome. The abductor hallucis and abductor digiti quinti should also be sampled to determine whether or not any fibrillation potentials are present.

The electrodiagnostic studies will also help to possibly rule out lumbar disk disease as the cause of the patient's pain.

Differential diagnosis

If the criteria previously stated are carefully followed in obtaining the history, eliciting the positive physical findings, and correlating these with the electrodiagnostic studies, there should be little doubt as to whether or not a true tarsal tunnel syndrome exists. As mentioned previously, if all three criteria are not present, the examiner should strongly consider a diagnosis other than tarsal tunnel syndrome. The boxed material on p. 207 presents a scheme for differential diagnosis of tarsal tunnel syndrome (Wilemon, 1979).

Treatment

The patient with tarsal tunnel syndrome should be treated conservatively by using antiinflammatory medications, or if the patient has severe hindfoot varus (Radin, 1983) or valgus, some type of orthosis to correct this may be of benefit. Occasionally, placing the extremity in a cast will bring about some relief. If the patient has a problem with edema, an elastic stocking may be of benefit.

If the patient's symptoms persist, however, consideration to releasing the tarsal tunnel should be given. In the patient who has a well-localized cause for the tarsal tunnel syndrome, a satisfactory clinical response can in most cases be expected, but if no specific cause can be identified, it has been my experience that approximately 75% of these patients are relieved by the surgery and about 25% obtain little or no relief (Mann, 1974). It is rare in my experience that a patient devel-

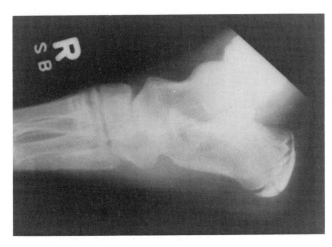

Fig. 9-36. Coalition of talus and navicular.

Its main importance is in differentiating it from other anatomic structures, as pointed out in Fig. 9-34.

Os subtibiale and os subfibulare. The os subtibiale and os subfibulare are located beneath the medial and lateral malleoli respectively. They may be confused as old avulsion fracture of either the medial or lateral mallolus, or dystrophic calcification within ligaments about these structure, suggesting an old sprain.

Bipartite first cuneiform. The bipartite first cuneiform is observed in approximately 1 out of 350 feet. It is usually asymptomatic, although it may be mistaken for a fracture (Fig. 9-35).

Failure of segmentation of navicular. Failure of the navicular to segment from the talus is extremely rare. Fig. 9-36 is an example of this.

REFERENCES
Sesamoid bones

Apley, A.G.: Open sesamoid, Proc. R. Soc. Med. **59:**120, 1966.

Bizarro, A.H.: On sesamoids and supernumerary bones of the limbs, J. Anat. **55:**258, 1921.

Caravias, D.E.: Osteochondritis of sesamoid bones, Br. J. Surg. **44:**623, 1957.

Gillette: Des os sesamoides chez l'homme, J. Anat. Physiol., pp. 506-538, 1872.

Helal, B.: Surgery of the forefoot, Br. Med. J. **1:**276, 1977.

Inge, G.A.L.: Congenital absence of medial sesamoid bone of great toe, J. Bone Joint Surg. **18:**188, 1936.

Inge, G.A.L., and Ferguson, A.B.: Surgery of sesamoid bone of great toe, Arch. Surg. **27:**466, 1933.

Jahss, M.H.: The sesamoids of the hallux, Clin. Orthop. **157:**88, 1981.

Kewenter, Y.: Sesamoid bones of human first metatarsophalangeal joint: a clinical, x-ray, and histopathological study, Acta. Orthop. Scand. [Suppl.] 2, 1936.

Lapidus, P.W.: Sesamoids beneath all metatarsal heads of both feet, J. Bone Joint Surg. **22:**1059, 1940.

Patterson, R.F.: Multiple sesamoids of hands and feet, J. Bone Joint Surg. **19:**531, 1937.

Pfitzner, W.: Die Sesamdiene des Menschen. In Schalbe, editor: Morphologische Arbeiten, vol. 1, Jena, Germany, 1892, Gustav Fischer Verlag, pp. 517-762.

Sarrafian, S.K.: Anatomy of the foot and ankle, Philadelphia, 1983, J.B. Lippincott Co., pp. 86-87.

Toepel, T.: Sesamoid bones: important factors in deformities of first metatarsophalangeal joint, J. Med. Assoc. Ga. **18:**499, 1929.

Trolle, D.: Accessory bones of the human foot: a radiological, histoembryological, comparative anatomical and genetic study, Copenhagen, 1948, Munksgaard, pp. 53, 150-151, 165.

Accessory bones

Bizarro, A.H.: On sesamoid and supernumerary bones of the limbs, J. Anat. **55:**256, 1921.

Chater, E.H.: Foot pain and the accessory navicular bone, Irish J. Med. Sci. **442:**471, 1962.

Dwight, T.: Variations of the bones of the hands and the feet: a clinical atlas, Philadelphia, 1907, J.P. Lippincott Co., pp. 14-23.

Faber, A.: Ueber das Os Intermetatarseum, Orthop. Chir. **61:**186, 1934.

Geist, E.S.: The accessory scaphoid bone, J. Bone Joint Surg. **7:**570, 1925.

Giannestras, N.J.: Foot disorders: medical and surgical management, Philadelphia, 1973, Lea & Febiger.

Harris, R.I.: Retrospect-peroneal spastic flat foot (rigid valgus foot), J. Bone Joint Surg. **47A:**1657, 1965.

Harris, R.I., and Beath, T.: Army foot survey: an investigation of foot ailments in Canadian soldiers (forms no. 1574, Rep. Nat. Res. Counc., Canada), Ottawa, 1947.

Henderson, R.S.: Os intermetatarseum and a possible relationship to hallux valgus, J. Bone Joint Surg. **45B:**117, 1963.

Hoerr, N.L., Pyle, D.I., and Frances C.C.: Radiologic atlas of skeletal development of the foot and ankle: a standard of reference, Springfield, Ill., 1962 Charles C Thomas, Publisher.

Holland, C.T.: The accessory bones of the foot, with notes on a few other conditions. In The Robert Jones birthday volume, London, 1928, Oxford University Press, pp. 160, 162-167, 170.

Kidner, F.C.: The prehalux (accessory scaphoid) in its relation to flatfoot, J. Bone Joint Surg. **11:**831, 1929.

Leonard, M.H., Gonzales, S., Breck, L.W., Bason, C., Palafox, M., and Kosicki, Z.W.: Lateral transfer of the posterior tibial tendon in certain selected cases of pes plano valgus (Kidner operation), Clin. Orthop. **40:**139, 1965.

McDougall, A.: The os trigonum. J. Bone Joint Surg. **37B:**257, 1955.

McKusick, V.A.: Mendelian inheritance in man: catalogues of autosomal dominant, autosomal recessive, and X-linked phenotypes, ed. 2, Baltimore, 1968, Johns Hopkins Press.

O'Rahilly, R.: A survey of carpal and tarsal anomalies, J. Bone Joint Surg. **35A:**626, 1953.

Pfitzner, W.: Beitrage zur Kenntniss des Menschlichen Extremitatenskelets: VI. Die Variatonen in Aufbau des Fusskelets. In Schwalbe, editor: Morphologische Arbeiten, Jena, Germany, 1896, Gustav Fischer, Verlag, pp. 245-527.

Trolle, D.: Accessory bones of the human foot (translated by E. Aagesen) Copenhagen, 1948, Munksgaard.

Wildervanck, L.S., Geodhard, G., and Meiier, S.: Proximal symphalangism of fingers associated with fusion of os naviculare and talus and occurrence of two accessory bones in the feet (os paranaviculare and os tibiale externum) in an European-Indonesian-Chinese family, Acta Genet. **17:**166, 1967.

Zadek, I.: The significance of the accessory tarsal scaphoid, J. Bone Joint Surg. **8:**618, 1926.

Zadek, I., and Gold, A.M.: Accessory tarsal scaphoid, J. Bone Joint Surg. **30A:**957, 1948.

10

Miscellaneous afflictions of the foot

ROGER A. MANN

FLATFOOT (PES PLANUS) IN ADULTS

Flatfoot, weak foot, or fallen arches, as the disorder is variously called, is difficult to classify. There is no known standard by which the longitudinal arch may be considered flat, normal, or high. Some primitive peoples in Africa and Australia are all flatfooted; when they have painful feet, it is only as a result of injuries. In our modern society, however, many people with so-called normal arches experience pain on weight bearing.

Many people with flatfoot can walk as comfortably and as easily as others who have so-called normal arches, yet for some reason a myth exists that people with flatfoot will have difficulty with their feet. During World War II, thousands of men were rejected from the U.S. Army because they had asymptomatic flatfoot. Athletes with flatfoot (some long-distance runners, particularly) are not impeded by the condition. With few exceptions, black people have flatfoot at an early age but later usually develop strong "normal" arches. Perhaps one out of 1,000 people with flatfoot will have pain from the condition because of congenital or acquired abnormalities (DuVries, 1967).

A precise classification of flatfoot deformities is difficult, but the following may be useful generally:

1. Flatfoot—congenital type
   a. Asymptomatic flexible flatfoot
   b. Symptomatic flexible flatfoot
   c. Peroneal spastic flatfoot
   d. Flatfoot secondary to an accessory navicular (prehallux)
   e. Old congenital deformity (e.g., congenital vertical talus)
   f. Associated with a generalized dysplasia (e.g., Marfan's syndrome)
2. Flatfoot—acquired type
   a. Trauma

(1) Dysfunction of the subtalar joint secondary to a fracture
(2) Rupture of the posterior tibial tendon
(3) Degenerative arthritis of talonavicular joint or metatarsocuneiform joint
   b. Generalized arthritic condition (e.g., rheumatoid arthritis)
   c. Neuromuscular imbalance (e.g., cerebral palsy, polio)
   d. Charcot foot

Flatfoot—congenital type

Asymptomatic flexible flatfoot. The asymptomatic flexible flatfoot does not require any treatment.

Symptomatic flexible flatfoot. It has always been somewhat puzzling to me why two feet that seem to be identical by both physical and x-ray examination can present two distinct clinical pictures. Why one flexible flatfoot is symptomatic and another is asymptomatic can be a perplexing and frustrating problem for the patient and the physician. This is particularly true if the patient has previously had an asymptomatic flatfoot. If, however, the patient gives a history of progressively recurring discomfort, it behooves the physician to make every effort to ascertain the etiology of the flatfoot condition.

Occasionally the patient will give a history of a radical change in work habits, such as increased standing for long periods of time on a hard floor or possibly having sustained an injury to the foot. As a result of some foot discomfort, the patient will often start to walk in an abnormal manner, which will secondarily cause a strain on other areas of the foot. This type of problem can occur in a normal foot as well as in a flatfoot, although the flatfoot seems to be somewhat more prone to becoming symptomatic.

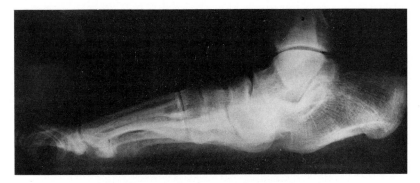

Fig. 10-1. Symptomatic severe flatfood (rocker-bottom foot); required stabilization.

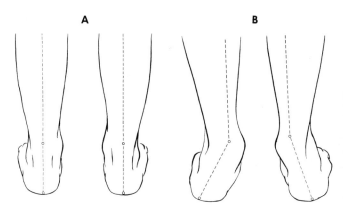

Fig. 10-2. A, Achilles tendon in vertical line. **B,** Valgus heel. Achilles tendon lies laterally behind lateral malleolus. **C,** Patient with valgus heel. (**C** courtesy Dr. Milton Lewis.)

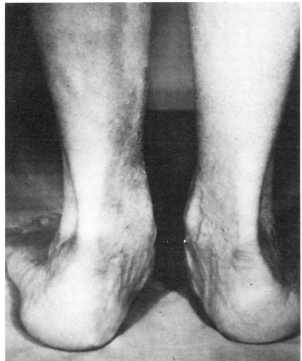

The history obtained from the patient is that the feet ache with weight-bearing of greater than 2 or 3 hours. The pain is dull and poorly localized. The symptoms are usually aggravated by prolonged weight-bearing and activities and relieved by getting off the feet.

The physical findings may demonstrate a normal-appearing arch when the patient is sitting on the examination table, but there is flattening of the longitudinal arch with weight-bearing (Fig. 10-1). An associated valgus of the heel (Fig. 10-2) and abduction of the forefoot are noted. When the patient is asked to stand on his toes, the heel inverts normally. The range of mo-

tion of the subtalar joint may be somewhat increased, particularly in eversion; and the range of motion of the transverse tarsal joint is likewise increased, particularly into abduction (Fig. 10-3). There may be a decrease in ankle dorsiflexion caused by tightness of the Achilles tendon. The motor function about the foot and ankle is normal.

Treatment of the symptomatic flexible flatfoot in adults should be conservative. It is most important to obtain an adequate shoe for the patient to wear. The use of a Thomas heel to support the talonavicular joint may be of benefit. Various other shoe corrections, such

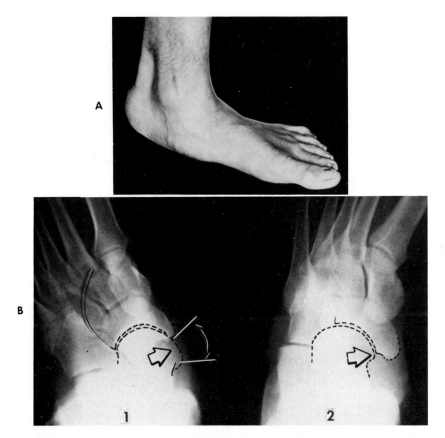

Fig. 10-3. A, Flatfoot with eversion and abduction of forefoot in 43-year-old man. **B,** Demonstration of, *1,* abduction and, *2,* extreme adduction in this man. Note excursion of navicular over head of talus.

as medial lift to help tilt the calcaneus into varus, may also be useful. Corrections within the shoes consist of felt, leather, metal, or plastic arch supports. Any shoe correction should be made gradually to allow the foot time to accommodate. It is ill-advised to start out hastily with an expensive plastic insert.

In some cases adhesive strapping to hold the foot in an adducted and inverted position along with a felt arch support will often give satisfactory results. Occasionally the use of a short leg cast with a well-molded arch will benefit the patient. Following the removal of the cast, the foot is placed into a University of California Biomechanics Laboratory (UCBL) type insert, which is fashioned to prevent the forefoot from going into an abducted position and to prevent the calcaneus from going into valgus, and which is well molded beneath the longitudinal arch. Before placing the foot into this position, it is important to evaluate the tightness of the Achilles tendon, because some patients with a chronic flatfoot will have developed a contracted heel cord that needs to be taken into account when placing the foot into a shoe. The patient may require some heel elevation or possibly a Achilles tendon lengthening.

If all methods of conservative treatment fail and the patient continues to be extremely symptomatic, consideration can be given to a double or triple arthrodesis. It should be kept in mind, however, that these procedures place increased stress on the ankle joint and this may become a source of further discomfort to the patient.

Surgical treatment of adult flatfoot. For the treatment of the symptomatic flexible flatfoot that has failed to respond to conservative management, DuVries used an arthrodesis of the talonavicular and calcaneocuboid articulations (Fig. 10-4). Although the technique is carried out infrequently, the overall results are satisfactory.

The technique consists of an incision over the talonavicular and calcaneocuboid joints. The articular cartilage is removed from the joints, and the foot is placed into a plantigrade position. This usually involves bringing the foot out of its somewhat abducted position into a neutral position. The talonavicular and calcaneocuboid joints are then fixed with staples. Postoperatively the patient is treated in a short-leg, non-weight-bearing cast for 6 weeks, followed by a short-leg walking cast for another 6 weeks (Fig. 10-5).

Occasionally these patients will complain of some an-

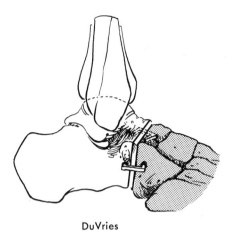

DuVries

Fig. 10-4. Arthrodesis of talonavicular and calcaneocuboid articulations for treatment of flatfoot with no osseous anomalies.

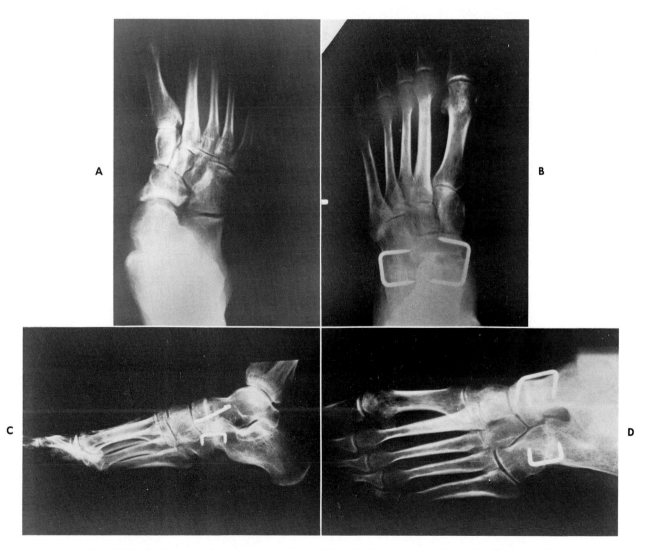

Fig. 10-5. A, Preoperative anteroposterior·radiograph demonstrating lateral subluxation of talonavicular joint. **B,** Postoperative radiograph following double arthrodesis, anteroposterior view. **C,** Lateral view. **D,** Oblique view.

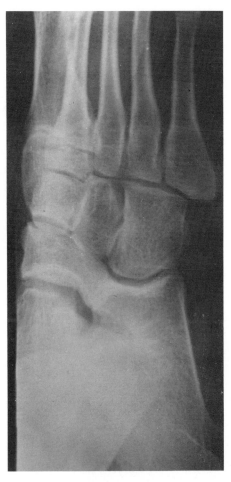

Fig. 10-6. Calcaneonavicular bar completely ossified (synostosis).

kle joint discomfort, probably secondary to the stress imposed on it by the double arthrodesis. No patient has complained of hindfoot pain caused by lack of fusion of the subtalar joint.

Peroneal spastic flatfoot

Etiology. The rigid type of peroneal spastic flatfoot in adults is often the end result of the flexible type.

Harris and Beath (1948) believed that the rigid type was always caused by an anomalous talocalcaneal bridge or by a calcaneonavicular bar (Figs. 10-6 to 10-8). Webster and Roberts (1951) supported this theory. A tarsal coalition can initially begin as a fibrous lesion and then in time progress to a cartilaginous, and finally to an osseous, lesion (Cowell, 1972). This is probably why some cases are initially flexible and then become rigid. There are also secondary bone changes in the subtalar and transverse tarsal joints that contribute to the progressive rigidity of the foot.

The etiology of the peroneal spasm per se is unknown except that it is probably a compensatory reflex spasm secondary to irritation of the subtalar joint mechanism.

We have seen several cases of acquired peroneal spastic flatfoot in adults in which no etiology could be found. In several of these patients, after failure of conservative treatment, a subtalar arthrodesis was undertaken. At the time of surgery, early degenerative changes were noted in the posterior facet of the subtalar joint; however, the etiology for the onset of this problem could not be identified.

Symptoms. The patient with a peroneal spastic flatfoot will usually complain of pain in the hindfoot associated with a flatfoot deformity. He rarely can relate

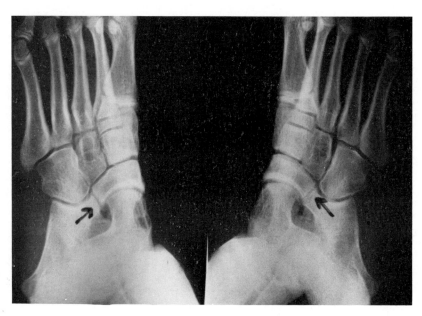

Fig. 10-7. Calcaneonavicular synchondrosis.

information that will aid in determining the etiology of the condition.

Physical examination. The physical findings demonstrate flattening of the longitudinal arch with eversion of the heel. When the patient is asked to stand on his toes, he is unable to invert the heel and it remains everted. The range of motion of the subtalar joint is either absent or considerably restricted. The calcaneus may be held rigidly in an everted position. Spasm of the peroneal tendon may be noted, and occasionally clonus can be elicited by strongly and sharply inverting the heel.

Treatment. The treatment in the adult patient whose foot can be brought back to neutral position or to slight varus is immobilization in a short-leg walking cast for a period of 6 weeks. Approximately 50% of patients will respond to this form of treatment, and in some cases it will have to be repeated. In patients whose foot cannot be brought to neutral, a general anesthetic is necessary for proper alignment and the application of a short-leg walking cast.

In the patient whose foot is very rigid with extensive secondary changes present in the subtalar and talonavicular joint, treatment by immobilization in a short-leg walking cast is much less successful. A molded leather ankle brace with medial and lateral metal stays to immobilize the foot and ankle or a polypropolene ankle-foot orthosis (AFO) may be of some benefit.

If conservative measures fail to give adequate relief, surgical intervention may be of benefit. If the coalition involves only the subtalar joint, and the secondary changes present in the talonavicular joint are minimal, then a subtalar arthrodesis may be of benefit. If there

is extensive involvement of the talonavicular joint, such as beaking or early degenerative changes, then a triple arthrodesis would be the treatment of choice.

In the patient with a symptomatic calcaneonavicular bar, strong consideration should be given to excision of the bar, even in the mature adult. I have seen a sufficient number of cases in which this has been successful in relieving the patient's pain, although not in regaining significant subtalar motion, that I consider it the treatment of choice. It is important, however, that the patient understand that a second procedure, namely a triple arthrodesis, may be necessary if the first procedure fails. When the calcaneonavicular bar is excised, the extensor digitorum brevis muscle should be inserted into the bony defect to help prevent reformation of bone (Fig. 10-9).

Flatfoot secondary to accessory navicular (prehallux). In some patients with a prehallux the normal support of the longitudinal arch by the posterior tibial tendon is insufficient. Kidner (1929) pointed out that this is because the posterior tibial tendon inserts into the prehallux, which is connected to the navicular by a fibrous union, and at other times the prehallux acts as an irritation to the posterior tibial tendon, causing it to reflexly lose function.

Symptoms. An accessory navicular becomes symptomatic much more frequently during adolescence than during adult life. In adults who have been previously asymptomatic, a history of trauma to the foot and ankle, usually in the form of a twisting injury, is elicited. The patient will complain of pain that is fairly well localized over the prominence on the medial side of the foot. The

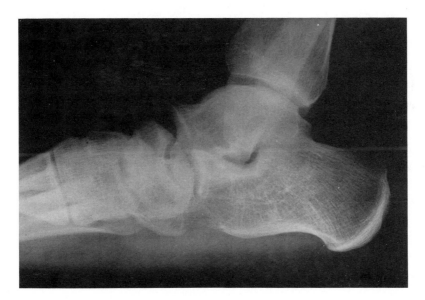

Fig. 10-8. Degenerative changes of talonavicular joint secondary to subtalar coalition.

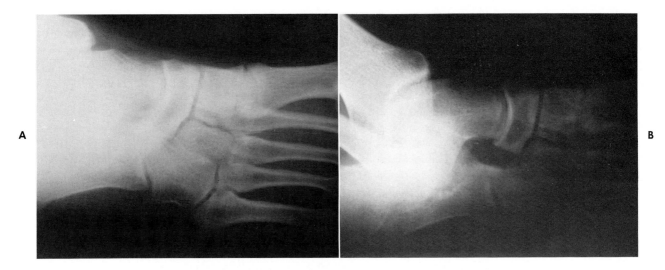

Fig. 10-9. Symptomatic calcaneonavicular coalition. **A,** Preoperative. **B,** Postoperative.

pain is often caused by the rubbing of the shoe against the prominence, but at times the patient experiences discomfort in the longitudinal arch.

Physical examination. The physical findings demonstrate a prominence on the medial side of the tarsal navicular bone. There is often local irritation of the skin, and a bursa is noted over the prominence. Approximately half the patients with an accessory navicular have a normal arch, and half demonstrate some loss of height of the longitudinal arch. Palpation usually causes discomfort. The function of the posterior tibial tendon, secondary to pain, is somewhat weak. When the patient stands, there may be further flattening of the longitudinal arch. The range of motion of the ankle, subtalar, and transverse tarsal joints is normal.

Treatment. Treatment of the symptomatic accessory navicular is initially conservative and consists of immobilization in a short-leg walking cast, use of antiinflammatory medications, and occasionally an injection of steroid into the area of maximum pain and tenderness. If conservative measures fail, a Kidner procedure will usually give a satisfactory result (p. 225).

Miscellaneous types of congenital flatfoot. The flatfoot deformity associated with an old congenital or generalized dysplasia rarely becomes sufficiently symptomatic to cause the patient to seek orthopaedic attention. If help is sought, however, the conservative measures just enumerated are applicable. If the foot remains symptomatic, some type of stabilization procedure is indicated.

Flatfoot—acquired type
Trauma

Dysfunction of subtalar joint. Occasionally following a fracture that extends into the posterior facet of the subtalar joint, a progressive flatfoot deformity will develop. Again the conservative treatment outlined earlier in this section should be applied; but if this fails, stabilization of the subtalar joint is indicated.

Rupture of posterior tibial tendon. From whatever cause, this usually leads to the rapid development of a severe symptomatic flatfoot deformity. The etiology should be suspected whenever a unilateral pes planus rapidly appears. These ruptures usually occur in middle-aged persons and are usually spontaneous although they may follow minor trauma or possibly an injection of steroids into the sheath of the posterior tibial tendon.

The physical examination will demonstrate that there is weakness of inversion of the foot. When the patient is asked to rise on his toes, he will find it difficult to do so on the involved side and there will be little or no inversion of the heel.

Treatment. The methods of treatment are dependent on the age of the patient and the acuteness of the rupture. In an active individual with an acute rupture, surgical correction consisting of repair or reconstruction of the posterior tibial tendon is indicated (p. 476).

Degenerative arthritis of tarsometatarsal joints. Following an injury to the tarsometatarsal joints, degenerative arthritis may ensue. This may result in an abduction deformity of the forefoot, which results in an acquired type of flatfoot deformity.

The physical examination may demonstrate marked abduction of the forefoot, often associated with osteophytic lipping of the tarsometatarsal joints. The deformity is often quite rigid and is difficult to passively realign.

The radiograph of the foot confirms the abduction deformity of the forefoot (Fig. 10-10).

143. If hyperextension is also present in the first metatarsophalangeal joint, a first-toe Jones procedure may be indicated (see p. 305).

Fixed clawtoe deformity. The fixed clawtoe deformity associated with a pes cavus presents a much more difficult problem than the dynamic flexible one previously described. In these patients, little or no active motor function is prsent at the metatarsophalangeal joint. It has been my experience in these cases that the problem can be handled either by carrying out an arthrodesis of the proximal interphalangeal joint of the lesser toes along with a dorsal capsulotomy, extensor tenotomy, and short and long flexor tenotomies. I have also experienced satisfactory results by carrying out a DuVries-type arthoplasty in which the distal portion of the proximal phalanx is generously removed, along with the aforementioned dorsal capsulotomy, extensor tenotomy, and flexor tenotomy. When this procedure is carried out, however, the toes should be stabilized by use of a small Steinmann pin in a neutral position for a period of 6 weeks. If all of the tendons about the toe are not released, the deformity often recurs.

Limited osteotomies. At times a specific bony abnormality is present with the pes cavus foot that significantly impairs the ability to obtain a plantigrade foot. The following three limited osteotomies are used either individually or occasionally together to correct the foot and obtain a more stable plantigrade foot.

First metatarsal osteotomy. Many times in patients with Charcot-Marie-Tooth disease the first metatarsal is significantly plantar flexed, which results in a forefoot valgus deformity. As a result of this, as the head of the first metatarsal contacts the ground, the forefoot is brought into an inverted position. If this is associated with varus of the calcaneus and/or a contracted plantar fascia, an extremely unstable situation results. To correct such a deformity, with or without the varus of the calcaneus, a dorsiflexion first metatarsal osteotomy is carried out. Good success has been obtained by a proximal closing wedge osteotomy to correct this deformity (Fig. 10-13).

Technique

1. Through a short dorsal incision, centered approximately 1 cm distal to the first metatarsocuneiform joint, the base of the metatarsal is exposed.

2. A closing wedge osteotomy is produced with the base located dorsally. Approximately 3 to 4 mm of bone is removed.

3. The osteotomy site is either fixed with a staple or a pin, and the patient ambulates in a wooden shoe until the osteotomy site is healed.

At times a plantar fascial release is carried out at the same time, and then a walking cast is used. Occasionally a Dwyer osteotomy is added if the patient has a fixed varus deformity of the heel.

The combination of relieving the forefoot varus, releasing the plantar fascia, and carrying out a lateral closing wedge osteotomy of the calcaneus changes an unstable foot to a stable one by permitting the weight-bearing line to pass medial to the subtalar axis.

Dwyer calcaneal osteotomy. Patient with a cavus foot, as mentioned previously, not infrequently have a fixed varus component to the hindfoot. If this varus hindfoot is too severe, then a lateral closing wedge osteotomy of the calcaneus can correct the problem. As mentioned previously, the Dwyer procedure is often carried out along with a plantar fascial release and first metatarsal osteotomy (Dwyer, 1959, 1975) (Fig. 10-14).

The technique for a Dwyer closing wedge osteotomy is described on p. 303.

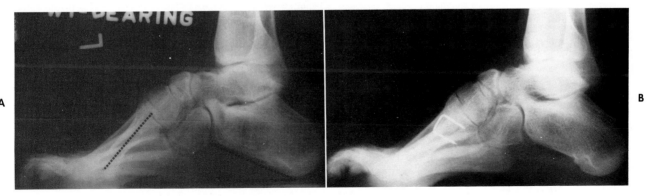

Fig. 10-13. A, Pes cavus deformity secondary to plantar flexion of first ray, preoperative. **B,** Postoperative radiograph following first metatarsal osteotomy correcting marked plantar-flexed position.

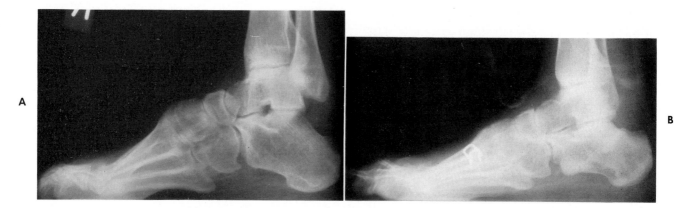

Fig. 10-14. **A,** Pes cavus foot with dorsiflexion of calcaneus and equinus of forefoot. **B,** Postoperative radiograph following Dwyer calcaneal osteotomy, plantar fascial release, and first and second metatarsal osteotomies to produce more plantigrade foot.

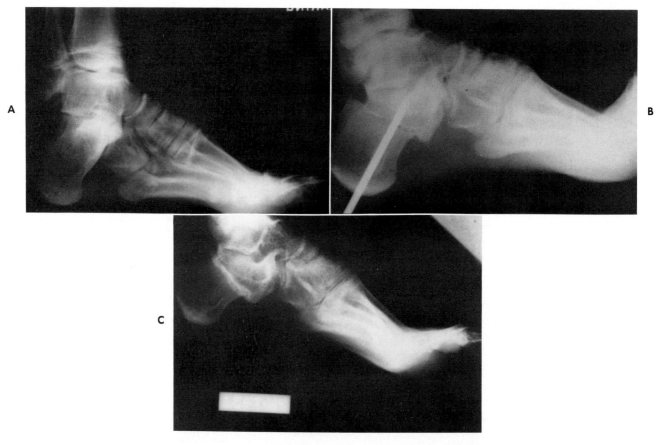

Fig. 10-15. **A,** Pes cavus deformity secondary to marked dorsiflexon of calcaneus and contracture of plantar aponeurosis. **B,** Postoperative radiograph following calcaneal osteotomy and plantar fascial release. **C,** Postoperative radiograph demonstrating satisfactory correction of pes cavus deformity.

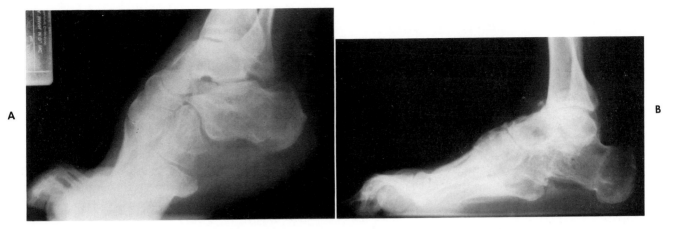

Fig. 10-16. A, Severe forefoot equinus, secondary to Charcot-Marie-Tooth disease. **B,** Post-operative radiograph following a beak type of triple arthrodesis that corrected marked forefoot equinus, producing plantigrade foot. (see p. 297)

Crescentic calcaneal osteotomy. In the patient who has an increase in the pitch of the calcaneus of greater than 30° and who has little or no varus deformity, the crescentic calcaneal osteotomy offers satisfactory realignment of the calcaneus (Samilson, 1976). It almost invariably is carried out in association with a plantar stripping (Fig. 10-15).

Technique

1. The calcaneus is exposed through a lateral oblique incision over the posterior half of the calcaneus, just behind the subtalar joint. Care is taken to identify the sural nerve.

2. The lateral aspect of the calcaneus is exposed, and the peroneal tendons are reflected slightly anteriorly. After the calcaneus is adequately exposed, a complete plantar fascial release is carried out.

3. A crescent-shaped osteotomy of the calcaneus is made. The posterior tuberosity is then shifted posteriorly and superiorly along the osteotomy cut to correct the pitch of the calcaneus.

4. The fragment is stabilized with a pin, and the foot is placed into a short-leg cast.

5. The pin is removed after 3 weeks, and the foot is then placed into a walking cast for another 3 weeks, following which weight bearing is permitted.

This procedure has been most satisfactory in relieving the pes cavus deformity that is brought about by the increased pitch of the calcaneus. The procedure along with the plantar fascial release significantly lowers the longitudinal arch and lengthens the foot.

Midfoot osteotomies. Various forms of midfoot osteotomies have been proposed for the patient who has a forefoot or anterior cavus deformity with an apex located at Chopart's joint. These include the Cole osteotomy (1940), which consists of removing a wedge of

bone from the navicular, cuneiforms, and cuboid. The resulting closing wedge will decrease the pes cavus deformity. The procedure is described on p. 304. A similar osteotomy, although somewhat more distal, has been proposed by Japas (1968), in which a V-osteotomy is made within the tarsal bones, with the distal portion being somewhat depressed to allow the forefoot to be brought out of its equinus position. A similar procedure, distally based, has been described by Jahss (1980). In this procedure, the osteotomy is carried out at the tarsometatarsal level. A truncated wedge is made, and a subsequent arthrodesis at that level is performed. Again, the principle of the procedure is to depress the osteotomy site to permit correction of the forefoot equinus.

I personally have little or no experience with these forefoot osteotomies and as such can only state that the literature supporting each of these authors' techniques seems to indicate that satisfactory realignment of the total forefoot equinus can be obtained.

It is important to appreciate that before such a procedure can be carried out, the forefoot needs to be carefully evaluated to be sure that indeed the entire forefoot is involved, not just plantar flexion of the first metatarsal. The obvious advantage of a midtarsal osteotomy is that any motion that is present in the hindfoot is preserved.

Bony stabilization. A bony stabilization is indicated when a rigid fixed deformity is present in the mature foot that is not correctable by carrying out limited osteotomies. Although various types of triple arthrodeses are used, I believe the one described by Siffert et al. (1966) and Siffert and del Torto (1983) should be strongly considered. This triple arthrodesis is carried out in such a way that the severe forefoot equinus is corrected by rotating the foot through the transverse tarsal joint, so as to place the navicular partially beneath the head of the talus. In so doing, the cavus deformity and forefoot equinus are corrected (Fig. 10-16).

HEEL PAIN

Pain about the plantar aspect of the heel is a multifaceted problem that at times can be a diagnostic enigma and a source of great frustration and discomfort to the patient. Proper treatment of heel pain is dependent on making as precise a diagnosis as possible so that the treatment modality can be directed at a specific problem rather than haphazardly trying various therapeutic modalities. As in any clinical problem, a careful history regarding the heel pain is important. It is important to discuss with the patient the onset, the precise location of the pain, whether or not the pain radiates, the activities that bring on the pain, and the activities that help to relieve it. An inquiry should be made toward what type of footwear and heel height may affect the symptom complex. It is important for the clinician to remember that heel pain may be a manifestation of other problems, such as degenerative disc disease or peripheral neuritis, or maybe associated with one of the collagen diseases, such as rheumatoid arthritis or Reiter's syndrome.

The following is a general outline of the basic etiologies of plantar heel pain:

1. Atrophy of the plantar fat pad
2. Plantar fasciitis at the origin of the plantar aponeurosis
3. Neurologic causes
   a. Sciatica
   b. Tarsal tunnel syndrome
   c. Medial calcaneal neuritis
   d. Lateral plantar nerve entrapment
4. Calcaneal spurs
5. Fractures about the calcaneus
   a. Stress fracture of the calcaneal spur
   b. Stress fracture through the body of the calcaneus
6. Miscellaneous causes
   a. Soft tissue trauma with or without fracture of the calcaneus
   b. Unstable heel pad secondary to cyst formation
   c. Generalized arthritide

Atrophy of fat pad. Atrophy of the plantar fat pad occurs beneath the heel just as it does beneath the metatarsal heads, particularly in older individuals. These individuals will usually complain of localized pain about the heel pad brought on by walking, particularly in hard-soled shoes. The physical examination demonstrates varying degrees of atrophy of the plantar fat pad so that the underlying tubercle of the calcaneus is read-

ily palpable beneath the skin. At times one almost gets the impression of a small bursa being formed between the skin and the calcaneal tubercle. In patients with this problem, treatment should be directed toward increasing the padding beneath the heel by using a soft-soled shoe, slight heel elevation, and at times an arch support centered underneath the talonavicular joint to move some of the weight bearing more anteriorly, off of the heel pad.

Fasciitis at origin of plantar aponeurosis. The patient with fasciitis may complain of chronic pain in the area of the origin of the plantar aponeurosis. At times the pain will be of an acute onset, occurring after the patient has missed a step or while he is participating in some athletic event. The pain is usually well localized and aggravated by activities. These patients will often note pain on arising in the morning and, after a period of "warming up," will usually note a lessening of the pain until later in the day. Then, if they have been on their feet for too long a period of time, the pain tends to recur. The physical examination demonstrates pain that is well localized in the area of the origin of the plantar aponeurosis and often extends distally for about 1 cm. Full dorsiflexion of the metatarsophalangeal joints, which places stress on the plantar aponeurosis, will often reproduce the patient's pain. The remainder of the plantar aponeurosis is usually not tender. Radiographs of the heel may demonstrate a large calcaneal spur, but usually they demonstrate only a normal-appearing calcaneal spur. The treatment should be directed toward relieving the fasciitis by using nonsteroidal antiinflammatory medications and soft shoes.

Injection of a steroid preparation into the area of maximum tenderness may be beneficial in patients with refractory pain. More than two or three injections into this area should not be undertaken because of possible damage to the plantar fat pad. Usually an arch support will be bothersome to this group of patients, because it tends to place pressure over the area of pain. At times taping the forefoot into some adduction will be of benefit in refractory cases.

Neurologic causes

Sciatica. Heel pain caused by sciatica is a result of pressure on the L5-S1 nerve root, which is represented about the heel area. These patients will often complain of heel pain, but on careful questioning they also report low back pain with radiation down the leg and calf to the heel, and sometimes radiation out into the foot. Occasionally there may be pain only in the low back or buttocks and the heel rather than along the entire sciatic nerve. The physical examination in these patients may reveal sensory or motor loss as well as evidence of tenderness over the sciatic nerve. Needless to say, once this diagnosis is made, the workup should be directed toward the cause of the problem, i.e., the back, rather than the heel.

Tarsal tunnel syndrome. The patient with heel pain secondary to tarsal tunnel syndrome will often complain of a tingling, burning, or numb feeling about the heel and foot. The pain is often aggravated by activities, although not infrequently it is present when the patient is in bed at night. These patients have difficulty in localizing the pain, as opposed to the patient with a fasciitis-type picture. The physical examination will often reveal a Tinel's sign, which can be elicited along the tarsal tunnel or over the lateral plantar or medial calcaneal nerve as it leaves the tarsal tunnel to pass behind the origin of the abductor hallucis. Rarely, there is a sensory loss associated with heel pain, which is caused by an entrapment of the posterior tibial nerve. The diagnosis should be confirmed by obtaining electrodiagnostic studies, which include both nerve conduction studies as well as examination for fibrillation potentials. The treatment is usually conservative in nature with antiinflammatory medications, but occasionally release of the tarsal tunnel may be of benefit (see p. 207).

Medial calcaneal neuritis. Medial calcaneal neuritis may be a manifestation of a tarsal tunnel syndrome in that the medial calcaneal nerves are branches of the lateral plantar nerve. In the patient with pure medial calcaneal neuritis, the pain is usually well localized to the medial side of the heel and the medial plantar half of the heel pad. It usually does not involve the entire foot as is seen with the patient with tarsal tunnel syndrome. In these patients percussion of the medial calcaneal nerves along the medial side of the heel will often reproduce the patient's symptom complex. Occasionally surgical release of the nerve, which becomes entrapped in a fibrous tunnel, may be indicated. Some authors have advocated neurectomy of the medial calcaneal nerve for this condition, but as a general rule I do not feel that these nerves should be disrupted, since a numb heel may be a very annoying condition that the patient does not tolerate very well.

Lateral plantar nerve entrapment. The patient with a lateral plantar nerve entrapment may complain of pain in the heel, with some radiation toward the lateral side of the foot. This pain is often aggravated by activities, but, again, as with other problems involving a nerve entrapment, pain may only be manifested when the patient is in bed at night. The pain is poorly localized and often difficult for the patient to pinpoint. The physical examination will demonstrate tenderness over the origin of the abductor hallucis muscle in the area where the lateral plantar nerve passes beneath it. Percussion or pressure on this area will often reproduce the patient's symptom complex. From a diagnostic standpoint, there may be a prolonged terminal latency of the lateral plantar nerve to the abductor digiti quinti, but often the nerve condition studies are normal. Whether this condition represents a true entrapment of the lateral plantar nerve beneath the abductor origin or possibly one of its branches as it passes over the medial edge of the plantar aponeurosis and along the calcaneal tubercle is difficult to state. The treatment should be conservative in nature. At times, in refractory cases, consideration of release of the abductor origin and careful exploration of the lateral plantar nerve and its various branches along the medial side and origin of the plantar aponeurosis may be indicated (Baxter and Thigpen, 1984) (Fig. 10-17).

Calcaneal spurs. The patient with an enlarged calcaneal spur will usually complain of a pain similar to that seen with a plantar fasciitis. The main question is whether the cause of the pain is truly the calcaneal spur or nothing more than a traction apophysis that has formed in response to the origin of the plantar aponeurosis. In my experience a calcaneal spur per se as the etiology of heel pain is infrequent and probably considerably overdiagnosed by some clinicians in lieu of carefully making a specific diagnosis of the heel pain. The physical findings will often include tenderness about the calcaneal spur, but I believe this usually represents a fasciitis of the origin of the plantar aponeurosis. The treatment of this problem should be directed toward the use of adequate padding about the heel, the use of an arch support to relieve the pressure on the area of the calcaneal spur, and occasionally slight elevation of the heel. I feel that further treatment, particularly excision of the spur, should be reserved for the occasional patient who truly has a marked enlargement of the calcaneal spur and has been shown to be refractory to a long course of conservative management. As an example of my conservatism regarding this condition, I have personally excised only one spur in the past 8 years. Unfortunately, I have seen many patients in consultation with persistent heel pain after excision of their calcaneal spur.

Fractures about the heel

Stress fracture of calcaneal spur. It has been demonstrated in a group of patients who have localized pain about the tubercle of the calcaneus that by obtaining multiple radiographs of the concave surface of the calcaneus, evidence of a fracture of the calcaneal tubercle can be seen (Graham, 1983). In patients in whom this specific diagnosis is made, treatment by a period of immobilization will often bring about resolution of the problem.

Stress fracture of the calcaneus. The patient with a stress fracture of the calcaneus usually will note progressive calcaneal pain. These patients almost invari-

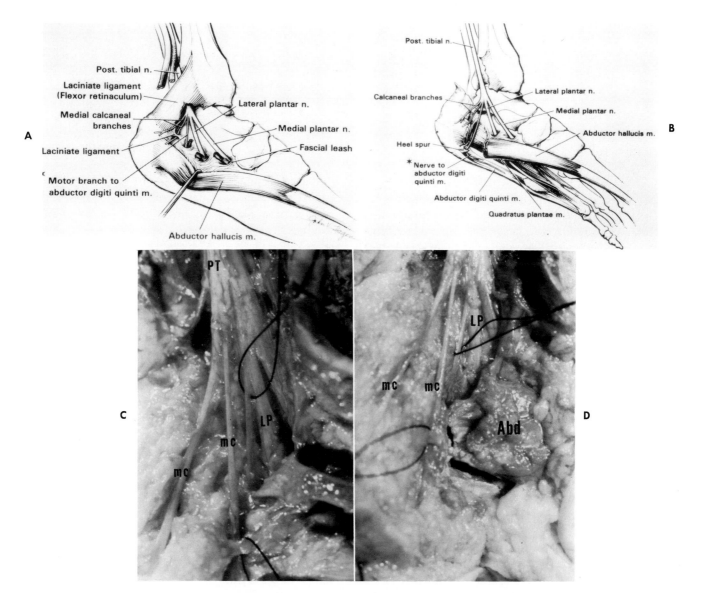

Fig. 10-17. A, Demonstration of the lateral plantar nerve and, just posterior to it, motor branch to abductor digiti quinti muscle as it passes behind origin of abductor hallucis muscle. **B,** Release of abductor hallucis origin decompresses nerve to abductor digiti quinti and lateral plantar nerve. **C,** Anatomic dissection demonstrating motor branch to abductor digiti quinti with silk loop around it. Note that it is just posterior to lateral plantar nerve *(LP)*. *PT,* posterior tibial nerve. *mc,* medial calcaneal branch. **D,** A magnified view of **C,** demonstrating lateral plantar nerve *(LP)* and, just posterior to it with silk ligature around it, motor branch to abductor digiti quinti. Note abductor hallucis *(Abd)* origin has been released, which decompresses nerves. (From Baxter, D., and Thigpen, M.: Foot Ankle **5:**16, 1984. © 1984, American Orthopaedic Foot Society.)

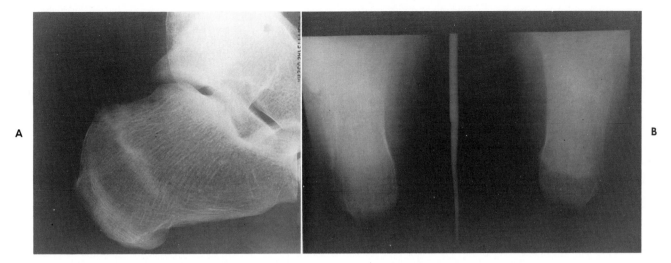

Fig. 10-18. A, Stress fracture through calcaneus. **B,** Stress fracture noted on tangential view of the calcaneus.

ably have a high level of athletic activity. The pain associated with a stress fracture of the calcaneus is quite disabling, and the diagnosis is made based on the history and the physical findings of generalized tenderness about the entire calcaneus, not just pain in the heel pad area. Although the initial x-ray film may be negative, follow-up x-rays will demonstrate a fracture line through the body of the calcaneus, which will confirm the diagnosis (Fig. 10-18). The treatment consists of immobilization until the fracture site has healed.

Miscellaneous conditions

Direct trauma. At times a patient will sustain direct trauma to the heel pad, which probably results in disruption of the well-organized fat pad that is present beneath the heel. This sometimes follows a motorcycle accident or falling onto a sharp object, etc. In these patients, the history obviously defines the etiology of the problem. The physical findings demonstrate generalized tenderness about the heel pad. From a clinical standpoint, as a rule, the pain will resolve with time, but occasionally this may be an extremely refractory condition. Treatment should be directed towards supportive measures, such as adequate padding, and occasionally cast immobilization. A similar problem can occur following a fracture of the calcaneus when there has been gross disruption of the calcaneus and probably the fibrous septum that makes up the specialized nature of the heel pad. The treatment should be the same as that outlined for the patient with direct trauma.

Loosened heel pad secondary to cyst formation. Occasionally patients will develop pain in their heel pad secondary to instability of the pad. They note that the heel pad has become distorted over a period of time so that any prolonged walking causes pain. The examina-

tion of patients with this rare conditoin demonstrates that indeed there is increased mobility of the heel pad. In my experience, this has been caused by a cyst that forms between the calcaneus and the heel pad, dissecting the heel pad off of the calcaneus. The treatment in these cases is difficult, but aspiration of the cyst with immobilization may be successful. If not, excision of the cyst and thin wafer off the plantar aspect of the calcaneal tubercle, followed by a compression dressing and adequate drainage, in an attempt to get the heel pad to become scarred to the calcaneus, may be considered.

Generalized arthritide. At times heel pain is secondary to a generalized arthritide. These patients may manifest other areas of joint involvement, but on occasions all the symptoms will be located about the heel. The physical findings in these cases usually demonstrate generalized tenderness about the entire heel pad that is poorly localized. The diagnosis is confirmed by a clinical suspicion and then obtaining laboratory studies to rule out these various conditions, which might include rheumatoid arthritis, Reiter's syndrome, psoriatic arthritis, or gout.

CALCANEAL PROBLEMS

Haglund's disease (prominent posterosuperior tuberosity of calcaneus) and related conditions

Haglund (1928) appears to have been the first to call attention to the possible relationship between the shape of the calcaneus and the appearance of pump bumps, Achilles tendon bursitis, retrocalcaneal bursitis, and small spurs at the attachment of the Achilles tendon. Saxl (1929) emphasized that if the upper surface of the tuberosity of the calcaneus was too prominent, the soft

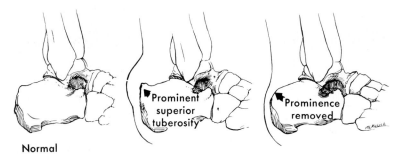

Fig. 10-19. Normally shaped calcaneus; prominent superior tuberosity (Haglund's disease) removal of posterior lip of calcaneus in Haglund's disease.

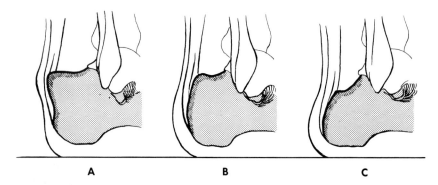

Fig. 10-20. Variations in shape of superior tuberosity of calcaneus. **A,** Hyperconvex (so-called Haglund's disease); **B,** normal; **C,** hypoconvex.

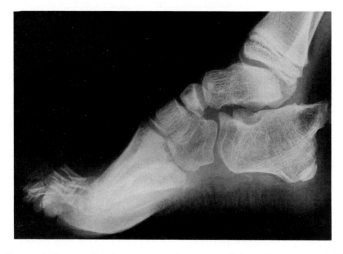

Fig. 10-21. Congenital anomaly of posterior tuberosity of the calcaneus; painful from pressure of shoes.

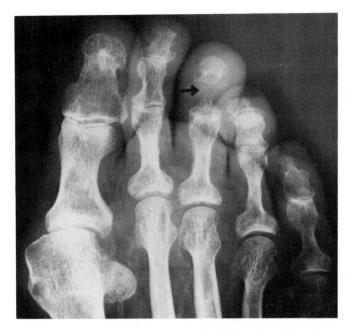

Fig. 10-41. Avascular necrosis of third middle phalanx.

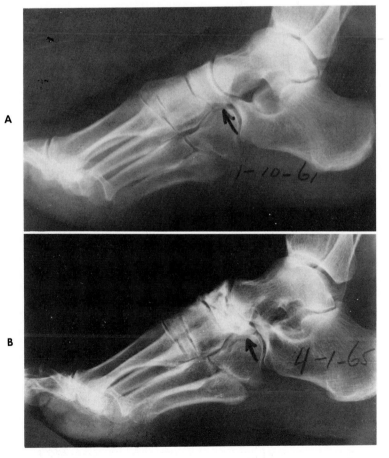

Fig. 10-42. Avascular necrosis of navicular in 42-year-old woman; pain in talonavicular joint. A, 1961, No osseous changes. B, 1965, Extensive dissolution of this bone; no underlying cause could be found.

may show signs of osteoporosis of disuse (Aegerter and Kirkpatrick, 1975). With a return of reparative vascular invasion and new bone apposition, the radiographic picture changes. Whereas the affected bone has a moth-eaten appearance and become atrophic with the invasion of granulation tissue, the new bone apposition manifests greater density (Bobechko and Harris, 1960). In the event that many bones are affected with avascular necrosis, a complete metabolic investigation must be performed to rule out the presence of systemic disease. Care must be taken not to mistake avascular necrosis for a tumor.

Avascular necrosis of the bones of the foot may occur secondary to trauma, particularly if fracture or dislocation has occurred and the blood supply has been interrupted (Fig. 10-41). The fractured talus is especially vulnerable to avascular necrosis.

In cases of avascular necrosis that cannot be ascribed to metabolic, infectious, or traumatic causes, congenital factors have been cited as etiologic agents. Shaw (1954) reported a particular case of avascular necrosis in which progressive destruction of one or more phalanges occurred in six generations of one family. "Idiopathic" avascular necrosis of the metatarsal heads and tarsal bones has been encountered, but reports of such cases are rare (10-42).

No rationale exists to explain the arrest of this condition. Except for the uncommon case in which destruction is permanent, treatment by supportive measures is indicated.

The term *bone infarct* designates a region of circulatory deprivation for bone that can occur in the metaphyseal or diaphyseal region of a tubular bone and may be asymptomatic. Both bone infarct and aseptic necrosis may describe the same condition.

REFERENCES
Flatfoot

Cowell, H.R.: Talocalcaneal coalition and new causes of peroneal spastic flatfoot, Clin. Orthop. **85**:16, 1972.

DuVries, H.L.: Five myths about your feet, Today's Health **45**:49, August 1967.

Harris, R.I., and Beath, T.: Etiology of peroneal spastic flat foot, J. Bone Joint Surg. **30B**:624, 1948.

Kidner, F.C.: The prehallux (accessory scaphoid) in its relation to flatfoot, J. Bone Joint Surg. **11**:831, 1929.

Webster, F.S., and Roberts, W.M.: Tarsal anomalies and peroneal spastic flatfoot, JAMA **146**:1099, 1951.

Pes cavus

Bentzon, P.G.K.: Pes cavus and the M. peroneus longus, Acta Orthop. Scand, **4**:50, 1933.

Brewerton, D.A., Sandifer, P.H., and Sweetnam, D.R.: "Idiopathic" pes cavus: an investigation into its aetiology, Br. Med. J. **2**:659, 1963.

Cole, W.H.: The treatment of claw-foot, J. Bone Joint Surg. **22**:895, 1940.

Duchenne, G.B.: Physiology of motion (translated and edited by E.B. Kaplan), Philadelphia, 1949, J.B. Lippincott Co. (Original French edition, 1867.)

Duchenne, G.B.: The physiology of motion (translated by E.B. Kaplan), Philadelphia, 1959, W.B. Saunders Co.

Dwyer, F.C.: Osteotomy of the calcaneum for pes cavus, J. Bone Joint Surg. **41B**:80, 1959.

Dwyer, F.C.: The present status of the problem of pes cavus, Clin. Orthop. **106**:254, 1975.

Hallgrímsson, S.: Pes cavus, seine Behandlung und einige Bemerkungen über seine Aetiologie, Acta Orthop. Scand. **10**:73, 1939.

Ibrahim, K.: Pes cavus. In Devarts, C.N., editor: Surgery of the musculoskeletal system. New York, 1983, Churchill Livingston, pp. 9-39.

Jahss, M.H.: Transmetatarsal truncated-wedge arthrodesis for pes cavus and equinovarus deformity of the forepart of the foot, J. Bone Joint Surg. **62A**:713, 1980.

Japas, L.M.: Surgical treatment of pes cavus by tarsal V-osteotomy, J. Bone Joint Surg. **50A**:927, 1968.

Samilson, R.L.: Proscentic osteotomy of the os calcis for calcaneocavus feet. In Bateman, J.E., editor: Foot science, Philadelphia, 1976, W.B. Saunders Co., p. 18.

Siffert, R.S., Forester, R.I., and Nachamle, B.: "Beak" triple arthrodesis for correction of severe cavus deformity, Clin. Orthop. **45**:101, 1966.

Siffert, R.S., and delTorto, U.: 'Beak' triple arthrodesis for severe cavus deformity, Clin. Orthop. **181**:54, 1983.

Steindler, A.: Operative treatment of pes cavus: stripping of the os calcis, Surg. Gynecol. Obstet. **24**:612, 1917.

Heel pain

Baxter, D., and Thigpen, M.: Heel pain—operation results, Foot Ankle **5**:16, 1984.

Graham, C.: Painful heel syndrome: rationale of diagnosis and treatment of, Foot Ankle **3**:261, 1983.

Haglund's disease

Fowler, A., and Philip, J.F.: Abnormality of the calcaneus as a cause of painful heel, Br. J. Surg. **32**:494, 1945.

Haglund, P.: Beitrag zur Klinik der Achillessehne, Z. Orthop. Chir. **49**:49, 1928.

Hohmann, K.G.G.: Fuss and Bein, ihre Erkrankungen und deren Behandlung, ed. 4, Munich, 1948, J.F. Bergmann.

Keck, S.W., and Kelly, P.J.: Bursitis of the posterior part of the heel: evaluation of surgical treatment of eighteen patients, J. Bone Joint Surg. **47A**:267, 1965.

Nissen, K.I.: Remodeling of the posterior tuberosity of the calcaneum. In Rob, C., and Smith, R., editors: Operative surgery, vol. 5, London, 1957, Butterworth and Co., Ltd.

Saxl, A.: Die Schiehgeschwalst der Ferse, Z. Orthop. Chir. **51**:312, 1929.

Morton's syndrome

Harris, R.I., and Beath, T.: The short first metatarsal: its incidence and clinical significance, J. Bone Joint Surg. **31A**:553, 1949.

Hawkes, O.A.M.: On the relative lengths of the first and second toes of the human foot from the point of view of occurrence, anatomy and heredity, J. Genet. **3**:249, 1914.

Jones, F.W.: Structure and function as seen in the foot, Baltimore, 1944, The Williams & Wilkins Co.

Morton, D.J.: The human foot, New York, 1935, Columbia University Press.

Morton, D.J.: Human locomotion and body form: a study of gravity and man, Baltimore, 1952, The Williams & Wilkins Co.

Hallux flexus

Lapidus, P.W.: "Dorsal bunion": its mechanics and operative correction, J. Bone Joint Surg. **22:**627, 1940.

Vascular disorders

Aegerter, E., and Kirkpatrick, J.A., Jr.: Orthopedic diseases, ed. 4, Philadelphia, 1975, W.B. Saunders Co.

Bobechko, W.P., and Harris, W.R.: The radiographic density of avascular bone, J. Bone Joint Surg. **42B:**626, 1960.

Braddock, G.I.F.: Experimental epiphysial injury and Freiberg's disease, J. Bone Joint Surg. **41B:**154, 1959.

Shaw, E.W.: Avascular necrosis of the phalanges of the hands (Thiemann's disease), JAMA **156:**711, 1954.

Waugh, W.: The ossification and vascularisation of the tarsal navicular and their relation to Köhler's disease, J. Bone Joint Surg. **40B:**765, 1958.

11

Conservative treatment and office procedures

ROGER A. MANN

Before discussing conservative means of treating some disorders of the feet, I should like to say a word about footwear and its influence on the functioning of the feet. As emphasized previously, shoes, especially women's shoes, have been responsible for a majority of the toe deformities physicians commonly encounter. Although men and women have worn and suffered the consequences of improper footwear since antiquity, contemporary society continues to perpetuate the use of ill-fitting shoes.

The deforming effects of improper shoes on a normal foot can cause hallux valgus, hammertoes, hard corns, and plantar keratoses. Properly fitted footwear should not crowd the forefoot but should allow the toes to extend fully as the person walks (Fig. 4-2, C). To ensure adequate length and width, shoes should always be fitted to the weight-bearing foot.

MODIFICATIONS OF THE SHOE

Numerous modifications can be made in the heel, shank, or sole areas of the basic shoe (separately or in combination) to treat specific disorders of the foot. Rather than recommend an "orthopaedic shoe" for all symptomatic feet, the clinician should prescribe shoe modifications that suit the individual needs of the patient.

Wedges and pads are used to accomplish shoe modifications. A wedge is usually made of leather and is placed on the exterior walking surface of the shoe or within the construction of the shoe. It is intended to alter the weight-bearing pattern of the foot. Unlike the wedge, the pad acts on a specific site. It is used for therapeutic purposes to relieve pressure and is in direct contact with the foot. It is usually made of felt, leather, or plastic.

The heel

Thomas heel. The most common heel modification is the Thomas heel (Fig. 11-1). This heel was originally designed to bring the calcaneus from a valgus position to a more neutral one and to support the medial aspect of the foot. Its use is indicated in cases of symptomatic flatfoot. It produces a varus tilt of the calcaneus and gives mechanical support to the collapsing talonavicular joint as well. In cases of hindfoot valgus it can be used to keep the calcaneus in a less valgoid position. A Thomas heel should not be used if the calcaneus is in a varus position.

Unfortunately, today most Thomas heels are not properly fitted. To be effective, a Thomas heel should extend from the midportion of the navicular on the medial side to a line that intersects the longitudinal axis of the fibula on the lateral side. The Thomas heel may be combined with an inner heel lift to help accomplish inversion of the calcaneus.

Heel lifts. A medial or lateral lift of 0.3 to 0.6 cm may be used to bring the heel out of a varus or valgus position (Fig. 11-2). Such a lift will transfer weight to the medial or lateral aspect of the foot.

Widened heels. Heels that have been widened are used to stabilize and thereby diminish painful subtalar motion. They are beneficial in the treatment of degenerative changes in the subtalar joint and to help stabilize the subtalar joint in cases of peroneal weakness.

SACH heel. A SACH heel is an elevated soft heel of soft compressible material that will cushion the impact of initial ground contact and help to permit the initiation for a rocker type of action during ground contact. It is useful for patients who have equinus contracture of the ankle or who have undergone ankle arthrodesis. The degree of the rockering effect can be altered de-

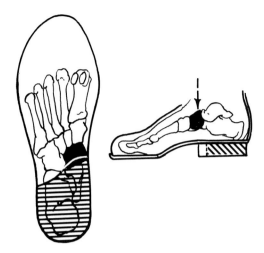

Fig. 11-1. Thomas heel; extends to midportion of navicular to provide support.

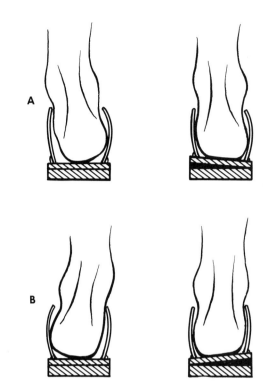

Fig. 11-2. Heel lifts. **A,** Medial heel wedge for correction of valgus heel deformity. **B,** Lateral heel wedge for correction of varus heel deformity.

pending on the height of the heel and the position of the forward area of the roll (i.e., under the arch, under the metatarsal head, or distally).

The shank

The shank of the shoe can be either flexible or rigid. In attempting to correct a postural abnormality of the foot by means of an external modification of the heel or sole, one usually recommends that the shank be flexible so the foot can respond to the areas being corrected. Conversely, if an appliance is to be placed within the shoe, the shank should be more rigid.

The sole

The sole of the shoe can be modified through the use of lifts to affect the regions of the great toe, the metatarsals, and the medial and lateral aspects of the foot. The sole material may be modified depending on the needs of the patient. The material can vary from a firm leather to a soft crepe. In patients with metatarsalgia I prefer initially to use a softer sole material to increase the cushion between the patient's foot and the environment. Some people, however, are not comfortable with a crepe sole and prefer a more rigid sole material with modification of the insole.

Lifts in region of great toe. Lifts in the region of the great toe make the toe less flexible and restrict the motion of the joint. This modification is useful in the treatment of hallux rigidus (Fig. 11-3). A rocker-bottom shoe will also diminish the motion in the metatarsophalangeal joint of the great toe and diminish pressure underneath the metatarsal heads.

Lifts in region of metatarsals. There are two devices for modifying shoes in the metatarsal area: a bar and an anterior heel.

The sole is often modified by a *metatarsal bar,* which transfers the weight usually borne by the metatarsal heads to a more proximal plantar area. The bar should be placed proximal to the metatarsal heads and may be either straight or curved (Fig. 11-4). Improper placement of the bar in relation to the metatarsal heads is the most common error made in using this type of appliance. If the bar is placed too far forward, the painful metatarsal condition will be aggravated. The insole of the patient's shoe should be examined to determine the weight-bearing area; marks should then be made on the sides of the sole just proximal to the metatarsal heads. In this way proper placement of the bar by the shoemaker is assured. The bar can be 0.3 to 1 cm thick, depending on the clinical picture.

The anterior *heel* is also effective in relieving pressure on the metatarsal region and is preferred by some clinicians to the metatarsal bar.

Both these appliances are used to relieve metatarsalgia caused by atrophy of the plantar fat pad, intractable plantar keratosis, Morton syndrome, trauma to the metatarsal heads, and other conditions that affect the metatarsal heads.

A great deal of progress has been made recently in the production of insole materials. There are now many materials that will permit the clinician in his office to

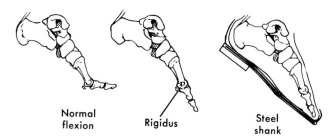

Fig. 11-3. Sole modification of treatment of hallux rigidus. Steel shank is incorporated to diminish motion at metatarsophalangeal joint.

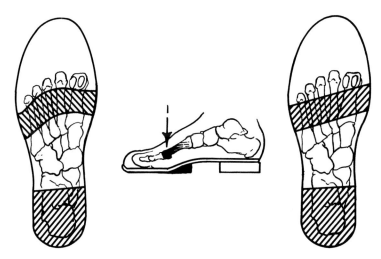

Fig. 11-4. Metatarsal bars. These appliances may be either straight or curved but must be placed proximal to metatarsal heads.

produce an insole that specifically relieves areas of pressure on the plantar aspect of the foot. Other materials such as Plastizote when placed in a shoe will mold to the pressure points exerted by the patient against the material and thus produce a total contact type of insole. When a total contact interface is established between the plantar skin and the insole, pressure is distributed over a broad area. When placing materials within the shoe, it is important that there is adequate room for the patient's foot after the insole material has been added. For this reason the extradepth shoe that has both a large toe box area and extra thickness to accommodate a Plastizote insole can be useful, particularly in treating patient with insensitive feet.

Lifts in medial and lateral regions of foot. Medial and lateral sole lifts (0.3 to 0.6 cm thick) may be used either alone or combined with a heel modification to help correct imbalances of the foot. A medial lift will transfer the weight to the outer border and can be used to accommodate forefoot varus or to help realign the foot after trauma. A lateral lift will transfer weight to the inner border of the foot, may be used to treat forefoot valgus, and will also help to realign the foot after

trauma (Fig. 11-5). In the treatment of flatfoot, the lateral lift is used to help correct the forefoot varus that often accompanies hindfoot valgus. A lateral lift is also frequently combined with a Thomas heel to help support a flatfoot deformity (Fig. 11-6).

Appliances

Felt pads. Felt pads are used primarily to relieve areas of abnormal pressure on the plantar aspect of the foot. They may also be used to support the longitudinal arch during the period when the clinician is attempting to determine which combination of supports is best suited for the patient. The pads may be cut by the physician (Fig. 11-7) or ready-made adhesive backed pads may be purchased in various sizes.

Placement of the felt pad in the shoe is often facilitated by carefully observing the insole of the patient's shoe. The insole beneath the area of a keratosis will have a dark stain, and this gives the clinician a clue about placing the metatarsal support, namely, just proximal to this mark. Correct placement and the indications for the most commonly used shoe pads are illustrated in Fig. 11-8. It is important when using a soft

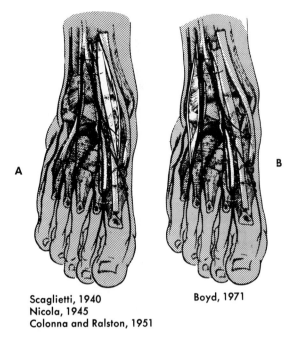

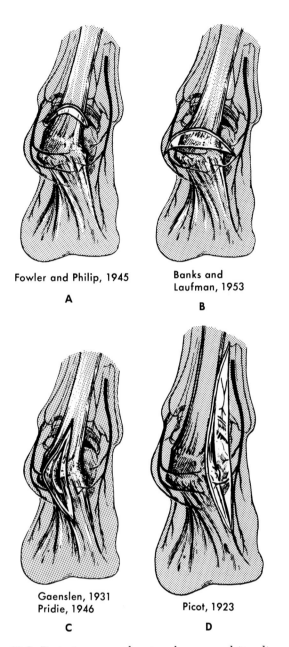

Fowler and Philip, 1945

A

Banks and
Laufman, 1953

B

Gaenslen, 1931
Pridie, 1946

C

Picot, 1923

D

Fig. 12-3. Posterior approaches to calcaneus and its adjacent structures.

Scaglietti, 1940
Nicola, 1945
Colonna and Ralston, 1951

Boyd, 1971

Fig. 12-4. Anterior approaches to ankle and its adjacent structures.

tinues distally to a point approximately 5 cm below the joint. The deep fascia is divided in line with the skin incision. The approach is usually developed in the interval between the extensor hallucis longus and extensor digitorum longus tendons; however, Scaglietti (1940) and Nicola (1945) advised using the interval between the tendons of the tibialis anterior and the extensor hallucis longus. The anterolateral, malleolar, and lateral tarsal arteries must be identified, isolated, and ligated. The dorsal artery of the foot and the deep peroneal nerve are carefully exposed and retracted. The periosteum, capsule, and synovium are incised in line with the skin incision, and the full anterior width of the ankle joint is exposed by subcapsular and subperiosteal dissection (Fig. 12-4, *A*).

EXPOSURE OF ANKLE JOINT INCLUDING SUBTALAR AND TRANSVERSE TARSAL ARTICULATIONS
Anterolateral approach

Exposure of the ankle, talocalcaneal, talonavicular, and calcaneocuboid articulations is best accomplished through an anterolateral approach. Boyd (1971), who has described this approach, has suggested that it may well be called a "universal incision" for many surgical procedures on the foot and ankle. It avoids major vessels and nerves, and it can be extended proximally to reveal the distal tibia or distally to expose the articulations between the cuboid and the fourth and fifth metatarsals. Through such an incision arthrodesis of the tarsal joints may be done and excision of the talus as well as various talar coalitions can be performed.

Achilles tendon to the level of its insertion. The superficial and deep fasciae are divided. A **Z**-plasty division and reflection of the Achilles tendon is done. The fat and areolar tissue in the space between the flexor hallucis longus and the peroneus brevis tendon are retracted medially to expose the distal tibia, the posterior ankle joint, and the posterior surface of the talus (Fig. 12-3, *D*).

Anterior approach

In the approach described by Colonna and Ralston (1951), the incision begins along the anterior aspect of the ankle 8 to 10 cm proximal to the joint line; it con-

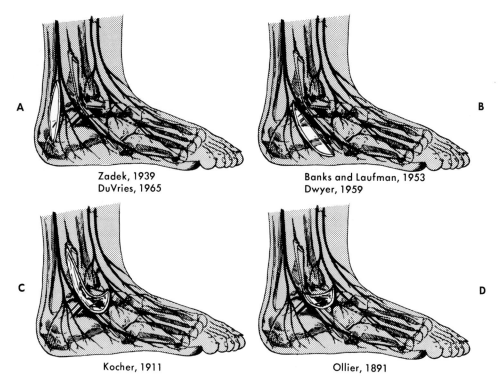

Fig. 12-5. Lateral approaches to calcaneus and subtalar joint.

The skin incision extends distally from a point 5 cm above the ankle joint and 1 cm in front of the anterior edge of the tibula toward the base of the fourth metatarsal. Here there is an overlap area supplied by twigs from the intermediate dorsal cutaneous peroneal branch and the superficial branches of the sural nerve.

If the intermediate dorsal cutaneous branch is exposed, it should be carefully preserved and retracted medially. The anterolateral malleolar artery will be encountered proximally and the lateral tarsal artery distally in the incision. Both may be sacrificed. The fascia and crural ligaments are incised, exposing the capsule of the ankle. The extensor digitorum brevis may be detached from its origin and reflected to uncover the talonavicular and calcaneocuboid regions and the region of the sinus tarsi (Fig. 12-4, *B*).

Lateral approaches to subtalar joint and adjacent structures

Approach to subtalar and talonavicular joints (Kocher, 1911). The approach described here is a classic one to the subtalar and talonavicular joints for subtalar or triple arthrodesis.

The incision begins about 2 cm proximal to the tip of the lateral malleolus, proceeds in a gentle curve around and below the malleolus, and terminates at the level of the talonavicular joint. The small saphenous vein and nerve should lie posteriorly. The anterior portion of the incision crosses the intermediate dorsal cutaneous

nerve. Both nerves should be protected. The deep fascia is incised to expose the peroneal tendons. They may be retracted posteriorly if necessary to gain a wider field, or they may be divided by a Z-plasty and later resutured. To gain access to the posterior facet of the subtalar articulation, the calcaneofibular ligament must be cut. If the lateral side of the ankle is to be explored, the anterior talofibular ligament must also be cut to permit dislocation of the talus medially (Fig. 12-5, *C*).

The disadvantage of this incision is that it necessitates the cutting of tendons and ligaments. Also, it is notorious for its poor healing. An anterolateral incision is preferable.

Lateral approach to sinus tarsi (Grice, 1952; Westin and Hall, 1957). Exposure of the sinus tarsi is readily performed through a short lateral curvilinear incision. This is the approach typically used in extraarticular arthrodesis of the subtalar joint in children.

The incision is 3 to 4 cm in length. It follows the skin creases from the tip of the lateral malleolus upward and forward and lies directly over the sinus tarsi. The peroneal tendons are located in the posterior extremity of the incision. Care should be taken to avoid cutting the intermediate dorsal cutaneous branch of the superficial peroneal nerve, which lies just at the anterior end of the incision. The cruciate ligament is incised and preserved to facilitate closure. The fat and the loose connective tissue are removed to expose the upper bony borders of the sinus tarsi. The origin of the extensor

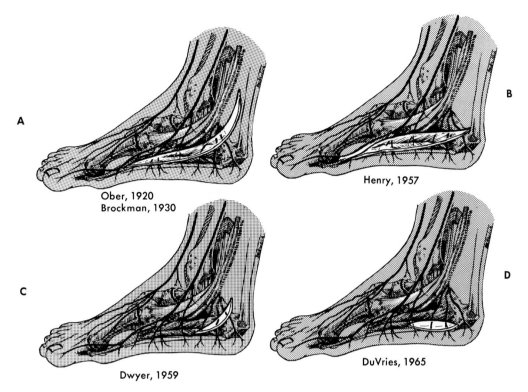

A
Ober, 1920
Brockman, 1930

B
Henry, 1957

C
Dwyer, 1959

D
DuVries, 1965

Fig. 12-6. Medial approaches to plantar structures.

digitorum brevis and the attachments of the interosseous talocalcaneal ligament appear at the floor of the sinus (Fig. 12-2, A).

Approach to subtalar joint (Ollier, 1891). The approach described here essentially uses only the anterior portion of the Kocher incision. It is slightly longer than the limited approach employed by Grice (1952) and Westin and Hall (1957) for extraarticular arthrodesis (Fig. 12-2, A). The approach is adequate for a subtalar or triple arthrodesis.

The incision commences 1 cm below the tip of the lateral malleolus and curves gently upward to terminate over the talonavicular joint. The intermediate dorsal cutaneous nerve crosses the anterior extremity of the incision and should be preserved. The peroneus tertius and long extensor tendons are exposed and must be retracted medially. The peroneal tendons lie distal and posterior to the lateral malleolus. They may be retracted inferiorly. The origin of the extensor digitorum brevis must be detached from its calcaneal attachment and is reflected distally (Fig. 12-5, D).

EXPOSURE OF CALCANEUS AND ADJACENT STRUCTURES
Medial approach to calcaneus (Dwyer, 1959)

The medial approach to the calcaneus can be used to expose the medial side of the calcaneus for osteotomy. It is also well suited for exposure of the soft tissue structures posterior to the medial malleolus and for de-

compression of the posterior tibial nerve in patients with tarsal tunnel syndrome or rupture of the posterior tibial tendon.

The incision begins at the superior aspect of the calcaneus and 1 cm posterior to the medial malleolus. It curves around and slightly distal to the malleolus and terminates at the tuberosity of the navicular. If the incision has been made properly, the saphenous vein and nerve will lie anterior to the incision. The posterior artery and venae comitantes and the posterior tibial nerve are located beneath the retinaculum between the tendons of the tibialis posterior and flexor digitorum anteriorly and the flexor hallucis posteriorly. In exposing the medial side of the calcaneus, the dissection may be carried down superficial to the retinaculum. The retinaculum must be incised to expose the tendons or neurovascular structures for exploration. Several branches of the medial calcaneal nerve course through this area. They should be searched for but unfortunately are rarely observed. These cut nerves will often produce a painful scar (Fig. 12-6, C).

Lateral approach to calcaneus (Banks and Laufman, 1953)

The lateral surface of the calcaneus is readily exposed through a curvilinear incision. This approach may be used for wedge osteotomies of the calcaneus (Dwyer, 1959), for osteomyelitis, or for excision of benign tumors.

The skin incision is 8 to 10 cm in length and parallels the underlying peroneal tendons. It begins at a point approximately 1 cm behind the lateral malleolus, curves with an upward concavity (just distal to the tip of the lateral malleolus), and terminates proximal to the base of the fifth metatarsal. Since the incision follows the course of the sural nerve, which lies in the subcutaneous tissue, the nerve should be sought, exposed, and protected. Occasionally the sural nerve divides into two trunks just past the tip of the lateral malleolus and should be looked for in this approach. The thick subcutaneous tissue may be undercut and reflected to expose the underlying bone (Fig. 12-5, *B*).

Posterior approaches to calcaneus

Circumferential heel incision (Banks and Laufman, 1953). The circumferential heel incision exposes the entire posterior aspect of the calcaneus. It may be employed in open reduction of an avulsion fracture, for osteotomy, or for partial excision of the calcaneus.

With the patient prone, a transverse incision approximately 15 cm long is made along one of the skin creases, extending equally on both sides of the midpoint of the heel. Skin flaps are undercut to permit wide separation of the wound. The entire posterior and inferior aspects of the calcaneus may be exposed (Fig. 12-3, *B*).

Split heel approach (Gaenslen, 1931; Pridie, 1946). The split heel approach has been employed for the complete or partial extirpation of the calcaneus in cases of osteomyelitis (Gaenslen, 1931) or in a markedly comminuted fracture (Pridie, 1946).

The incision is made in the midline of the heel and begins 2 to 3 cm above the attachment of the Achilles tendon to the calcaneus. It extends to the plantar surface of the heel and ends at the level of the calcaneocuboid articulation. The Achilles tendon is split in line with the skin incision for a distance of 2 to 3 cm, as is the plantar aponeurosis. With an osteotome or saw, the calcaneus is cut longitudinally and the two halves are separated. Curettement of abscesses can be done or excision of the calcaneus may be accomplished by shelling out the fragments of bone. The superficial fibers of the Achilles tendon and periosteum, which pass over the bone to become continuous with the plantar fascia, should be preserved (Fig. 12-3, *C*).

Exposure of Achilles tendon

Exposure of the Achilles tendon can be readily accomplished by a straight linear incision placed medially, laterally, or directly posteriorly. A medial approach is generally recommended, however, since cosmetically a scar on the medial side is less apparent. As a rule, the direct posterior approach to the Achilles tendon should be avoided to prevent a scar that would be irritated by shoewear.

Exposure of adventitious Achilles bursa

Normally a bursa is present at the attachment of the Achilles tendon to the calcaneus, which lies between the tendon and the posterosuperior edge of the calcaneus. An adventitious bursa may be present between the skin and the tendon. This superficial bursa is readily approached through a transverse or longitudinal incision. A curved transverse incision located above the edge of the counter of the shoe is perhaps the preferable approach.

Resection of the deep bursa, without an osteotomy of the calcaneus, may be accomplished through a posteromedial or a posterolateral approach.

Posteromedial approach (Fowler and Philip, 1945). A curved transverse incision is made with an upward convexity that is sufficiently high to prevent pressure from the counter of a shoe. The flap is reflected downward. A superficial bursa is readily exposed and if a deeper bursa is to be resected, the upward skin flap may be undermined and retracted upward to expose the Achilles tendon. The tendon is split for a distance of 4 cm and is separated to expose the bursa. A sharp posterior edge of the calcaneus can be rounded, but a transverse osteotomy cannot be performed with ease through this incision (Fig. 12-3, *A*).

Posterolateral approach (Zadek, 1939). A longitudinal incision 5 to 6 cm in length is made lateral to and parallel with the Achilles tendon. The bursa is readily isolated and removed. In addition, any sharp edge of the calcaneus can be smoothed off. If an excisional wedge is to be removed from the calcaneus, the wedge can be taken by extending this incision distally (Fig. 12-5, *A*).

EXPOSURE OF PLANTAR STRUCTURES
Medial approaches to plantar structures

Henry (1957). Since the foot is essentially a half hemisphere that is open medially, structures in the plantar surface are most conveniently approached from the medial side. The skin incision should be located in the overlap area between the medial dorsal cutaneous nerve and the saphenous nerve. The incision begins at the first metatarsophalangeal articulation, proceeds in a smooth curve, passes just below the tuberosity of the navicular, and terminates anterior to the attachment of the Achilles tendon to the calcaneus.

The key to exposure of all the deep structures is the abductor hallucis. By isolating its tendon distally and following the tendon proximally, the surgeon carefully detaches the muscle from its attachments extending from the navicular tuberosity to the inner tuberosity of the calcaneus. The nerve supply to the abductor enters the muscle on its deep side and should be exposed and preserved. The muscle is hinged downward with the plantar flap, thus exposing most of the deep structures in the foot (Fig. 12-6, *B*).

DuVries (1965). A simple and direct approach to expose the tuber portion of the calcaneus and the attachment of the plantar aponeurosis was described by DuVries (1965). It may be employed for a fasciotomy of the aponeurosis, removal of a calcaneal spur, or resection of a benign tumor.

An incision approximately 5 cm long begins just short of the heel and is carried forward along the line of the junction of the thick plantar skin and the side of the heel. The skin with its fascia is slightly undermined to permit retraction, and the deep fascia is exposed. The deep fascia is incised, and the abductor hallucis, plantar fascia, and anteroinferior aspect of the calcaneus are exposed (Fig. 12-6, *D*). Occasionally terminal branches of the medial calcaneal nerve become caught in the scar; this makes the scar quite sensitive and most frequently occurs in the posterior portion of the scar.

Combined posteromedial and plantar exposure (Ober, 1920; Brockman, 1930). It is sometimes necessary to expose the posterior aspect of the ankle and subtalar articulation together with structures on the medial and plantar surfaces of the midfoot. An approach with such exposure is appropriate for a posterior and medial release in resistant clubfoot. The incision is a combination of the posteromedial and medial exposures of the plantar structures.

The incision begins 5 to 6 cm proximal to the medial malleolus and midway between the border of the tibia and the Achilles tendon. It is carried distally, curves around the medial malleolus and along the medial side of the foot, and terminates in the region of the medial cuneiform. The saphenous vein and saphenous nerve lie anteriorly. The posterior flap is reflected to expose the Achilles tendon; the anterior flap is reflected to expose the posterior tibial tendon beneath the deep fascia. From this stage on, the extent of the deep dissection depends on the surgical procedure to be performed. Whatever the procedure, the posterior tibial nerves and vessels must be carefully exposed and retracted if the surgeon wishes to expose the posteromedial aspect of the ankle and subtalar joints. To expose the deep plantar structures, the abductor hallucis must be dissected free of its attachments to the fascia, the navicular, and the calcaneus (Fig. 12-6, *A*).

EXPOSURE OF STRUCTURES OF FOREFOOT

Many incisions are available for the exposure of specific structures on the dorsum of the foot. Since most of these are essentially subcutaneous, only cutaneous nerves, tendons, and certain vessels need be considered. Surgeons generally agree that surgical exposure of the extensor tendons and the metatarsals can be adequately obtained through longitudinal incisions over-

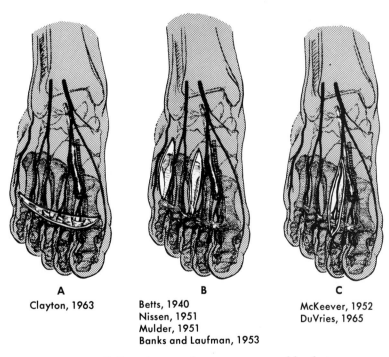

A
Clayton, 1963

B
Betts, 1940
Nissen, 1951
Mulder, 1951
Banks and Laufman, 1953

C
McKeever, 1952
DuVries, 1965

Fig. 12-7. Dorsal approaches to structures of forefoot.

lying and roughly paralleling the appropriate structures (Fig. 12-7, B).

The choice of a surgical approach when dealing with abnormalities in the area of the metatarsophalangeal articulations is not unanimously agreed on among surgeons. Some express grave misgivings concerning the placement of a skin incision on the weight-bearing surface of the foot; others recommend such approaches with impunity, stating that surgical exposure is the important criterion. Neither group has presented unequivocal evidence to cause the widespread adoption of a standard approach. Therefore the individual surgeon must base his choice upon his own experience and upon reports in the literature. I believe that plantar incisions should be avoided when possible.

The most common indications for the use of surgical procedures in this area of the foot are such disorders of the forefoot as dislocation of the metatarsophalangeal articulations (hammertoes), metatarsalgias, and perineural fibromas.

Approaches to metatarsal heads for resection

Resection of the metatarsal heads is a procedure that has proved to be of value in cases of marked deformities of the forefoot caused by the ravages of rheumatoid arthritis. These deformities consist of depression of the metatarsal heads, dorsal luxations at the metatarsophalangeal articulations, and hammertoes. The indication for surgical correction is incapacitating pain on weight bearing. When multiple metatarsal heads are to be resected, I prefer the following incisions: dorsal centered over the first metatarsophalangeal joint, dorsal web space between the second and third metatarsals, and dorsal web space between the fourth and fifth metatarsals. The other incisions are presented for completeness of the discussion.

Transverse plantar approach (Hoffmann, 1911). Hoffmann was one of the first surgeons to perform resections of the metatarsal heads. After experimenting with dorsal approaches, he proposed a plantar incision. A single transverse curved plantar incision is made just proximal to the web of the toes. A plantar flap of fascia and skin is reflected proximally, immediately exposing the metatarsal heads.

The same approach has been recommended by Kaplan (1950) for exposure of the plantar digital nerves, since they lie between the metatarsal heads. The advantage of this incision is its exposure of digital nerves in several interspaces through a single incision (Fig. 12-8, A).

Transverse dorsal approach (Clayton, 1963). After trying many dorsal incisions, Clayton proposed a single transverse dorsal approach to the metatarsal heads. The skin incision is made over the metatarsal heads and curves slightly proximally on the medial side to overlie

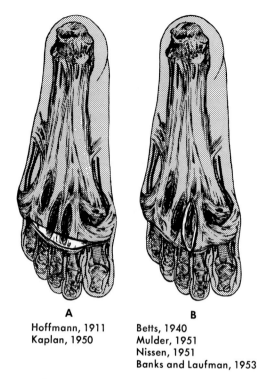

A	B
Hoffmann, 1911	Betts, 1940
Kaplan, 1950	Mulder, 1951
	Nissen, 1951
	Banks and Laufman, 1953

Fig. 12-8. Plantar incisions for exposure of structures in area of metatarsophalangeal articulations.

the first metatarsophalangeal joint. The extensor tendons are exposed and may be retracted or, if markedly contracted, cut in the line of the incision. The incision is opened by depressing the toes and the bases of the proximal phalanges; the metatarsal heads are thereby delivered into the wound. The metatarsals are osteotomized at the junction of the shaft to the head, and the metatarsal heads are dissected free. Only subcutaneous tissue and skin are sutured. If the tendon of the extensor hallucis has been cut, it is resutured (Fig. 12-7, A).

Approaches to digital nerves for removal of perineural fibromas

Longitudinal plantar approach (Betts, 1940). The longitudinal plantar incision was originally proposed as a direct approach to the digital nerves for the removal of perineural fibromas. It offers an excellent view of the digital nerve and preserves the transverse metatarsal ligament. The disadvantages of the incision are (1) it places the scar on the weight-bearing surface and (2) it provides an exposure that is limited to a single metatarsal interspace. This incision is recommended by Mulder (1951), Nissen (1951), and Banks and Laufman (1953).

A straight longitudinal incision is made on the plantar surface of the foot extending from the web between the toes proximally for 3 cm. It is placed midway between the metatarsal heads (Fig. 12-8, B).

Transverse plantar approach (Kaplan, 1950). To avoid placing the scar over the metatarsal pads and to permit exposure of more than a single digital nerve without section of the transverse metatarsal ligament, a transverse incision was proposed for the removal of perineural fibromas. This approach is similar to the one suggested by Hoffmann (1911) for excision of the metatarsal heads.

The incision is placed transversely, slightly distal to the interdigital folds, and may extend from the medial side of the first toe to the lateral side of the fifth toe. The subcutaneous plantar fat is cut in the line of the skin incision to expose the digital extensions of the plantar fascia. The skin with superficial fascia is retracted, exposing the flexor tendon sheaths that lie superficial to the tendons of the lumbrical muscles and transverse metatarsal ligament (Fig. 12-8, A).

Longitudinal dorsal approach (McKeever, 1952; DuVries, 1965). Because of aversion to plantar incisions, many surgeons employ a dorsal approach. Although this avoids placing a scar on the weight-bearing surface, the exposure of the nerve requires deeper dissection and cutting of the transverse metatarsal ligament. Cutting the transverse metatarsal ligament has not been shown to cause any significant postsurgical problems, however.

A skin incision is made between the proper metatarsals, extending proximally from the web for 3 cm. With a hemostat, blunt dissection is achieved between the metatarsal heads. To separate the metatarsal heads adequately for exposure of the digital nerve, the transverse metatarsal ligament must be incised. Firm pressure under the metatarsals will present the nerve. To permit sufficient proximal sectioning of the nerve, it may have to be grasped with a hemostat and delivered into the wound (Fig. 12-7, C).

For exposure of a metatarsophalangeal joint, a skin incision is made between the proper metatarsals starting in the web space and continuing obliquely until centered over the metatarsal head and shaft to be exposed. A direct longitudinal incision over the dorsal aspect of a metatarsophalangeal joint should be avoided because of possible contracture of the scar, which would cause the toe to be held dorsally so it would not touch the ground.

REFERENCES

Banks, S.W., and Laufman, H.: An atlas of surgical exposures of the extremities, Philadelphia, 1953, W.B. Saunders Co.

Betts, L.O.: Morton's metatarsalgia: neuritis of the fourth digital nerve, Med. J. Aust. **1**:514, 1940.

Boyd, H.B.: Surgical approaches. In Crenshaw, A.H., editor: Campbell's operative orthopaedics, ed. 5, vol. 1, St. Louis, 1971, The C.V. Mosby Co.

Brockman, E.P.: Congenital club-foot (talipes equinovarus), Bristol, England, 1930, J. Wright & Sons, Ltd.

Broomhead, R.: Discussion on fractures in the region of the ankle-joint, Proc. R. Soc. Med. **25**:1082, 1932.

Clayton, M.L.: Surgery of the lower extremity in rheumatoid arthritis, J. Bone Joint Surg. **45A**:1517, 1963.

Colonna, P.C., and Ralston, E.L.: Operative approaches to the ankle joint, Am. J. Surg. **82**:44, 1951.

DuVries, H.L.: Surgery of the foot, ed. 2, St. Louis, 1965, The C.V. Mosby Co.

Dwyer, F.C.: Osteotomy of the calcaneum for pes cavus, J. Bone Joint Surg. **41B**:80, 1959.

Fowler, A., and Philip, J.F.: Abnormality of the calcaneus as a cause of painful heel: its diagnosis and operative treatment, Br. J. Surg. **32**:494, 1945.

Gaenslen, F.J.: Split-heel approach in osteomyelitis of os calcis, J. Bone Joint Surg. **13**:759, 1931.

Gatellier, J., and Chastang: La voie d'accès juxtarétropéronière dans le traitement sanglant des fractures melléolaires avec fragment marginal postérieur, J. Chir. **24**:513, 1924.

Grice, D.S.: An extra-articular arthrodesis of the subastragalar joint for correction of paralytic flatfeet in children, J. Bone Joint Surg. **34A**:927, 1952.

Henry, A.K.: Extensile exposure, ed. 2, Baltimore, 1957, The Williams & Wilkins Co.

Hoffmann, P.: An operation for severe grades of contracted or clawed toes, Am. J. Orthop. Surg. **9**:441, 1911.

Jergesen, F.: Open reduction of fractures and dislocations of the ankle, Am. J. Surg. **98**:136, 150, 1959.

Kaplan, E.B.: Surgical approach to the plantar digital nerves, Bull. Hosp. Joint Dis. **11**:96, 1950.

Kocher, T.: Textbook of operative surgery, ed. 3 (translated by H.J. Stiles and C.B. Paul), London, 1911, A. & C. Black.

McKeever, D.C.: Surgical approach for neuroma of plantar digital nerve (Morton's metatarsalgia), J. Bone Joint Surg. **34A**:490, 1952.

McLaughlin, H.L., and Ryder, C.T.: Open reduction and internal fixation for fractures of the tibia and ankle, Surg. Clin. North Am. **29**:1523, 1949.

Mulder, J.D.: The causative mechanism in Morton's metatarsalgia, J. Bone Joint Surg. **33B**:94, 1951.

Nicola, T.: Atlas of surgical approaches to bones and joints, New York, 1945, The Macmillan Co.

Nissen, K.I.: The etiology of Morton's metatarsalgia, J. Bone Joint Surg. **33B**:293, 1951.

Ober, F.R.: An operation for the relief of congenital equino-varus deformity, J. Orthop. Surg. **2**:558, 1920.

Ollier, L.: Traité des résections et des opérations conservatrices qu'on peut practiquer sur le système osseux, vol. 3, Paris, 1891, G. Masson.

Patrick, J.: A direct approach to trimalleolar fractures, J. Bone Joint Surg. **47B**:236, 1965.

Picot, G.: L'intervention sanglante dans les fractures malléolaires, J. Chir. **21**:529, 1923.

Pridie, K.H.: A new method of treatment for severe fractures of the os calcis: a preliminary report, Surg. Gynecol. Obstet. **82**:671, 1946.

Scaglietti, O.: Tecnica e risultati dell'artrodesi della tibiotarsica, Chir. Organi Mov. **26**:244, 254, 1940.

Westin, G.W., and Hall, C.B.: Subtalar extra-articular arthrodesis: a preliminary report of a method of stabilizing feet in children, J. Bone Joint Surg. **39A**:501, 1957.

Zadek, I.: An operation for the cure of achillobursitis, Am. J. Surg. **43**:542, 1939.

13

Major surgical procedures for disorders of the ankle, tarsus, and midtarsus

ROGER A. MANN

THE ANKLE
Open reduction of fractures about the ankle

If closed reduction fails to reposition all articular surfaces of the ankle mortise accurately, open reduction and internal fixation are indicated.

Fractures of internal malleolus. The saphenous nerve crosses the medial malleolus midway between the anterior and posterior borders of the malleolus. The nerve can be palpated by passing one's fingernail across the skin. The nerve is felt as a taut cord between the fingernail and the underlying bone. It should be avoided, since its injury or section may produce annoying symptoms. To avoid the nerve, either a posteromedial or an anteromedial approach can be used (Chapter 12).

In the posterior approach, care should be taken not to open the sheath of the posterior tibial tendon or to lacerate the tendon. The posterior approach will avoid the saphenous nerve but affords a less satisfactory view of the interior of the ankle joint. The anteromedial approach, if extended distally, is more likely to interrupt the saphenous nerve, but this approach provides a better view of the interior of the ankle joint and enables the surgeon to check the accuracy of the reduction.

The distal fragment of the medial malleolus is usually slightly displaced anteriorly. After the fracture site is exposed, soft tissue imposition should be looked for and any tissue found should be removed. The malleolar fracture can be reduced and fixed with a towel clip while a screw or pin is placed through the distal tip of the malleolus into the shaft of the tibia.

Fractures of lateral malleolus. The sural nerve passes along the posterior border of the lateral malleolus and can be palpated beneath the skin between the

examiner's fingernail and the underlying bone. Preliminary palpation will help avoid interruption of this nerve.

The lateral malleolus is exposed through a direct longitudinal incision placed over the malleolus. Fractures of the lateral malleolus are usually spiral in nature and occur at the level of the joint or above the joint in the distal shaft. In the latter case the examiner should suspect a possible tibiofibular diastasis. The fracture can usually be reduced with ease and fixed with an intermedullary pin or screw.

Fractures of posterior lip of tibia (trimalleolar fracture; Cotton's fracture). An isolated fracture of the posterior lip of the tibia occurs infrequently; however, it is a common fracture in conjunction with fractures of the malleoli with posterior dislocation of the ankle joint. More than any other type of fracture, it is one that requires open reduction and an accurate realignment of the fragments. Usually the fracture occurs on the lateral side of the plafond; the talus is rotated and displaced backward and laterally.

The posterior aspect of the ankle joint can be approached through a posterolateral or posteromedial incision. A 10 cm linear incision is made 1.5 cm medial or lateral to the Achilles tendon. The tendon is retracted either laterally or medially. The dissection is carried down through the loose fatty areolar tissue until the posterior aspect of the joint is encountered. The tendon of the flexor hallucis longus is located as it crosses the posterior capsule from the lateral side toward the medial side. The tendon is retracted medially, and the posterior aspect of the ankle joint is exposed. By keeping lateral to the tendon of the flexor hallucis longus, the surgeon avoids the posterior tibial vessels and the nerve. The fracture can be readily located, and the upwardly displaced posterior lip of the tibia is corrected with a towel clip. After visual confirmation of the reduction, the surgeon may fix the reduction by the insertion of a stainless steel nail or a screw. Since accurate alignment is mandatory, radiographs should be taken after reduction and before closure.

Fractures of anterior lip of tibia. Fractures of the anterior tip of the tibia require accurate reduction. The anterior aspect of the tibia is best exposed through an anteromedial approach. The incision is made in the space between the anterior tibial tendon and the extensor tendons; the tendons are displaced medially to expose the anterior aspect of the joint.

After reduction is carried out, the fragments may be fixed with stainless steel pins or screws.

Arthrodesis of the talocrural (ankle) joint

Many methods to arthrodese the ankle have been reported in the literature. The selection of one particular procedure over others has been influenced by such factors as the type of pathologic process present, the preconceived ideas of individual surgeons, and the kind of fusion indicated.

Extraarticular fusions have been done for septic arthritis, particularly for tuberculous destruction of the joint. They have also been used when the surgeon has felt that simultaneous fusion of the ankle and subtalar joints was necessary because of the presence of lesions involving both articulations. Such cases fall into a special category and are discussed separately.

In arthrodeses of the ankle joint alone, the objective is to accomplish good bony apposition between the body of the talus and the mortise; after removal of the articular cartilage from the surfaces of the joint, a loose and sloppy articulation is left. To ensure firm contact between the bony surfaces and to stabilize the joint during the time required for union, various procedures have been employed, including packing bone chips into the space between the bones, using bone grafts to span the joint, and performing osteotomies of one or both of the malleoli to narrow the mortise. Any combination of these methods has been used, with or without additional internal fixation with metal pins, rods, and screws.

Most of the basic operations were introduced by the pioneers in orthopaedic surgery at the beginning of this century. An excellent historical review with an extensive bibliography of earlier operative procedures was published in 1946 by Schwartz. Only minor modifications have been introduced by individual surgeons who felt that their contributions either improved the chances of fusion or decreased the time required to achieve a firm union.

The methods used to arthrodese the ankle joint may be divided into the four categories listed below. Figs. 13-1 through 13-4 offer a pictorial summary of the various procedures.

1. Intraarticular bone graft
2. Malleolar osteotomy
3. Anterior tibial graft
4. Compression arthrodesis

Intraarticular bone graft. The ankle joint has been exposed through various incisions—including a lateral J-shaped incision (Schwartz, 1946), the anterolateral approach (Anderson, 1945; Cramer, 1910; Hallock, 1945; Lasker, 1923; Vahvanen, 1969), and the approach that employs two linear incisions, one along the anterior border of the lateral malleolus and a second along the anterior margin of the medial malleolus (Barr and Record, 1953).

After denuding all cartilage from the articular surfaces to expose bleeding bone, the surgeon fills the joint space with bone chips either "fish-scaled" from the tibial and talar surfaces (Hallock, 1945) or secured from the iliac crest or the anterior surface of the tibia (Fig. 13-1, A). Chuinard and Peterson (1963) inserted a wedge graft taken from the iliac crest between the plafond of the tibia and the talus (Fig. 13-1, B). This method of arthrodesis is particularly applicable to young persons, whose epiphyses are still open.

Malleolar osteotomy. The need to achieve a snug fit between the trochlea of the talus and the mortise after removal of the articular cartilage was recognized early.

Goldthwait (1908) proposed narrowing the mortise by performing an osteotomy of the fibula and displacing the fibula medially. Several modifications of this procedure have appeared (Adams, 1948; Horwitz, 1942). Glissan (1949) and Cordebar (1956) osteotomized the medial malleolus. Mead (1951) osteotomized both malleoli. Wilson (1969) osteotomized only the anterior halves of both malleoli to avoid possible injury to or malfunction of the tendons of the peroneal and posterior tibial muscles (Fig. 13-2).

Various incisions were employed by the several surgeons, depending on the required exposure.

Anterior tibial graft. The anterior tibial graft has been an old and popular method of arthrodesis (Fig. 13-3). It appears to have been first employed by Cramer (1910), Lasker (1923), and Campbell (1929).

The ankle joint is exposed through an anterior approach. After denuding the articular cartilage from the joint surfaces and correcting the deformity, the surgeon cuts a bone graft from the anterior aspect of the tibia, places it across the joint, and affixes it to the talus and the tibia with screws (Fig. 13-3, A). A modification of this procedure proposed by Hatt (1940) was popularized by Brittain (1942), in which the tibial graft is embedded

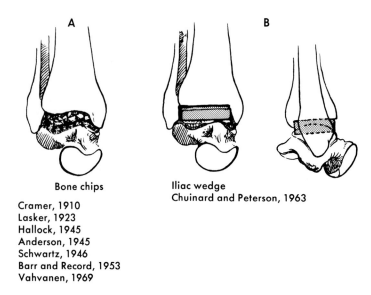

Bone chips

Cramer, 1910
Lasker, 1923
Hallock, 1945
Anderson, 1945
Schwartz, 1946
Barr and Record, 1953
Vahvanen, 1969

Iliac wedge
Chuinard and Peterson, 1963

Fig. 13-1. Arthrodeses of talocrural joint using intraarticular bone grafts. **A,** Denuding articular surfaces of cartilage and packing interval with bone chips. **B,** Insertion of single bone graft between plafond and the talus.

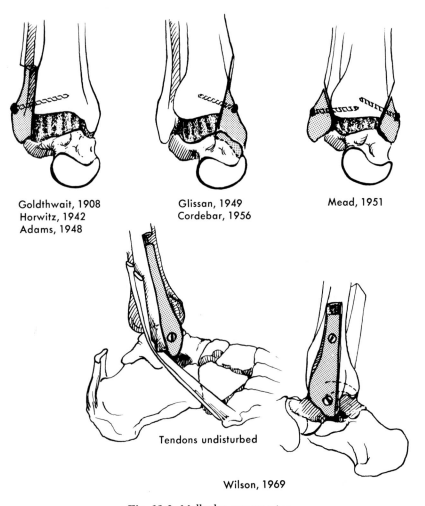

Goldthwait, 1908
Horwitz, 1942
Adams, 1948

Glissan, 1949
Cordebar, 1956

Mead, 1951

Tendons undisturbed

Wilson, 1969

Fig. 13-2. Malleolar osteotomies.

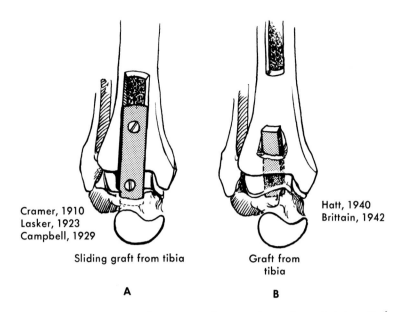

Cramer, 1910
Lasker, 1923
Campbell, 1929

Sliding graft from tibia

A

Hatt, 1940
Brittain, 1942

Graft from
tibia

B

Fig. 13-3. Anterior tibial bone grafts. Anterior bone graft supplements intraarticular fusion.

into the body of the talus through a hole in the plafond (Fig. 13-3, *B*).

Compression arthrodesis. Although Anderson (1945) used an external metal appliance to retain the bones in position and White, in discussing Hallock's (1945) paper, stated that he had been placing pins through the tibia and the calcaneus, which were connected by rubber bands to maintain compression, it was Charnley (1959) who popularized compression arthrodesis (Fig. 13-4).

Charnley employed a transverse incision across the anterior aspect of the ankle joint extending 1 cm above the tip of each malleolus. The extensor tendons were divided, the vessels were ligated and cut, and the nerves were severed. The extensor tendons were resutured during closure. Ratliff (1959), in a review of 55 ankles repaired by Charnley's technique, reported a high percentage of fusion. However, minor complications and disabilities also occurred. These residual conditions included extensor tendons adherent to the scar, persistent mild edema of the foot distal to the incision, persistent numbness over the dorsum of the foot, and a decrease in the power of dorsiflexion of the toes. If this approach is used, the nerves should be preserved.

Jansen (1962) approved the concept of compression arthrodesis but felt that the tranverse incision was unnecessary. He combined compression with the medial and lateral approach of Anderson (1945) and reported 24 out of 25 solid fusions. Dahmen and Mleyer (1965) published an extensive and critical review of their experience with the various methods of fusion of the talocrural joint.

Recommended procedure. In my experience a

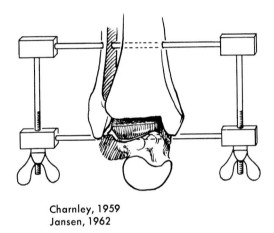

Charnley, 1959
Jansen, 1962

Fig. 13-4. Compression arthrodesis. After removal of articular cartilage from joint surfaces, joints are continuously compressed by means of pins, threaded rods, and wing nuts.

Charnley-type arthrodesis through the anterior approach using an anterior sliding tibial graft has been most successful in the ankle. To avoid the possibility of a thick scar over the anterior aspect of the ankle, the anterior approach should be a lazy **S** skin incision. Extreme caution should be exercised in the anterior approach to be sure the superficial branches of the peroneal nerve are identified and retracted.

The position of choice for an ankle arthrodesis is neutral for dorsiflexion and plantar flexion in men and up 5° of plantar flexion in women. When considering varus and valgus, one must place the ankle in 0° to 5° of valgus. When considering the position at the time of surgery, one must keep in mind the overall alignment of

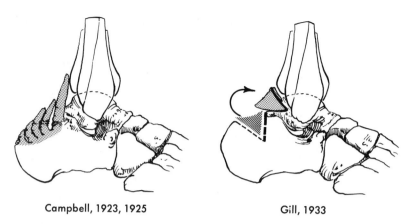

Campbell, 1923, 1925   Gill, 1933

Fig. 13-5. Posterior bone blocks of ankle joint for stabilization of foot.

the entire lower extremity and not just the relationship of the talus to the distal tibia.

Posterior bone blocks

Posterior bone blocks have been employed as supplementary techniques for the stabilization of the foot. The procedures of Campbell (1923, 1925) and Gill (1933) are illustrated in Fig. 13-5. A case of paralytic dropfoot treated by means of the Gill procedure is illustrated in Fig. 13-6.

Indications for these procedures and the Inclan (1949) procedure have been recorded in detail by Branch (1939), Inclan (1949), Ingram and Hundley (1951), and Wheeldon and Clark (1936). When used in conjunction with triple arthrodesis and a lateral stable talotibial joint, the posterior bone block limits plantar flexion by contact with the inferior and posterior articular surfaces of the tibia.

Soft tissue procedures

Surgical repair of ankle ligaments. Severe ligamentous injuries of the ankle often masquerade as sprains. For adequate evaluation, radiographs of the ankle in stressed position must be taken; occasionally, arthrograms are necessary as well.

Collateral ligaments. Complete tears of the collateral ligaments necessitate surgical exploration and repair. In acute cases direct surgical repair of the torn ligaments is possible (Ruth, 1961) (Fig. 13-7). In old cases of instability of the ankle, repair of the old tear, particularly of the anterior talofibular ligament (Broström, 1966), or reconstruction of the collateral ligaments is necessary. Broström has pointed out that even after several years it is possible to adequately dissect out and suture the torn end of ankle ligaments. In a few cases in which the ligamentous tissue was inadequate for direct repair, the anterior talofibular ligament was reconstructed using a flap from the lateral talocalcaneal ligament.

Reconstruction of lateral collateral ligament. The lateral collateral ligament of the ankle is composed of three separate structures. With forceful inversion of the ankle, the susceptibility to rupture of each component appears to be as follows (Francillon, 1962): The anterior talofibular ligament is most likely to be torn. This will usually occur with the ankle in plantar flexion when the anterior talofibular ligament is in line with the fibula. With further inversion, disruption of the calcaneofibular ligament occurs in addition to the tear of the anterior talofibular ligament (Ruth, 1961). Isolated tears of the calcaneofibular ligament are infrequent and occur only if the foot is inverted while in a position of full dorsiflexion. In full dorsiflexion the calcaneofibular ligament is in line with the fibula. This ligament is usually torn when the person steps in a hole, which forces the ankle into a dorsiflexed position. Tears of the posterior talo-fibular ligament seem to occur rarely if at all (Anderson and LeCocq, 1954; Ashhurst and Bromer, 1922).

Various procedures for the reconstruction of the lateral collateral ligament have been employed. Elmslie (1934) attempted to replace the injured ligaments anatomically with a strip of fascia lata (Fig. 13-8). His procedure demonstrated an appreciation of the mechanical relationships that exist between the arrangement of the ligaments and the axes of motion of the ankle and subtalar joints. Some surgeons have questioned the durability of fascia for the repair and have preferred to use tendon. Kelikian (1980) used the plantaris tendon to anatomically reconstruct the torn ligaments.

The obvious availability of the peroneal tendons led to their use in these procedures, which differed only according to the personal ingenuity of the surgeon who employed the handy structures. Unfortunately the anatomic arrangements resulting from these procedures placed the newly formed collateral ligaments in such a position as to always compromise the subtalar motion. The Chrisman and Snook (1969) reconstruction fairly

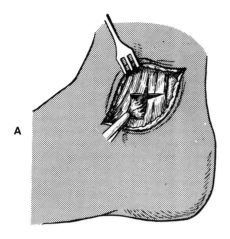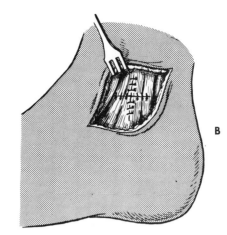

DuVries, 1965

Fig. 13-11. DuVries' technique for reconstruction of deltoid ligament. **A,** Vertical incision into ligament bisected at center by transverse incision. Resulting four right-angular flaps of ligament are denuded and freed from bone. **B,** Four flaps sutured to form cross-shaped scar, which stabilizes ankle.

the muscle is at its rest length. If the muscle is activated when it is shorter or longer than its rest length, it will generate less force. Rest length can be determined by gently pulling the tendon and estimating the increase in passive resistance to further stretching. The rest length is the point at which passive resistance can first be determined by the surgeon. Thus the tendon should be implanted in bone with only minimum tension and with the skeletal part in the position of maximum function.

Because of the multiplicity of factors that must be considered, each case presents a unique problem that the surgeon must consider carefully before he attempts a solution by means of a tendon transfer.

Synovectomies. Synovectomies have had a long and variegated history. The reader interested in an excellent historical review may consult the article by Geens (1969).

London (1955) rekindled enthusiasm for synovectomy of the knee in rheumatoid arthritis, and the literature since then has been copious. With the increasing popularity of synovectomy of the knee, the procedure has been applied to almost every joint. This operation is useful for relieving pain in the active stages of the disease before joint destruction has occurred. Heywood (1967), Jakubowski (1970), Murray (1972), Vahvanen (1968), and Whitefield (1967) reported on the use of this procedure on the ankle joint.

The most satisfactory approach is the anterolateral, which permits excision of most of the synovial membrane lining at the front and sides of the joint. As much of the synovial membrane in the posterior part of the joint as possible is removed with pituitary rongeur.

Tendon dislocations and subluxations in ankle region. There are several tendons in the region of the ankle that are subject to partial or complete dislocation. These dislocations usually result from twisting injuries to the ankle, but they have been reported to occur spontaneously. The peroneals are by far the most frequently injured tendons.

Mounier-Kuhn and Marsan (1968) published a careful review of 44 cases of tendon dislocation in the ankle. They divided the cases into five groups according to etiology, pathology, and treatment. In readily reducible acute dislocations that are stable after reduction, conservative treatment consisting of reduction and immobilization of the foot in a cast for 6 to 8 weeks may be used. If the reduction is unstable—as in an osteoperiosteal avulsion (Murr, 1961) or a complete tear of the tendon sheath—surgical repair will be indicated.

Several procedures have been employed. Kelly (1920) and Watson-Jones (1955) displaced an osteoperiosteal graft from the malleolus posteriorly (Fig. 13-12, A). DuVries (1965) cut a wedge-shaped bone graft from the malleolus, displaced it posteriorly, and fixed it with a screw. At the same time the redundant sheath of the peroneal tendons was excised and the tendon sheath repaired (Fig. 13-12, B). These procedures deepened the sulcus and prevented recurrences of the dislocation.

Daimant-Berger (1971) and Mounier-Kuhn and Marsan (1968) plicated and resutured the tendon sheath. Weigert (1969) tightened the sheath by suturing its border to the fibula through drill holes in the malleolus. Bogutskaia (1970) and Folschveiller (1967) reinforced the sheath with a falp of periosteum that was reflected from the fibula and sutured over the repaired tendon sheath. In chronic dislocations and habitually dislocat-

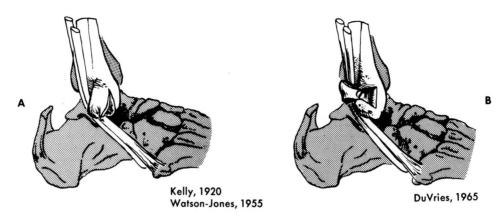

Kelly, 1920
Watson-Jones, 1955

DuVries, 1965

Fig. 13-12. Method of deepening sulcus for prevention of recurrent dislocations of peroneal tendons.

ing tendons, osteotomies of the malleolus are required.

Jones (1932) stabilized the peroneal tendons by reconstructing the retinacular ligament with a flap of Achilles tendon. This is carried out by developing a strip of Achilles tendon, measuring approximately 0.5 × 5 cm, along the lateral aspect. This is left attached to the calcaneus and brought through a drill hole through the widest portion of the fibula. The tendon is then sutured back onto itself.

The posterior tibial tendon may be dislocated from its sulcus behind the medial malleolus, although such an occurrence appears to be quite rare. Muralt (1956) was the first to describe a case. Scheuba (1969), in reporting two cases, stated the opinion that a habitually dislocating posterior tibial tendon may be more common than is indicated from the literature. He pointed out that when individuals complain of instability and pain in the area of the medial malleolus, the possibility of dislocation of the posterior tibial tendon should be kept in mind.

Because of the lack of reported cases, no standard operative procedure has emerged. Based on the experience gained from peroneal dislocations, however, an osteoperiosteal flap from the medial malleolus similar to that in the procedure used by Kelly and Watson-Jones on the lateral malleolus seems indicated.

THE TARSUS
Posterior tarsus

Subtalar and triple arthrodeses. During the first two decades of the twentieth century, the problem of treatment of the deformed or flail foot occurring as a sequela to poliomyelitis occupied the attention of the orthopaedist. The necessity of stabilizing the articulations of the posterior tarsus was apparent.

The surgical solution to this problem was attempted with two ideas in mind: one was to achieve greater stability by obliterating or limiting ankle and subtalar mo-

tion; the other was to displace the foot posteriorly so the body weight would pass more nearly through the midfoot. A variety of surgical procedures were proposed and carried out by different surgeons, ranging from talectomy to pantalar arthrodesis. The majority of the operations were intended to correct pes cavus and to stabilize the subtalar and transverse tarsal articulations (Davis, 1913; Dunn, 1928; Hoke, 1921; Jones, 1908; Ryerson, 1923). Numerous modifications, with adjuvant procedures such as tendon transfers, have been used. Some of these procedures have withstood the test of time; others have been abandoned.

Subtalar and triple arthrodeses are now done less frequently, since the deformities resulting from poliomyelitis no longer constitute a major part of the practice of orthopedics. Excellent reviews and discussions concerning surgical arthrodeses, particularly in poliomyelitis, have been presented (Crego and McCarroll, 1938; Hart, 1937; Hallgrímsson, 1943; Schwartz, 1946).

Although the need for a variety of procedures to deal with the multiplicity of disabilities resulting from poliomyelitis is currently not so great, indications for subtalar and triple arthrodeses in specific cases still remain. From the numerous methods employed in the past, two have proved useful and have become accepted as standard procedures.

Most of the triple arthrodeses carried out today are performed to correct the residuals of trauma. In the majority of these the trauma was a fracture of the calcaneus that extended into the subtalar and transverse tarsal joints. If only the subtalar joint is involved following a fracture of the calcaneus, then only a subtalar arthrodesis need be performed. The transverse tarsal joint can always be added later if it becomes necessary. Thus far, in more than 40 subtalar arthrodesis, I have not found it necessary to add the transverse tarsal joint. In patients in whom little or no correction of the position of the foot is required, the arthrodeses can be car-

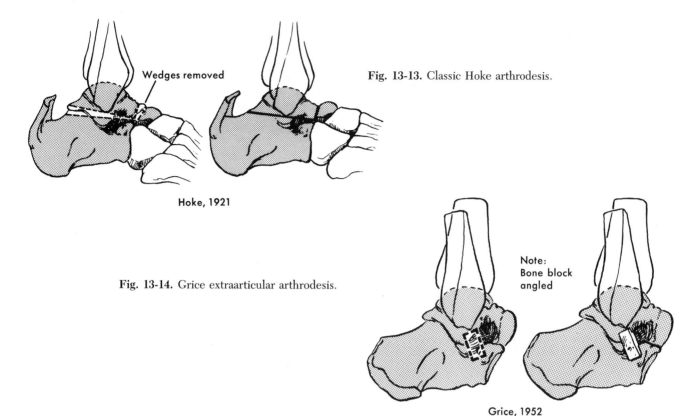

Hoke, 1921

Fig. 13-13. Classic Hoke arthrodesis.

Fig. 13-14. Grice extraarticular arthrodesis.

Note:
Bone block
angled

Grice, 1952

ried out by using inlays of bone graft into the tarsal joints to effect adequate stabilization and eventual fusion. When a triple arthrodesis is carried out, stabilization of the joints should be achieved by the use of staples, pins, or other fixation devices. In this manner the foot can be well aligned at the time of the surgical procedure, which will ensure the patient a plantigrade foot.

When carrying out a triple arthrodesis, two incisions permit better visualization of the arthrodesis sites. The first incision is a lateral approach that is made from the tip of the fibula to the base of the fourth metatarsal. This straight-line incision provides adequate exposure to the subtalar joint and the calcaneocuboid joint. The medial or dorsomedial incision is centered over the talonavicular joint, which permits adequate exposure of this area. When carrying out a triple arthrodesis, the addition of bone should be left to the discretion of the surgeon and depends on the type of fusion that is being attempted. I do not find it necessary to add bone when doing a subtalar or triple arthrodesis, since taking down the joint surfaces creates good bony apposition. If an inlay technique is being used to perform the arthrodesis, then bone graft material is necessary.

Occasionally a specific type of arthrodesis is indicated to correct a certain bony abnormality. The Beak triple arthrodesis, as advocated by Siffert et al. (1966, 1983),

is useful in correcting a severe pes cavus deformity. The procedure is discussed in detail on p. 297.

The first of the previously mentioned triple arthrodeses that has become a standard procedure is the Hoke arthrodesis, with numerous modifications (Fig. 13-13). It is an intraarticular arthrodesis and is useful for painful arthritic processes involving the subtalar and transverse tarsal articulations.

The second is the extraarticular arthrodesis of Grice (Fig. 13-14), which is useful in blocking subtalar motion in patients who have no gross skeletal deformities but have instability of the hindfoot. The Grice arthrodesis is particularly applicable in children, since there is little interference with future growth of the foot.

In the Grice extraarticular arthrodesis, the operative technique is relatively simple. The region of the sinus tarsi is exposed through a short curvilinear incision extending from the peroneal tendons to the extensor tendons. The ligamentous structures and adipose tissue are removed from the sinus tarsi. The origin of the extensor digitorum brevis is dissected from the calcaneus and reflected distally, allowing complete visualization of the interval between the talus and the calcaneus. With an osteotome, slots are cut in the inferior surface of the talus and the superior surface of the calcaneus. The surgeon should recall the direction of the axis of the subtalar joint; the graft, to provide adequate stabilization,

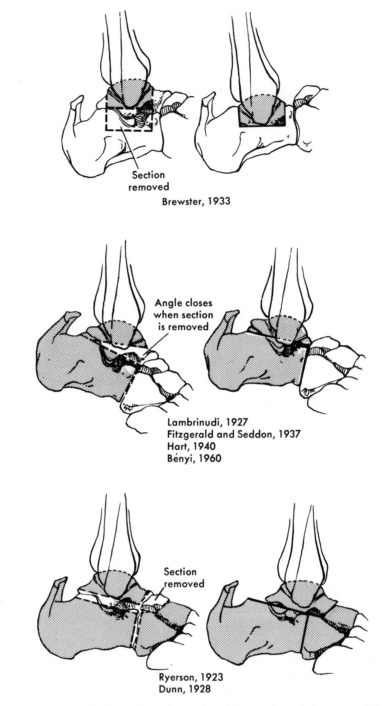

Section
removed

Brewster, 1933

Angle closes
when section
is removed

Lambrinudi, 1927
Fitzgerald and Seddon, 1937
Hart, 1940
Bényi, 1960

Section
removed

Ryerson, 1923
Dunn, 1928

Fig. 13-15. Arthrodeses formerly employed for paralytic deformities of foot.

must lie in a plane that is perpendicular to this axis (Fig. 13-14). Thus the graft should run distally and anteriorly; otherwise it will not block motion of the subtalar joint and may become displaced. The graft may be taken from the anterosuperior surface of the tibia or from the iliac crest.

There are several other surgical methods of arthrodesing the articulations of the hindfoot. These pro-cedures were formerly employed for paralytic deformities and are depicted in Fig. 13-15. The surgeons advocating each procedure are indicated. The *beak* triple arthrodesis as advocated by Siffert et al. (1966, 1983) is most useful for correction of a severe cavus deformity (Fig. 13-16).

Combined talonavicular, talocrural, and pantalar arthrodesis. Orthopaedic surgeons disagree as to the

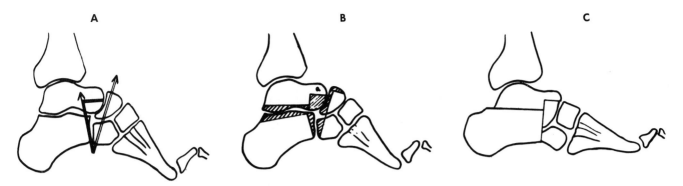

Fig. 13-16. **A,** In beak triple arthrodesis a large wedge is planned as in routine triple arthrodesis. Only inferior cortex of talus is osteotomized, however, and surgeon must be careful not to disturb dorsal talar soft tissues. **B,** Hatching indicates bone removed in procedure. **C,** Final position after forefoot has been displaced downward and navicular has been locked under talar beak with flattening of foot. (From Siffert, R.S., et al.: Clin. Orthop. **45:**101, 1966.)

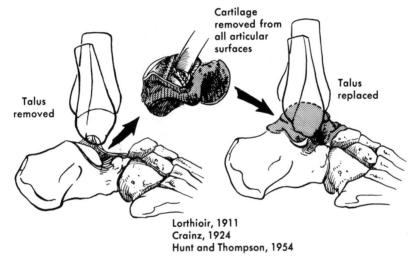

Fig. 13-17. Pantalar arthrodesis accomplished by removing entire talus, denuding it of all its articular cartilage, and reinserting it as a graft.

indications for an arthrodesis of the joints of the posterior tarsus. Furthermore, once the decision has been made to perform such an extensive fusion, there is further disagreement as to the best procedure to follow.

Lorthioir (1911), who originally reported the results of such an operation, extirpated the entire talus and replaced it as a free graft to achieve a pantalar arthrodesis. The same procedure (Fig. 13-17) was reported by Crainz (1924) and by Hunt and Thompson (1954); however, most orthopaedic surgeons appear to have been fearful of the possibility of necrosis of the talus when it is employed as a free graft and have used other methods (Marek and Schein, 1945). Whereas Crainz (1924), Hamsa (1936), Hunt and Thompson (1954), Lorthioir (1911), Steindler (1923), and Waugh et al. (1965) did their fusions in a single stage, Liebolt (1939) and Pat-

terson et al. (1950) believed fewer complications resulted when the fusion was performed in two stages, with either the subtalar or the talocrural joint being fused first.

Various approaches have been recommended, depending on the surgical procedure to be used. If a single-stage arthrodesis is to be performed, the most popular surgical incisions appear to be the anterolateral or the Kocher incisions. When an anterior bone graft and/or a posterior bone graft are being considered, the preferred combination seems to be the anterolateral and posterolateral incisions.

The methods employed to achieve bony stabilization of both the talocrural and the subtalar articulations may be divided into two general categories: (1) those that are essentially intraarticular, in which the cartilage is

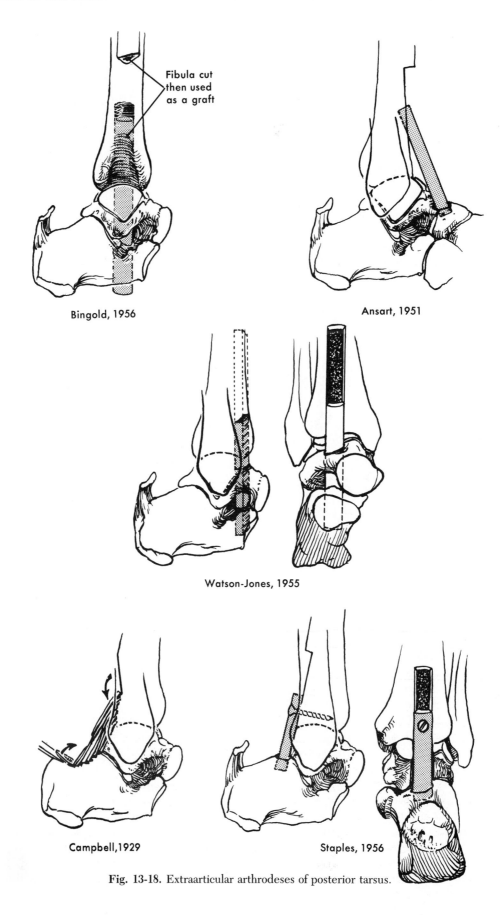

Fibula cut then used as a graft

Bingold, 1956

Ansart, 1951

Watson-Jones, 1955

Campbell, 1929

Staples, 1956

Fig. 13-18. Extraarticular arthrodeses of posterior tarsus.

denuded from all articular surfaces of the respective joints, and (2) those that are extraarticular, depending on various types of bone grafts to span the joints. The procedures employed are summarized in Fig. 13-18. Names of the surgeons are indicated under each drawing.

Talectomy (astragalectomy). Talectomy is a surgical procedure that has been performed for many years. The first talectomy was done in 1608, probably by Fabricius Hildanus, for a compound fracture. After that time the procedure was mainly used for fracture or disease.

In 1901 Whitman published a report of 13 cases of paralytic talipes of the calcaneus type that he had managed by telectomy. For 20 years the procedure gained popularity in treatment of calcaneus and calcaneal valgus feet. It was also found useful in flail feet, especially when caused by poliomyelitis and not associated with varus or equinus deformities. The reason for the apparent success of talectomy was that it provided enough laxity of the tissues in both the equinus and the varus deformities to permit correction without tension. Furthermore, the false joint between the mortise and the calcaneus was sufficiently stable when the foot was plantigrade to permit weight bearing.

Following a peak of popularity during the late 1920s, the enthusiasm for this procedure began to wane. Dunn (1930) stated that "the operation of astragalectomy should not now be taught or practised for the treatment of any type of paralytic deformity of the foot." Commendatory reports continued to appear in the orthopaedic literature, however. Thompson (1939), in an excellent review, surveyed 2066 records and reported on a sample of 100 patients who had undergone talectomy. His conclusions were that the foot can be corrected and stabilized by removal of the talus, that in children the deformity is apt to recur with growth, and that disabling pain is likely to occur in patients over 15 years of age. Tompkins et al. (1956) stated that "astragalectomy does not deserve either wholesale condemnation or unqualified praise."

With proper application and indications, talectomy remains an excellent procedure. Besides having been used for the correction of paralytic deformity, it has also been employed for diverse pathologic conditions such as osteoblastoma or osteoid osteoma, osteogenic sarcoma, giant cell tumor, Ewing sarcoma, tuberculosis, fracture and posttraumatic arthritis, and occasionally osteomyelitis. Excision of the talus for traumatic fracture or fracture-dislocation has been done, and the procedure has been used for spina bifida and arthrogryposis multiplex congenita (Menelaus, 1971), for the correction of untreated clubfoot in adults, and for rheumatoid arthritis (Murray, 1972).

With the increasing interest in prosthetic replacement of skeletal parts, talectomy for aseptic necrosis following fractures of the talus has been performed. Sohier (1952, 1952-1953), Boron and Viarnaud (1958), and Queinnec and Quinnec (1971) replaced the excised talus with a plastic reproduction and reported favorable results.

The criteria for a good result with talectomy are (1) even weight distribution on the plantar surface in both stance and gait, (2) good lateral stability, (3) an ankle axis that is forward and at a right angle to the long axis of the foot, (4) limited ankle motion, especially in dorsiflexion, (5) no pain, (6) no necessity for external support, and (7) a good appearance of the foot.

A talectomy may be performed by one of several methods. Whitman (1901) approached the talus through a curved posterolateral incision extending from the attachment of the Achilles tendon, passing below the lateral malleolus, and terminating over the head of the talus. The two peroneal tendons were freed and were either retracted distally or divided. The lateral collateral ligaments of the ankle were cut and the foot was inverted, exposing the talus, which was extracted with comparative ease after the inferior talocalcaneal (interosseous) ligament was severed.

More recently, as talectomy has been employed in avascular necrosis and rheumatoid arthritis, the anterolateral approach has been widely used. In such an approach the talus is readily extirpated with minimum disruption of the supporting soft tissue structures. After the dorsal capsule has been detached and the inferior talocalcaneal ligament in the sinus tarsi cut, the talus is scooped out totally with a curved gouge. To achieve a better fit between the mortise and the superior surface of the calcaneus in cases in which no prosthetic replacement is being considered, it may be necessary to remove a portion of the malleoli and reshape the posterior facet of the calcaneus so the tibial plafond contacts the calcaneus below and the navicular in front.

Although many surgeons prefer arthrodeses and/or tendon transfers for stabilization of a paralytic foot, these procedures are not universally accepted because they often give unpredictable results. The method of talectomy described by Whitman was once judged the best procedure for the stabiization of a paralytic foot by the American Orthopaedic Surgery Committee.

External rotation of the foot not compensated for by internal rotation of the leg in gait can be corrected by osteotomy of the tibia as a secondary procedure, but it is rarely necessary. An important point in the surgical technique is to avoid aligning the foot with the patella, for doing so may lead to an unstable foot with a varus deformity.

The calcaneus

Open reduction and bone grafting for calcaneal fractures. It is well known that the prognosis for fractures involving the articular surfaces of the calcaneus is unfavorable. Accurate realignment of the displaced fragments is mandatory and often can be achieved only under direct vision by an open reduction.

Palmer (1948) stated that in approximately 50% of cases a major longitudinal fracture line through the calcaneus occurs. It extends from the medial side upward and laterally, splitting the calcaneus into two major fragments. The fracture passes through the posterior facet of the calcaneus. The lateral fragment is usually found displaced, and a "ledge" or "step" is produced in the articular surface of the posterior facet. Such fractures are amenable to open reduction and bone grafting. To select the proper cases for such a procedure requires the closest cooperation between the surgeon and the radiologist.

Hazlette (1969), Vestad (1968), and Widén (1954), reported favorable results with open reduction and bone grafting for suitable cases.

The surgical procedure is relatively simple. The calcaneus is approached through a curvilinear incision approximately 15 cm long extending from the back of the calcaneus, passing just below the lateral malleolus, and terminating at the calcaneocuboid articulation. The sheath of the peroneal tendons is incised, and the tendons are displaced forward. The talocalcaneal ligament is divided, and the posterior facet of the talocalcaneal (subtalar) joint is exposed. The heel is carefully inverted to reveal the articular surface of the calcaneus; this allows inspection and assessment of the extent of the injury. With a traction pin through the tuber of the calcaneus and with judicious use of an elevator, the joint surfaces may be realigned. However, the reduction is usually very unstable and a large defect, formed by compression of the cancellous bone, is present. A bone graft from the iliac crest is shaped and driven into the defect and acts as a key to hold the reduction. Hazlette (1969) found it necessary in some cases to use screws to supplement the graft and secure reduction of the major fragments. The degree of stability of the reduction should indicate to the surgeon whether or not the transfixing pin should be incorporated into the cast to ensure that the reduction is maintained during the early stages of healing.

Osteotomies of calcaneus. In the so-called normal or average foot the superincumbent body weight is transmitted through a vertical plane to the talus and thence to the tuberosity of the calcaneus. The axes of the subtalar and ankle joints, when projected onto a transverse plane, intersect in the center of the trochlea (Isman and Inman, 1969). The body of the calcaneus has a medial curve, which brings the tuberosity under the weight-bearing line of the leg. With such an arrangement a metastable state is created that requires minimum muscular effort to maintain. The variations in the position of the axis of the subtalar joint and the variability of the anatomic structure of the calcaneus may cause the weight-bearing line of the leg to fall outside the reaction point on the heel. A moment is thus created that, if not resisted by muscular effort, will cause the foot either to pronate or to supinate.

This situation has been recognized for many years and has led to the development and use of shoe modifications and different types of appliances. Surgical procedures designed to bring the weight-bearing line of the leg within the reaction point on the heel and thus improve alignment have also been devised and are of interest historically. Trendelenburg (1889), in cases of flatfoot, moved the weight-bearing line of the leg laterally by carrying out a supramalleolar varus osteotomy of the tibia and fibula. Gleich (1893) osteotomized the calcaneus, moving its posterior segment downward and to retain the motions of the joints and preserve the elasticity of the foot (Fig. 13-19). Operations that fused the midtarsal region of the foot, popular at that time, sacrificed these elements.

Since the pioneering efforts of certain surgeons, osteotomy of the calcaneus has been used for a variety of deformities of the foot including cosmetic improvement in cases of flatfoot, treatment of congenital flaccid flatfoot, and correction of deformities resulting from spastic or paralytic states. Osteotomy has been employed in pes cavus and pes planus and has consisted of both closing and opening wedges, with and without lateral or medial displacement of the posterior portion of the calcaneus. The purpose of all the osteotomies is to improve the alignment of the weight-bearing structures of the hindfoot; nevertheless, one should be aware that these procedures may also alter the function of the effective lever arms of the muscles acting on the calcaneus. Unfortunately, the effects have not been adequately studied; but in the reported cases supplementary tendon lengthening and transplants have often been necessary.

The calcaneus may be easily approached from either the medial or the lateral side. Gleich (1893) used a "stirrup" incision passing under the heel to expose the inferior aspect of the calcaneus. Few surgeons have employed this, however, since it places a scar on the weight-bearing surface. An opening wedge tends to increase the normal posterior projection of the heel slightly and may make skin closure more difficult. In employing an opening wedge, many surgeons have be-

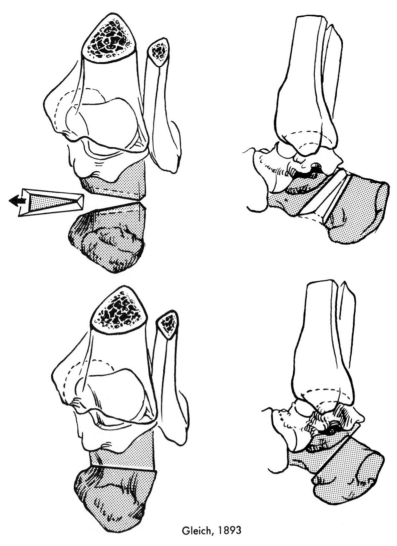

Gleich, 1893

Fig. 13-19. Original osteotomy of calcaneus for correction of flatfoot.

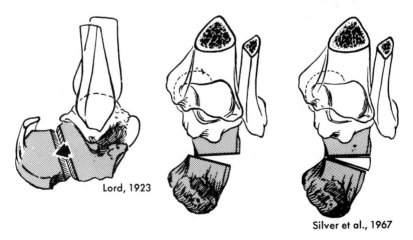

Lord, 1923

Silver et al., 1967

Fig. 13-20. Displacement osteotomies for treatment of flatfoot.
Continued.

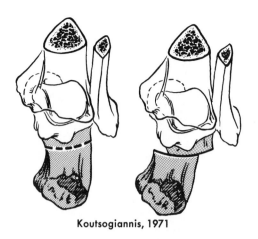

Koutsogiannis, 1971

Fig. 13-20, cont'd. Displacement osteotomies for treatment of flat foot.

lieved the defect must be filled with some type of bone graft. Closing wedges that retain a precise contact of the surfaces are technically a little more difficult to achieve. Furthermore, a closing wedge tends to shorten the heel slightly.

The various types of osteotomies of the calcaneus may be roughly divided into three categories: (1) those that are used to treat valgus deformities (Figs. 13-19 to 13-21), (2) those that are employed to improve cavus feet (Fig. 13-22), and (3) those that are used for specific pathologic conditions.

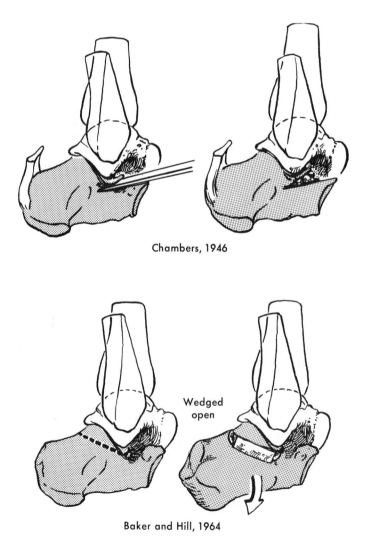

Chambers, 1946

Wedged open

Baker and Hill, 1964

Fig. 13-21. Procedures to restrict pronatory motion without resorting to arthrodesis.

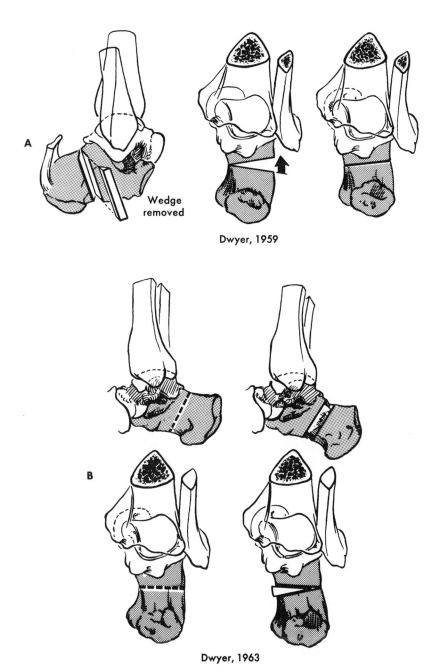

Dwyer, 1959

Dwyer, 1963

Fig. 13-22. Osteotomies for inverted heel and pes cavus. **A,** Original procedure: closing osteotomy on lateral side. **B,** Opening wedge with graft on medial side. Procedure was proposed by Dwyer to replace closing osteotomy, which shortened heel.

THE MIDTARSUS

The surgical correction of some deformities of the foot has been achieved by means of wedge osteotomies or fusions in the area of the midtarsus. Such procedures have been employed in cases of marked pes cavus or pes planus, with or without accompanying adduction or abduction of the forefoot, and in cases in which operative procedures on the hindfoot are not indicated because of the absence of an appreciable varus or valgus of the heel.

Pes cavus

Cole (1940) employed a transverse midtarsal osteotomy to treat pes cavus in patients for whom all types of conservative treatment (e.g., soft tissue releases, manipulations, tendon transfers, casts, and external appliances) had failed. The procedure consisted of the removal of a wedge of bone from the navicular, the cuneiforms, and the cuboid (Fig. 13-23, A); closing of the wedge led to the correction of the deformity. When adduction of the forefoot accompanied the cavus deformity, as in persistent or untreated clubfoot, the direction of the wedge of bone could be changed to correct this added deformity (Fig. 13-23, B).

Pes planus

The term peroneal spastic flatfoot has been loosely applied to the type of flatfoot in which passive correction of the deformity is resisted by contracture and reflex spasm of the peroneal muscles (i.e., a rigid flatfoot). Such resistance is indicative of an irritative lesion in the hindfoot or midfoot. These lesions are frequently found in arthritic processes involving the subtalar and transverse articulations and in various types of tarsal coalition. Since the proper remedial procedure must be based on the precise pathologic condition, a careful physical and radiographic examination of the foot is mandatory.

If the condition is caused by the presence of a calcaneonavicular bar, DuVries has found that excision of the bar through a lateral approach to the sinus tarsi will often relieve the disorder, especially in adolescents (Fig. 13-24). If arthritic changes in the subtalar or transverse tarsal articulations are the etiologic factor, subtalar or triple arthrodesis may be the indicated treatment.

The only kind of flexible flatfoot that requires treatment is symptomatic flatfoot. The cosmetic appearance of the foot is not an indication for surgical procedures. Conservative measures (appliances, e.g., heel wedges, higher heels, shoe inserts) may be employed to improve the appearance of the foot and reduce the concomitant deformation of the shoe.

In most cases of flexible flatfoot, an accompanying valgus position of the hindfoot is present. Since inversion of the heel by various means both improves the appearance of the foot and relieves symptoms, the majority of surgical procedures have been done on the hindfoot (e.g., osteotomies of the calcaneus and subtalar fusions). In some individuals, however, pes planus appears to manifest itself as a vertical collapse of the longitudinal arch without a valgus heel, and in these individuals stabilization procedures of the midfoot are indicated.

Hoke (1921, 1931) and Miller (1927) found that the instability of the medial side of the longitudinal arch appeared to be caused by the malfunctioning of a series of individual articulations between the first metatarsal, the first cuneiform, the navicular, and the head of the talus. Both men believed that stability of the longitudinal arch could be restored without undue loss of mo-

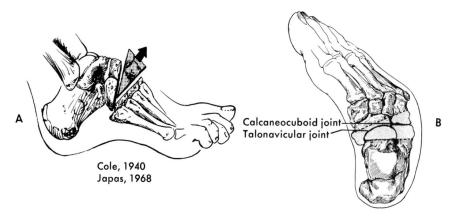

Cole, 1940
Japas, 1968

Calcaneocuboid joint
Talonavicular joint

Fig. 13-23. Midtarsal osteotomies. **A,** For correction of pes cavus. **B,** For correction of pes cavus with adduction of forefoot. (From Crenshaw, A.H., editor: Campbell's operative orthopaedics, ed. 5, vol. 2, St. Louis, 1971, The C.V. Mosby Co.)

bility by arthrodesing some of these articulations. Hoke arthrodesed the naviculocuneiform articulations, using an inlay tibial graft after removing the articular cartilage (Fig. 13-25, *A*). Miller resected the articular cartilage between the navicular and the first cuneiform and, in more severe cases, also between the first cuneiform and the base of the first metatarsal. In such a procedure any abduction of the forefoot could be corrected by removing various sizes of wedges of bone (Fig. 13-25, *B*).

L'Episcopo and Sabetelle (1939) reported their observations of 16 patients with flatfoot after operation by Hoke's procedure; 68% obtained good results and 32% fair results. Butte (1937) reported on 76 feet operated on by Hoke's procedure; results were satisfactory in about 50%. Jack (1953) performed Hoke's operation for flatfoot in 46 cases and obtained satisfactory results in 82%.

Clawing of the great toe—Jones' tendon transfer

In the case of a congenital hammered great toe, the articular surface of the interphalangeal joint is abnormal and soft tissue repair alone will not permanently reduce the deformity. Arthrodesis of the joint as described in Jones' technique without transference of the extensor hallucis longus will usually best correct this condition.

In patients who have developed hyperextension of the metatarsophalangeal joint of the great toe secondary to a combination of weakness of ankle dorsiflexors but with a normally functioning extensor hallucis longus, the Jones technique for transferring the tendon of the extensor hallucis longus and arthrodesing the interphalangeal joint still offers the best results. Forrester-Brown (1938) and Wagner (1934).

1. Make an elliptical transverse incision centered

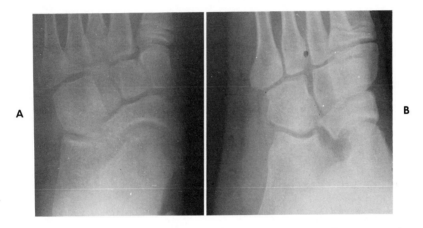

Fig. 13-24. Excision of calcaneonavicular bar. **A,** Preoperative; **B,** postoperative.

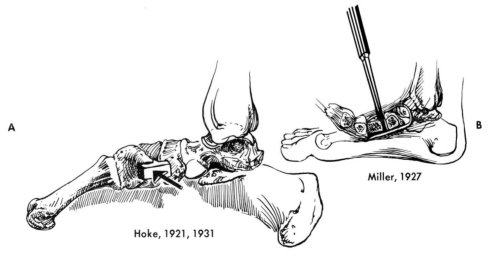

Miller, 1927

Hoke, 1921, 1931

Fig. 13-25. Stabilization procedures. **A,** Bone graft of naviculocuneiform joints. **B,** Arthrodesis of talonavicular joint and cuneiform and first metatarsal without graft.

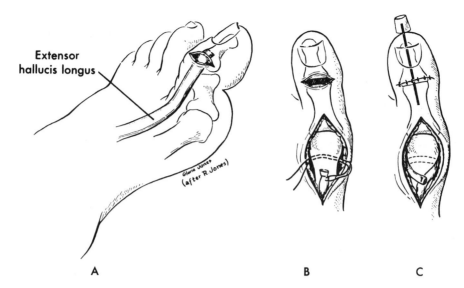

Fig. 13-26. Jones reduction for static clawed great toe. **A,** Incision for cut and release of tendon. **B,** Phalangeal joint denuded of cartilage and tendon threaded through drill hole. **C,** Tendon sutured to itself and pin inserted into arthrodesed phalangeal joint. Exposed pin is covered with cork.

over the interphalangeal joint of the great toe and carry it down through the extensor tendon to bone (Fig. 13-26, *A* and *B*).

2. Remove all articular cartilage from the head of the proximal phalanx and base of the distal phalanx, shortening the former enough to correct any deformity at the interphalangeal joint. The arthrodesis site is then fixed with two threaded Steinmann pins.

3. Make a second longitudinal incision along the border of the extensor hallucis longus tendon, starting at the level of the metatarsophalangeal joint and extending proximally to the middle of the first metatarsal shaft (Fig. 13-26, *B*).

4. Dissect out the extensor hallucis longus tendon both proximally and distally and pull it into the proximal wound.

5. Drill a transverse hole through the first metatarsal just proximal to the metatarsal neck.

6. Thread the extensor tendon through the hole and then, pushing the foot into as much dorsiflexion as possible, suture the extensor tendon back onto itself using interrupted 0 silk sutures (Fig. 13-26, *C*).

7. Close the wounds in a routine manner and place the patient in a short leg cast for a period of 6 weeks.

8. After 6 weeks of immobilization, the tendon transfer has healed but the interphalangeal joint usually requires about 1 month of healing time. We allow the patient to walk in a wooden shoe the last 4 weeks until the interphalangeal joint has become arthrodesed.

REFERENCES

Adams, J.C.: Arthrodesis of the ankle joint: experiences with the transfibular approach, J. Bone Joint Surg. **30B:**506, 1948.

Anderson K.J., and LeCocq, J.F.: Operative treatment of injury to the fibular collateral ligament of the ankle, J. Bone Joint Surg. **36A:**825, 1954.

Anderson, R.: Concentric arthrodesis of the ankle joint: a transmalleolar approach, J. Bone Joint Surg. **27:**37, 1945.

Ansart, M.B.: Pan-arthrodesis for paralytic flail foot, J. Bone Joint Surg. **33B:**503, 1951.

Ashhurst, A.P.C., and Bromer, R.S.: Classification and mechanism of fractures of the leg bones involving the ankle: based on a study of three hundred cases from the Episcopal Hospital, Arch. Surg. **4:**51, 1922.

Baker, L.D., and Hill, L.M.: Foot alignment in the cerebral palsy patient, J. Bone Joint Surg. **46A:**1, 1964.

Barr, J.S., and Record, E.E.: Arthrodesis of the ankle joint, N. Engl. J. Med. **248:**53, 1953.

Bényi, P.: A modified Lambrinudi operation for drop foot, J. Bone Joint Surg. **42B:**333, 1960.

Bingold, A.C.: Ankle and subtalar fusion by a transarticular graft, J. Bone Joint Surg. **38B:**862, 1956.

Bogutskaia, E.V.: Privychnyy vyvikh sukhzuliy malobyertsovykh myshts u sporsmyenov [Habitual dislocation of fibular muscles of athletes], Khirurgiia **46:**83, 1970.

Boron, R., and Viarnaud, E.: Une observation de prothèse astragalienne en acrylique, Mem. Acad. Chir. **84:**549, 1958.

Branch, H.E.: Drop-foot: end results of a series of bone-block operations, J. Bone Joint Surg. **21:**141, 1939.

Brewster, A.H.: Countersinking the astragalus in paralytic feet, N. Engl. J. Med. **209:**71, 1933.

Brittain, H.A.: Architectural principles in arthrodesis, Baltimore, 1942, Williams & Wilkins.

Broström, L.: Sprained ankles. VI. Surgical treatment of "chronic" ligament ruptures, Acta Chir. Scand. **132:**551, 1966.

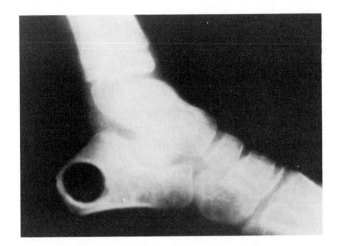

Fig. 14-14. Radiograph taken at time of surgery; dramatically illustrates donor site. Bone debris from subtalar joint is inserted in defect in os calcis, and area rapidly fills in by time patient is ready for weight bearing. (Courtesy S.L. Alban, M.D.)

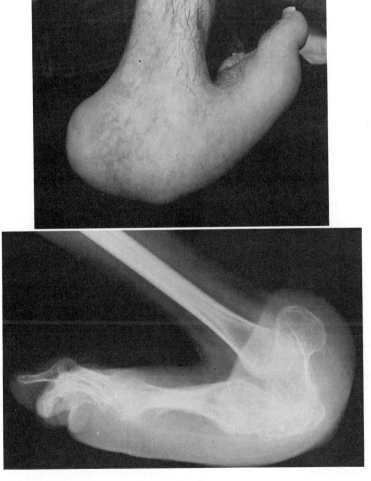

Fig. 14-15. Vertical talus deformity (equinovalgus) can cause pressure areas over prominent head of talus and is impossible to shoe when severe.

ple methods were used. Extensive surgery is necessary, regardless of the method. This is because the deforming tendons must be released and transferred, the contracted ligaments must be released (as in a medial plantar release), and the navicular must be placed in the proper position to the talus (as with equinovarus). Differentiation must be made from those feet correctable by plantar flexion.

Sharrard's technique (1977) requires an interosseus ligament release from the lateral side; lengthening of the Achilles tendon, toe extensors, peroneus tertius, and peroneus longus; and transfer of the peroneus brevis posteriorly to the posterior tibial tendon and of the tibialis anterior to the talar neck. Pins are placed across the talonavicular joint and across the reduced subtalar joint through the heel. The navicular has been excised in some techniques (Clark et al., 1977) to reduce the medial column to obtain reduction. This has not been necessary in my limited series. Menelaus (1980) describes extraarticular subtalar fusion for patients without a functioning anterior tibialis. He states that occasionally the deformity may be seen in feet without any functioning muscle.

In the older more rigid foot, talectomy and calcaneocuboid reduction are performed.

Cavus foot and clawtoes

The cavus foot has a prominent middorsal area with metatarsal heads protruding on the plantar surface and dorsally displaced toes with clawing. In similar sensitive feet, painful callosities develop on the plantar surface and corns arise on the dorsal surface of the toes. In the insensitive foot, these areas become intractable ulcers and special protective shoes must be worn to avoid ulceration. The deformities are usually seen in low-level spinal lesions, notably the sacral level, in patients who have active long toe flexors and extensors but not intrinsic musculature. Occasionally, spastic intrinsic muscles are present in an otherwise paralyzed foot to give a cavus deformity.

Treatment is directed at balancing the forces of the foot, releasing spastic muscles, and correcting the bony deformity. These are generally the feet most successfully treated (Sharrard and Grosfeld, 1968).

The treatment is quite variable, depending on the deformity and its cause. In early childhood, before fixed bony deformities are present, the foot can be treated by release of the plantar fascia and short flexors at the heel and transfer of the long toe flexors to the extensor hood to provide metatarsophalangeal flexion and interphalangeal extension (the Girdlestone procedure of splitting the flexor tendons and bringing half up each side of the proximal phalanx) (Taylor, 1951). I have been transferring the entire flexor tendon to the medial side of the lesser toes to save time and avoid the pos-

sibility of complete neurovascular damage to the toe. This has been successful without causing toe deviation. Sharrard (1976) prefers tenodesis of the flexor tendon of the first toe; however, the Girdlestone transfer has been successful in my hands over the last 8 years without late deformity, and I have performed it in patients of all ages from infancy to adulthood. The extensor tendon may be transferred to the neck of the first metatarsal in older patients at the same time if there is plantar flexion of the first metatarsal or the lesser metatarsals. Rarely is sufficient muscle power present to change the midfoot deformity so that osteotomy of the metatarsals or cuneiform cuboid is required.

Spastic intrinsic muscles can be denervated by cutting the plantar nerves, if the foot is insensitive, or by the Garceau-Brahms (1956) technique of cutting only the motor branches, if sensory nerves are to be spared.

Bony deformities are corrected by cuneiform cuboid osteotomies and, if calcaneus deformities are present, the crescentic osteotomy of Samilson (1976) (Fig. 14-16). The latter must be done in conjunction with release of the plantar ligament.

Plantar ulcers will heal if the bony prominence is removed. This is accomplished by the appropriate correction of the deformities. If chronic infection is present around the metatarsal heads, the cure is excision of the offending metatarsal head and placement of a large metatarsal bar on the bottom of the shoe. The bar gives a rocker effect to the bottom of the shoe, distributing the weight on the sole and decreasing the metatarsophalangeal dorsiflexion on roll-off.

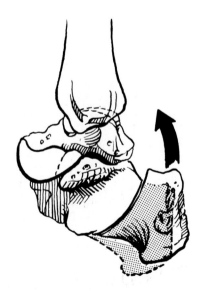

Fig. 14-16. Crescentic osteotomy of Samilson corrects calcaneus deformity and improves posterior lever arm of calcaneus. Healing is as rapid as for closing-wedge osteotomy. (From Samilson, R.: In Bateman, J.E., editor: Foot science, Philadelphia, 1976, W.B. Saunders Co.)

The foot in cerebral palsy

M. MARK HOFFER

A thorough understanding of orthopaedic surgery and cerebral palsy is required before plans are made on a cerebral palsy patient's foot (Banks, 1975; Basset, 1971). It is important to ascertain whether the patient is a potential ambulator. Foot deformities rarely affect the child enough to prohibit ambulation. Neurologic balance is the key to ambulation. If the child has not achieved that balance by the first 6 years of life, he rarely will walk later. Retention of perinatal reflexes in an obligatory fashion over the first few years of life also bodes poorly for the ambulatory or potentially ambulatory child with cerebral palsy. Adults with cerebral palsy, especially those who walk very little, have poor tissue circulation in their feet. One should be very cautious about suggesting reconstructive surgery in these adults, for the complication rates far exceed the rates in children.

The child with motion disorders (athetosis, ataxia, dyskinesia) will have foot deformities that are difficult to analyze. This is because the deformities are inconsistent, are never fixed, and seem to depend to a large degree on writhing postures. Deformities caused by spasticity are easier to analyze, and the results of surgery are more predictable. It is important to differentiate fixed from flexible deformities in the spastic child. The increased tone in the muscles of spastic feet initially results in dynamic deformity, but eventually soft tissue and joint contracture occur.

In the diplegic child with bilateral involvement, the most frequent combination of deformities seems to be equinovalgus; in the hemiplegic spastic child, equinovarus is most often found.

EQUINUS DEFORMITIES

Equinus deformities should not be overtreated, for this may result in the more disabling calcaneus (Banks and Green, 1958). In these children I usually perform stretching exercises; I use progressive walking plasters and braces before resorting to surgical procedures.

Equinus deformities have often been analyzed by the two-joint muscle test (Fig. 14-17). This test uses the

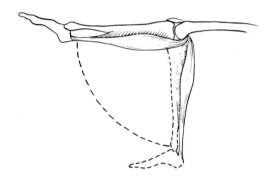

Fig. 14-17. Classic two-joint muscle test to differentiate gastrocnemius contracture from gastrocsoleus contracture.

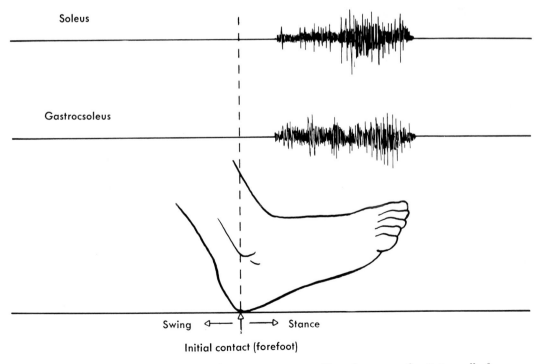

Fig. 14-18. EMG tracing of normal triceps surae gait. Note the onset of activity well after heel strike.

supposed difference in gastrocnemius contracture from gastrocsoleus contracture. I believe most children with cerebral palsy have a positive differential test clinically but not when tested by electromyography (Perry et al., 1974). Electromyograms in gait usually show increased activity of both gastrocnemius and gastrocsoleus in the child with equinus deformities (Figs. 14-18 and 14-19). Therefore I usually advise an Achilles tendon lengthening rather than a gastrocnemius slide.

When performing an Achilles tendon lengthening procedure, I prefer the three-levels cuts—distal and proximal on the medial side and central laterally (Fig. 14-20). I bring the ankle up to neutral only and do not overcorrect. I find this operative procedure works more consistently than the two-level operation, because of the variation in the spiraling of the Achilles tendon fibers from individual to individual. For fear of contracting scars, I do not ever use longitudinal posterior inci-

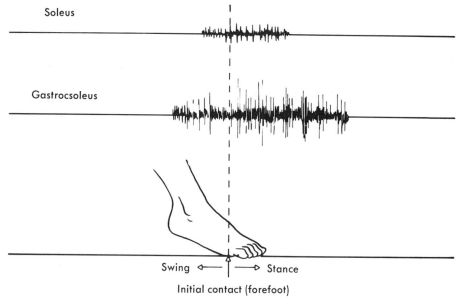

Fig. 14-19. EMG tracing of cerebral palsy equinus gait. Note onset of activity before initial floor contact.

Fig. 14-20. Method of Achilles tendon lengthening through three short transverse skin and tendon incisions.

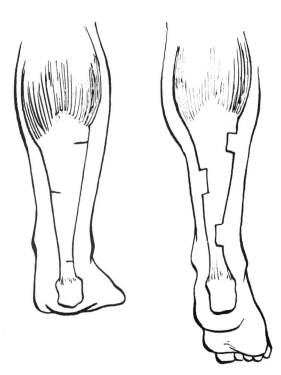

sions. I generally use multiple transverse incisions. The foot is immobilized with a short leg walking cast. The plaster is removed in 4 weeks and a brace is continued for at least a year.

VARUS DEFORMITIES

Varus deformities that are flexible may be caused by overactivity of any of the muscles medial to the ankle joint. The triceps surae and the posterior tibial and anterior tibial muscles are most often implicated. These spastic deformities do not respond well to orthoses or inserts. My general policy is to determine the dynamic deforming force by gait electromyography and perform either anterior tibial or posterior tibial surgery combined with Achilles tendon lengthening if necessary (Figs. 14-21 to 14-23).

The overactive anterior tibial muscle in stance and swing requires a split anterior tibial tendon transfer (Hoffer et al., 1974) (Fig. 14-24). The anterior tibial tendon is split longitudinally from its insertion to the ankle joint by two separate incisions. It is then transferred subcutaneously to the cuboid. Immediate ambulation in a short-leg plaster cast is permitted, and a brace is applied at 4 weeks to be worn for at least 1 year.

The overactive posterior tibial muscle in stance and swing requires lengthening at the musculotendinous junction (Root and Frost, 1971). In the rare situation when a posterior tibial muscle is active exclusively in swing, the muscle is transferred anteriorly (Bisslar and Lewis, 1975; Root, 1971). Here short leg plaster is used and removed in 4 weeks when therapy is begun. When good muscle function occurs (usually 6 to 8 weeks), weight bearing in a brace begins and is continued for at least 1 year. Unfortunely, overcorrection can occur with this posterior tibial tendon transfer (Schneider et al., 1977). Another approach to the problem of varus by split posterior transfer has recently been suggested (King and Hensinger, 1983).

When varus deformities have been allowed to become fixed, calcaneal osteotomy in addition to the aforementioned procedures is advised (Silver et al., 1967).

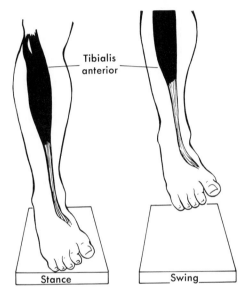

Fig. 14-21. Continuous anterior tibial activity in varus cerebral palsy foot. Here split anterior tibial tendon transfer is performed.

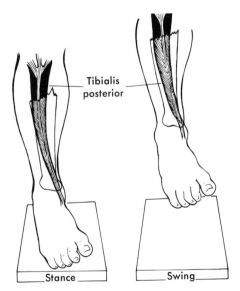

Fig. 14-22. Continuous posterior tibial activity in varus cerebral palsy foot. Here lengthening of muscle is advised.

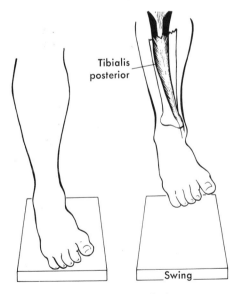

Fig. 14-23. Swing phase posterior tibial activity in varus cerebral palsy foot. Here posterior tibial tendon transfer forward is advised.

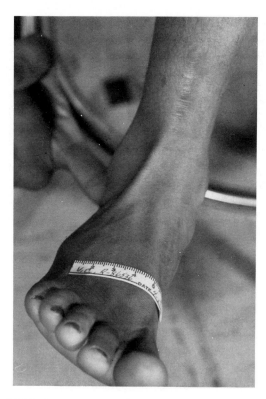

Fig. 14-24. Postoperative appearance of properly performed split anterior tibial tendon transfer. (From Hoffer, M.M., et al.: Orthop. Clin. North. Am. **5**:31, 1974.)

VALGUS DEFORMITIES

Flexible valgus deformities may be caused by hyperactivity of the triceps surae and/or peroneal muscles or to the position of the hips and knees. The adducted hip–valgus knee combination forces weight bearing on the medial aspect of the foot. The surgeon must be especially careful to get proper alignment and balance of these proximal joints before beginning treatment of the valgus of the foot.

Ankle-foot orthoses, especially polypropylene insert molded shells, can control minor flexible valgus of the hindfoot; but with increased tone these orthoses become ineffective. Heel cord lengthening and peroneal release-and-transfer have been suggested for the flexible hind part of the foot valgus (Sharrard, 1972). I have performed eight such peroneal tendon procedures. Six resulted in either overcorrection or undercorrection. I hope that dynamic electromyography will give more predictable results. At this point I advise that the hind part of foot valgus be treated with extraarticular subtalar arthrodesis. Currently I use iliac crest bone placed in the denuded sinus tarsi with talocalcaneal pin fixation. The smooth pin is removed at 8 weeks, when ambulation is allowed in a walking plaster. At 10 to 12

weeks, a molded polypropylene brace is applied below the knee and used for 1 year.

The procedure of extraarticular arthrodesis was first described using tibial bone (Grice, 1952); some surgeons use fibula. I do not use tibia or fibula, for fear of pathologic fracture in the first case and growth disturbances of the fibula in the second. An excellent method has been described using the calcaneus as a source of graft (Alban and Alban, 1975) (Fig. 14-14).

Triple arthrodesis is rarely indicated in cerebral palsy. For the mature foot with fixed valgus or varus deformity that interferes with function, however, triple arthrodesis is advised. Staples should be used for the joints in these spastic feet, and an attempt should be made to release deforming muscle forces to prevent recurrence. Although triple arthrodesis may correct deformity and decrease pain, it rarely increases ambulatory ability. Occasionally, marginal ambulators will stop walking after this surgery.

Calcaneovalgus feet are extremely rare in cerebral palsy. I have seen them after posterior tibial and Achilles tendon surgery. Calcaneal osteotomies, triple arthrodesis, and staged tendon transfers may be necessary to correct the mature deformed foot (Bradley, 1981). In the younger child, I suggest an Alban-Grice hindfoot stabilization with release of the anterior tibialis and transfer of the peroneals to the calcaneal defect (Fig. 14-25, A to C).

Operative procedure

An oblique incision is made in the lateral dorsum of the foot in line with the skin folds halfway between the lateral malleolus and the fifth metatarsal base. The incision extends from the extensor tendon to the tip of the calcaneus. The tight anterior extensor tendons are released. The sinus tarsi is excised of its contents and reamed with a Cloward bone plug remover, with the foot in the foot in the corrected position. A Cloward plug of bone is removed from the calcaneus and placed in the sinus tarsi defect with the foot in the corrected position. A staple is placed across the talocalcaneal fusion area. The peroneus brevis and longus are released as far distally as possible. The brevis is transferred to the calcaneal defect through a subcutaneous lateral route. The longus is transferred to the defect medially by way of a second proximal incision above the lateral malleolus and a subcutaneous passage around the back of the calf. The tendons are connected to each other with a nylon suture at tension, which holds the foot in maximum obtainable equinus.

FOREFOOT DEFORMITIES

The valgus hind part of the foot is often associated with a hallux valgus deformity of the first metatarsopha-

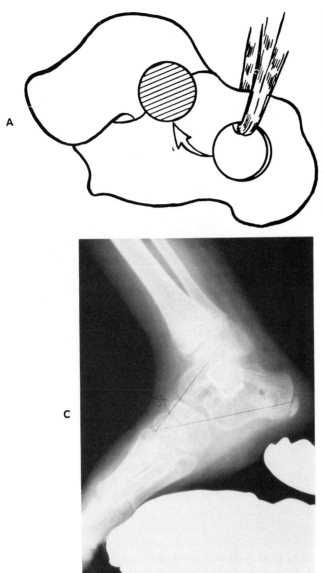

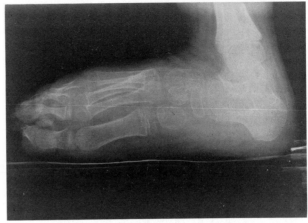

Fig. 14-25. A, Alban-Grice hindfoot stabilization. Cloward plug is removed from calcaneus and placed in sinus tarsi defect. This is stapled in place. Peroneals are transferred subcutaneously, medially, and laterally and sutured together in defect. **B,** An 8-year-old with calcaneal valgus after posterior tibial tendon transfer and Achilles tendon lengthening. **C,** Patient in **B,** 1 year postoperatively.

langeal joint (Fig. 14-26). Here I advise that, during correction of the valgus hindfoot, release of the adductor hallucis insertion and plication of the medial metatarsophalangeal joint capsule be performed. Pin fixation of the corrected metatarsophalangeal joint should be maintained for 6 weeks. Recurrence will happen if the hindfoot valgus is not corrected.

The long toe flexors are often spastic in cerebral palsy feet, but the contractures rarely become fixed. By contrast, a child with acquired brain damage will frequently develop severe toe flexor spasticity. Release of spastic toe flexors is easily accomplished by tenotomies in the proximal segment of the toes, a much more predictable procedure than lengthening these tendons at

the ankle level. Before Achilles tendon lengthening in a spastic child, it is wise to study the activity of the toe flexors during barefoot gait. Even mild spasticity of these muscles can become significant after the lengthened Achilles tendon permits increased stretch. Therefore simultaneous Achilles tendon lengthening and toe flexor tenotomies may be necessary in appropriate cases.

Occasionally in cerebral palsy the great toe extensor will work selectively as a foot dorsiflexor more effectively than the anterior tibial muscle. Tohen et al. (1966) suggested that these muscles be transferred together to the dorsum of the foot.

It should be emphasized again that, although the

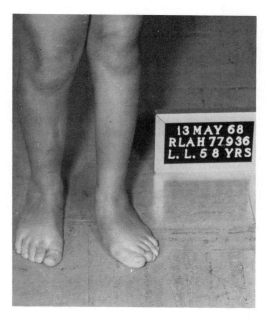

Fig. 14-26. Child with cerebral palsy and valgus hindfoot. He has also developed spastic hallux valgus. (From Proceedings of Foot Society, 1977.)

procedures are not difficult technically to perform, they should be reserved for surgeons well indoctrinated in the care of the cerebral palsy child.

Foot surgery in motor unit disease
JOHN D. HSU

Motor unit disease consists of neuropathies and myopathies, diseases traditionally known as neuromuscular diseases. The term *motor unit disease* defines the area better, although there are many instances in which neuromuscular diseases cross the motor unit barrier and become influenced by the spinal cord at the higher centers.

Neuropathies are generally stable conditions and involve the motor unit from the anterior horn cell to the neuromuscular junction. Nonprogressive examples include spinal muscular atrophy, Charcot-Marie-Tooth disease, and poliomyelitis. Landry-Guillain-Barré-Strohl disease represents a form of neuropathy in which progressive recovery of motor weaknesses is seen.

Myopathies, by contrast, are diseases that are directly attributable to degeneration of the muscle fiber. These conditions are generally progressive. Progression can be rapid, as in Duchenne pseudohypertrophic muscular dystrophy, to which a victim succumbs in his early 20s; or slowly progressive, as in fascioscapulohumeral or limb-girdle muscular dystrophy, which are fairly stable conditions (Fowler and Nayak, 1983). In certain congenital muscular dystrophies, no progression of weakness can be seen.

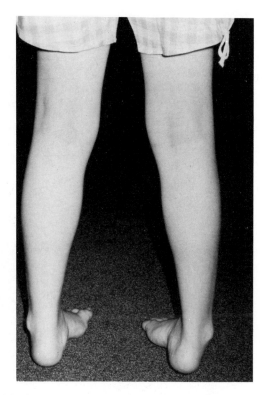

Fig. 14-27. DMD patient, age 10 years; varus and adductus deformity of foot in late walking phase.

It is out of the scope of this section to discuss general identification or clinical manifestations of these diseases; rather, the foot changes that accompany these diseases will be described and current treatment methods summarized.

GOAL IN TREATMENT

The goal in treatment of the foot deformities in motor unit disease is to maintain function and comfort. The resultant position of the foot is the effect of a fine balance between agonist and antagonist muscle groups. Because of selective weaknesses, one group of muscles can become overpowering. Gravity, positioning, and adaptation to equipment may also help direct the foot into abnormal positions. Soft tissue contractures can occur, resulting in the development of an abnormal position. When this happens, additional factors may set up a vicious cycle of deformity production, causing further loss of balance and function (Roy and Gibson, 1970).

DUCHENNE PSEUDOHYPERTROPHIC MUSCULAR DYSTROPHY (DMD)
Walking phase—early

The young child with DMD does not show any deformity. Early, there is anterior tibial weakness. The gastrocnemius-soleus muscle remains strong. Coupled with gravitational forces in sitting and walking, there is a natural tendency for the ankle to be in equinus. Early

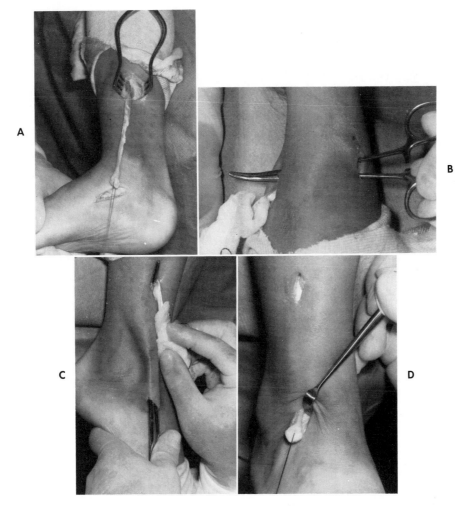

Fig. 14-28. Our procedure for posterior tibial tendon transfer anteriorly through interosseous membrane. **A,** Exposure of posterior tibial tendon and removal from medial side of foot. **B,** Incisions used to bring tendon anteriorly through interosseous membrane. **C,** Tendon passer used to bring tendon to dorsum of foot. **D,** Tendon ready for anchoring.

management should include stretching, generally taught by the physician or the physical therapist to the family, and the use of long-leg night splints to hold the knee and the ankle in a neutral position.

Walking phase—late

As the child with DMD gets older (between 7 and 8 years of age), walking becomes more difficult (Sutherland et al., 1981). Weakness in the hip extensors, the quadriceps, and the anterior tibial muscles is significant, and the child rises and walks on his tiptoes. The posterior tibial muscle generally remains strong, turning the forefoot into varus and adductus (Fig. 14-27). Dynamic walking electromyographic studies show leg muscle activity to be out of phase and, in many instances, continuous (Melkonian et al., 1980). To prolong ambulation, correction of the deformities followed by bracing is necessary.

Correction of equinus deformity. If equinus is the predominant deformity, lengthening of the Achilles tendon percutaneously is the method of choice. Frequently, this is used in conjunction with bracing and other procedures.

Correction of varus and adductus deformity. In the patient with DMD, the deformity of varus and adductus is generally caused by the pull of the relatively strong posterior tibial muscle. The posterior tibial tendon is transferred anteriorly through the interosseous membrane (Hsu, 1976; Spencer, 1973). A simplified method for the accomplishment of this surgical procedure is illustrated in Fig. 14-28. I favor this method in patients with DMD, because it minimizes surgical trauma and achieves a satisfactory result (Hsu and Hoffer, 1978; Williams, 1976).

Postsurgical management. After surgical correction has been made, lightweight casts made of fiberglass

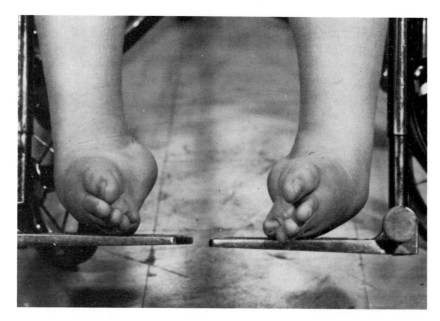

Fig. 14-29. DMD patient, age 13 years; equinovarus deformity in nonwalking patient.

have been routinely used in my clinic. The patients are generally standing the day after surgery and walking in 3 to 4 days with training. Casts are allowed to remain approximately 6 weeks and are then removed in favor of prefitted bilateral long-leg braces (knee-ankle-foot orthoses [KAFOs]) (Miller et al., 1982).

Late stages—wheelchair patients

If preventive measures have not been instituted or corrections have not been made earlier, progressive foot deformity is frequently seen in the older patient with DMD (Fig. 14-29). I believe this is attributable to previous deformity and to poor wheelchair adaptation and design. The feet do not reach the pedal, and gravitational forces pull the foot into further equinus. In the extreme varus position, pressure sores can occur on the dorsal and lateral aspects of the foot. In these cases, corrective measures need to be taken, including tendon and contracture releases. The following procedure can be used: (1) Achilles tendon lengthening, (2) release of the contracted medial structures, and (3) posterior and anterior tibial release. Generally all these procedures can be done percutaneously and followed by immobilization in the corrected position in short leg casts. After removal of the casts (3 to 4 weeks), short leg braces (e.g., a plastic-type ankle-foot orthosis) can be used. Bracing is mandatory, otherwise the deformities will recur (Hsu and Jackson, 1984).

CHARCOT-MARIE-TOOTH DISEASE

Charcot-Marie-Tooth disease is an inherited condition involving peripheral motor neurons and showing progressive muscular atrophy of the feet and legs first (Dyck et al., 1975). Fig. 14-30 illustrates the foot deformities seen in an involved family. The condition is classified as a heriditary motor and sensory neuropathy (HMSN). The general pattern of weakness occurs with wasting of the leg muscles, peroneal weakness, pes cavus, hammertoes, and clawing of the toes. This results in a steppage gait and shuffling of the feet. Foot drop and selective progressive muscle atrophy cause fixed deformities and contractures to occur in the feet (Jacobs and Carr, 1950; Mann and Missirian, 1983).

Initial treatment should be directed at support with splinting. When foot deformities persist, a careful assessment of the muscle strength by selective muscle testing is necessary. Frequently with the patient at an early age, correction of the foot deformities can be made by appropriate tendon transfers to maintain balance. The anterior tibial tendon can be transferred to the midfoot or lateral side, or the posterior tibial tendon can also be transferred anteriorly through the interosseous membrane (Hsu, 1980).

As the deformity increases, the foot develops into abnormal positions. With fixed bony deformities, wedge corrected followed by triple arthrodesis is indicated and should be made at a time when bone growth has nearly ceased.

SPINAL MUSCULAR ATROPHY

Spinal muscular atrophy represents a neuropathy caused by selective degeneration of the anterior horn cells. It is a stable condition in most cases (Munsat et al., 1969). The primary feature is muscle atrophy; as the

The basic surgery in the past consisted of bone procedures, but deformities often recurred if there was not appropriate tendon transfer. In the child, even if the disease is progressing, soft tissue procedures may be performed and will minimize structural bony deformities. A plantar fasciotomy and Achilles tendon lengthening may be indicated early in the disease. A transfer of the long toe flexors into the extensors (Girdlestone-Taylor procedure) prevents the hyperextension deformity of the metatarsophalangeal joints and fixed flexion deformity of the interphalangeal joints. Early tendon transfers may prevent later bony procedures. The peroneus longus may be transferred to the peroneus brevis to prevent varus and diminish flexible cavus. If the patient has fixed equinovarus, bony changes may already be present. This gives the tibialis posterior an added mechanical advantage, and it may also become a deforming force. If varus of the heel is fixed or is detected with standing, the posterior tibial tendon may require lengthening or sectioning. The tibialis posterior may be transferred anteriorly to the middle or lateral aspect of the forefoot, depending on the degree of varus. In the presence of fixed bone deformity subtalar or triple arthrodesis is performed. The SPLATT procedure may rarely be employed to balance the forefoot. The tibialis anterior is usually involved and is therefore not always a strong muscle for transfer.

Once a stationary point of the progession of the disease is achieved, bone procedures can be undertaken with or without soft tissue procedures. The triple arthrodesis, frequently with an Achilles tendon lengthening and plantar fasciotomy, is the most common procedure to correct these deformities. A modification of the triple arthrodesis, such as the Lambrinudi procedure, may be indicated when the anterior muscles are weakened and foot drop is present.

In the adult foot, cavus and toe clawing are the most frequent deformities. The cavus may be corrected by a triple arthrodesis, a tarsal osteotomy, or osteotomies of the metatarsals, depending on the location and severity of the deformity. A V-osteotomy on the tarsi rather than an anterior wedge osteotomy is recommended, since the foot is not shortened by the former. Plantar fasciotomy is usually performed at the same time. Correction of a mild varus sometimes lessens the associated toe deformity. If toe clawing is present and not fixed, a Girdlestone-Taylor procedure is indicted. The ideal patient for a Girdlestone-Taylor procedure does not have callosities under the metatarsal heads and bears weight on the end of his toes. Metatarsalgia or callosities under the metatarsal heads usually are not corrected by the Girdlestone-Taylor procedure alone. Tarsal osteotomies, proximal transfer of extensor tendons with interphalangeal fusion, or partial phalangectomies will be required for this deformity. If the foot remains balanced but equinus develops after the bone procedure, a polypropylene orthosis is indicated.

PERONEAL NERVE PALSY

The outlook for significant recovery of motor function following transection and repair of the peroneal nerve in adults is poor. Even when the nerve stroma remains intact following stretch injuries, the prognosis is variable unless recovery occurs in the early stages. After compression injuries, full return may be anticipated if the compressive force is identified early and removed.

It is difficult to predict the chances for recovery based on results recorded in the literature. Outcome is often expressed as the time elapsed between injury and initial motor recovery. The return of some voluntary motion, however, does not always lead to sufficient recovery of strength to prevent injury. If there is no advancing Tinel sign at 6 months or some voluntary motion, however, does not always lead to sufficient recovery of strength to prevent injury. If there is no advancing Tinel sign at 6 months or some voluntary contraction in 9 months, minimal chance for significant functional recovery exists.

Despite uncertainty regarding recovery of nerve function following acute injury, correction of foot drop can be initially obtained by a plastic shoe insert–type orthosis. Custom-fitted polypropylene orthoses fabricated over a positive mold of the patient's foot and ankle may be worn without discomfort. Shoes may be interchanged as long as they have approximately the same heel height. Objections to orthoses as a permanent method of correcting foot drop have been less frequent since the introduction of cosmetic plastic material that enables one to conceal the orthosis in socks, slacks, or trousers. These orthoses are superior to traditional orthoses with metal uprights. Consequently, the cosmetic orthosis may also be the treatment of choice for many patients with temporary foot drop.

Posterior tibial tendon transfer may be considered as a means of eliminating the need for an orthosis. The limitations of surgery, however, should be carefully considered. Despite favorable reports in the literature the following problems have been encountered after this tendon transfer: failure of automatic response of the tibialis posterior in the swing phase of gait, gradual passive stretching of the tibialis posterior, and increasing pronation in patients with preexisting pes planus.

In our experience the posterior tibial tendon restores "active voluntary dorsiflexion" and demonstrates activity in the swing phase only when the patient makes a conscious effort to contract it with each step. When the patient ambulates with unconscious effort the posterior tibial muscle reverts to its normal stance phase activity instead of the desired swing phase. Apparent good results occur initially when the tendon is transferred and tightly secured, acting mainly as a tenodesis. Later the patient may voluntarily dorsiflex the foot and not demonstrate a foot drop if, during ambulation, he consciously makes an effort to dorsiflex the foot. However, because of the tenodesis effect, careful questioning of the patient's family will reveal that during routine walking foot drop is usually present. The reason for this paradoxic response lies in the organization of the CNS. Direct corticospinal tracts enable the normal patient with an intact cerebral cortex to consciously contract the tibialis posterior in the swing phase. The basic locomotor mechanisms responsible for walking, however, are located subcortically. These mechanisms normally enable normal muscle activity to occur without conscious effort. Despite intensive therapy, it is generally not possible to reprogram the tibialis posterior to be a swing-phase muscle in all patients.

Since the tibialis posterior is normally inactive at heel strike, it is subject to tensile forces that stretch out the passive elements of the muscle beyond their normal length. This occurs when resultant body weight forces pass anterior to the point of heel contact. Consequently, most patients examined several years after surgery display foot drop unless they make a conscious effort to dorsiflex the foot. Greater correction can be usually obtained with an orthosis.

Patients with pes planus may not tolerate any loss of hindfoot varus support. If the tibialis posterior is transferred, planovalgus may increase (associated with increased pronation), and collapse of the medial arch may occur and become symptomatic.

When performing tendon transfer, we prefer to transfer the flexor hallucis longus and flexor digitorum longus rather than the tibialis posterior. This is based on the fact that the combined cross-sectional area of these two muscles and their combined strength is greater than the area and strength of the tibialis posterior alone. It is also our opinion that these muscles more easily convert to automatic swing-phase activity, although this has not occurred in all patients. The two tendons are passed through the interosseous membrane and inserted into the second cuneiform via the same surgical approaches as described for stroke patients.

SCIATIC AND POSTERIOR TIBIAL NERVE PALSY

As with damage to the peroneal nerve, the outlook for functional motor recovery following complete sciatic or posterior tibial nerve palsy is poor unless early recovery occurs after a compression or stretch injury. Although recovery of motor function is usually poor following surgical repair of complete transection, recovery of some protective sensation is of considerable benefit. Consequently, we recommend exploration of sciatic and posterior tibial nerve injuries if there is no recovery of sensation distal to the site of injury. Treatment consists of prescription of a rigid AFO to provide ankle stability. Particular emphasis is placed on teaching the patient the importance of three-times-a-day foot inspection for signs of excessive pressure. Once pressure ulceration occurs and the normal protective covering of the foot pad is scarred, prevention of pressure sores becomes increasingly difficult. Patients with an intact peroneal nerve and adequate ankle dorsiflexion may not require an AFO.

Extreme care should be taken in the use of plastic orthoses. These devices rely on direct skin contact and must be fitted with extreme precision to avoid excessive skin pressure.

Pantalar arthrodesis is mentioned only to be condemned. The patient with complete sciatic palsy will have near-normal gait and walking tolerance with a well-fitted orthosis to correct foot drop. Although the foot is held within the orthosis, some ankle and subtalar motion occurs. This motion is important and helps the foot adapt to the sole of the shoe and underlying terrain. Pantalar arthrodesis robs the patient of this important adaptive mechanism and increases both pressure and shear stress on the insensitive skin.

HEREDITARY SPINOCEREBELLAR ATAXIA

Friedreich's ataxia is the most common type of spinocerebellar degeneration. Degeneration can be found in the Purkinje cells of the cerebellum, the spinocerebellar tracts, the posterior column, and the corticospinal tracts. The exact etiology is unknown, but the condition is transmitted by an autosomal recessive gene.

Clinical findings. The onset occurs during childhood and adolescence and may be insidious. Difficulty in ambulation (ataxia) is the major complaint. Foot problems and scoliosis are frequently present. As the disease progresses, ataxia is detected in the upper extremity and an intention tremor may be present. Speech abnormalities, nystagmus, and cardiac abnormalities can also become evident. With further progression, a generalized hypotonia is noted, and death may occur when the patient is in his 30s.

The most common foot deformity is a symmetric cavus with or without clawtoes. The great toe also demonstrates the clawtoe deformity. Equinus may be present, sometimes only involving the forefoot. Muscle imbalance, both intrinsic and extrinsic, must cause these deformities. Peroneal muscle weakness is the most common muscle abnormality. Weakness of the tibialis anterior is a less consistent finding. The knee and ankle jerks are usually absent, and a positive Babinski sign may be elicited. Two-point discrimination along with position and vibration sense may be diminished.

Surgery. Since cavus and toe clawing are the most common deformities, the majority of the surgical procedures are directed toward correcting them. Surgery should be performed early in the milder cases to prevent further deformity. Since the disease may be nonprogressive, an aggressive surgical approach may be undertaken. A well-balanced, stable foot will often aid in ambulation and lessen the effects of ataxia.

The most common operation is directed toward correcting the cavus deformity. Depending on the degree of the deformity and the surgeon's preference, a triple arthrodesis, a tarsal osteotomy, or metatarsal osteotomies may be performed. A plantar fasciotomy frequently is required at the same time.

Toe clawing is the second most common problem. For the great toe deformities, transfer of the long toe extensor to the first metatarsal and fusion of the interphalangeal joint (Jones procedure) is often indicated. If the deformities are not fixed, a Girdlestone-Taylor procedure can be employed on the other toes. For metatarsalgia or fixed clawtoe deformities, a Girdlestone-Taylor procedure is not indicated, since it will not correct these deformities. Metatarsal osteotomies, transfer of the extensor tendons proximally, interphalangeal fusion, or resection are indicted for this problem.

The cavus and clawtoe deformities are secondary to intrinsic and extrinsic muscle imbalance. The toe clawing may be accentuated by a weakened tibialis anterior, since the common toe extensors aid in foot dorsiflexion.

A review by Makin (1953) stated that a frequently used procedure for this deformity was transfer of the extensor digitorum longus to the dorsum of the foot. Of 18 patients, however, 16 subsequently developed hammertoes, and 8 required interphalangeal arthrodesis. This is to be expected, because the intrinsic muscles must be weak or the deformity would not develop. A Girdlestone-Taylor procedure would seem to be more logical. If foot drop were the problem, the extensor of the great toe could be transferred to the dorsum of the foot with interphalangeal fusion of the great toe.

A polypropylene orthosis should be employed for proprioceptive loss or weakened anterior muscles or to aid in ankle stability.

REFERENCES

Allen, W.: Relation of hereditary pattern to clinical severity as illustrated by peroneal atrophy, Arch. Intern. Med. **63**:1123, 1939.

Garland, D.E., Lucie, R.S., and Waters, R.L.: Current uses of open phenol nerve block for adult-acquired spasticity, Clin. Orthop. **165**:217, 1982.

Jacobs, J.E., and Carr, C.R.: Progressive muscular atrophy of the peroneal type, J. Bone Joint Surg. **32A**:27, 1950.

Makin, M.: The surgical management of Friedreich's ataxia, J. Bone Joint Surg. **35A**:425, 1953.

Perry, J.: Lower extremity management in stroke. Examination: a neurologic basis for treatment. In American Academy of Orthopaedic Surgeons: Instructional course lectures, St. Louis, 1975, The C.V. Mosby Co., p. 21.

Perry, J., Giovan, P., Harris, L.J., Montgomery, J., and Azaria, M.: The determinants of muscle action in the meiparetic lower extremity. Clin. Orthop. **131**:71, 1978a.

Perry, J., Waters, R.L., and Perrin, T.: Electromyographic analysis of equinovarus following stroke, Clin. Orthop. **131**:47, 1978b.

Twitchell, T.E.: The restoration of motor function following hemiplegia in man, Brain **74**:448, 1951.

Waters, R.L., Garland, D., Jordan, C., and Perry, J.: Electromyographic gait analysis before and after operative treatment for hemiplegic equinus and equinovarus deformity, J. Bone Joint Surg. **64A**:284, 1982.

16

Affections of the foot

JAMES O. JOHNSTON

TUMOROUS CONDITIONS OF THE SOFT TISSUES AND BONES OF THE FOOT

In this discussion of tumor and tumorlike conditions occurring in the foot and ankle area, it should first be stated that malignant tumors of the foot (and incidentally of the hand) are rare conditions and that soft tissue tumors are more common. Therefore when one is uncertain whether a lesion is benign or malignant, it is better to assume the benign condition and treat accordingly rather than perform an unnecessary amputation for a pseudomalignant condition.

Generally most of the neoplastic conditions occurring in the foot are seen more typically in other parts of the body and are not specific problems of the foot. There is, however, an important difference in clinical prognostication of like tumors located in different parts of the body. For example, when one considers cartilaginous tumors in the pelvis or proximal large bones of the extremity, one must be extremely cautious because of the known potential of these tumors for malignancy and tendency to metastasize. By contrast, the same type of cartilaginous tumor located in the foot is almost always benign. This has a direct bearing on treatment: cartilaginous tumors in the proximal part of the body should be aggressively resected whereas smaller lesions in the hand or foot can usually be handled by conservative resection. The giant cell tumor is another good example of a tumor with variable prognosis depending on its location. Surgical treatment for the giant cell tumor can therefore also vary.

Benign tumors of the soft tissues

Fibroma. Fibromas are benign soft tissue lesions seen in all parts of the body, in soft tissue and in bone. They are well-localized lesions in most cases with well-defined borders. Fibromas are frequently subcutaneous in location and firm to palpation. They grow very slowly and are usually asymptomatic and nontender to palpation.

Fig. 16-1 shows a typical, firm, and well-circumscribed subcutaneous fibroma resected from the tarsal sinus area of the foot. The lesion can be cut like a piece of hard rubber, and the exposed surfaces are white with the gross appearance of a cut Achilles tendon.

Microscopically this tumor is composed of well-differentiated fibroblasts producing large amounts of dense collagen fiber that contributes to its physical characteristics.

A fibroma can be easily resected, and there is very little chance of local recurrence.

Fig. 16-2 shows a patient with surfer's knobs. These fibromatous lesions are found on the dorsum of the foot as the result of repeated physical trauma to this area (e.g., many hours spent on a surfboard).

Keloid. Keloid is the clinical name given to dense hypertrophic dermal fibrous tissue that forms in excess as a response to skin lacerations or surgical incisions. Keloids are familial and are firmly fixed in the genetic makeup of fibroblasts all through the body. It is difficult therefore to avoid keloid formation in certain patients when making surgical wounds for reconstructive purposes.

To reduce the chance of a disfiguring or disabling scar, one should at least be aware of this potential before performing surgery. It is well known that dark-skinned people are generally more prone to keloid formation whereas light-skinned races or individuals with hyperelastic skin rarely form keloids but instead tend to form flat scars that spread.

The best treatment for keloid formation is prevention if possible. For this reason it is best to make surgical incisions parallel with skin creases or skin lines (in the

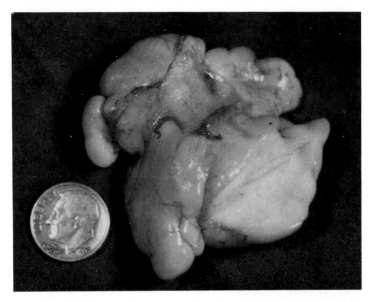

Fig. 16-1. Well-circumscribed firm subcutaneous fibroma removed from foot.

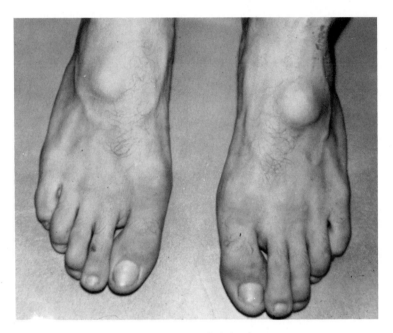

Fig. 16-2. Surfer's knobs.

extremities, a transverse incision). It is also wise to use good subcutaneous closures and avoid surface stitches completely. Skin tapes left in place for several weeks and splinting of wounds near joints are helpful. The use of gamma irradiation or steroids to inhibit fibrosis is considered controversial and is probably best left in the hands of a plastic surgeon who has experience with these modalities.

Fig. 16-69 is a classic picture of a keloid scar formed as the result of a longitudinal incision made along the heel cord and across the ankle joint (p. 376).

Plantar fibromatosis (Keller and Baez-Giangreco, 1975). Plantar fibromatosis is a locally aggressive idiopathic proliferative fasciitis of the plantar aponeurosis that is usually bilateral and frequently seen in children and young adults. In older people it is often associated with Dupuytren's contracture of the palmar fascia of the hand. The basic microscopic pathology of Dupuytren's and plantar fibromas is about the same. However, in children the microscopic picture is much more worrisome and can be misdiagnosed as a malignant fibrosarcoma. Fig. 16-3 shows the typical nodularity of this fibroma in the long plantar ligament.

If the nodules are small and cause little trouble, they can be left alone. If they grow large and cause pain or

pressure on an adjacent nerve, however, it is best to perform aggressive resection. Pedersen and Day (1954) advised a longitudinal incision along the medial plantar aspect of the first metatarsal proximally to the tarsal navicular. Skin flaps are developed to expose the fibroma and plantar fascia. The fibrotic lesion is aggressively excised, with removal of much of the normal-appearing adjacent plantar fascia. It is important to perform aggressive resection because of the high incidence of local recurrence when only the fibroma is removed. The skin flaps are then tacked down to prevent hematoma, and Hemovac brand suction tubes are placed beneath the skin as well. A firm compression dressing is also helpful in preventing hematoma formation.

Neurilemoma. The neurilemoma is a benign neurogenic tumor of nerve sheath origin that is well encapsulated, usually solitary, and found on the surface of a peripheral nerve. Fig. 16-4 shows a typical lesion resected from the surface of the medial plantar nerve. This tumor is easy to resect and rarely causes damage to its nerve of origin because of its eccentric location. It rarely recurs or becomes malignant.

Neurofibroma. The most common neurogenic tumor is the neurofibroma. This tumor can be solitary (Fig. 16-5) or multicentric and quite diffusely invasive, as in the plexiform type seen in the dysplastic condition known as von Recklinghausen disease (neurofibromatosis) with associated tan-pigmented café-aulait spots on the skin. The neurofibroma is more disabling because of its central location in a peripheral nerve. As a result it interferes with nerve function and, if resected, the entire nerve is frequently removed with the tumor. The

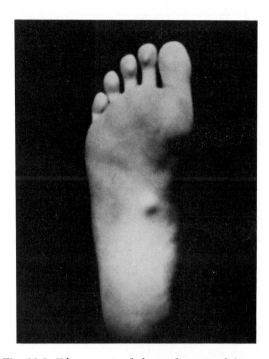

Fig. 16-3. Fibromatosis of plantar fascia in adolescent.

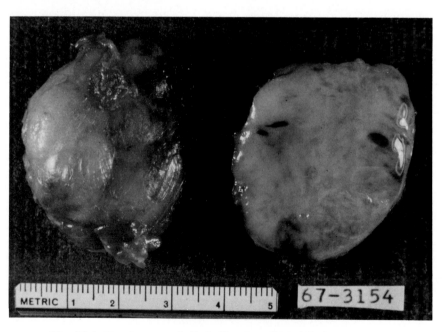

Fig. 16-4. Neurilemoma shelled off surface of medial plantar nerve.

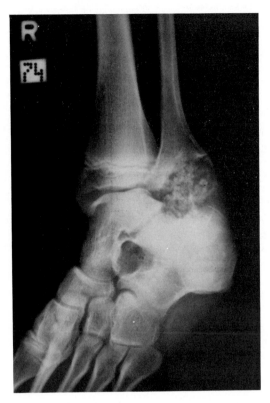

Fig. 16-27. Chondroblastoma in distal fibular epiphysis of 12-year-old boy.

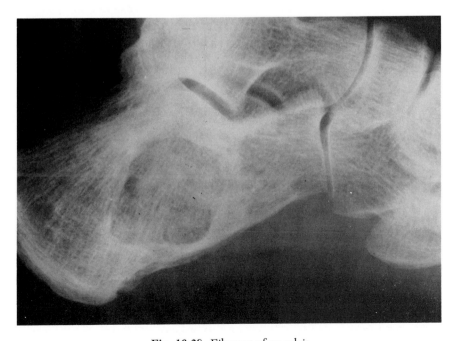

Fig. 16-28. Fibroma of os calcis.

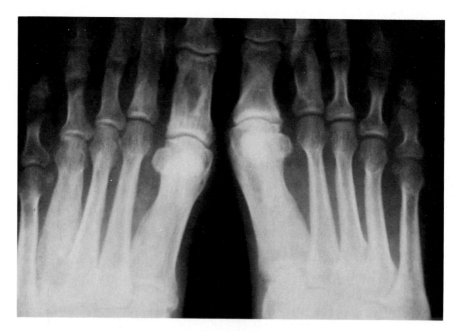

Fig. 16-29. Polyostotic fibrous dysplasia involving both feet.

bone seen in the os calcis. Notice the sharp geographic appearance, which suggests a benign condition. These lesions are usually asymptomatic until the time of a possible pathologic fracture. They are frequently seen in children and young adults in metaphyseal bone. If treatment is necessary because of recurrent fracture or threat of fracture, it consists of simple curettement and grafting.

At times a patient is found to have multiple bony involvement with fibromas of bone in the feet; this condition is referred to as *polyostotic fibrous dysplasia* (Fig. 16-29). There is chronic dilation of the first and fourth metatarsal shafts. The condition tends to amplify on one side of the body more than on the other, with a resultant leg length discrepancy caused by bowing of the femur.

Another benign variation of fibrous defects in bone is the so-called *chondromyxoid fibroma* (Fig. 16-30). This tumor has about the same radiographic appearance as the nonossifying fibroma and can be treated the same way, i.e., with simple curettement and possible grafting. The distinguishing histologic characteristic of this rare lesion is the presence of myxoid and chondroid tissue.

Sarcoidosis. Sarcoidosis is a generalized systemic granulomatous disease of unknown cause that acts in many ways like a low-grade lymphoma. It involves structures of the lymphoid system (including bone marrow), especially in blacks. Bones most typically involved are located in the hands and feet. Fig. 16-31 is a typical radiograph of a sarcoid foot with granuloma-

tous changes in the distal first metatarsal that might suggest gout. However, the smaller, more centrally located lesions in the phalanges suggest sarcoidosis. These patients have subcutaneous nodularities overlying the bony changes that could suggest a rheumatoid process.

Melorheostosis. Melorheostosis is an idiopathic condition seen typically in the bones of the lower extremities. It is usually picked up as an incidental finding from a radiograph obtained for some other reason. Fig. 16-32 provides an example of this abnormality of enchondral ossification involving the tibia, talus, and first ray to the tip of the great toe. The flowing appearance on the radiograph accounts for the name given this condition, which can sometimes occur across joints and result in stiffening.

Tarsoepiphyseal aclasis. Tarsoepiphyseal aclasis is a rare and localized epiphyseal dysplasia of a hypertrophic nature seen usually in bones about the ankle of one leg only. Its characteristic deformed enlargement of the talus is well demonstrated in Fig. 16-33, where it might suggest other conditions such as fibrous dysplasia or neurofibromatosis. The talus is the most common place to find this defect, but it can occur in a growing child on the medial side of the knee with enlargement of the medial femoral condyle. Early recognition should lead to early surgical treatment.

Stippled epiphyses. Conradi disease (chondrodysplasia punctata) is a rare form of congenital dwarfism seen at birth with the clinical manifestations of achondroplastic dwarfism. However, on radiographic examination,

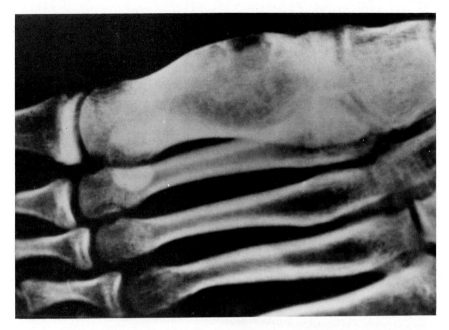

Fig. 16-30. Benign chrondromyxoid fibroma of first metatarsal.

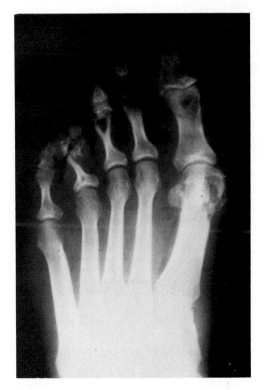

Fig. 16-31. Lytic-appearing granulomas in sarcoidosis of foot.

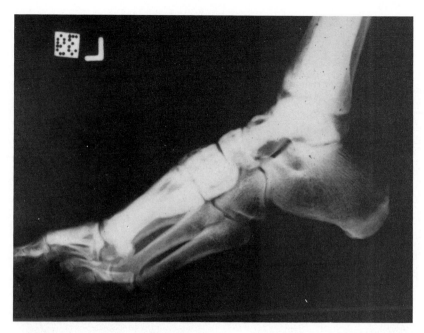

Fig. 16-32. Melorheostosis; flowing hyperostosis down inner aspect of foot and ankle.

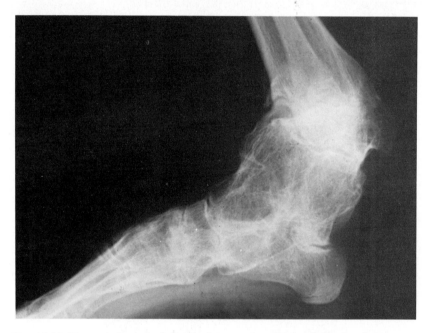

Fig. 16-33. Tarsoepiphyseal aclasis involving entire talus, with localized gigantism.

the diagnostic features of stippled epiphyses appear (Fig. 16-34). There is extensive calcific stippling around the major epiphyseal ossification centers of the tarsal areas of the foot. This is a dystrophic form of calcification in the germinal cartilage that gradually disappears with time and growth. In many cases the dwarfism clears up, and the older child may enjoy a fairly normal physical appearance.

Bone islands. Bone islands are common findings on bone radiographs. These represent small, well-circumscribed areas of increased bone density secondary to a failure of proper remodeling of bone in the metaphyseal areas of the growing skeleton. If multiple lesions are seen (Fig. 16-35), the condition is referred to as osteopoikilosis; it is usually observed in radiographs of the asymptomatic hands and feet. Lesions located more

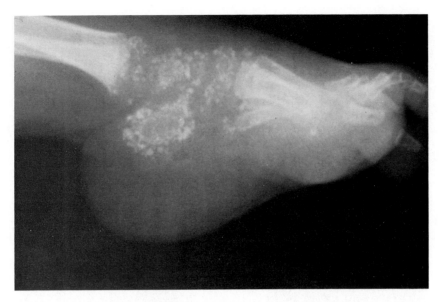

Fig. 16-34. Stippled epiphyses seen in newborn dwarf.

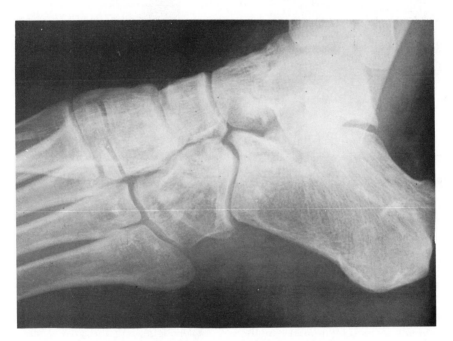

Fig. 16-35. Osteopoikilosis or multiple bone islands in foot.

proximally may suggest the possibility of osteoblastic metastatic disease. An isotopic bone scan can help clear this differential diagnostic point in most cases.

Malignant tumors of bone

Malignant tumors of the hand or foot are unusual; when they do occur, they tend to behave less aggressively than the same tumor in a more proximal portion of the extremity in larger bones. For this reason, when the pathologist is uncertain as to the exact nature of a lesion of the hand or foot at biopsy, it is frequently good judgment on the part of the clinician to assume a benign diagnosis and elect conservative local resection. The general statement can also be made that malignant tumors of the hand and foot will tend to metastasize rather late in the course of the disease.

Osteosarcoma. The osteogenic sarcoma is a highly malignant tumor, usually seen in the metaphyseal areas of fast-growing bones in children such as the tibia or femur. Most of these are seen in boys, and they are

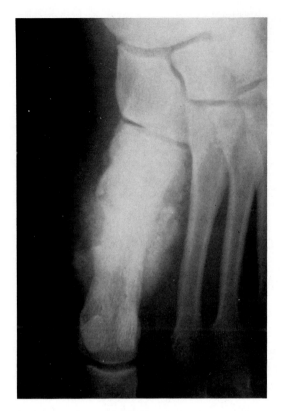

Fig. 16-36. Malignant osteosarcoma in first metatarsal of young man.

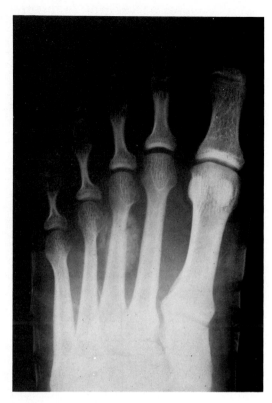

Fig. 16-37. Stress fracture in third metatarsal, presenting as pseudotumor.

common about the knee joint. Bones of the feet are involved in less than 1% of all cases, which makes this diagnosis rare. Fig. 16-36 shows one of these rare cases of an osteosarcoma in the first metatarsal of a young man. The combination of lytic destruction of the subadjacent cortex and exuberant and chaotic production of neoplastic osteoid around the entire shaft of the metatarsal points strongly toward a malignant diagnosis of a bone-forming sarcoma.

At the present time the best method of treatment is amputation. Since about 1972, however, adjunctive chemotherapy has greatly improved the prognosis. The drugs used most commonly include high-dosage methotrexate with citrovorum factor rescue and adriamycin in combination with other chemotherapeutics such as vincristine.

One of the newest chemotherapy programs today is the T-10 Protocol used by the Sloan-Kettering Institute (Rosen, 1982). This is a combined preoperative and postoperative multidrug therapy that claims an 80% cure rate for this tumor.

Pulmonary metastasis from this tumor was at one time considered a fatal condition, and nothing further was done for the patient. However, Spanos et al. (1976) have presented encouraging results with resection of metastatic lesions. They report a 28% 5-year survival

without recurrence. The new chemotherapy programs may well improve this figure.

It should be mentioned that radiotherapy has been dropped as a therapeutic modality for this tumor. Immunotherapy may hold some promise for the future.

Because the osteosarcoma is such a rare lesion in the foot, it might be wise to include a few pseudotumors that masquerade as malignant lesions. Fig. 16-37 is a radiograph of such a pseudotumor in the third metatarsal of a 19-year-old track runner that demonstrates the typical callus formation seen in a stress fracture. These lesions frequently show no fracture line across the involved bone, and the patient may give no definite history of any single injury to the foot. Biopsy generally shows aggressive osteoid production that might suggest to the pathologist a malignant diagnosis. Such a mistaken diagnosis could then tragically lead to treatment by amputation for a benign process.

Another example of a pseudotumor is seen in Fig. 16-38 in a young patient with factor VIII–type hemophilia. This occurs in the form of a highly lytic and aneurysmal lesion of the os calcis that could easily pass for an aggressive sarcoma of some type.

Ewing sarcoma. Ewing sarcoma is also a childhood tumor seen more typically in long bones of the lower extremities or in the pelvis. However, according to

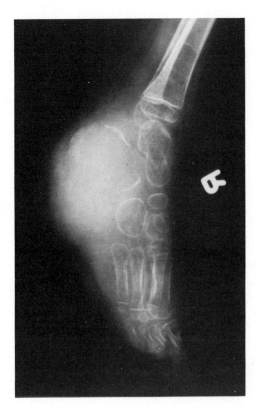

Fig. 16-38. Pseudotumor of hemophilia in os calcis of young boy.

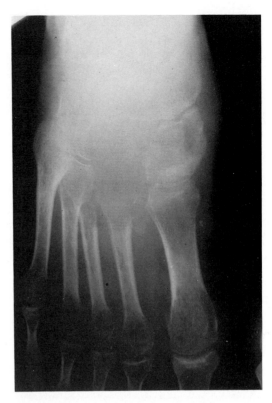

Fig. 16-39. Ewing's sarcoma in midtarsal area of young man.

Pritchard et al. (1975) at the Mayo Clinic, about 5% are located in the foot area. It carries the worst prognosis for survival of any of the primary sarcomas of bone. It probably is a very primitive mesenchymal tumor of the round cell variety, similar to the reticulum cell tumor seen in adults.

Fig. 16-39 shows the typical radiographic appearance of Ewing sarcoma seen in the midtarsal area of a young man. This lesion is purely lytic in nature, and its high degree of bony permeation suggests an infectious process such as tuberculosis. It is also quite necrotic and, when cut into, may drain a liquid necrotic material that suggests purulence to the operating surgeon.

Fig. 16-40 illustrates another Ewing sarcoma in the area of the first cuneiform bone of a 35-year-old man that displays extensive lytic destructive changes that might also suggest an infectious process. This patient was treated by amputation.

In the past, the traditional therapy for Ewing sarcoma has been irradiation therapy with 5,000 to 6,500 rad to the entire bone. There is a current trend away from this, however, because of the advent of the newer chemotherapeutic programs that have increased the short-term prognosis for survival up to 60% (Tepper et al., 1980).

At the Mayo Clinic, Pritchard et al. (1975) have re-

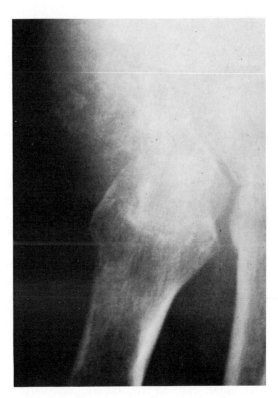

Fig. 16-40. Ewing's sarcoma of first cuneiform.

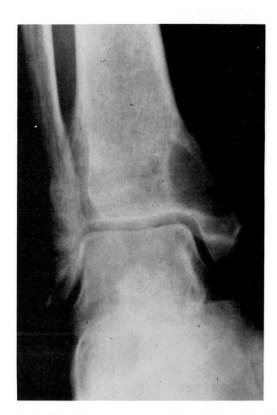

Fig. 16-41. Chondrosarcoma in medial malleolus of middle-aged man.

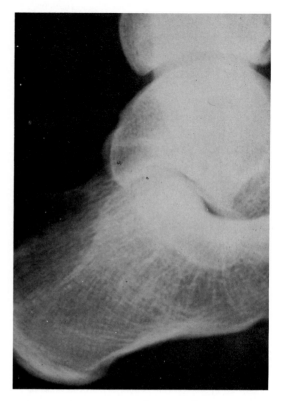

Fig. 16-42. Giant cell tumor of os calcis.

ported a 45% 5-year survival following amputation, compared with a 13% survival after irradiation therapy alone. They therefore are suggesting amputation with adjunctive chemotherapy for extremity lesions. Lewis et al. (1977) also advise amputation for extremity lesions, especially those of the foot and ankle.

Chondrosarcoma. Like the osteosarcoma, chondrosarcoma is rare in the foot. About 1% of all cases are seen in the foot or tarsal area and usually occur as primary lesions in middle-aged adults. The usual site for this tumor is the pelvis. The tumor is slow growing and late to metastasize to the lung. Fig. 16-41 is a radiographic film of a chondrosarcoma seen in the medial malleolus of a 50-year-old man. Unlike the benign cartilage tumors, the malignant chondrosarcoma usually involves symptoms of pain. In the large study of these tumors of the foot by Dahlin and Salvador (1974), it was shown that local curettement is not beneficial. Treatment is by excision of the entire bone involved with the tumor. This gives very little chance of recurrence or metastasis.

Giant cell tumors (Goldenberg et al., 1970). Giant cell tumors are low-grade malignant lesions that are rarely seen in the hand or foot. If discovered in the foot, this tumor may, in fact, be an aneurysmal bone cyst (which has a similar clinical appearance). Fig. 16-

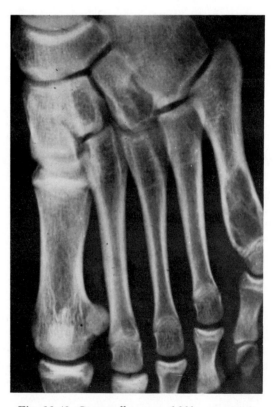

Fig. 16-43. Giant cell tumor of fifth metatarsal.

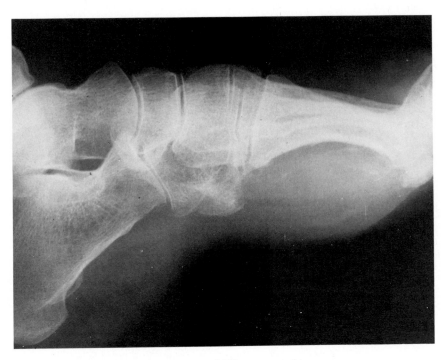

Fig. 16-44. Fibrosarcoma of fifth metatarsal in young man.

42 shows a giant cell tumor in the os calcis with typical lytic appearance and fairly aggressive permeative edge suggesting malignancy. Fig. 16-43 presents a more benign-appearing giant cell tumor of the fifth metatarsal in a 16-year-old boy; this tumor has the slightly aneurysmal appearance typical of giant cell tumors. Most experts agree that giant cell lesions in the hand or foot carry a much better prognosis than do giant cell tumors of long bones. For this reason the accepted treatment for the first occurrence is usually local curettement and bone grafting, if needed. Radiotherapy is contraindicated because of possible transformation into an irradiation sarcoma.

Fibrosarcoma (Larsson et al., 1976). The fibrosarcoma as a primary bone tumor of the foot is extremely rare. Fig. 16-44 is an example of the fibrosarcoma seen in the fifth metatarsal of a young adult man. This tumor occurs in about the same locations as the osteosarcoma, and the recommended treatment is amputation of the entire foot. Adjunctive chemotherapy could be considered for grade 3 to 4 lesions.

Metastatic tumors to foot. It is generally unusual to find a metastatic carcinoma in the bones of the hand or foot, or even distal to the elbow or knee. Of the metastatic group in this rare location, the bronchogenic carcinoma of the lung is perhaps the most common. Fig. 16-45 is a radiograph of a metastatic carcinoma of the lung to the lateral malleolus with lytic destructive changes and periosteal lifting that might well suggest a primary sarcoma such as the Ewing tumor seen more

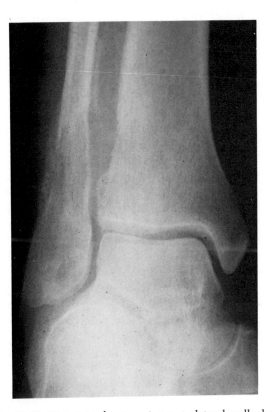

Fig. 16-45. Metastatic lung carcinoma to lateral malleolus.

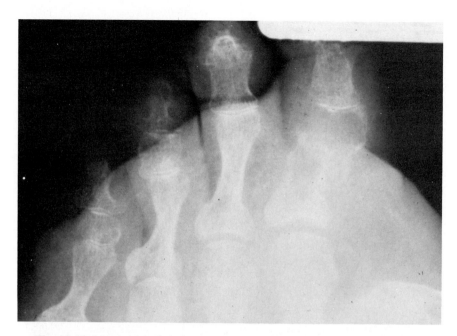

Fig. 16-46. Metastatic colon carcinoma to second toe with pathologic fracture.

typically in this location. Another example of a metastatic lesion in the foot is seen in Fig. 16-46, where a carcinoma of the colon has metastasized to the second toe, with a pathologic fracture through the proximal phalanx. Conservative treatment for these lesions must be considered, with local resection followed by irradiation of the part to prevent local recurrence.

METABOLIC BONE DISEASE

Just as an internist looks at the chest radiograph for evidence of generalized disease process, a physician who deals with hand or foot problems should become familiar with generalized radiographic changes in the structure of bone. Much can be learned about the general metabolic state of the entire patient based on the various changes that take place in bone for one reason or another. In this section I will introduce some of the major categories of metabolic bone disease and present examples of these disease states as we recognize them on routine radiographs of the foot.

Osteoporosis. Osteoporosis is not a disease state but, in fact, is a condition of bone seen in many diseases in which there occurs a total decrease in bone volume that results in a decreased bone density and an increased bone porosity associated with decreased physical strength.

The most common cause for an osteoporotic change in normal bone is through the simple process of disuse. Just as muscle loses its volume with lack of exercise, so bone decreases in volume by weight if not physically stressed with activity. A good example of disuse osteoporosis is seen in Fig. 16-47, a radiograph of a foot that has been in a non–weight-bearing cast for 6 weeks. The greatest degree of bone loss occurs in the metaphyseal-epiphyseal areas, where metabolic changes are seen early, as opposed to cortical bone, in which more time is needed to show thinning or increased porosity. The simple solution to this form of osteoporosis is removal of the cast as soon as possible to begin stressing the bone once again. Even weight bearing in a cast will help avoid unnecessary osteoporosis from inactivity.

Another example of osteoporosis related to the disuse type is *Sudeck's atrophy* (reflex sympathetic dystrophy) (Arieff et al., 1963), sometimes referred to as sympathetic dystrophy of bone. This is a painful type of osteoporosis frequently seen in (often neurotic) women who sustain a minor injury to their foot that causes them to overreact to their injury by not using the foot for a prolonged period. The result is a radiographic picture like that seen in Fig. 16-48, with characteristic spotty porosis throughout the midtarsal area. At first, the radiograph might suggest the infiltrative process of an inflammatory disease such as osteomyelitis. The foot may look cold and sweaty or at other times hot and swollen. These appearances have been attributed to some reflex instability of the autonomic system controlling the capillary flow of blood through the tissues of the foot. The best treatment for this chronic painful condition is to motivate the patient to exercise the foot and begin weight bearing as soon as possible. Sometimes lumbar sympathetic blocks are useful to decrease the pain so weight bearing can begin.

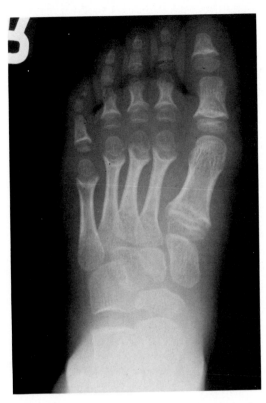

Fig. 16-55. Schmid form of metaphyseal chondrodysplasia that mimics rickets.

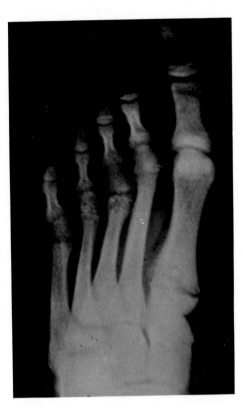

Fig. 16-56. Osteomalacic bone in adolescent with primary hyperparathyroidism.

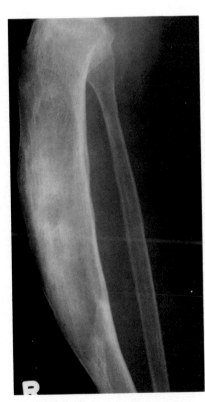

Fig. 16-57. Brown tumor of hyperparathyroidism giving appearance of Paget's disease.

this metabolic state continues for a long time, the bones take on an osteomalacic appearance like those in Fig. 16-56, of a 14-year-old girl with a parathyroid adenoma. The bones look washed out, and there is a very specific tapering of the terminal tufts of the distal phalanges. One of the secondary complications of hyperparathyroidism is the production of pseudotumors of bone called brown tumors. These lytic aneurysmal lesions of bone are loaded with giant cells and can appear much like a giant cell tumor of bone but are not neoplastic in any way. Fig. 16-57 is a typical radiograph of a large brown tumor of the tibia giving the appearance of Paget disease of the tibia.

Another interesting parathyroid disease of bone that frequently presents the radiographic appearance of hyperparathyroidism but exhibits low serum calcium levels is a disease known as *pseudohypoparathyroidism*. Fig. 16-58 is the radiograph of a patient with this disease. Metatarsals two through five are short, with hypoplastic distal phalanges. Subcutaneous ectopic bone also is seen. This disease results because of a heritable defect in the renal tubule that is resistant to the normal or elevated levels of parathormone in these patients.

Paget disease. Most people still consider Paget disease of bone to be an idiopathic inflammatory disease state that initially produces a spotty hyperemic osteo-

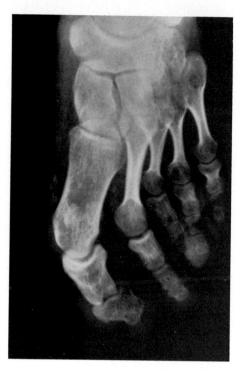

Fig. 16-58. Pseudohypoparathyroidism.

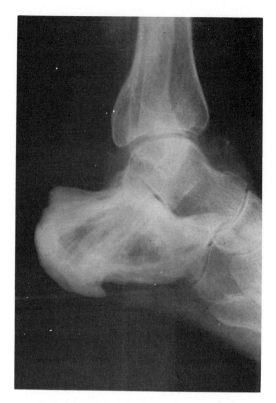

Fig. 16-59. Paget's disease of os calcis.

lysis associated with pain and an elevated alkaline phosphatase level in the blood. The bone becomes weakened because of the lytic process, and deformity results (e.g., bowing of the legs and widening of the skull). Then as a healing response by the patient, osteoblastic activity occurs, and the involved bones become very dense-appearing on x-ray examination. Fig. 16-59 shows a good example of the late blastic changes seen in a pagetoid os calcis. The coarsened trabecular pattern and the chronic external enlargement of the bone shell are evident, as is the prominent calcaneal spur, following the early softening phase of this disease that is similar to osteomalacia. This disease has been known to progress into a sarcoma; in the case of the hand or foot, such progression would be very unusual.

Gout. Gout is a heritable disease seen mostly in older men with a clinical picture of hyperuricemia associated with synovitis and the presence of urate deposits in soft tissue. The exact cause for the peripheral tissue production of excessive uric acid is still unknown. The condition frequently appears for the first time in the area of the first metatarsal heads with an acute intermittent cellulitis that eventually turns into a granulomatous process involving the juxtaarticular structures about the first metatarsophalangeal joint (Fig. 16-60). There is geographic erosion on the medial aspect of the first metatarsal head and on the base of the proximal phalanx. As time progresses, the arthritic process develops

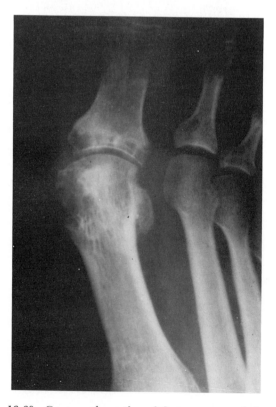

Fig. 16-60. Gouty arthropathy of first metatarsophalangeal joint.

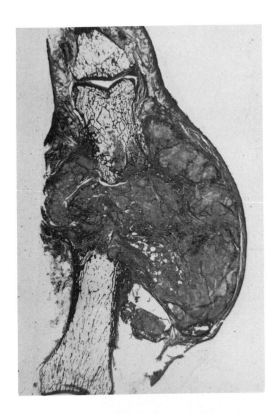

Fig. 16-61. Tophaceous gouty arthropathy of first metatarsophalangeal joint.

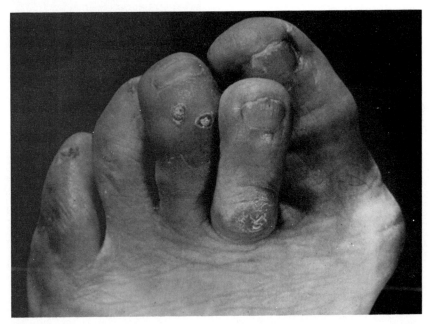

Fig. 16-62. Gouty ulcerations on dorsum of third toe.

into a tophaceous condition with accumulation of urate deposits around the joint like those seen in the macroscopic section (Fig. 16-61). Extensive destructive changes can be seen in the first metatarsophalangeal joint. Sometimes the presence of small cutaneous ulcerations with uric acid crystals at the center that can be scraped with a knife and viewed under the microscope confirm the clinical diagnosis of gout. Fig. 16-62 shows a gouty foot with two diagnostic ulcers on the dorsum of the third toe. Fig. 16-63 shows more extensive gouty arthritic changes throughout the entire midtarsal area and first ray. Tophaceous gout can produce extensive soft tissue tumor masses beneath the skin, which might suggest neurofibromatosis (as seen in Fig. 16-64 in a 45-

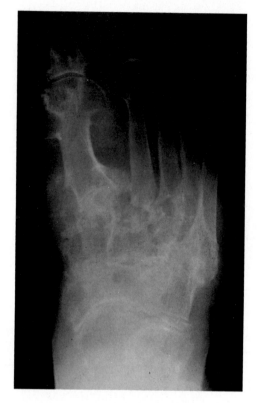

Fig. 16-63. Extensive gouty arthropathy of midtarsal area.

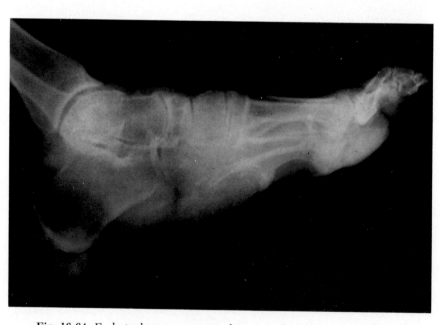

Fig. 16-64. Early tophaceous gout involving mainly subcutaneous tissues.

year-old with minimum arthritic changes). However, as time passes, the joints also become involved and the tophaceous material calcifies as seen in Fig. 16-65 in a much older patient. This radiograph takes on the appearance of the radiograph of a neuropathic foot. Balasubramanian and Silva (1971) suggest debridement of the tophi and bone grafting, if necessary.

Acromegaly. In acromegaly there is an overproduction of pituitary hormone after adult life is reached. This produces generalized hypertrophy of all somatic tissues including bone and soft tissues overlying the bones. Fig. 16-66 shows an example of the thickening seen in the heel pad of such a patient. More characteristic of this disease state is the generalized hypertrophy of bone about the face and jaw (Fig. 16-67). Large air sinuses and a "Dick Tracy" mandible are evident, and the sella turcica is enlarged as a result of the pituitary adenoma.

Hypercholesterolemia. Another metabolic disease state relating to the foot and ankle area is hypercholesterolemia, which can lead to the life-threatening problems of coronary artery disease and myocardial infarction. In the ankle area, however, one commonly sees evidence of dystrophic calcification in the heel cord associated with weakening of the cord, pain, and microscopic tearing in the weakened structure. Fig. 16-68 shows the typical radiographic appearance of the calcification seen in a patient's heel cord associated with a fusiform enlargement of the cord that could even suggest a tumor mass.

These tendons should never be injected with cortisone, for this could increase the possibility of the patho-

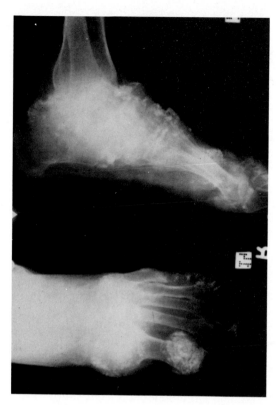

Fig. 16-65. Advanced calcific tophaceous gout in elderly patient.

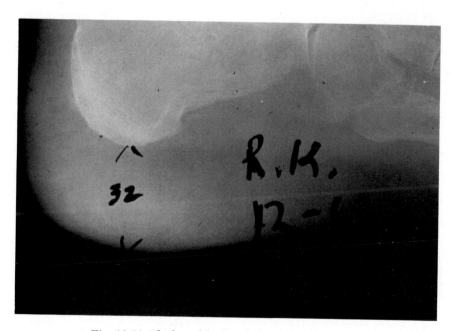

Fig. 16-66. Thickened heel pad in acromegalic patient.

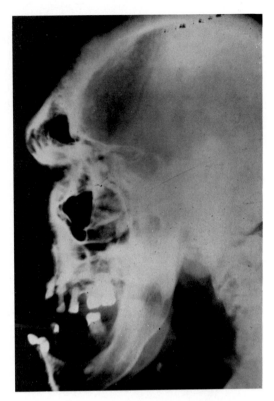

Fig. 16-67. Typical acromegalic skull and face.

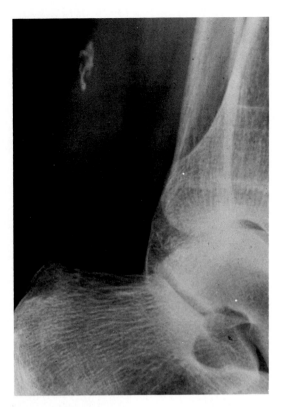

Fig. 16-68. Dystrophic calcification in heel cord of patient with hypercholesterolemia.

logic rupture that occurs in a fair number of such patients. In one of my own patients both heel cords ruptured, and large deposits of cholesterol were found in and around the area, requiring multiple debridements. It was eventually necessary to completely remove both heel cords because of advanced degenerative changes that frustrated any attempt at a reconstructive approach to her mechanical problem. Fig. 16-69 is a photograph of this patient's heels after multiple surgical procedures.

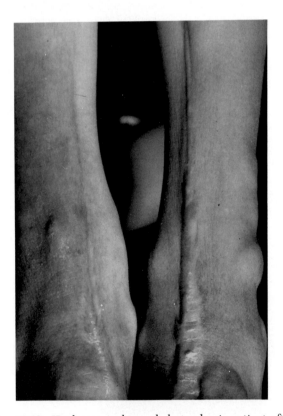

Fig. 16-69. Heel area in hypercholesterolemic patient after complete debridement of both heel cords.

REFERENCES
General

Ackerman, L.V., and Spjut, H.J.: Tumors of bone and cartilage, Washington D.C., 1962, Armed Forces Institute of Pathology.

Aegerter, E., and Kirkpatrick, J.A., Jr.: Orthopedic diseases, ed. 4, Philadelphia, 1975, W.B. Saunders Co.

Dahlin, D.C.: Bone tumors, ed. 2, Springfield, Ill., 1967, Charles C Thomas, Publisher.

Enzinger, F.M., and Weiss, S.W.: Soft tissue tumors, St. Louis, 1982, The C.V. Mosby Co.

Geiser, M., and Trueta, J.: Muscle action, bone rarefaction and bone formation, J. Bone Joint Surg. **40B:**282, 1958.

Greenfield, G.B.: Radiology of bone diseases, Philadelphia, 1969, J.B. Lippincott Co.

Jaffe, H.L.: Tumors and tumorous conditions of the bones and joints, Philadelphia, 1958, Lea & Febiger.

Spjut, H.J., Dorfman, H.D., Fechner, R.E., and Ackerman, L.V.: Tumors of bone and cartilage, Atlas of tumor pathology, Ser. 2, Fasc. 5, Washington, D.C., 1971, Armed Forces Institute of Pathology.

Stout, A.P., and Lattes, R.: Tumors of the soft tissues. Atlas of tumor pathology, Ser. 2, Fasc. 1, Washington, D.C., 1967, Armed Forces Institute of Pathology.

Specific

Ackerman, L.V.: Surgical pathology, ed. 4, St. Louis, 1968, The C.V. Mosby Co.

Arieff, A.J., Bell, J.L., Tigay, E.L., and Kurtz, J.F.: Reflex physiopathic disturbances, J. Bone Joint Surg. **45A:**1329, 1963.

Balasubramanian, P., and Silva, J.F.: Tophectomy and bone-grafting for extensive tophi of the feet, J. Bone Joint Surg. **53A:**133, 1971.

Cameron, H.U., and Kostuik, J.P.: A long-term follow-up of synovial sarcoma, J. Bone Joint Surg. **56B:**613, 1974.

Capanna, R., Dal Monte, H., Gitelis, S., and Campanacci, M.: The natural history of unicameral bone cysts after steroid injection, Clin. Orthop. **166:**204, 1982.

Cowie, R.S.: Benign osteoblastoma of the talus, J. Bone Joint Surg. **48B:**582, 1966.

Dahlin, D.C., and Salvador, A.H.: Chondrosarcoma of bones of the hands and feet: a study of 30 cases, Cancer **34:**755, 1974.

Das Gupta, T.K., Patel, M.R., Chaudhuri, P.K., and Briele, H.A.: The role of chemotherapy as an adjuvant to surgery in the initial treatment of primary soft tissue sarcomas in adults, J. Surg. Oncol. **19:**193, 1982.

Eisenstein, R.: Giant-cell tumor of tendon sheath, J. Bone Joint Surg. **50A:**476, 1968.

Giannestras, N.J., and Diamond, J.R.: Benign osteoblastoma of the talus: a review of the literature and report of a case, J. Bone Joint Surg. **40A:**469, 1958.

Goldenberg, R.R., Campbell, C.J., and Bonfiglio, M.: Giant cell tumor of bone, J. Bone Joint Surg. **52A:**619, 1970.

Jones, F.E., Soule, E.H., and Coventry, M.D.: Fibrous xanthoma of synovium (giant-cell tumor of tendon sheath, pigmented nodular synovitis), J. Bone Joint Surg. **51A:**76, 1969.

Keller, R.B., and Baez-Giangreco, A.: Juvenile aponeurotic fibroma: Report of three cases and a review of the literature, Clin. Orthop. **106:**198, 1975.

Larsson, S.E., Lorentzon, R., and Boquist, L.: Fibrosarcoma of bone: a demographic, clinical and histopathological study of all cases recorded in the Swedish Cancer Registry from 1958 to 1968, J. Bone Joint Surg. **58B:**412, 1976.

Lewis, G.M.: Practical dermatology, ed. 3, Philadelphia, 1967, W.B. Saunders Co.

Lewis, R.J., Marcove, R.C., and Rosen, G.: Ewing's sarcoma-functional effects of radiation therapy, J. Bone Joint Surg. **59A:**325, 1977.

Makely, J.: Personal communication, 1982.

McNeill, T.W., and Ray, R.D.: Hemangioma of the extremities: a review of 35 cases, Clin. Orthop. **101:**154, 1974.

Pedersen, H.E., and Day, A.J.: Dupuytren's disease of the foot, JAMA **154:**33, 1954.

Pritchard, D.J., Dahlin, D.C., Dauphine, R.T., Taylor, W.F., and Beabout, J.W.: Ewing's sarcoma: a clinicopathological and statistical analysis of patients surviving five years or longer, J. Bone Joint Surg. **57A:**10, 1975.

Rosen, G., Capanos, B., Huvos, A.G., Koslof, C., Nirenberg, A., Cacavio, A., Marcove, R.C., Lane, J.M., Mehta, B., and Urban, C.: Preoperative chemotherapy for osteosarcoma: selection of postoperative adjutant chemotherapy based on the response of the primary to preoperative chemotherapy, Cancer **49:**1221, 1982.

Simon, M.A., and Enneking, W.F.: The management of soft tissue sarcomas of the extremities, J. Bone Joint Surg. **58A:**317, 1976.

Smith, R.W., and Smith, C.F.: Solitary unicameral bone cyst of the calcaneus: a review of twenty cases, J. Bone Joint Surg. **56A:**49, 1974.

Smyth, M.: Glomus-cell tumors in the lower extremity: report of two cases, J. Bone Joint Surg. **53A:**157, 1971.

Soren, A.: Pathogenesis and treatment of ganglion, Clin. Orthop. **48:**17, 1966.

Spanos, P.K., Payne, W.S., Ivins, J.C., and Pritchard, D.J.: Pulmonary resection for metastatic osteogenic sarcoma, J. Bone Joint Surg. **58A:**624, 1976.

Stening, W.S.: Primary malignant tumours of calcaneal tendon, J. Bone Joint Surg. **50B:**676, 1968.

Tepper, J., Glaubiger, D., Lichter, A., Wachenhut, J., and Glatstein, E.: Local control of Ewing sarcoma of bone with irradiation therapy and combined chemotherapy, Cancer **46:**1969, 1980.

17

Infectious disorders of the foot

STANFORD F. POLLOCK

An understanding of infectious disorders of the foot is important for two reasons:

1. Foot infections are among the most common conditions seen in the practice of medicine and podiatry.
2. A patient with generalized systemic illness, which makes him more susceptible to any infection, may first seek medical attention because of the symptoms of that infection. Thus the patient with unrecognized diabetes mellitus, arterial insufficiency, venous insufficiency, or systemic mycobacterial or fungal infection may have presenting complaints referable only to an infection of the foot.

The following outline offers a convenient guide for considering infections of the foot.

1. Bacterial infections
   a. Infections of soft tissues
      (1) Cellulitis
      (2) Lymphangitis
      (3) Felon
      (4) Tenosynovitis
      (5) Bursitis
   b. Infections involving bone
      (1) Pyogenic osteomyelitis
         (a) Acute
         (b) Chronic
         (c) Special types
            (i) Brodie's abscess
            (ii) Garré's osteomyelitis
      (2) Mycobacterial infection
         (a) Tuberculosis
         (b) Leprosy
      (3) Clostridial infection
      (4) Syphilis
2. Fungal infections
   a. Infections of skin and nails
      (1) Tinea pedis
      (2) Onychomycosis
   b. Infections involving deep structures including bone
      (1) Coccidioidomycosis
      (2) Mycetoma (madura foot)
         (a) Actinomycotic mycetoma
         (b) Maduromycosis

BACTERIAL INFECTIONS
Infections of soft tissues

Superficial pyogenic infections are often induced or aggravated by footwear. The distal portion or segment of the toe is susceptible to a felon similar to that which occurs in the finger. The troublesome, ubiquitous, tinea pedis organisms may combine with other bacterial organisms to infect the foot by means of neglected minor scratches, irritations caused by friction, or injury from such instruments as scissors. In the presence of such infection, continued wearing of shoes and weight bearing may lead to extension of the infection into the fascial planes, tendon sheaths, or lymphatic channels. Pyogenic organisms may invade any part of the foot through an abrasion in the skin surface. The abrasion may be microscopic, and the patient may be completely unaware of its presence.

Cellulitis. Cellulitis can result from the entrance of pyogenic bacteria to the tissues underlying the epidermis. The most commonly encountered organism is *Staphylococcus*, and the most common sites of entry of the organism are the numerous hair follicles. Continued irritation such as that caused by the eyelets of the shoe over the dorsum of the first metatarsocuneiform joint, generally the highest point on the dorsum of the midfoot, may aggravate the condition.

Cellulitis is best treated by complete bed rest, elevation of the foot, continual hot compresses, and appropriate systemic antibiotics. If pus is allowed to accu-

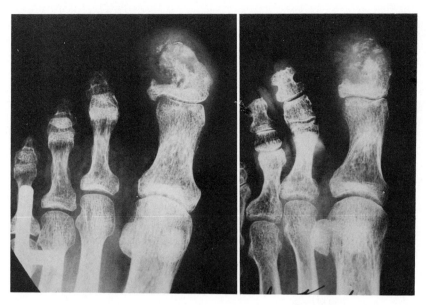

Fig. 17-1. Felon of great toe with involvement of distal phalanx.

mulate in a localized area, adequate drainage is mandatory.

Lymphangitis. Lymphangitis is generally caused by staphylococcal or streptococcal organisms that penetrate small wounds or abrasions.

The onset of symptoms of lymphangitis is sudden; a history of injury or abrasion may or may not be present. Pain and tenderness are experienced over a local point; chills often occur, followed by a rapidly rising temperature. Within 12 to 24 hours, bright red streaks may appear along the course of the lymphatic channels; inflammation and edema surround the streaks. The lymph glands proximal to the focus of infection become swollen, painful, and inflamed. Symptoms of general toxicity may be severe, out of all proportion to the appearance of the local lesion. In a few cases, organization of pus takes place at the focus of infection. Occasionally the infection spreads rapidly despite treatment until general septicemia develops. Koch (1934) has contributed a long study of the disease as it applies to the hand.

Treatment. Patients with lymphangitis should be hospitalized and kept at complete bed rest. The leg should be elevated, and moist hot compresses should be applied to the entire foot and leg continuously. High blood levels of appropriate antibiotics should be maintained. Close attention should be paid to such complications of toxemia as dehydration and electrolyte imbalance. Incision and drainage are rarely indicated and may even be harmful (Koch, 1929; Kanavel, 1939). Even if there is evidence of partial organization, it is better to err on the conservative side by not incising. The only indication for incision and drainage is the

presence of localized loculated areas of material. That condition is manifested by the presence of a blister or fluctuant mass directly under the skin, which ordinarily occurs at the focal point of infection but occasionally appears along the course of the lymphatic channels or in the area of the regional lymph nodes.

Felon. A felon, or whitlow, is a septic infection of the pulp space of the distal phalanx of the finger or toe (Fig. 17-1). Purulent material collects in the pulp space and may develop considerable pressure, causing accompanying severe throbbing pain. The pressure may cause decrease or obliteration of the blood supply to bone, which results in necrosis and sequestration. Osteomyelitis of the distal phalanx and interphalangeal joint is a common complication of a felon (Fig. 17-2).

The distal segment of the toe becomes indurated, swollen, and throbbing 24 to 48 hours following the onset of infection. Pain may be severe, with sleep impossible. The discrepancy between objective observations and the severity of the pain is characteristic of a felon. After several days the pain diminishes as necrosis of bone progresses. Radiographic examination at the time may disclose early osteomyelitis of the distal phalanx.

Treatment. Local and systemic measures, which include bed rest, elevation of the foot, and warm compresses, should be instituted immediately. Appropriate systemic antibiotics tend to localize the infectious process and should also be started immediately.

Except during the early stages in the development of a felon, incision and drainage are mandatory under general anesthesia or adequate regional block. The pulp space should be opened widely by a semicircular (fishmouth) incision extending from one side of the toe to

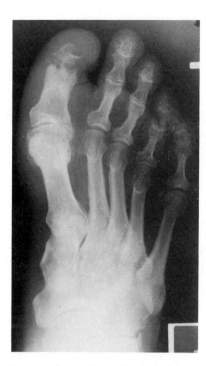

Fig. 17-2. Osteomyelitis of first distal phalanx and heads of proximal phalanges after injury.

the other and encircling the distal half of the distal phalanx. Secondary vertical incisions may be made into the pulp space to facilitate drainage. If sequestra are present, they may be removed. In most cases the process subsides in 2 to 3 weeks, and the bone regenerates. If the bone of the distal phalanx has sequestered completely, the sequestrum is occasionally better left in position in the hope that it will serve as a scaffold for the new bone formation and thereby conserve the contour of the toe. In most cases, however, the entire sequestered bone should be removed.

On occasion, the infection will progress so rapidly and with such local destruction of bone and tissues that amputation of the distal phalanx or of the entire digit is necessary. This destructive process is generally seen in diabetes or peripheral small-vessel disease. When amputation is necessary, the skin flaps should be left open for free drainage and subsequent secondary closure.

Infectious tenosynovitis. Infectious tenosynovitis is a bacterial inflammation of tendon sheaths that may be acute or chronic. It is always caused by invasion of the bacteria into the involved tendon sheaths. The course of the disease depends largely on the virulence of the invading organism and the extent of invasion of the tendon sheaths.

Acute infectious tenosynovitis (Christie, 1956) is caused by a spread of infection from adjacent tissues by accidental laceration (direct inoculation) or by contamination from an incision made because of a subcutaneous infection. The laceration or puncture may be microscopic. Occasionally the infection spreads to other parts of the body.

The invader in most cases is one of the common pyogenic organisms, although infections from other more unusual organisms have been reported.

Diagnosis is based on the classic signs of inflammation along the course of the tendon. The inflammation produces extreme pain, especially severe at the insertion of the tendon (even though the active infection may be distant from it) because the infected tendon is immobilized. Any tendon or tendon sheath may be involved, but the extensor tendons of the foot are most commonly affected. Sliding of the tendon or tendons is a complication that may lead to extreme contracture.

Treatment consists of complete bed rest and prompt administration of appropriate antibiotics. Continuous, hot, moist compresses should be applied, and when fluctuation gives evidence of the organization or localization of purulent material, surgical drainage should be carried out promptly. The local injection of antibiotics into the tendon sheath will occasionally reduce the necessity for incision and drainage but should not be relied on to the exclusion of surgical drainage.

Chronic infectious tenosynovitis is caused by a specific disease such as syphilis or tuberculosis. It may be the only manifestation of active tuberculosis. Chronic infectious tenosynovitis is rare, but when it occurs, it involves the sheaths of the extensors and peroneal tendons around the ankle joint.

Treatment consists of immobilization of the affected tendons and general treatment of the underlying systemic disease. Surgical repair of the gliding mechanism may be necessary when injury to the tendon and its sheath is severe.

Bursitis. Infectious bursitis includes two types: acute septic and retrocalcaneal.

Acute septic bursitis is inflammation of an adventitial bursa caused by the invasion of pyogenic organisms. It is often accompanied by pus formation. Usually a wound such as a small abrasion or laceration in the vicinity of the bursa causes acute septic bursitis. The condition may also follow a simple acute or traumatic bursitis resulting from the implantation of organisms from the circulatory system during a period of transient bacteremia.

Treatment consists of complete rest, hot compresses, appropriate antibiotics, and incision and drainage if localization or loculation has occurred. After the acute stage subsides, the patient may be ambulatory, provided pressure has been completely removed from the affected area.

Retrocalcaneal bursitis is an inflammation of the only

consistent anatomic bursa of the foot. This bursa is situated between the posterosuperior surface of the calcaneus and the Achilles tendon. The condition is usually acute but may be chronic and may or may not suppurate.

Etiology. Tension from a tight heel, friction, and pressure from the shoe counter, with ensuing secondary infection, are ordinarily the causative factors. Infection may be metastatic. Because the bursa is enclosed in a limited area, the infected area is under pressure. The symptoms of swelling and inflammation above the posterosuperior portion of the calcaneus, pain, and tenderness to touch may be acute. Dorsiflexion of the foot increases the pain.

Treatment. In the acute stage of retrocalcaneal bursitis, treatment is the same as for acute cellulitis: complete rest, hot packs, and antibiotics. If the infection becomes organized, drainage should be instituted. In chronic or recurrent cases the heel cords must be stretched or lengthened and the bursa may need to be excised; however, such excision is at times followed by lengthy and painful convalescence because of the difficulty of occluding the dead space left by removal of the bursa.

For a more complete discussion of the surgical procedures done in cases of infectious bursitis, see Chapter 13.

Infections involving bone

Pyogenic osteomyelitis. The term *osteomyelitis* implies infection of bone. Particular subtypes, based on objectively determined variations, are placed within this broad definition and include acute, subacute, and chronic osteomyelitis and special types of infectious diseases, such as mycotic infections of bone.

Acute osteomyelitis. Acute osteomyelitis may occur at any age by means of either local bacterial invasion or bacteremia with secondary seeding.

An intact bone in a healthy individual is resistant to infection, and although bacterial infection of soft tissues will often spare the skeleton, massive tissue injury may lower resistance to bacterial invasion. In some cases this lowered resistance is accompanied by a decreased blood supply to the bones as well. Many systemic illnesses lower intrinsic resistance, and subsequent infection of bone, which necessitates radical treatment, may occur.

Acute hematogenous osteomyelitis was encountered more frequently during the preantibiotic era than it is today. Antibiotics have significantly diminished the problems of osteomyelitis.

In 1936 Wilson and McKeever reported that they had found 10 out of 90 foci of infection caused by hematogenous osteomyelitis in the bones of the foot. In the

10 cases the infection was distributed among the following sites: calcaneus, 5; metatarsals, 3; phalanges, 2.

The use of antibiotics may alter an acute osteomyelitis. For example, when antibiotics are administered in a random manner, a chronic smoldering infection may result and bypass the acute stage of the condition. The most common source of blood-borne bacterial seeding is *Staphylococcus aureus* (Clawson and Dunn, 1967).

The clinical picture of acute osteomyelitis varies according to the causative factors involved. Local bacteria invasion by hematogenous seeding produces a regional tissue response, with adjacent thrombosis, leukocytosis, and an attempted walling of the inoculum. The peculiarity of bone and its resistance to physical deformation render spontaneous drainage and tissue contractability impossible; consequently, the infectious process will develop rapidly by means of intramedullary extension until the entire bone may become involved. Acute hematogenous spread is associated with localized pain, erythema, edema, fever, and systemic signs of toxicity. A positive blood culture will confirm the diagnosis.

Infection caused by local inoculation, or contamination caused by the loss of bony integrity resulting from a compound fracture, may not produce the extreme picture of acute hematogenous osteomyelitis because an immediate drainage pathway is available in these instances. However, the attendant tissue destruction and decreased vascularity do provide a medium that perpetuates the acute infection.

The radiographic picture of acute osteomyelitis can change. At the time of onset, no positive findings may appear; later, rarefaction caused by hyperemia and disuse, soft-tissue swelling, periosteal thickening, medullary cloudiness, and loss of trabeculation may be evident. Radiographic findings are sometimes suggestive of greater bone destruction than actually exists (Fig. 17-3).

If left untreated, acute osteomyelitis will ultimately lead to chronic osteomyelitis or, in some instances, to one of the variant forms of osteomyelitis. The complementary relationship of the resistance of the host and the virulence of the invading agent bear a direct relationship to the ultimate resolution of the condition.

Treatment. The principles of treatment for acute bacterial osteomyelitis are basically the same as for pyogenic infection in other tissues of the body. Prompt identification of the infecting agent and antibiotic treatment, with correctly timed surgical drainage, are paramount. Needle aspiration through aseptically prepared skin into the suspected area, with immediate culture implantation, has proved to be the most successful technique for identifying the agent of infection. Selection of the antibiotic is best determined by the use of in vitro sensitivity studies and is confirmed by checking

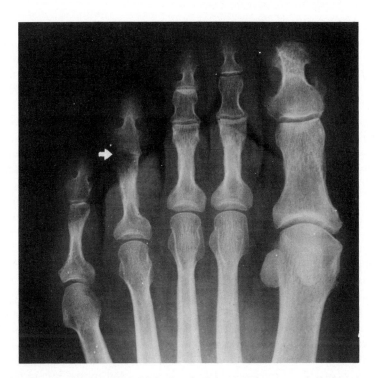

Fig. 17-3. Acute osteomyelitis of the head of the fourth proximal phalanx (arrow).

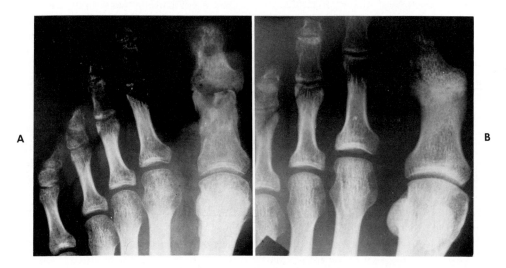

Fig. 17-4. A, Osteomyelitis of entire hallux. B, After healing.

bactericidal serum levels with subcultures in the laboratory (Jawetz, 1962).

It should be mentioned that in many instances an effective concentration of the antibiotic of choice may be hazardous to other organ systems of the body. Care must be taken to anticipate this danger and detect such damage promptly (Benner, 1967). Studies of renal function and electrolytic and audiometric studies may be indicated for debilitated patients before antibiotic treatment is initiated.

Surgical drainage may be accomplished by direct incision of the abscess, with open packing and delayed closure, or by the insertion of a tube for aspiration. In most areas of infection, tubal aspiration may be performed alternately with topical instillation of the antibiotic (Jergesen and Jawetz, 1963). The primary goals of drainage are to relieve the pressure of the pus and to curtail the spread of the infectious process. Once adequate drainage is established, the systemic findings will regress (Fig. 17-4).

ing out that approximately 1,900 cases of leprosy existed between 1950 and 1969.

Clinical course and types of lesions. Jacobson and Trautman (1976) have outlined the classification of forms of leprosy as follows: An individual coming in contact with *M. leprae* may develop no disease or may develop an indeterminate form of leprosy. This form is characterized by a macular skin lesion with or without sensory nerve loss. From the indeterminate form the patient may, in the absence of treatment, go on to develop the tuberculoid form, the lepromatous form, or the borderline form existing in various mixtures of the tuberculoid and lepromatous forms.

TUBERCULOID. The lesions in tuberculoid leprosy consist of areas of asymmetric lesions from tubercles containing epithelial cells, giant cells, lymphocytes, and plasma cells with few or no bacilli present. The lepromin skin test is positive in patients with this form of leprosy.

LEPROMATOUS. The lesions in lepromatous leprosy are characterized by the formation of lepromas, nodules that are made up of large macrophages that contain numerous bacilli and fat droplets. This is considered the most advanced stage of the disease, and the lepromin skin test is negative in individuals with this form of leprosy.

BORDERLINE. Borderline leprosy (known in the United States as intermediate or dimorphous) is characterized by the presence of lesions that demonstrate mixtures of both the tuberculoid and the lepromatous types, and an entire spectrum of pathologic findings between the two types and may be encountered. The skin test is variable, tending to be positive in patients exhibiting lesions of the tuberculoid type and negative in patients exhibiting lesions more consistent with the lepromatous type.

It would appear that the cellular immunity to *M. leprae* is highest in the tuberculoid form and lowest in the lepromatous form.

Effects of leprosy on feet. The foot may be affected in several ways: (1) leprous lesions may develop in the feet directly; (2) lepromatous involvement of the peripheral nerves may result in anesthetic feet; and (3) involvement of the peroneal nerve may result in foot drop.

Harris and Brand (1966) indicated two distinct methods of destruction of the foot once pain sensibility is lost. The first is slow erosion and shortening associated with perforating ulcers under the distal, weight-bearing end of the foot. The second is a proximal disintegration of the tarsus in which mechanical forces often determine the onset and progress of the condition.

The treatment of such feet is as follows:

1. The patient must be educated to use the feet only for gentle walking.

2. Immobilization of the feet in plaster or complete bed rest is necessary for the treatment of ulcers.

3. One should be alert to signs of tarsal disintegration. The earliest signs may be local warmth, swelling, or both. When these signs occur, gait analysis should be carried out and suitable shoe adjustment should be made until the patient can walk a limited distance without developing abnormal tarsal heat at points of stress.

4. When definite bone damage is seen, full immobilization is imperative.

5. In cases in which joints are disintegrating, surgical fusion should be performed without delay.

Warren (1971), in a study of tarsal bone disintegration in over 1,500 leprosy patients treated at the Hong Kong Leprosarium during a 12-year period, found that early detection and treatment by immobilization permitted healing with minimal deformity or disability and that feet with advanced lesions could be similarly treated without amputation.

Involvement of the common peroneal nerve frequently results in foot drop. Carayon et al. (1967) described promising results in the correction of this deformity with a dual transfer of the posterior tibial and flexor digitorum longus tendons.

Treatment. The current management of leprosy is primarily by chemotherapeutic means with dapsone (DDS, diaminodiphenylsulfone), clofazimine, and rifampin used in combination or alone as the drugs of choice.

Jacobson and Trautman (1976) have reviewed the use of these drugs and the reactions that may be seen to the treatment of leprosy. The reactions to treatment include the (1) reversal reaction, in which a more lepromatous form tends to revert to a more tuberculoid form accompanied by fever, edema, and ulceration, and (2) erythema nodosum leprosum. The reversal reaction is best treated by the administration of systemic corticosteroids and erythema nodosum leprosum by the administration of thalidomide.

Surgical procedures continued to play an important role in the treatment of neurologic manifestations of leprosy.

Clostridial infection (gas gangrene). Anaerobic bacteria of the genus *Clostridia* may be found in wounds in three situations: as saprophytic contaminants, in clostridial cellulitis, and in clostridial myonecrosis (true gas gangrene).

Sim (1975) has pointed out that examination of stained smears of nearly all fresh wounds caused by violent trauma reveals clostridial organisms. Despite the high incidence of contamination, clostridial infections

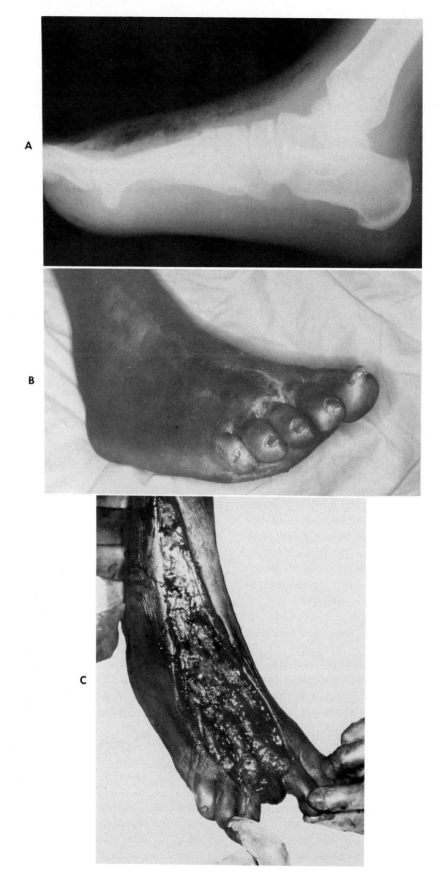

Fig. 17-9. Gas gangrene of foot. **A,** Lateral view showing gas formation in subcutaneous tissue on dorsum as result of clostridial cellulitis. **B,** Clostridial cellulitis of dorsum of foot. Note fluctuant swelling of subcutaneous tissue. **C,** At time of wide incision and drainage; necrotic tissue excised.

do not occur often. When the anaerobic clostridial organism multiplies in tissues devitalized by wounding without significant production of toxin, saprophytic contamination is felt to be present, and no specific treatment other than the general measures applicable to all contaminated wounds is necessary.

Clostridial cellulitis is a septic process usually caused by *Clostridium perfringens* and is often mistakenly diagnosed as gas gangrene (clostridial myonecrosis). It is an infection of the subcutaneous tissues and fascial planes rendered susceptible by ischemia or crush injury. In this case, muscle is generally not affected; the patient exhibits only mild toxemia and profuse crepitation in the subcutaneous tissues of the involved areas.

Gas gangrene or clostridial myonecrosis is characterized by clostridial invasion of normal uninjured muscle with necrosis of muscle cells rapidly extending in every direction from the site of injury. The patient is extremely toxic, probably as a result of the production by the clostridia of the alpha toxin or lecithinase. Gas production may be minimal in myonecrosis, and the course of the disease may be extremely rapid. In the foot clostridial cellulitis is more commonly encountered because, compared with the leg or thigh, the foot has relatively little muscle tissue (Fig. 17-9). The most common causative organisms are *Clostridium perfringens*, *C. novyi*, and *C. septicum*.

Diagnosis. The possibility of clostridial infection should be considered whenever there is a crush injury with devitalized tissue of even a small amount. This is especially true if there has been the possibility of contamination by foreign body, soil, or feces.

The diagnosis is made essentially by physical examination. The characteristic picture of gas gangrene is tissue edema, necrosis, discoloration, characteristic autopsy room odor, brown exudate, and crepitation caused by gas formation in the soft tissues. Care should be taken, however, not to assume that any infection associated with gas formation is clostridial; many other organisms can produce gas, or air can be trapped in the soft tissues as a result of open injury. Diagnosis is confirmed by the findings of characteristic gram-positive bacilli on exudate or debrided soft tissue. Cultures are rarely of value in making the diagnosis because of the prolonged delay.

Treatment. Gas gangrene is almost always preventable. The most important single aspect in the prevention of gas gangrene is thorough, adequate debridement of all dead avascular tissue. The wound must be debrided back to bleeding tissue and, in the case of muscle, to the point at which the muscle contracts when gently pinched. Prophylactic use of antibiotics is of some value; generally penicillin in very high doses is the drug of choice. It must be pointed out, however, that no antibiotic can prevent gas gangrene in the absence of thorough surgical debridement.

The use of polyvalent gas gangrene antitoxin is controversial; probably it should not be used prophylactically. Its value in treatment remains questionable. Also used in treatment is hyperbaric oxygen (3 atmospheres), which is probably a helpful adjunct. However, hyperbaric oxygen should not be considered a substitute for adequate thorough surgical treatment. Despite adequate local debridement and the use of antibiotics and hyperbaric oxygen, occasionally the infection cannot be controlled without amputating the involved limb.

Syphilis

Syphilitic neuropathy. Until the advent of antibiotics, latent syphilis was the most common destroyer of the joints of the body (Figs. 17-10 and 17-11). Although the late manifestations of syphilis have now become rare, the sexually transmitted disease rate for both syphilis and gonorrhea has continually increased throughout the world. Charcot's joint was frequently encountered as a result of syphilis; but its predilection was for the knee rather than the foot, although the ankle was often affected and other joints were not affected. Antibiotics and antianemia therapy have greatly diminished the incidence of arthropathies caused by syphilis and anemia.

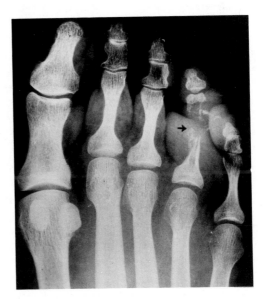

Fig. 17-10. Necrosis of fourth digit in latent syphilis.

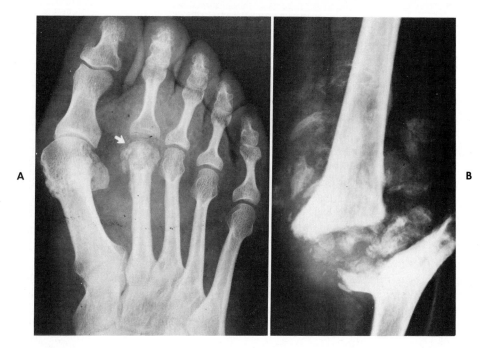

Fig. 17-11. Charcot's joints in latent syphilis. **A,** Second metatarsophalangeal. **B,** Knee. Note bizarre destruction and new bone formation.

FUNGAL INFECTIONS
Infections of the skin and nails

Tinea pedis (athlete's foot, dermatophytosis, ringworm). Tinea pedis is perhaps the most common infection of the foot. Spores of one or more strains of trichophytes are commonly harbored between the toes and under the nails, but they may also invade any part of the foot. Chronicity and recurrence are common. The spores of the organisms may lie dormant for months or years before they mature and multiply under favorable conditions such as excessive moisture, friction, pressure, or trauma either accidentally or iatrogenically.

When the disease is active, it assumes various forms and degrees from minute fissures between the toes to a vesicular scaly dermatitis over large areas on the entire foot (Fig. 17-12). It varies from a low-grade inflammatory process to a violent infection, although serious illness is rare. The most common causative organisms are *Trichophyton mentagrophytes* and *T. rubrum*. In severe cases secondary bacterial infection may be present.

Treatment is directed at relieving the severe itching and other signs of local irritation. Frequent changes of dry socks, use of foot powders, and drying thoroughly between toes after bathing are of importance. For severe cases an article in *Medical Letter* recommends the drugs clotrimazole and miconazole applied locally ("Drugs for Athlete's Foot," 1976). Griseofulvin taken systemically for many months has been useful in sup-

pressing the infection but is probably *not* indicated, since there is some question as to the carcinogenicity of griseofulvin.

The condition known as pustular acrodermatitis enters into the differential diagnosis, for it may have an identical appearance. Microscopic examination of potassium hydroxide–treated scrapings from suspected lesions, however, will show the typical mycelia of a true fungal infection.

Onychomycosis. Onychomycosis represents a condition in which there is fungal infection of the toenail and nail bed. This is most commonly caused by *Trichophyton rubrum* and secondly to *T. mentagrophytes*. Other cases have been caused by *Candida albicans*. In this condition thick accumulations of keratinous material appear under the nail; the nail is often discolored to a yellowish tint and grows erratically.

Treatment is generally with keratolytic agents. Topical treatments such as Castellani's paint and gentian violet along with nail debridement appear to be the most useful in controlling but not eradicating the condition. In cases caused by *Candida albicans*, underlying systemic illness may be suspected. In severe cases nail avulsion is indicated.

Infections involving the deep structures including bone

Coccidioidomycosis. *Coccidioides immitis*, a specific fungus, gains entrance through the respiratory tract or

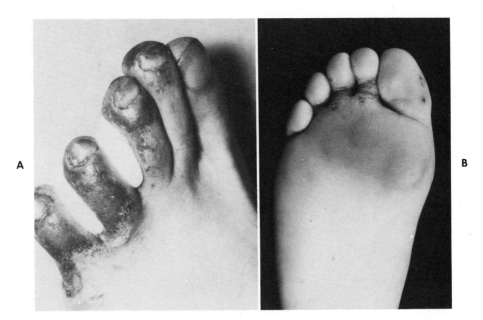

Fig. 17-12. Dermatophytosis. **A,** Acute, of toes. **B,** Chronic, in plantar creases of toes.

skin and is disseminated through the blood or lymph channels or is spread by direct extension. Spores settle in cancellous bone, and bone lesions form. The resulting infection is usually chronic and shows clinical and radiographic changes similar to those in chronic osteomyelitis.

McMaster and Gilfillan (1939) reported 24 cases of coccidioidal osteomyelitis with multiple foci involving various parts of the body, including the foot. The average age of their patients, who were predominantly men, was 32 years. Thirteen of the patients died; all were proved to have had an associated active pulmonary involvement.

Grebe (1954) reported a case of monostotic coccidioidal infection in which the bone lesion occurred in the left calcaneus. Evidence of disease or injury had not been observed. There was no response to wide excision of the bone lesion, but rapid healing was accomplished by treatment with hydroxystilbamidine isethionate.

More recently, the use of amphotericin B as described by Winn (1955, 1963) has produced encouraging results in cases that might previously have been fatal. Amphotericin B has been particularly useful in preventing massive dissemination of the disease in patients who undergo surgical procedures for coccidioidal lesions. A fall in the coccidioidal complement fixation titer indicates successful treatment and may occur after surgical removal of the infected tissue. Although treatment with amphotericin B has effectively reduced the toxicity of the disease, it should also be noted that amphotericin B is an extremely toxic drug and that *Coccidioides immitis* is among the most resistant of fungal infections to the drug.

Mycetoma (madura foot)

Actinomycotic mycetoma and maduromycosis. Mycetoma is a chronic granulomatous disease (Fig. 17-13) found mainly in tropical countries, especially in some districts of India. Etiologically mycetoma can be separated into actinomycotic mycetoma, caused by several species of *Streptomyces* and *Nocardia*, and maduromycosis, caused by large filament-producing species of higher fungi such as *Madurella, Leptosphaeria senegalensis, Allescheria boydii, Monosporium apiospermum,* and others.

The clinical picture is the same whether the condition is actinomycotic in origin or produced by the higher fungi. The disease begins as a granuloma, generally subcutaneous in location (Fig. 17-14). The deep structures are involved only late in the course of the disease (Oyston, 1961). New tumors form while old ones soften, and the foot increases enormously in size, becoming deformed.

Franz and Albertini (1954) found extensive osteoporosis of the tarsal bones in one of their patients. Primary mycetoma of bone is a more uncommon condition. According to Majid et al. (1964), all primary intraosseous infections that have been studied mycologically are caused by *Madurella mycetomi.*

A similar condition indigenous to the United States is caused by *Actinomyces bovis,* a gram-positive, non-acid-fast, nonmotile filamentous organism related to true bacteria but resembling fungi.

The characteristic lesion in this condition is a firm, relatively nontender, abscess with central necrosis that may drain to the surface. Consequently, the sinus tract produced has little tendency to heal spontaneously.

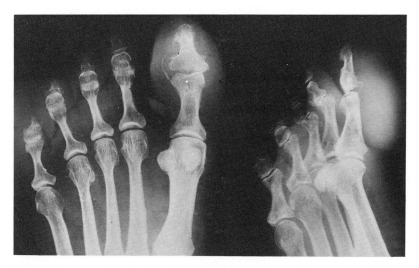

Fig. 17-13. Massive granuloma of great toe; result of mycotic infection acquired in tropical country.

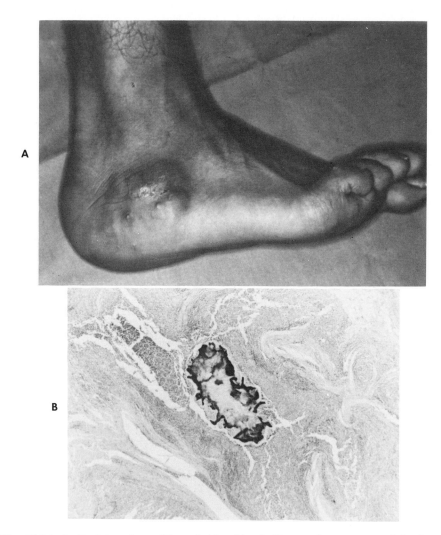

Fig. 17-14. A, Draining sinus of lateral side of heel. Biopsy of extensive nodular lesion of soft tissues revealed *Nocardia*. **B,** *Nocardia* colony with chronic inflammation; sulfur granule of lesion in **A.**

Identification of the organisms and appropriate antimicrobial sensitivity studies are important, since treatment may depend to some degree on the use of antimicrobial agents. Atinomycotic mycetoma may be sensitive to penicillin, tetracycline, erythromycin, and chloramphenicol and sulfones. Even restoration of diseased and partially destroyed bones has been reported with chemotherapy in the treatment of mycetoma caused by *Streptomyces madurae* by Kamalam et al. (1975).

Mycetomas caused by *Madurella* types of organisms are fairly resistant to antimicrobial therapy. Although Neuhauser (1955) reported promising therapeutic results with diaminodiphenylsulfone, Wilson (1975) has stated that he knows of no chemotherapeutic agent, including amphotericin B, effective against infections with such organisms as *Allescheria boydii*. In spite of the results of antimicrobial treatment, surgery often is necessary. In all these conditions early excision of superficial lesions lead fairly often to cure. In advanced cases amputation above the disease area may be necessary.

REFERENCES

Aegerter, E., and Kirkpatrick, J.A., Jr.: Orthopedic diseases, ed. 3, Philadelphia, 1968, W.B. Saunders Co.

Benner, E.J.: Use and abuse of antibiotics J. Bone Joint Surg. **49A**:977, 1967.

Carayon, A., Bourrel, P., Bourges, M., and Touzé, M.: Dual transfer of the posterior tibial and flexor digitorum longus tendons for drop foot: report of thirty-one cases, J. Bone Joint Surg. **49A**:144, 1967.

Christie, B.G.B.: The diagnosis and treatment of tenosynovitis, Br. J. Clin. Pract. **10**:677, 1956.

Clawson, D.K., and Dunn, A.W.: Management of common bacterial infections of bones and joints, J. Bone Joint Surg. **49A**:164, 1967.

Drugs for athlete's foot and tinea cruris, Med. Lett. Drugs Ther. **18**:101, 1976.

Feldman, R.A., and Sturdivant, M.: Leprosy in the United States 1950-1969: an epidemologic review, South. Med. J. **69**:970, 1976.

Franz, A., and Albertini, B.: Sul micetoma primitivo del piede: piede di Madura, Chir. Organi Mov. **40**:412, 1954.

Friedman, B., and Kapur, V.N.: Newer knowledge of chemotherapy in the treatment of tuberculosis of bones and joints, Clin. Orthop. **97**:5, 1973.

Grebe, A.A.: Monostotic coccidioidal infection: report of a case successfully treated with 2-hydroxystilbamidine, J. Bone Joint Surg. **36A**:859, 1954.

Greenfield, G.B.: Radiology of bone diseases, Philadelphia, 1969, J.B. Lippincott Co.

Harris, J.R., and Brand, P.W.: Patterns of disintegration of the tarsus in the anaesthetic foot, J. Bone Joint Surg. **48B**:4, 1966.

Jacobson, R.R., and Trautman, J.R.: The diagnosis and treatment of leprosy, South. Med. J. **69**:979, 1976.

Jawetz, E.: Assay of antibacterial activity in serum, Am. J. Dis. Child. **103**:81, 1962.

Jergesen, F., and Jawetz, E.: Pyogenic infections in orthopedic surgery: combined antibiotic and closed wound treatment, Am. J. Surg. **106**:152, 1963.

Kamalam, A., Premalatha, S., Augustine, S.M., and Saravanamuthu, A.: Restoration of bones in mycetoma, Arch. Dematol. **111**:1178, 1975.

Kanavel, A.B.: Infections of the hand, ed. 7, Philadelphia, 1939, Lea & Febiger.

Koch, S.L.: Felons, acute lymphangitis and tendon sheath infections: differential diagnosis and treatment, JAMA **92**:1171, 1929.

Koch, S.L.: Acute rapidly spreading infections following trivial injuries of the hand, Surg. Gynecol. Obstet. **59**:277, 1934.

Majid, M.A., and Mathias, P.F., Seth, H.N., and Thirumalachar, M.J.: Primary mycetoma of the patella, J. Bone Joint Surg. **46A**:1283, 1964.

McMaster, P.E., and Gilfillan, C.: Coccidioidal osteomyelitis, JAMA **112**:1233, 1939.

Miltner, L.J., and Fang, H.C.: Prognosis and treatment of tuberculosis of the bones of the foot, J. Bone Joint Surg. **18**:287, 1936.

Neuhauser, I.: Black grain maduromycosis caused by *Madurella grisea*, Arch. Dermatol. **72**:550, 1955.

Oyston, J.K.: Madura foot: a study of twenty cases, J. Bone Joint Surg. **43B**:259, 1961.

Reeves, J.D.: Differential diagnosis in case 44122: presentation of the case, N. Engl. J. Med. **258**:612, 1958.

Rowling, D.E.: The positive approach to chronic osteomyelitis, J. Bone Joint Surg. **41B**:681, 1959.

Sim, F.H.: Anaerobic infections, Orthop. Clin. North Am. **6**:1049, 1975.

Trueta, J.: The three types of acute haematogenous osteomyelitis: a clinical and vascular study, J. Bone Joint Surg. **41B**:671, 1959.

Warren, G.: Tarsal bone disintegration in leprosy, J. Bone Joint Surg. **53B**:688, 1971.

Wilson, J.C., and McKeever, F.M.: Bone growth disturbance following hematogenous osteomyelitis, JAMA **107**:1188, 1936.

Wilson, J.W.: Discussion of transactions of the Los Angeles Dermatological Society: *Nocardia brasiliensis* mycetoma, Arch. Dermatol. **11**:1371, 1975.

Winn, W.A.: The use of amphotericin B in the treatment of coccidioidal disease, Am. J. Med. **27**:617, 1955.

Winn, W.A.: Coccidioidomycosis and amphotericin B, Med. Clin. North Am. **47**:1131, 1963.

18

Dermatology and disorders of the toenails

JERRAL S. SEIBERT and ROGER A. MANN

In many specialties of medicine there is overlapping of subject matter; such is the case concerning orthopaedic and skin foot problems. It behooves the practitioner to have some knowledge of the allied fields because frequently patients unknowingly will seek advice concerning symptoms and conditions of the other specialty. The following cutaneous entities commonly found on the feet are discussed. By no means is this listing complete for all the dermatologic conditions affecting the feet. That is beyond the scope of the present chapter; the reader is referred to further complete treatises such as those of Costello and Gibbs (1967) and Gibbs (1974).

An important corollary should be reemphasized for examining skin lesions of the feet: the clinician should always check the hands and occasionally other parts of the integument because many afflictions involving the feet will also be present on the palms or other areas of the skin.

CORNS, CALLUSES, AND WARTS

Discrete hyperkeratotic skin lesions on the feet are perhaps the most common complaint and it is important to distinguish the exact identity of the lesion for successful therapy.

Calluses develop at sites of pressure, usually under the bony prominences of the feet. They tend to be the largest, and corns the smallest, and the hyperkeratotic lesions. To differentiate these plantar lesions, one must pare away the hyperkeratotic coverings so the distinguishing clinical characteristics are evident. Calluses have wide papillary lines that do not diverge from their normal direction. The margins of calluses are rather diffuse whereas those of corns and warts are sharply de-

marcated. Corns and warts have deviating papillary lines or lines that are interrupted by a sharply marginated lesion. Calluses have no cores and no visible blood vessels. Corns have papillary lines diverging around a sharply marginated translucent core devoid of blood vessels. Warts have the fine capillaries that diagnostically rise perpendicularly to the surface. Pain may be a distinguishing feature with the various lesions. Calluses are usually not painful until they become large and extensive. Corns, particularly the neurovascular and soft types, are quite painful. Warts may be painful, depending on the type and location (Fig. 18-1). Lateral pressure elicits pain in the wart; direct pressure causes pain in the corn.

Treatment of a callus usually requires that the pressure causing it be removed. This requires the patient to wear correctly fitted shoes or use corrective protective pads to distribute the body weight evenly over the weight-bearing portions of the foot. To reduce the callus formation, periodic paring plus use of 40% salicylic acid plasters is effective.

Corns also result from friction and pressure localizing especially on the bulb of the great toe or on the sides, tips, and tops of other toes; under bony prominences, and in the metatarsal area. Treatment consists of paring periodically plus application of a 40% salicylic acid plaster with a felt pad fashioned to fit around the corn to relieve the pressure. Protective padding is required to keep the corn from recurring; the padding or cushion can be incorporated into a supportive insole in the shoe. Again, it is important to emphasize that properly fitted shoes should be worn to prevent recurrences. In this regard, as Montgomery points out, properly fitted shoes are an important part in the treatment of any

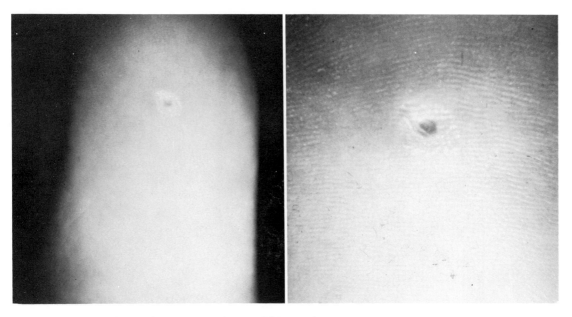

Fig. 18-1. Plantar clavus (corn). This painful lesion developed on heel of adolescent girl who suspected a wart. Inspection of her "everyday shoes" revealed protruding nail at site of hyperkeratosis.

plantar keratotic lesions. Too narrow a shoe squeezes the toes together and may cause soft corns; too short a shoe may cause corns to form on the tips and tops of the toes; too high a heel interferes with the proper distribution of the body weight across the foot and may cause painful calluses, corns, or warts.

The second type of corn, neurovascular corn, is notable for it is usually painful and frequently mistaken as a verruca. It is usually situated on the plantar surface under the first or fifth metatarsal head and appears as a small (1 to 3 mm) lesion with a diffuse translucent core that fades into the surrounding tissues. At the periphery of the corn, small dried up capillaries appear, some of which lie parallel with the skin rather than perpendicular as do the vessels in warts. Treatment of neurovascular corn consists of weekly paring and application of caustic such as 50% silver nitrate. Further thinning by application of keratolytic such as 40% salicylic acid plaster can further thin down this tissue. Adequate padding, again, is essential. Excising these painful lesions is inadvisable, for a resolving scar may occur that is more painful than the original corn. Orthopaedic surgery is sometimes required for removal of the plantar condyle of the metatarsal head for resistant cases.

A third type of corn affects the intertriginous aspects of the toes and is sometimes misdiagnosed as tinea pedis. The soft corn is painful and appears as a flat white soggy area on the opposing surfaces of adjacent toes usually in the fourth interdigital web. Other interdigital spaces may be involved, for the condition occurs whenever the condyle of a phalanx of one toe presses against the condyle of the head of the adjacent metatarsal. Paring away the superficial material reveals two small cores opposing each other. Sometimes for chronic cases a sinus tract with purulent exudate will be present. Treatment of the soft corn may be simply separating the toes with a cushion such as lamb's wool or a thin piece of foam rubber, or other measures may be tried such as keeping the corn thin by paring and by application of a keratolytic such as salicylic acid plaster. Again, proper fitting shoes that give the toes room to spread apart should be worn. If these conservative measures fail, excision of the prominent condyle will effect a cure.

Plantar warts or "papillomas of the sole" are frequent lesions seen in a dermatology office. They can occur on any part of the foot; when they occur under pressure points, they give rise to tenderness and localized pain. Fig. 18-2 presents the histologic difference between a wart and a keratotic lesion (e.g., a callus). Warts are caused by a DNA virus belonging to the papovavirus group. The first step in treatment is to pare away the superficial keratin surface. A sharply marginated lesion appears with many capillary dots that rise perpendicular to the surface of the skin.

Plantar warts are usually grouped into one of three types:

1. A single or solitary wart surrounded by callus tissue with the papillary lines diverging around it. Depending on its location, if it is located under a

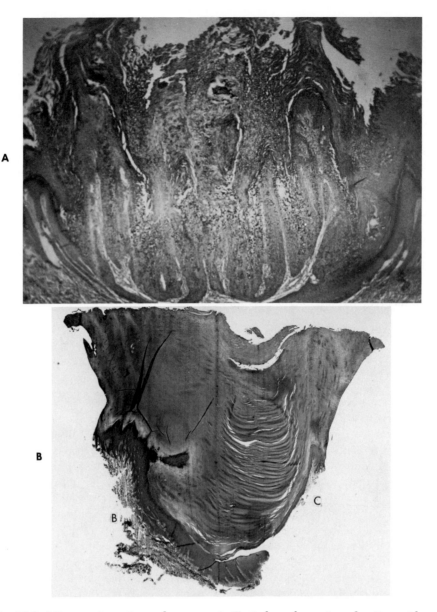

Fig. 18-2. Microscopic sections of verruca. **A,** Typical mushrooming of entire epidermis. Note thickening of rete pegs with some fusion at base and degeneration at top. **B,** Compression of subdermal living epithelium. Hyperkeratinization of uppermost layers of epidermis, with flushing of rete Malpighi (B and C), is shown.

bony prominence, it may be painful (Fig. 18-3).

2. Mutiple warts, a second type, are characterized by a large "mother" wart surrounded by tiny "daughter" warts that appear as blister satellites nearby (Fig. 18-4). When these tiny lesions are pared, a minute capillary usually is found.

3. The mosaic wart, which is usually painless, is commonly mistaken for a callus. These warts may be quite large (several centimeters in diameter) and may be present for years appearing as patches of individually coalescent cores resembling a mosaic (Fig. 18-5).

Treatment of plantar warts vexes most dermatologists, since these viral lesions show a strong tendency to recur. Nonscarring measures are preferable because of the tendency of the scars to be painful. Use of 40% salicylic acid plaster when applicable sometimes reduces the warts and occasionally cures them. Other measures, like the application of 10% formalin and then covering with 40% acid plaster and tape nightly, a measure devised by Tromovitch and Kay (1973), will cure many plantar warts, Cryosurgery with liquid nitrogen is frequently effective for small plantar warts. Blunt dissection of the plantar warts (Pringle and Helms, 1973)

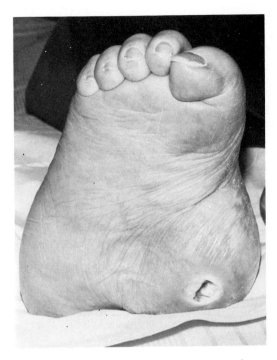

Fig. 19-18. Severe Charcot joint destruction; ulcer under apex of weight-bearing deformity.

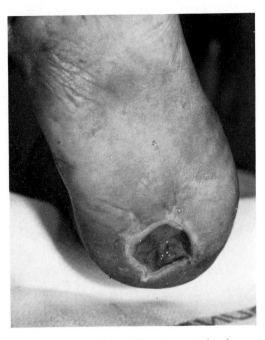

Fig. 19-19. Recurrent ulcer following partial calcanectomy. The patient walked without AFO for protection.

Neuropathy

The diabetic diathesis includes involvement of the nervous system (Lamontagne and Buchtal, 1970). The exact mechanisms are not known but appear to be part of the metabolic disorder and probably involve the sorbitol pathway (Chopra et al., 1969). Autopsy studies show loss of anterior horn cells, reduction in number of axons, and abnormalities of the Schwann cells (Greenbaum et al., 1964). The autonomic system is also involved and can affect the limbs.

Chronic sensory neuropathy is the most common form seen in our clinic. There is loss of ankle reflex, diminution or loss of vibratory sense, diminution in position sense, and diminution in pain appreciation. Symptoms of dysesthesia, hyperesthesia, and muscle and limb pains will be described variously as burning, aching, gnawing, ants crawling on the skin, or hot liquid flowing on the skin. These disappear as loss of sensation progresses.

Trophic and autonomic changes result in brittle hyperkeratotic skin, thickened deformed nails, atrophy of fat in the sole, and loss of function in the sebaceous and sweat glands.

The motor loss resembles an intrinsic muscle palsy. The metatarsophalangeal joints become extended and the proximal interphalangeal joints flexed, and typical clawed toes result. The plantar fat pad shifts distally, and the metatarsal head is covered with skin and subcutaneous tissue less able to withstand direct and shear pressures.

Treatment of the neuropathy itself is usually not successful. There is some indication that strict diabetic control and B-complex vitamins can give temporary relief in a case that has resulted from poor diabetic control. Cases with some regression of symptoms have been followed and have eventually shown progression of the neuropathy despite good control of the diabetic state. All patients who have had diabetes mellitus for 20 years manifest signs of diabetic neuropathy.

In my experience, ulcerative lesions occur mainly at bony prominences such as at the heel, under deformities, or at depressed metatarsal heads (Figs. 19-18 and 19-19). Ulcers can occur at other sites, but usually only after some traumatic incident such as penetration of a foreign object. Many of these patients have no signs of vascular impairment. Prophylactic removal of bony prominences after healing of the ulcer can protect a patient from further breakdown. The usual onset of a plantar ulcer follows the formation of a thickened plantar callosity under a metatarsal head. The neuropathic foot is especially prone to the development of extra-thick callosities. These callosities can act as foreign bodies and traumatize the tissues between the callus and the underlying bony prominence, with the ultimate production of an ulcer. Exudate from the ulcer breaks through, and the patient is first aware of the lesion

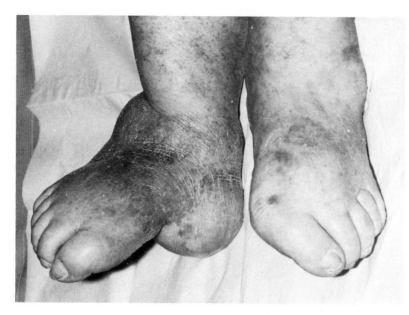

Fig. 19-20. Severe Charcot changes of right foot with ulcer under prominence of talus following lateral dislocation of tarsus. Grade 1 left foot "at risk" with bunion and hammered toes.

when he notices moisture on his stocking. Trimming of the overlying callus can also reveal an undiscovered ulcer. Pressure-relieving shoe inserts, rocker bottom shoes, and similar devices can help the ulcer heal and prevent recurrence. However, if this is not successful, removal of the intrinsic bony pressure point by osteotomy or ostectomy is indicated.

If the ulcer progresses despite treatment, it may eventually reach deeper tissues and produce an abscess or osteomyelitis. Further treatment would be indicated as outlined in the treatment diagrams.

Diabetic arthropathy and osteopathy. Bone and joint changes are seen accompanying diabetic neuropathy. The arthropathy first described by Charcot was seen mainly with tabes dorsalis or locomotor ataxia caused by late syphilis. Other causes of neuropathic joints have been described associated with loss of nerve function from various etiologies. Now diabetes mellitus is the most common cause of neuropathic bone and joint disease in the Western world (Jacobs, 1958; Jordan, 1936). Hansen's disease is more common in Africa, Asia, and countries in the equatorial belt.

There are five patterns of diabetic arthropathy and osteopathy; and each requires different treatment or there is no known treatment.

Osteoporosis (osteopenia). Osteoporosis is usually first seen in the bones of the forefoot. It also can occur as generalized demineralization without a period of immobilization or other causative event. It seldom causes a clinical problem unless fracture occurs. No treatment is usually required unless pain and swelling are pres-

ent. Fractures may also occur with minimal sprains. They may not be painful because of sensory loss and are usually discovered when swelling does not regress and radiographic examination is performed.

Osteolysis. Osteolysis can result in virtual disappearance of bones with narrowing of the entire shaft. The advanced cases may include subluxation, fractures at the metatarsal and phalangeal joints, and disruption of the joint. Cast treatment may lead to reappearance of the bone.

Hyperostosis. Increased bone formation is usually seen adjacent to a Charcot joint. Unless the excessive bone threatens ulceration, treatment is usually not necessary. If the foot is warm and swollen, it must be treated with a cast until it is cool.

Spontaneous subluxation or dislocation. Subluxation or dislocation can occur spontaneously to the foot and ankle joints without bony disruption. Joint instability is lost through capsular and ligamentous destruction. Surgical arthrodesis may be necessary if long-term casting does not stabilize the joint.

Charcot joints. Charcot joints are the most common major manifestation. They are seen more frequently in the midfoot, but can involve other joints (Fig. 19-20 and 19-21). They are less common in the ankle. The onset may involve minor trauma, alteration of the mechanics of the foot following surgery, or fractures (Kristiansen, 1980). With spontaneous onset, there is frequently heat, swelling, and redness around the ankle and distal leg. I have seen many cases treated for weeks as infections or phlebitis until radiographic examination

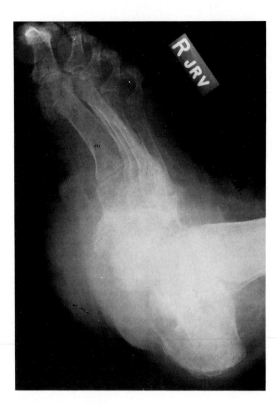

Fig. 19-21. Severe diabetic Charcot changes in right foot; virtual dissolution of midtarsal structures.

revealed the true nature of the bony process. Periarticular fractures are common and joint stability is lost. Complete destruction and disintegration may result unless cast treatment is begun. The repair process may lead to callus formation, appearance of periosteal new bone, and even spontaneous fusion of joints. Ulcers may form under the local protuberances that are formed as a result of joint dislocation or bone healing. Treatment is carried out in four phases, as follows:

1. Protection against deformity must be provided during the active phase. Bed rest may sometimes be necessary before a cast is applied if the swelling is severe. A nonwalking cast provides rest and stabilization in a functional position. When warmth and swelling have disappeared, protection with an ankle-foot orthosis (AFO) is continued until full healing is seen by radiographic examination.
2. Following cast and brace treatment, any deformity must be protected with forgiving shoewear. If the deformity is severe, it should be corrected with osteotomies and fusions as necessary.
3. If ulceration is present under a bony prominence, the prominence should be removed surgically.
4. Arthrodesis may be necessary if bony stability has not occurred or if the deformity is so severe that

weight bearing is not possible. Triple arthrodesis has been successfully performed in very early lesions before destruction is too severe. Prolonged casting is necessary. Late cases as seen in Fig. 19-18 may sometimes require a two-stage Syme amputation because of infection, deformity, and loss of stability.

Bacteriologic studies in infected diabetic feet

Multiple organisms are usually cultured from infected diabetic gangrene and diabetic ulcers (Williams et al., 1974). Enteric gram-negative bacilli and enterococci have been incriminated in infection accompanied by subcutaneous gas (Bessman and Wagner, 1975; Di Gioia et al., 1977). In these studies the material for culture was obtained at the bedside from the draining lesion. With a mixed flora and varied bacterial sensitivities, it is difficult to set up an antibiotic treatment program.

In an attempt to identify the pathogenic bacteria in the infected lesions, superficial wound exudates were contrasted with material dissected aseptically from the surgically excised specimen. Our study showed little agreement between cultures of the deep and superficial material. There was complete concordance in only 10 patients (17%). In this group antibiotic therapy directed against all of the organisms failed to eradicate them.

In the majority of cases most but not all of the causative bacteria can be isolated at the bedside. The most common organisms are the Enterobacteriacae, enterococci, and staphylococci. Relatively few anaerobes are isolated, and no anaerobes have been isolated in pure culture. *Staphylococcus epidermidis* and *Corynebacterium* were cultured from both superficial and deep areas but were never isolated as the sole causative organisms.

Antibiotic treatment is selected not to eradicate the deep infection but to reduce and minimize the surrounding cellulitis. Gangrenous tissue, deep abscess, and osteomyelitis must be surgically drained or excised in the diabetic patient. A penicillin-type antibiotic with an aminoglycoside appears to provide the best all-around results until cultures and sensitivities indicate a change. Since the aminoglycosides are ototoxic and nephrotoxic, close attention must be paid to hearing and kidney function.

Control of blood glucose in surgery

A high percentage of diabetic patients will undergo surgical procedures in their lifetimes. Most of these patients will be under the care of an internist, but occasionally a previously undiagnosed patient will be found to have the disease during his surgical course. It is not within the scope of this chapter to discuss the medical care of the diabetic patient, but the surgeon should be aware of problems in the perioperative period. A short time with a practical article should give him a good approach to blood glucose control in case of emergency. An especially good article is one by Rossini and Hare (1976).

Surgical techniques

Amputations. Ablative procedures are discussed more thoroughly in the section on amputations (p. 441).

Metatarsal osteotomies. Pressure from and pressure on the metatarsal heads can be relieved by a number of procedures that shorten the metatarsal and/or change the angle of the shaft.

Osteotomies close to the metatarsal head tend to develop hypertrophic callus in the diabetic patient. This callus can then become as much of a pressure point as the metatarsal head and lead to an ulcer. Osteotomies in the midshaft are more prone to nonunion and the development of Charcot-like changes in the nonunion, which can lead to pressure points from the amount of bone formed.

Osteotomies in the cancellous bone at the metatarsal base appear to be superior. With relief of pressure on one head, transfer of pressure to the adjacent head is common. Palpation of the adjacent head at surgery will give an indication of its prominence and the probable necessity to osteotomize, shorten, or angulate the shaft to about 50% of the correction obtained with the first osteotomy.

If the protuberance of the fifth metatarsal head is especially large, it is best corrected by excision of the distal half of the metatarsal through an oblique osteotomy. Removal of the base of the proximal phalanx prevents a pressure point from the flare. Syndactylization of the fourth and fifth toes prevents proximal migration of the fifth. Partial fifth metatarsal head resection has frequently resulted in an unstable joint and further deformity and is no longer used.

Clawtoe and hammertoe repair. If clawtoes or hammertoes are not too severe, they can be corrected by dorsal capsulotomy, tendon lengthening, and proximal interphalangeal joint fusion. These procedures work in early cases with minimal deformities. Late cases may show initial correction but almost all recur. Clawtoe surgery will not be considered for the usual patient unless ulcers have recurred or the deformity is severe enough to interfere with the wearing of shoes. In older patients it is almost a truism that some bone must be removed and soft tissue procedures will not succeed.

Metatarsal head resection (Hoffman-Clayton procedure). Although the Hoffman-Clayton procedure was originally described for severe arthritic deformities with marked joint destruction, it is finding use in the dia-

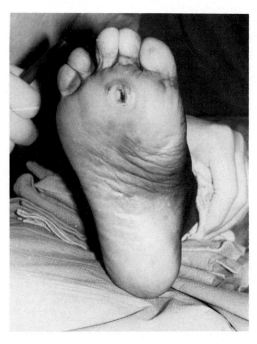

Fig. 19-22. Foot with severe ulcer under second metatarsal head, disruption of metatarsophalangeal joints, and previous resection of first metatarsal head for osteomyelitis.

betic patient with plantar callosities and ulceration (Figs. 19-22 to 19-27).

Single-head resection is performed for plantar ulceration. If the adjacent heads feel prominent at surgery, a dorsal wedge osteotomy of the adjacent shafts will prevent transfer lesions. To prevent hypertrophic callus near the head or distal shaft, the osteotomy is best performed at the base. The foot must be protected in a walking cast for about 8 weeks to prevent neuropathic breakdown of the tarsometatarsal and midtarsal joints. I now advocate resection of the proximal portion of the proximal phalanx to further shorten the bony structures and thus provide relative lengthening of the soft tissue structures. This minimizes the tendency for the toes to be pulled dorsally as healing progresses. Pressure from the prominence of the flare is also avoided. Intramedullary Kirschner wires aid in toe and shaft alignment postoperatively and help prevent excessive toe retraction. If there has been recent infection, the wires are not used. Most of these patients have a flat-footed gait preoperatively and continue with the same gait in ordinary shoes. A rocker bottom stiff-soled shoe adds motion that converts the gait to an almost normal heel-toe progression.

Bunionectomy. The medial aspect of the first metatarsophalangeal joint is susceptible to pressure if hallux valgus is more than a few degrees. Once ulceration and scarring have occurred, the skin is especially prone to recurrent ulcers.

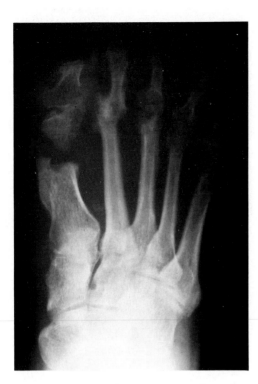

Fig. 19-23. Foot in Fig. 19-22; resection of previous osteomyelitis of first metatarsal and breakdown of metatarsophalangeal joints.

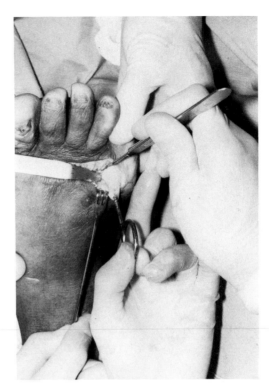

Fig. 19-24. Use of screw to hold metatarsal head during sharp dissection for removal of head.

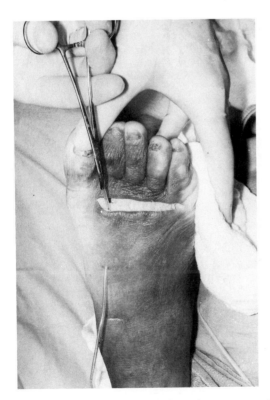

Fig. 19-25. Placing irrigation tube through separate stab incision.

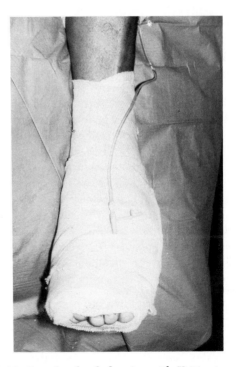

Fig. 19-26. Completed soft dressing with Kritter type irrigation system. Fluid exits through incision.

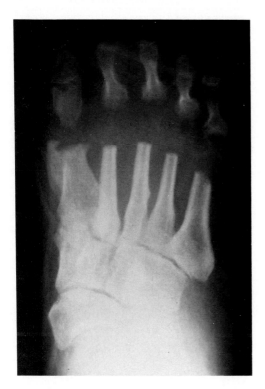

Fig. 19-27. Completed Hoffman procedure.

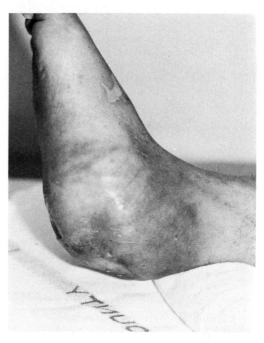

Fig. 19-28. One year after partial calcanectomy. Patient walked without orthosis and caused new ulcer.

The Keller resection provides excellent relief of local pressure. Attachment of the flexor hallucis brevis to the base of the resected proximal phalanx aids in preventing hyperextension of the great toe.

Resection of bony prominences

Calcaneus. Enforced bed rest during an illness, following a cerebrovascular accident, or during convalescence from surgery such as open reduction and internal fixation of hip fracture frequently leads to pressure sores under the prominences around the heel.

If the ischemic index is over 0.45, the ulcer and underlying bone are removed to allow closure of the ulcer (Figs. 19-28 and 19-29). If the ischemic index is under 0.45, a below-knee amputation usually must be performed. Postoperative drainage of the cavity is essential. After healing, a polypropylene AFO allows almost normal gait. The patient must use the orthosis for all weight bearing.

Calcaneocuboid, cuboid–fifth metatarsal, and midtarsal joints. Charcot involvement of these joints can lead to disintegration with plantar angulation and subsequent bony protuberances, rapidly causing ulcers (Figs. 19-18 and 19-19).

Resection of the bone is accomplished through separate medial or lateral incisions approaching the protuberance subperiosteally. The prominence is resected flush with the surrounding bone. Walking-cast treatment is started 10 to 12 days postoperatively and is con-

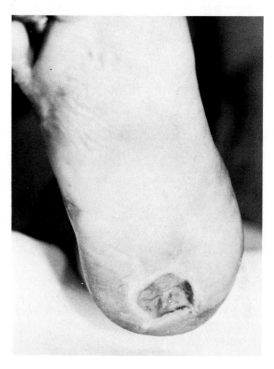

Fig. 19-29. Removal of remainder of calcaneus is necessary to heal ulcer.

tinued until the surrounding bone is healed. This may take up to 6 months.

Summary

The number of diabetic patients is increasing. An infected foot is the most common septic problem requiring hospitalization of the diabetic patient. To aid in establishing treatment programs, diabetic foot lesions have been graded from 0 (intact skin) through 5 (gangrene of the whole foot). A flow chart has been constructed for each grade to indicate treatment at progressive stages.

An ischemic index has been developed to aid in assessment of vascular potential. Local healing, healing of operative procedures, and healing of amputations are all dependent on sufficient blood supply (Williams et al., 1974). The ischemic index represents the value obtained by dividing the various lower extremity systolic pressures by the brachial artery pressure. The leg pressures are obtained by transcutaneous Doppler ultrasound used as a sensitive stethoscope. If the ischemic index is over 0.45, 93% + healing has occurred following surgical procedures.

Standard reconstructive procedures can be performed in the diabetic foot to relieve deformities and prevent breakdown of skin over bony protuberances. Partial-foot and Syme's amputations have been performed in a large number of diabetic patients, with a high success rate.

Diabetic neuropathy is present to some degree in all patients with diabetes of 20 or more years' duration. Charcot arthropathy can be triggered by minor trauma or can be completely insidious in onset. Absolute rest followed by protection with walking casts may result in healing of juxtaarticular fractures and even fusion of affected joints. Surgical fusion can be successful if performed early enough.

It is believed that the team approach with close cooperation between the medical and orthopaedic staffs has contributed to our low mortality rate and high healing rate.

FOOT AMPUTATIONS

Amputation is described as the process of cutting off (*ambi*, around; *putare*, to prune), especially by surgery of a portion of the body. In the lower extremity the causes, in descending order of frequency are as follows:

1. Peripheral vascular disease (with diabetics forming the greater percentage of these patients)
2. Trauma (becoming more frequent in younger male patients)
3. Tumors
4. Chronic infection (e.g., osteomyelitis not responding to usual treatment)
5. Congenital and acquired deformities (e.g., fibular hemimelia)
6. Cosmesis (rare)

Level selection in foot amputations

In trauma, tumors, chronic infection, and congenital deformities, the level selection is usually dictated by the underlying pathologic process. All length is saved—as determined by skin viability in trauma, degree of malignancy of the tumor, or remaining function in the extremity with a congenital defect. Traumatic lesions that require prolonged casting can leave the patient with a stiff and painful partial foot. This is especially true at the Chopart and Lisfranc levels.

If a walkable partial foot is not possible by 6 months, serious consideration should be given to ablation as a reconstructive procedure. Longer delay raises false hope in the patient and frustration in the surgeon. Amputation should not be considered a procedure to hide failure of previous treatment; rather it is a further step in treatment of a badly injured foot. It should be done as a plastic procedure to provide a new interface between the patient and his new environment—the prosthesis.

In dysvascular patients new diagnostic procedures are aiding the assessment of healing at various levels. Noninvasive techniques are of major importance, for penetration of the diabetic or dysvascular foot can precipitate an acute infection or local thrombosis. Radioactive xenon has been reported to give reliable results (Moore, 1973) but frequently is not available in smaller hospitals. Transcutaneous Doppler ultrasound is being used as a sensitive stethoscope to assess blood flow in dysvascular limbs (Barnes et al., 1976; Carter, 1973; Mackereth and Lennihan, 1970; Yao, 1970). The procedure is described at the beginning of the chapter. In the nondiabetic patient healing can occur with an ischemic index of 0.35.

Specific amputations

Toes. Loss of a part or all of the toe can usually be compensated by shoe correction, especially the rocker bottom shoe (Fig. 19-30). Partial amputation of a lesser toe may be necessary for gangrene of diabetes, arteriosclerosis, congenital deformity, tumor, or trauma.

Surgical techniques. Flaps may be of any shape, size, or description; they must only be long enough to close without tension. They may be long-dorsal, long-plantar, side-to-side, or fish-mouth; however, their length must not be over 50% greater than the width at the base. The flaps should be tested before suturing and the stump palpated to be sure that no bony prominence is present. Bone must be removed and angular areas rounded to relieve internal pressure and palpable ex-

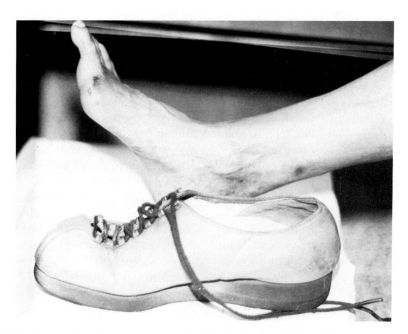

Fig. 19-30. Amputation of great toe; gait aided by thickening of sole and moderate rocker of sole.

ternal pressure. Flaps must close without tension. If such closure is not possible, more bone must be removed (Wagner, 1977).

Terminal amputation of hallux and toenaill (terminal Syme). Deformity of the great toenail and recurrent severe infections may not respond to simple treatment. Partial phalangectomy and removal of the nail and matrix from the dorsum allow primary closure of the distal flap. If the closure is under tension, more bone must be removed (Fig. 19-31).

Amputation of great toe. The base of the proximal phalanx of the great toe is saved, if at all possible, to preserve the action of the flexor hallucis brevis. This appears to pull the fat pad and the proximal phalanx over the distal portion of the first metatarsal head to provide cushioning at roll-off. If disarticulation is necessary, plantar skin should be used over the metatarsal head. In the lesser toes no distinction is made between amputating through a phalanx and disarticulating at the joints. Again, flaps must close without tension. If there is a contracture of a joint that would leave a protruding stump, this must be corrected.

Amputation of toes and metatarsal rays. Any or all of the lateral toes and rays can be taken through an oblique incision, leaving a remarkably effective foot. The flap must be wide and long enough to close without tension. Antibiotic solution lavage is brought into the wound and exits between the sutures. This aids in the evacuation of hematoma and debris (Kritter, 1973). A Plastizote filler is used to compensate for the loss of the lateral toes (Fig. 19-32).

Resection of osteomyelitis bone without amputation. A satisfactory toe stub may result if osteomyelitic bone is excised leaving the soft tissue behind. This is usually indicated in the great toe and fifth toe. A medial or lateral incision is made along the extent of the infected bone. The bone is then dissected extraperiosteally. The wound either is packed open with povidone, iodoform, or similar packs or is closed over antibiotic irrigation tubes. The residual soft tissue shrinks as it heals and provides a pad for the metatarsal head.

Transmetatarsal amputation. McKittrick et al. (1949) outlined the indications for a transmetatarsal amputation in the diabetic patient. Their criteria are as valid today as they were then:

1. Gangrene of all or part of one or more toes, provided the gangrene and accompanying infection have become stabilized and the gangrene has not involved the dorsal or plantar aspect of the foot
2. A stabilized infection or open wound involving the distal portion of the foot, when total excision of the infected area with primary or delayed closure can be accomplished
3. An open infected lesion in a neurogenic foot as a curative procedure when the entire area of anesthesia can be excised or as a delayed procedure when the area of infection can be excised but the line of incision is through the area of anesthesia

In dysvascular patients the addition of the ischemic index obtained with the transcutaneous Doppler ultrasound has allowed selection of the level of amputation more easily than could be done by clinical means alone.

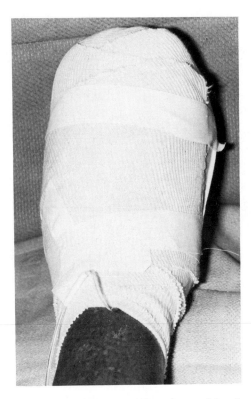

Fig. 19-40. Soft dressing is used until wound has healed.

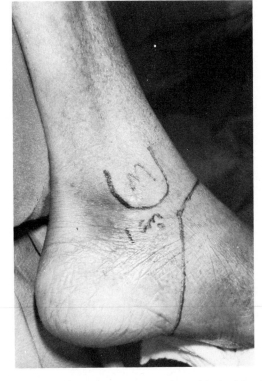

Fig. 19-41. Syme's two-stage amputation; skin incision 1 cm anterior and 1 cm distal to midpoint of malleoli.

An alleged advantage of Lisfranc and Chopart amputations is that ordinary shoes can be used. In general, we have found most patients require some sort of stiffening in the sole and/or a special toe block arrangement to wear ordinary shoes. A polypropylene AFO has been of great help.

Syme's amputation. Since the heel pad is part of the foot and the function of a Syme amputee approximates more closely that of a partial-foot amputee (Syme, 1843; Waters et al., 1976), the Syme amputation is considered a partial foot in our clinic.

Indications. Any patient with a deformed, traumatized, dysvascular, or infected foot is a possible candidate for a Syme amputation. Congenital defects that produce shortened limbs and equinus deformity of the foot frequently do better with an amputation than with multiple attempts at reconstruction. A Syme prosthesis is far more functional and cosmetic than a shoe with a 5- or 6-inch platform and a severe equinus built in to gain length. Patients with fibular hemimelia, proximal focal femoral deficiencies, and congenital pseudarthrosis of the tibia frequently benefit from a Syme amputation.

Surgical technique. In noninfected cases the surgical technique should be that described by Harris (1956, 1961). In children the malleoli are not removed unless

pressure problems occur (Wood et al., 1965). Then they are removed below the epiphyseal lines so as not to cause growth disturbances.

Spittler et al. (1954) described a two-stage method for infected forefeet following war wounds. This method has been modified with a simpler second stage for diabetic and dysvascular gangrene and infection (Wagner, 1977). Doppler transcutaneous ultrasound is used to obtain an ischemic index. If the index is above 0.45 in diabetics and 0.35 in arteriosclerotics, over 93% of the amputations have healed.

With one exception, the Syme amputation technique is the same for a single-stage procedure as for the first stage of a two-stage method. In the two-stage method the incisions are 1 to 1.5 cm more anterior and distal than described by Syme to allow for the extra volume of the malleoli, which are not removed in the first stage. The incision starts medially 1 to 1.5 cm below and anterior to the midpoint of the medial malleolus (Fig. 19-41).

The incision then swings dorsally directly over the ankle joint to a point about 1.5 cm below and anterior to the lateral malleolus. The two malleolar points are connected by an incision directly across the sole. This incision goes down to bone usually across the os calcis or near the calcaneocuboid joint. On the dorsum the

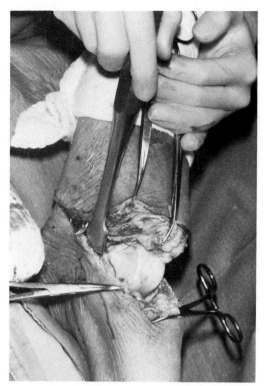

Fig. 19-42. Incision carried directly to bone; subperiosteal dissection of os calcis begun.

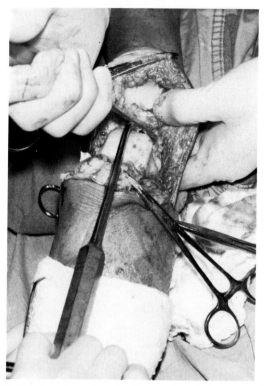

Fig. 19-43. Bone hook in talus for traction. Subperiosteal dissection to os calcis continues.

incision is carried down to the dome of the talus (Fig. 19-42).

Tendons are pulled down, severed, and allowed to retract. Vascular structures are identified and ligated or electrocoagulated. The medial and lateral ligaments are severed from the body of the talus, allowing the talus to be dislocated anteriorly and downward. There is no preferred sequence of cutting; the exact method differs in each patient depending on which structures are tightest. Division of the collateral ligaments is alternated from side to side. Dissection of the body of the calcaneus is started subperiosteally on the lateral side (Figs. 19-42 to 19-44).

The superior surface of the os calcis is denuded subperiosteally. Traction through a bone hook in the talus aids as the dissection is continued around the os calcis (Fig. 19-45).

The two major danger points were well described by Syme. (1) The *neurovascular bundle* courses between the flexor hallucis longus and the flexor digitorum longus (Fig. 19-46). It is at danger when the knife is pushed in medially to sever the medial collateral ligaments. The flexor hallucis longus is first identified and used to protect the nerve and artery until the medial surface of the os calcis is dissected free. (2) The second danger point is at the immediate *subcutaneous attachment of the Achilles tendon*. Piercing of the posterior

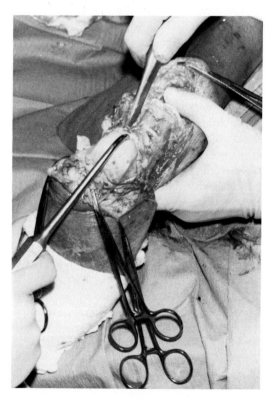

Fig. 19-44. Top of os calcis denuded. Bone hook in talus aids in control of foot.

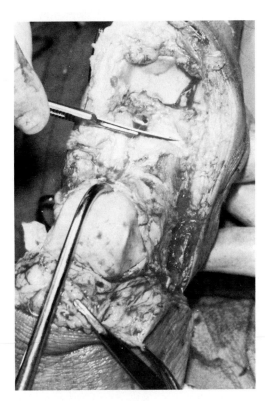

Fig. 19-45. Attachment of Achilles tendon sectioned with scalpel; dome of ankle joint just above scalpel.

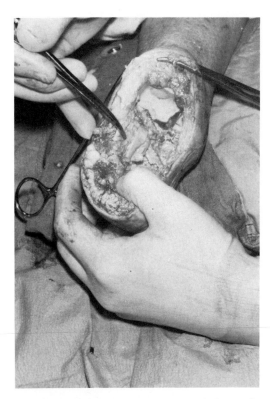

Fig. 19-46. Neurovascular bundle at tip of clamp; dome of ankle just above clamp.

skin at this thin point jeopardizes healing. The operation failed in most of the few cases in which skin was inadvertently cut. Careful sharp dissection of the tendon and further subperiosteal dissection allow complete removal of the os calcis and talus. Minor bits of debris are removed, and hemostasis secured.

A Shirley drain is drawn into the cavity through a separate stab wound made over the tip of a hemostat pushed out posterolaterally (Fig 19-15). The air filter is removed to allow antibiotic solution to be irrigated through the wound by gravity drainage (Wagner, 1977). This is done for 48 hours unless there is further sign of infection in the wound. Late removal is based on clinical appearance of the wound. At removal the tip of the tube is cut off aseptically and sent for culture. Closure of the wound is begun by suturing the plantar aponeurosis to the deep fascia over the front of the tibia (Fig. 19-47).

If either malleolus produces skin pressure, a stab incision into the fat pad produces a cavity that allows nesting of the malleolus into the fat and relief of the pressure. The skin is closed with nylon or similar suture (Figs. 19-48 and 19-49).

A soft dressing is used for 7 to 10 days (Fig. 19-50). A plaster cast is then applied, and the patient discharged if general health permits. If the heel pad is especially tough, a walking heel is added and the patient allowed to walk (Fig. 19-51).

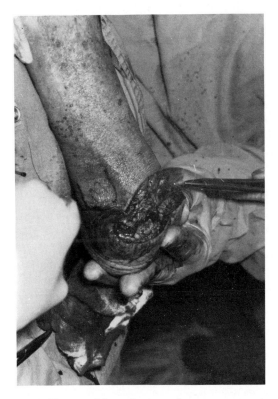

Fig. 19-47. Closure of deep fascia to plantar aponeurosis.

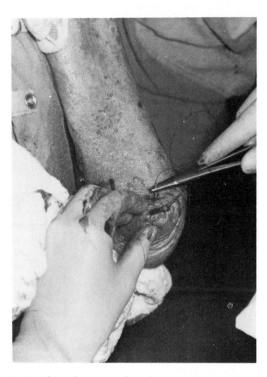

Fig. 19-48. Skin closure with nylon or other nonabsorbable suture.

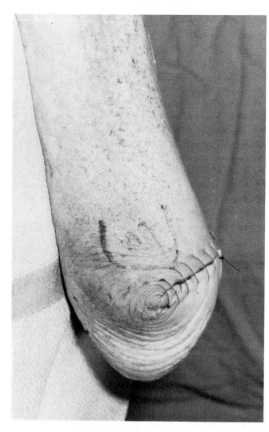

Fig. 19-49. Closed incision with dog ears; good base of posterior skin. This would be sacrificed if dog ears were removed.

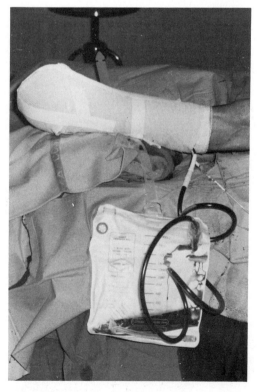

Fig. 19-50. Soft dressing applied in surgery. Wound irrigation is to gravity drainage.

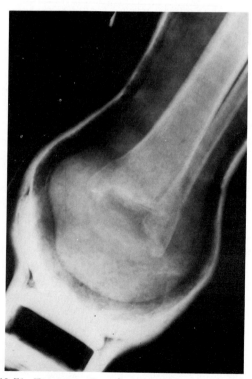

Fig. 19-51. First-stage Syme's amputation in weight-bearing cast. Felt pads with the center cut out are used over malleoli and dog ears to relieve pressure.

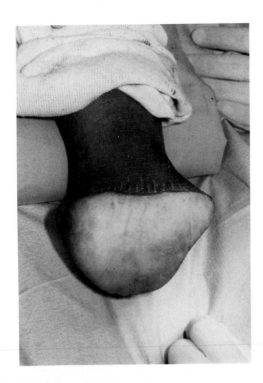

Fig. 19-52. Second-stage Syme's; healed first stage ready to have dog ears and malleoli removed.

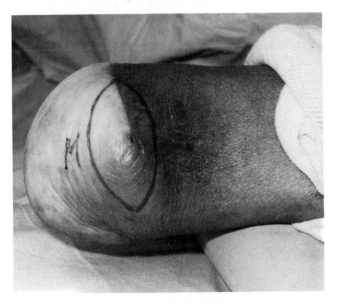

Fig. 19-53. Second-stage Syme's; elliptical incision over the medial malleolus. Volume of this wedge should equal volume of the malleolus.

Felt pads are cut out in the center and placed over the dog ears to protect them from pressure in the cast.

In noninfected and traumatic cases the procedure is performed in one stage. The incisions start at the midpoint of each malleolus and go directly to and through the sole. They then course obliquely across the ankle joint anteriorly. After disarticulation is complete, the malleoli and 1.5 cm of the distal tibia are exposed. The tibia must not be cut too short. Transection is done so a circle of about 3 cm of cartilage is left in the center of the plafond. Several drill holes are made around the periphery and the pad sutured in place. If the medial

and lateral flares are too prominent or sharp, they are rounded. Closed irrigation and drainage are carried out for 48 hours. A cast is applied after the drain is removed. Walking is started at 10 to 12 days.

In two-stage procedures the second stage is performed at 6 weeks if healing is secure (Fig. 19-52). The dog ears are removed through medial and lateral elliptical incisions (Fig. 19-53). The malleoli are removed flush with the ankle joint (Fig 19-54). A small portion of the flare is removed from the tibia and fibula to narrow the stump and eliminate pressure points (Fig. 19-55). If the pad is loose at this stage, more soft tissue is

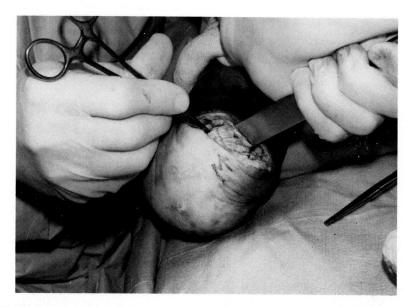

Fig. 19-54. Second-stage Syme's; removal of medial malleolus flush with dome of ankle joint. Articular cartilage is not removed.

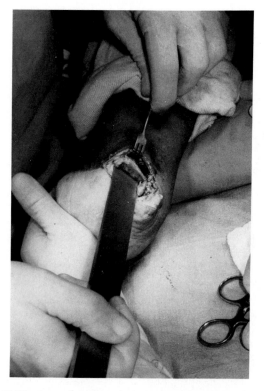

Fig. 19-55. Second-stage Syme's; removal of flare of tibia to relieve bony prominence.

removed from the elliptical incision. I have not found it necessary to remove the articular cartilage because the pad has already begun to fibrose in place. For further fixation the fascia of the pad is sutured to the bone through drill holes (Fig. 19-56). Skin closure is with nylon or similar suture (Fig. 19-57). At 7 to 10 days the patient is placed in a walking cast (Fig. 19-58). The patient is usually ready for prosthetic fitting in about 6 weeks.

Syme's stumps have been long lasting and relatively free of trouble. Very few have become loose as atrophy progressed. These were returned to surgery and tightened up by removal of appropriate tissue wedges and suturing of the pad to the bone through drill holes. Late complications have been mainly related to progression of arteriosclerotic vascular lesions and have resulted in whole leg gangrene unrelated to any local problem in the Syme stump.

In patients amputated at the Syme level for breakdown of Charcot joints in the foot, hypertrophic joint-like tissues have formed resulting in hypermobile pads. Removal of the excess tissue through wedge incisions has resulted in firm pads.

Syme's amputation in two stages for diabetic and dysvascular gangrene and infection. There has been some criticism of the two-stage technique, which requires a second hospitalization and a second anesthetic and surgical procedure. Other centers have not performed many Syme amputations in this type of patient because of the relatively high failure rate when performed in a single stage (Sarmiento and Warren, 1969). I believe that the articular cartilage left by disarticula-

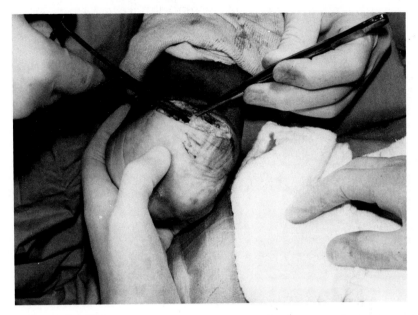

Fig. 19-56. Deep fascia drawn together to test stability of pad. More soft tissue is excised if pad is too loose.

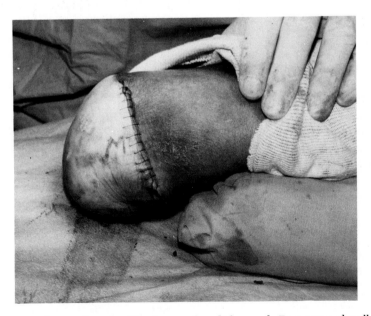

Fig. 19-57. Second-stage Syme's; skin closure of medial wound. Dog ears and malleoli have been removed.

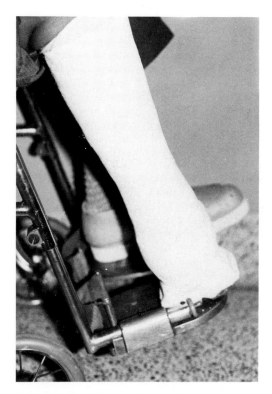

Fig. 19-58. Second-stage Syme's in walking cast. This cast is used until the stump has matured enough for definitive prosthesis.

tion acts as a barrier to the spread of infection from the forefoot through cancellous bone channels. The irrigation drainage system also appears to aid in removal of potentially infected hematoma from the cavity left by disarticulation.

Studies show the Syme amputation to be superior in function to below-knee and above-knee levels in velocity, stride length, cadence, and oxygen-per-meter consumption (Waters et al., 1976). This is of importance because the diabetic patient is especially prone to amputation of the opposite limb within 18 to 36 months (Goldner, 1960). Approximately 50% of our amputees are bilateral. Most with a Syme amputation on one side and a higher level on the opposite state their wish to have had both at the Syme level.

Syme's amputation for crushing injuries. Heel pain has been a late disabling factor in a large group of non-diabetic patients with industrial crushing injuries of the foot. They have been unable to wear standard prostheses, and a substantial number have required further amputation to a below knee level. Review of these cases has disclosed the presence of preamputation heel pain in all. The postamputation pain was not that of the usual amputation neuroma or phantom pain but appeared more like that of a tarsal tunnel or a sympathetic dystrophy.

The amputation surgeon is urged to watch preoperatively for this type of heel pain in crushing foot injuries which may otherwise be suitable for a Syme amputation. If there is such pain, a low calf level should be chosen.

PROSTHETIC CARE

Toe and partial foot amputations rarely require prosthetic replacement. Shoe correction in the form of sole stiffeners and rocker bottoms appear to be of more value. Room temperature–vulcanizing foam is an excellent material for filling a shoe. It is especially valuable when all of the lateral toes and rays have been removed and the first metatarsal and great toe remain. Plastizote and similar foams can be shaped easily for shoe fillers.

Syme's prosthesis

Prostheses with windows, straps, buckles, and other loose pieces tend to break down faster and require more maintenance than do those with no loose structures. The double-wall prosthesis, with an elastic inner wall to provide suspension, appears to be most satisfactory. The single-action cushion heel (SACH) allows near normal gait. In bilateral amputees in whom length is not a problem, five-way ankles and similar mechanisms can be installed to aid in torque and other pressure relief.

Physical therapy

The Syme amputee appears to walk as a partial-foot amputee in his prosthesis. Most require no training except in the procedures for donning and doffing. Most have used a walking cast between stages, and all have done so following the second stage. The transition to a prosthesis is smooth. Most require no instruction and their daily use rapidly habituates them to their new relatively "stiff foot."

REFERENCES

Barnes, R.W., Shanik, G.D., and Slaymaker, E.E.: An index of healing in below-knee amputation: leg blood pressure by Doppler ultrasound, Surgery **79**:13, 1976.

Bessman, A.N., and Wagner, F.W.: Nonclostridial gas gangrene: report of 48 cases and review of the literature, JAMA **233**:958, 1975.

Burgess, E.M., and Marsden, F.W.: Major lower extremity amputation following arterial reconstruction, Arch. Surg. **108**:655, 1974.

Carter, S.A.: The relationship of distal systolic pressures to healing of skin lesions with arterial occlusive disease with special reference to diabetes mellitus, Scand. J. Clin. Lab. Invest. (suppl. 128) **31**:239, 1973.

Chopra, J.A., Hurwitz, L.J., and Montgomery, D.A.D.: The pathogenesis of sural nerve changes in diabetes mellitus, Brain **92**:391, 1969.

Collens, W.S., Vlahos, E., Dobkin, G.B., Neuman, E., Rakow, R.K., Altman, M., and Siegman, F.: Conservative management of gangrene in the diabetic patient, JAMA **181**:692, 1962.

DiGioia, R.A., Kane, J.G., and Parker, R.H.: Crepitant cellulitis and myonecrosis caused by Klebsiella, JAMA **237**:2097, 1977.

Ecker, M.D., and Jacobs, B.S.: Lower extremity amputations in diabetic patients, Diabetes **19**:189, 1970.

Goldner, M.: The fate of the second leg in diabetic amputees, Diabetes **9**:100, 1960.

Glattly, H.: A statistical study of 12,000 new amputees, South. Med. J. **57**:1373, 1964.

Greenbaum, D., Richardson, P.C., Salmon, M.V., and Urich, H.: Pathological observations on six cases of diabetic neuropathy, Brain **87**:201, 1964.

Gundersen, J.: Diagnosis of arterial insufficiency with measurement of blood pressure in fingers and toes, Angiology **22**:191, 1971.

Harris, R.I.: Syme's amputation; the technical details essential for success, J. Bone Joint Surg. **38B**:614, 1956.

Harris, R.I.: The history and development of Syme's amputation, Artif. Limbs **6**:4, 1961.

Harris, W.R., and Silverstein, E.A.: Partial amputations of the foot: a follow-up study, Can. J. Surg. **7**:6, 1964.

Holstein, P.: Distal blood pressure. A guidance in choice of amputation level, Scand. J. Clin. Lab. Invest. (suppl. 123) **31**:245, 1973.

Jacobs, J.E.: Observations of neuropathic (Charcot) joints occurring in diabetes mellitus, J. Bone Joint Surg. **30A**:1043-1057, 1958.

Jacobs, R.: Personal communication, 1977.

Jordan, W.R.: Neuritic manifestations in diabetes mellitus. Arch. Intern. Med. **57**:307, 1936.

Kahn, O., Wagner, F.W., and Bessman, A.N.: Mortality of diabetic patients treated surgically for lower limb infection and/or gangrene, Diabetes **23**:287, 1974.

Kirkendall, W.M., Burton, A.C., Epstein P.H., and Freis, E.D.: Recommendations for human blood pressure determination by sphygmomanometers, Circulation **36**:980, 1967.

Kramer, D.W., and Perilstein, P.K.: Peripheral vascular complications in diabetes mellitus. A survey of 3,600 cases, Diabetes **7**:384, 1958.

Kristiansen, B.: Ankle and foot fractures in diabetics provoking neuropathic joint changes, Acta Orthop. Scand. **51**:975-979, 1980.

Kritter, A.E.: A technique for salvage of the infected diabetic gangrenous foot, Orthop. Clin. North Am. **4**:21, 1973.

Kunin, C.M.: Urinary tract infections flow charts (algorithms) for detection and treatment, JAMA **233**:458, 1975.

Lamontagne, A., and Buchtal, F.: Electrophysiological studies in diabetic neuropathy, J. Neurol. Neurosurg. Psychiatry **33**:442, 1970.

Louie, T.J., Bartlett, J.G., Tally, F.P., and Gorbach, S.L.: Anaerobic bacteria in diabetic foot ulcers, Ann. Intern. Med. **85**:461, 1975.

Mackereth, M., and Lennihan, R.: Ultrasound as an aid in the diagnosis and management of intermittent claudication, Angiology **21**:704, 1970.

McKittrick, L.S., McKittrick, J.B., and Risley, T.S.: Transmetatarsal amputation for infection of gangrene in patients with diabetes mellitus, Ann. Surg. **130**:826, 1949.

Medical Staff Conference, University of California, San Francisco: Diabetic micro-angiopathy, West. J. Med. **121**:404, 1974.

Mooney, V., Wagner, F.W., Jr.: Neurocirculatory disorders of the foot, Clin. Orthop. **122**:53, 1977.

Moore, W.S.: Determination of amputation level measurement of skin blood flow with xenon (Xe133), Arch. Surg. **107**:798, 1973.

Pratt, T.C.: Gangrene and infection in the diabetic, Med. Clin. North Am. **49**:987, 1975.

Rossini, A.A., and Hare, J.W.: How to control the blood glucose level in the surgical diabetic patient, Arch. Surg. **111**:945, 1976.

Romano, R.L., and Burgess, E.M.: Level selection in lower extremity amputations, Clin. Orthop. **74**:177, 1971.

Sarmiento, A., and Warren, W.D.: A re-evaluation of lower extremity amputations, Surg. Gynecol. Obstet. **129**:799, 1969.

Senn, N.: Principles of surgery, Philadelphia, 1890, F.A. Davis & Co.

Spittler, A.W., Brenner, J.J., and Payne, J.W.: Syme amputation performed in two stages, J. Bone Joint Surg. **36A**:37, 1954.

Stabile, B.E., and Wilson, S.E.: The profunda femoris-popliteal artery bypass, Arch. Surg. **112**:913, 1977.

Syme, J.: Amputation at the ankle joint, Mon. J. Med. Sci. **2**:93, 1843.

Wagner, F.W., Jr.: Amputation of the foot and ankle—current status, Clin. Orthop. **122**:62, 1977.

Waters, R.L., Perry, J., Antonelli, D., and Hislop, H.: Energy costs of walking of amputees: the influence of level of amputation, J. Bone Joint Surg. **58A**:42, 1976.

Williams, H.T.G., Hutchinson, K.J., and Brown, G.D.: Gangrene of the feet in diabetics, Arch. Surg. **108**:609, 1974.

Wood, W.L., Zlotsky, N., and Westin, G.W.: Congenital absence of the fibula. Treatment by Syme amputation—indication and techniques, J. Bone Joint Surg. **47A**:1159, 1965.

Yao, S.T.: Haemodynamic studies in peripheral arterial disease, Br. J. Surg. **57**:761, 1970.

20

Traumatic injuries to the soft tissues of the foot and ankle

Ligamentous injuries
DONALD E. BAXTER

A sprain is a wrenched or twisted joint. A strain is a condition of overuse or stretching of muscles, tendons, or ligaments in which there is no significant tear.

Sudden injuries of the foot may be grouped as those that occur during violent accidents and those that occur during the normal use of the foot. Sudden injury as the result of an accident includes any degree of crushing, tearing, or breaking of one structure or a group of structural components of the foot and ankle. Sudden injuries that take place during normal use usually involve the ligaments. Often ligaments are torn from their attachments along with a small fragment of bone. These injuries are termed sprains or avulsion chip fractures.

The foot and ankle are more subject to sprains than any other part of the body. Injuries vary from mild to severe, depending on the force involved, and may best be classified in degrees, as found in the Standard Nomenclature of Athletic Injuries (1966). A first-degree sprain is considered a mild injury, a second-degree sprain is a moderate injury, and a third-degree sprain is a severe injury. The third-degree injury therefore is a complete rupture of the involved ligaments, tendons, or muscles. A sprain of the lateral aspect of the foot and ankle is, by far, the most common.

ANATOMY

The distal end of the tibia and fibula forms the ankle mortise that maintains the trochlear surface of the talus and permits a hinge motion in this joint. The lateral malleolus lies posterior to the medial malleolus, thereby placing the foot in slight external rotation with relation to the tibia. The articular surface of the talus is wider anteriorly. Inman (1976) has shown that the mal-

leolar surfaces of the tibia closely approximate the sides of the talus in all positions from full plantar flexion to full dorsiflexion. Contrary to previous belief, there is no appreciable instability when the ankle is in full plantar flexion.

The ligaments about the ankle joint maintain the anatomic mortise. There are three groups of ligaments: (1) medial collateral ligament (deltoid), (2) lateral collateral ligament, and (3) inferior tibiofibular ligament (syndesmosis) (Fig. 20-1).

The medial collateral (deltoid) ligament originates from the medial malleolus and extends anteriorly to attach to most of the medial aspect of the talus and the sustentaculum tali, with some filaments inserting into the navicular.

The lateral collateral ligament is composed of three separate and distinct fascial bands: the posterior talofibular ligament, the anterior talofibular ligament, and the calcaneofibular ligament. These are the collateral ligaments commonly affected in an ankle sprain.

According to Brostrom (1964), the ligament most frequently injured, to be exact, in two thirds of the cases, is the anterior talofibular. Next in order of frequency of injury is the combined anterior talofibular and calcaneofibular ligaments, occurring in one fifth of the cases. Other lesions are rare.

BIOMECHANICS OF ANKLE LIGAMENTS (p. 24)

Although the foot may assume varying positions of plantar flexion or dorsiflexion at the time a sprain injury is incurred, either inversion or eversion is the principal mechanism initiating the ligamentous injury. Normally the thrust of the body weight in motion is transmitted through the foot to the supporting surface. When the foot is turned suddenly in extreme inversion or eversion, which may happen during walking or running, the

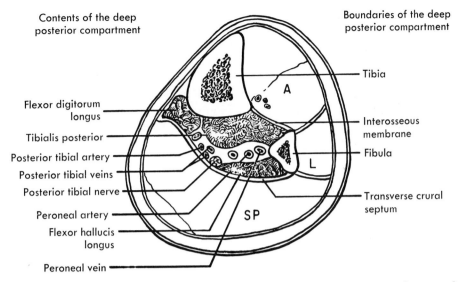

Contents of the deep
posterior compartment

Boundaries of the deep
posterior compartment

Flexor digitorum
longus

Tibialis posterior

Posterior tibial artery

Posterior tibial veins

Posterior tibial nerve

Peroneal artery

Flexor hallucis
longus

Peroneal vein

Tibia

Interosseous
membrane

Fibula

Transverse crural
septum

Fig. 20-26. Osteofascial compartments of leg. Deep posterior compartment is shown in detail; superficial compartments are represented by letters: *A* (anterior), *L* (lateral), and *SP* (superficial posterior). (From Matsen, F.A., III, and Clawson, D.K.: J. Bone Joint Surg. **57A:**34, 1975.)

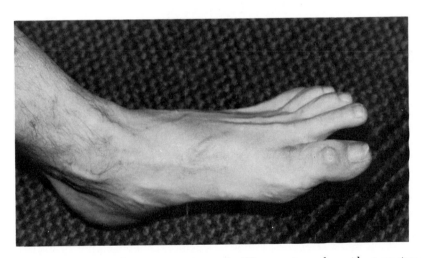

Fig. 20-27. Crush injury to deep compartment of calf from motorcycle accident causing contracture of flexor hallucis longus muscle and resultant claw hallux deformity.

partment syndrome often severely affects the flexor hallucis longus (Fig. 20-27). There may be associated loss of sensation in the sole of the foot. A clawfoot deformity results, and the foot cannot be dorsiflexed against unopposed contracted extrinsic flexors. The structure of the superficial posterior compartment of the leg with the gastrosoleus muscle complex is unconstrained. This protects it from developing the syndrome.

Peroneal compartment syndrome

The peroneal compartment syndrome is uncommon. If the syndrome occurs, however, fascial release pre-serves muscle viability. Neurolysis of the common peroneal nerve is not as successful as with other nerves because of its sensitive exposed position at the fibular neck and the region from which the deep peroneal branch originates (Whitesides, 1982). If contractures of the peroneal muscles occur, a mild equinus and abduction deformity results. Tenotomy may be necessary with an orthosis to control foot alignment and equinus.

Anterior compartment syndrome

Isolated anterior compartment syndrome with loss of the deep branch of the peroneal nerve results in a drop foot gait. Calcaneus deformity of the foot can also occur following contracture of the same muscles with infarction of all the musculature. Tenotomy is indicated with an appropriate orthosis. If indicated, tibialis posterior tendon transfer is performed to aid in ambulation.

The treatment of compartment syndromes is based on early recognition. Respect for soft tissues during surgical procedures is important. Surgery including fasciotomy at the time high tibial osteotomy is performed is an important prophylactic measure. The leg should be elevated postoperatively as a standard of good orthopaedic care. if symptoms of the syndrome occur, constrictive dressings should be completely divided and the limb rewrapped more loosely. If a cast is present, it should be split widely along with the underlying cast padding so that the skin is clearly visible throughout the length of the cast. If these measures are not effective and symptoms persist, fasciotomy should be performed to prevent development of a Volkmann's ischemic contracture. Since compartment syndromes develop rapidly and their results can be disastrous, close observation at frequent intervals is important so that a decision may be made before the viability of a limb is threatened.

If a single compartment is involved, fasciotomy over the specific area is performed. This is either through a single incision or through the method described by Kelly and Whitesides (1967) whereby through a single incision a partial fibulectomy is performed, thereby decompressing all four compartments.

TRAUMATIC ULCERS

A traumatic ulcer can occur as a result of sudden trauma such as a laceration, crush injury, or thermal or chemical injury. Often the injury is great enough to produce destruction of a large area of skin and subcutaneous tissue, which destroys circulation. These ulcers are the result of sudden insult followed by an immediate reaction of the tissue with death, demarcation, and sloughing of the involved tissue, leaving a raw healing surface beneath. Often tendons, muscles, vessels, nerves, and bone are exposed. Early evaluation will determine if the tibialis posterior or dorsalis pedis arteries have been injured. The physician must determine if the injury has compromised the major vessels of the foot. Since overlying tissue may have lost its circulation, vein graft may be necessary to reestablish circulation to the distal foot and prevent ischemia.

Early treatment includes cleansing and observation with the leg elevated at 30° to promote drainage. If there is gross tissue loss as a result of avulsion injury, temporary split-thickness or full-thickness skin grafting covers the wound until the limits of injury have demarcated and reconstructive surgery is performed to reestablish appropriate soft tissue cover, particularly over weight-bearing areas.

Traumatic ulcers often occur in older patients in whom tissue vitality may be compromised. If the injury occurs over a bony prominence that normally has thin non-weight-bearing skin, the injury takes considerable time to heal. The healing of an ulcer is limited by the general condition of the patient and is affected by such diseases as diabetes mellitus and peripheral neuropathy.

Treatment of small traumatic ulcers may be affected by excision of hypertrophic callus, debridement, and cauterization of the depth of the ulcer to permit fresh granulation tissue to grow. Occasionally, excision of the painful ulcerous lesion is necessary with mobilization of the skin and primary closure (Fig. 20-28).

Murray and Goldwyn (1966) treated 15 patients with intractable plantar ulcers by using split-thickness skin graft, pedicle flap, or both. In 13 patients the procedures were completely successful. Large defects about the foot require specialized techniques to provide a soft tissue and weight-bearing surface with sensation. Sensory innervated musculocutaneous free flaps have been reported to be successful in children (Argamaso et al., 1973; Bennett and Kahn, 1972; Furnas, 1976). Drabyn and Avetian (1979) report using a buttock flap for coverage of a large ankle lesion in a young child.

Mladick (1969) reported a technique for coverage of a large defect of the foot in children. Simple debridement of the injured area without application of a skin graft is performed. Ten days later a full-thickness ipsilateral buttock flap including the fascia just superficial to the flap is elevated through two transverse incisions. After 14 days the flap is elevated using a medial longitudinal incision just superficial to the gluteal fascia. Two weeks later the medial side of the flap is incised, elevating the medial third. In 10 days the knee is flexed, and the free end of the flap is attached to the heel and foot. The donor site is covered with a split-thickness skin graft. A splint holds the knee in the flexed position. Two weeks later the pedicle is partially divided, and 5 days subsequent to that complete division of the flap is made and sutured over the defect. This technique is more effective in young children who tolerate the extreme position of the knee and ankle. Bocca and Baruffaldi (1983), Dabb and Conklin (1981), and Maxwell (1979) reported the use of free musculocutaneous grafts with neurovascular pedicle for covering large defects of the lower leg. Dabb (1981) insists that complete anatomic evaluation of the pathologic anatomy is necessary because positioning the free graft may require appropriate vein grafting and a musculocutaneous flap transfer to maintain circulation. The use of such covering techniques requires specialized meticulous care in handling of the wound and may require additional split

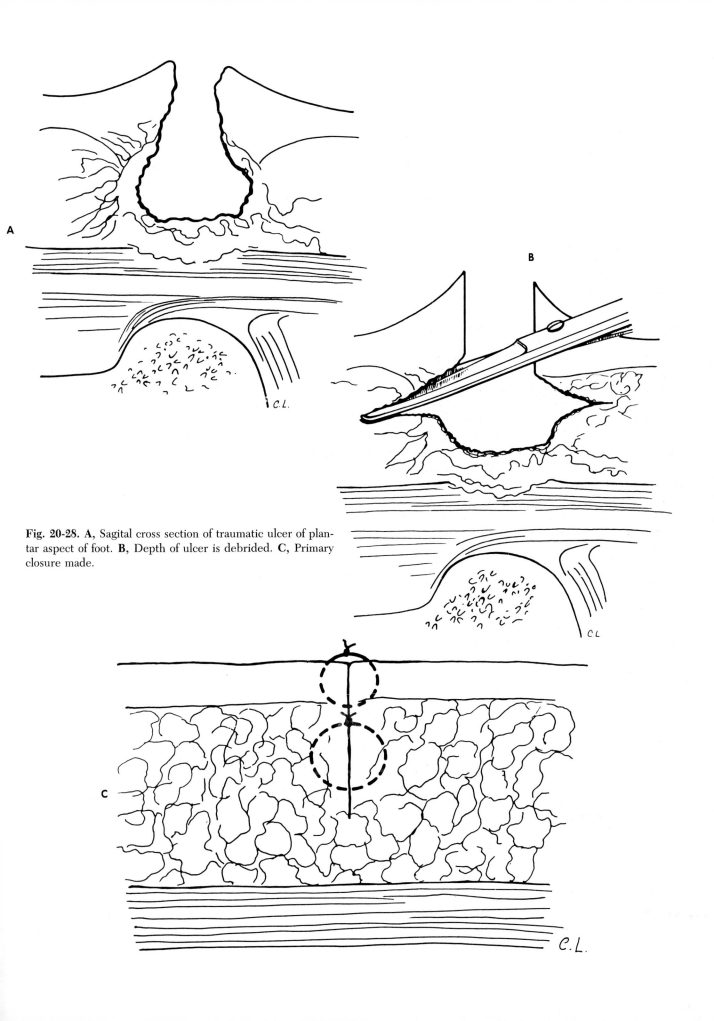

Fig. 20-28. A, Sagital cross section of traumatic ulcer of plantar aspect of foot. **B,** Depth of ulcer is debrided. **C,** Primary closure made.

thickness skin grafting in those areas that cannot maintain circulation. Recovery takes several months.

COLD INJURY

Cold injury to the foot is common. Not only does it occur in mountainous areas, arctic climates, and during warfare, but many injuries occur in temperate climates with the victims unaware of or unprepared for the weather. The body's response to cold is variable and therefore the extent of injury unpredictable. There are two types of freezing injuries, those caused by wet and those caused by cold (Hermann et al., 1963). Frostbite is caused by freezing cold. A combination of wet and cold causes immersion foot. Freezing injuries have been classified as burns by the degree of severity, but this classification has not been found to be a reliable indicator for treatment and prognosis.

Temperature regulation of the extremities is an important factor in regulating the temperature of the body. Fifty percent of the body's surface lies on the extremities. The vasculature is arranged to be an effective heat exchanger so that the hands and feet are kept at the best working temperature. Normally there is a high blood flow to the toes. This is ensured by numerous arteriovenous shunts that pass warm arterial blood from arteries to superficial veins. From there the blood flows centrally. During this passage heat is exchanged from the blood to the surrounding tissue that then ensures a higher temperature to the deeper structures such as the supporting tissues and nerves. Even in a very cold environment a person with a positive heat balance exhibits temperatures in the toes higher than those found proximally in the same extremity. When the temperature of the body core is threatened, these distal anastomoses are closed, which minimizes heat loss. This reduction in blood flow is so rapid that the local temperatures in the toes fall at a rate similar to that seen with arterial occlusion under the same environmental conditions (Vanggard, 1969). Local cooling above the level of freezing can cause local vasoconstriction. This does not cause injury if the patient is in positive heat balance. After some minutes a reactive vasodilation occurs, giving the sensation of prickling heat, the so-called Lewis Hunting reaction (Lewis, 1930). If cold prevents the normal body temperature from being maintained, the arteriovenous anastomoses close, leading to irreversible changes. It is impossible to produce boots that will prevent a freezing injury. The insulation of a boot only determines the rate of fall of temperature in the foot, not the final result. When the local temperature drops to 50° F (10° C), sensory nerves are inhibited from making the victim aware of ensuing frostbite. At 28.4° F (−2° C) tissue freezes. Some of the extracellular water is transformed into ice, increasing the hypertonicity of the remaining fluids and thus dehydrating cells in the toes. The longer the period of increasing dehydration, the more severe the injury. Rapid cooling tends to decrease the amount of this damage.

Frostbite

Frostbite is a specific type of cold injury that occurs between the actual freezing of all tissue and an immersion foot (Bigelow, 1942; Browrigg, 1943). Frostbite of the foot is common. Blair (1964) reported that of 100 cases of frostbite seen during the Korean war, 89 occurred in the foot and 11 in the hand. The most common form of frostbite is superficial. A white patch of frozen skin is all that may be visible and, in fact, this heals within a few days without tissue damage. Frostbite of the foot is considered a serious injury, since there is only a small margin between the superficial and the deep type (Fig. 20-29). When deep frostbite occurs, those portions of the foot become stiff and brittle. Symptoms and signs may be similar to those of a burn. Radiographic changes in bone resulting from frostbite have also been noted (Vinson and Schatzki, 1954). Pathologic evaluation of tissue includes tissue necrosis. Edwards and Leeper (1952) analyzed 71 cases and noted that the extent of necrosis was in direct relation to the duration of freezing following onset of symptoms. Contributing factors associated with cold injuries include hyperhidrosis, chronic vasospasm, and possibly smoking. Simeone (1960) noted a proliferation of adventitial cells in the capillaries of smaller vessels, clotting of the vascular tree with fibrin-poor clots typically seen in stagnant blood, and mural hemorrhage in the vessel walls. He noted that most changes were thought to be a result of vascular occlusion.

Residual symptoms caused by severe freezing include cold and numbness in the feet, pain, hyperhidrosis, deformed toenails, scarring, and mutilation of the terminal phalanges (Blair et al., 1957; Lewis, 1941).

Treatment includes the principle of rewarming of the foot and local care to maintain the surviving tissue. Rapid warming is recommended. A frozen foot should be placed in a water bath between 104° and 108° F (40° and 42° C) (Knize et al. 1969; Owens, 1970; Washburn, 1962). When general hypothermia is present, the normal body temperature should be restored before thawing the frozen foot. Analgesics may be necessary during the rewarming period. Strict cleanliness and asepsis of the feet are maintained during the first 7 to 10 days following the rewarming. The foot is splinted in neutral position, but a flexibility program with active range of motion is encouraged even if gangrene is present. Intravenous low molecular weight dextran has been used in an attempt to reverse the tendency to intravascular sludging at low flow rates (Weatherly-White et al., 1965). Hyperbaric oxygen has been reported to be beneficial (Okuboye and Ferguson, 1968; Washburn,

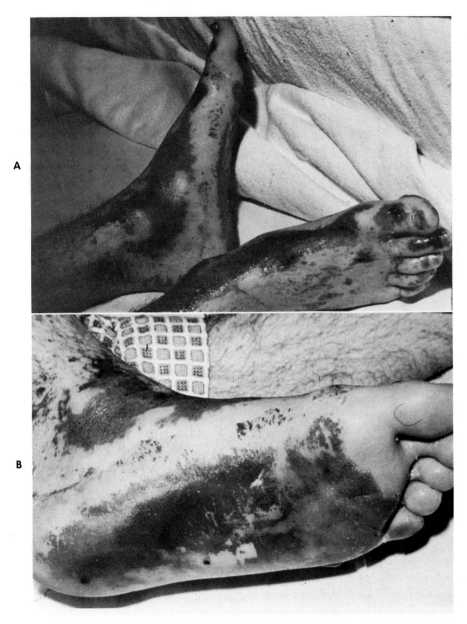

Fig. 20-29. A, Severe frostbite of feet. **B,** Plantar aspect of foot. Surgical debridement was withheld until clear demarcation of necrotic tissue developed. (Courtesy of Dr. J. Cranley.)

1962), but some have found no benefit (Gage et al., 1969). Following thawing of the injured foot, observation is important. After demarcation of necrosis has been well established 2 to 3 weeks later, debridement of tissue is performed. Immediate amputation should not be performed, however, as long as there is motion and a chance for revitalization of the foot and toes (Holm and Vanggard, 1974).

Injuries in which deep frostbite has been thawed and refrozen behave like a deep burn. It is suggested that only 3 weeks of observation be made before definitive debridement and reconstructive surgery so that muscle wasting is held to a minimum and rehabilitation is not delayed. Spontaneous arthrodesis has not been found following frostbite. The bones of the foot show signs of demineralization probably as a result of immobilization. This appears to be transient and reverses as the patient becomes active (Tishler, 1972).

Immersion foot and trench foot

Prolonged contact of the foot with subfreezing temperatures while activity is limited causes cold injury. If the feet are not removed from boots and stockings and allowed to dry and warm with regular intervals of massaging, along with a change into dry clothes, a change in the metabolism at the cellular level begins to occur

(Lyons, 1972). Metabolic changes present for long periods lead to irreversible damage. This condition was observed in survivors from sinking ships or aircraft downed over water. Webster (1942) and Fausel and Hemphill (1945) studied large numbers of cases that also occurred in soldiers during combat. Symptoms tend to increase when boots are removed and the feet are dried and warmed. A dusky cyanosis with blanching is first observed followed by a rapid swelling. The feet then become hyperemic and red. The temperature of the feet becomes markedly elevated, but there is no evidence of sweating. Tibial pulses are palpable. Subsequently, cyanosis with blebs, ecchymosis, and an obvious vasodilation develops. This is most dramatic over the medial aspect of the foot along the hallux and the medial portion of the longitudinal arch. If the foot has been immersed in water for a long time such as with survivors of a sinking ship, there is greater maceration of skin than seen in trench foot. This is associated with greater edema of the foot and leg.

The principles involved in treating immersion foot include preservation of living tissue and supportive measures to prevent further injury by infection or trauma. Rewarming should be at temperatures between 104° and 108° F (40° to 42° C). This is the maximum allowable temperature without causing injury from heat, which is a serious possibility when rewarming the foot. Additional treatment includes bed rest and active motion of the feet with elevation. Massage and walking are not recommended (Ungley, 1943). The use of heparin is not helpful. Pathologic studies of blood clots within blood vessels indicate that these appear to be caused by stasis with little fibrin present. Low molecular weight dextran intravenously with hydration of the patient may be of benefit. Surgical debridement of the areas that appear necrotic is not recommended for several weeks following treatment. Areas of skin and deep tissue that initially appear dead often become revitalized, particularly in younger individuals. Debridement and amputation are reserved for areas that have become necrotic and clearly demarcated after 2 to 3 weeks. Sympathectomy is reserved for those patients who have clear evidence of increased sympathetic tone. This usually becomes clear several weeks after injury and is seen more frequently in patients with immersion foot or trench foot rather than other types of cold injury (Dinep, 1975).

Because most cases of trench foot and immersion foot occur in victims who have little or no control over the environmental circumstances in which they are found, prophylaxis is difficult. However, regular drying and warming of the feet when possible, carrying extra socks when on expeditions into wilderness country, and recognizing early symptoms of cold injury are important for prevention of this syndrome.

Chilblain

Chilblain (lupus pernio) is a neurocirculatory disturbance of the skin of the feet (Lewin, 1941). It occurs in subfreezing weather from exposure (often repeated) to cold in a wet or dry environment. Symptoms include dermatitis and occasionally ulceration of skin. Microscopic examination of the tissues reveals a perivascular infiltration and intimal proliferation of vessels. Often subcutaneous tissue and skin show a chronic inflammatory reaction, and there may even be fat necrosis (Mennell, 1969). Chilblain has often been considered as the same as a milder form of frostbite. Hauser (1939) notes that it occurs where the circulation is poorest, such as on the dorsal aspect of the toes, the heads of the first and fifth metatarsals, and the posterior surface of the heel. Lake (1938) noted that chilblain tends to be more common in children than adults. If exposure to cold is repeated and prolonged, the fibrotic changes around the blood vessels and in tissues sensitize the foot to future exposure to cold. Chilblain tends to appear in cold weather and disappear in dry summer months. In some patients, however, symptoms may persist year-round. Excessively tight footwear aggravates symptoms.

Treatment includes avoiding tight-fitting shoes, wearing comfortable socks that are appropriately thick for cold weather, and avoiding remaining in wet footwear for a long period. Workers in cold environments including meat cutters, frozen food handlers, and workmen whose occupations require them to be outside for a long time during the winter are particularly prone to this condition.

BURNS

Thermal injury to the foot is common. Burns can be caused from heat, chemicals, radiation, and electricity. It is important to properly diagnose the injury, institute immediate measures to prevent further injury, begin definitive care as early as possible, and rehabilitate the patient on a regular schedule so that total disability will be at a minimum.

Burns caused by fire and contact by hot objects are less common because the foot is often covered. They are seen more often in patients with severe burns on other parts of their body (Artz and Mancrief, 1969).

Injury to the foot from electric burns is related to the duration and force of the insult. Alternating current injuries tend to produce tissue necrosis deep to the skin, much more than is visible on observation. Early observation is important, and treatment may require long skin incisions to thoroughly debride the dead deep tissues.

Isolated burns of the feet produced by hot liquids are common and often may occur from spills. It has been noted that most burns of the feet are caused by domes-

most glass objects may be visible. Cultures should be taken of any wound, and an appropriate history of tetanus immunization should be obtained to ensure proper antitetanus therapy. In locating a nonradiopaque foreign body, it is often prudent to wait up to 72 hours following the onset of symptoms so that body reaction will help the surgeon determine the position of the foreign body by tissue reaction.

REFERENCES

Ligamentous injuries of the foot and ankle joints

Anderson, K.J., and Lecocq, J.F.: Operative treatment of injury to the fibular collateral ligament of the ankle, J. Bone Joint Surg. 36A:825, 1954.

Anderson, K.J., Lecocq, J.F., and Lecocq, E.A.: Recurrent anterior subluxation of the ankle joint: a report of two cases and an experimental study, J. Bone Joint Surg. 34A:853, 1952.

Berridge, F.R., and Bonnin, J.G.: The radiographic examination of the ankle joint, including arthrography, Surg. Gynecol. Obstet. 79:383, 1944.

Bromstrom, L.: Sprained ankles. I. Anatomic lesions in recent sprains, Acta Chir. Scand. 128:483, 1964.

Bromstrom, L., Liljeehl, S.O., and Lindval, N.: Sprained ankles. II. Arthrographic diagnoses of recent ligament ruptures, Acta. Chir. Scand. 129:485, 1965.

Fordyce, A.J.W., and Horn, C.V.: Arthrography in recent injuries of ligaments of the ankle, J. Bone Joint Surg. 54B:116, 1972.

Glick, J.M.: Traumatic injuries to the soft tissues of the foot and ankle. In Mann, R.A., editor: DuVries surgery of the foot, ed. 4, St. Louis, 1978, Mosby Co.

Gordon, R.B.: Arthrography of the ankle joint, J. Bone Joint Surg. 52A:1623, 1970.

Henry, J.H.: Lateral ligament tears of the ankle: one to six-years follow-up study of 202 ankles, Orthop. Rev. 12(10):31, 1983.

Inman, V.T.: The joints of the ankle, Baltimore, 1976, Williams & Wilkins.

Kelly, R.P.: Ankle injuries, J. Ky. Med. Assoc. 50:281, 1952.

Komprda, J.: Le syndrome du sinus du tarse, Ann. podologie, 1:11317, 1966.

Leach, R.E.: Acute ankle sprains: vigorous treatment for best results, J. Musculoskel. Med. 1(1):68, 1983.

McMaster, P.E.: Treatment of ankle sprain: observations in more than 500 cases, JAMA 122:659, 1943.

Meyer, J.M., and Lagier, R.: Post-traumatic sinus tarsi syndrome, Acta Orthop. Scand., 48:121, 1977.

O'Connor, D.: Chicago 1958, American Academy of Orthopaedic Surgeons.

O'Connor, D.: Sinus tarsi syndrome: a clinical entity, J. Bone Joint Surg. 40A:720, 1958.

Percy, E.C., Hill, R.O., and Callaghan, J.E.: The sprained ankle, J. Trauma 9:972, 1969.

Subcommittee on Classification of Sports Injuries, American Medical Association, Committee on the Medical Aspects of Sports: Standard nomenclature of athletic injuries, Chicago, 1966, American Medical Association.

Taillard, W., Meyer, J., Garcia, J., and Blanc, Y.: The sinus tarsi syndrome, Int. Orthop. 5:117, 1981.

Tendon injuries

Brahms, M.A.: Common foot problems, J. Bone Joint Surg. 49A:1653, 1967.

Burman, M.S.: Subcutaneous rupture of the tendon of the tibialis anticus, Ann. Surg. 100:368, 1934.

Cohen, H., and Reid, J.B.: Tenosynovitis crepitans associated with oxaluria, Liverpool Med. Chir. J. 43:193, 1935.

Dickinson, P.H., Coutts, M.B., Woodward, E.P., and Handler, D.: Tendo achillis bursitis, J. Bone Joint Surg. 48A:77, 1966.

Els, H.: Ueber eine Abrissfraktur des Tibialisanticus-Ansatzes, Dtsch. Z. Chir. 106:610, 1910.

Floyd, D.W., Heckman, J.D., and Rockwood, C.A.: Tendon lacerations in the foot, Foot Ankle 4:8, 1983.

Ghormley, R.K., and Spear, I.M.: Anomalies of the posterior tibial tendon: a cause of persistent pain about ankle, Arch. Surg. 66:512, 1953.

Goldner, J.L., Keats, P.K., Bassett, F.H., and Clippinger, F.W.: Progressive talipes equinovarus due to trauma or degeneration of the posterior tibial tendon and medial plantar ligaments. Orthop. Clin. North Am. 5:39, 1974.

Griffiths, J.C.: Tendon injuries around the ankle, J. Bone Joint Surg. 47B:686, 1965.

Gunn, D.R.: Stenosing tenosynovitis of the common peroneal tendon sheath, Br. Med. J. 1:691, 1959.

Hann, J.B.: L.D. Howard technique of Achilles tendon repair: a post-humous tribute, Presented at the Western Orthopaedic Association Meeting, Honolulu, 1974.

Hamilton, W.G.: Stenosing tenosynovitis of the flexor hallucis longus tendon and posterior impingement upon the os trigonum in ballet dancers, Foot Ankle 3:74, 1982.

Inglis, A.E., Scott, W.N., Sculco, T.P., and Patterson, A.H.: Ruptures of the tendo Achillis: an objective assessment of surgical and nonsurgical treatment, J. Bone Joint Surg. 58A:990, 1976.

Jahss, M.H.: Spontaneous rupture of the tibialis posterior tendon: clinical findings, tenographic studies, and a new technique of repair, Foot Ankle 3:158, 1982.

Keck, S.W., and Kelly, P.J.: Bursitis of the posterior part of the heel, J. Bone Joint Surg. 47A:267, 1965.

Kettelkamp, D.B., and Alexander, H.H.: Spontaneous rupture of the posterior tibial tendon, J. Bone Joint Surg. 51A:759, 1969.

Lapidus, P.W.: Indirect subcutaneous rupture of the anterior tibial tendon: report of two cases, Bull. N.Y. Hosp. Joint Dis. 2:119, 1941.

Lapidus, P.W., and Seidenstein, H.: Chronic nonspecific tenosynovitis with effusion about the ankle, J. Bone Joint Surg. 32A:175, 1950.

Lipscomb, P.R.: Nonsuppurative tenosynovitis and paratendinitis. In American Academy of Orthopaedic Surgeons, Instructional Course Lectures, vol. 7, Ann Arbor, 1950, J.W. Edwards.

Lipscomb, P.R., and Kelley, P.J.: Injuries of the extensor tendons in the distal part of the leg and in the ankle, J. Bone Joint Surg. 37A:1206, 1955.

Mensor, M.C., and Ordway, G.L.: Traumatic subcutaneous rupture of the tibialis anterior tendon, J. Bone Joint Surg. 35A:675, 1953.

Parvin, R.W., and Ford, L.T.: Stenosing tenosynovitis of the common peroneal tendon sheath, J. Bone Joint Surg. 35A:1352, 1956.

Puddu, G., Ippolito, E., and Postacchini, F.: A classification of Achilles tendon disease, Am. J. Sports Med., 4:145, 1976.

Rorabeck, C.H.: The surgical treatment of exertional compartment syndrome in athletes, J. Bone Joint Surg. 65A:1245, 1983.

Sammarco, G.J., and Miller, E.H.: Partial rupture of the flexor hallucis longus in classical ballet dancers, J. Bone Joint Surg. 61A:149, 1979.

Trevino, S., Gould, N., and Korson, R., Surgical treatment of stenosing tenosynovitis at the ankle, Foot Ankle, 2:37, 1981.

Williams, R.: Chronic non-specific tendovaginitis of tibialis posterior, J. Bone Joint Surg. 45B:542, 1963.

Miscellaneous soft tissue injuries

Argamaso, R.V., Lewin, M.L., Baird, A.D., et al.: Cross-leg flaps in children, Plast. Reconstr. Surg. 51:662, 1973.

Artz, C.P., and Reiss E.: The treatment of burns, Philadelphia, 1957, W.B. Saunders Co.

Artz, C.P., and Moncrief, J.A.: The treatment of burns, ed. 2, Philadelphia, 1969, W.B. Saunders Co.

Becktold, F., and Lipin, R.J.: Differentiation of full thickness and partial thickness burn with the aid of fluorescein, Am. J. Surg. 119:436, 1965.

Bennett, J.E., and Kahn, R.A.: Surgical management of soft tissue defects of the ankle-heel region, J. Trauma 12:696, 1972.

Bigelow, W.G.: The modern conception and treatment of frostbite, Can. Med. Assoc. J. 47:529, 1942.

Blair, J.R., Schatzki, R., and Orr, K.D.: Sequelae to cold injury in one hundred patients, JAMA 163:1203, 1957.

Blair, J.R.: Proceedings of Symposium on Arctic Medicine and Biology, Vol. 4, Frostbite, Ft. Wainwright, Alaska, 1964, Actic Aero Medical Laboratory.

Bocca, M., and Baruffaldi, M.: La chirurgia plastica degli arti inferiori: lembi miocutanei. Muscolo tensore della fascia lata, gracile, peroniero lungo e breve, Estratto da Minerva Chirurgica 38:317, 1983.

Brownrigg, G.M.: Frostbite in shipwrecked mariners, Am. J. Surg. 59:232, 1943.

Burny, F.L.: Elastic external fixation of tibial fractures: study of 1421 cases. In Brooker, A.F., and Edwards, C., editors: External fixation: the current state of the art, Baltimore, 1979, The Williams & Wilkins Co.

Connes, H.: Le fixateur externe d'Hoffman: technique, indications, resultats, Paris, 1977, Editians GEAD.

Dabb, R.W., and Conklin, W.T.: A sensory innervated latissimus dorsi musculocutaneous free flap: case report, J. Microsurg. 2:289, 1981.

Dahlback, L.O.: Effects of temporary tourniquet ischemia on striated muscle fibers and motor end plates, Scand. J. Plast. Reconstr. Surg. (suppl. 7), 1970.

Dinep, M.: Cold injury: a review of current theories and their application to treatment, Conn. Med. 39:8, 1975.

Drabyn, G.A., and Avedian, L.: Ipsilateral buttock flap for coverage of a foot and ankle defect in a young child, Plast. Reconstr. Surg. 63:422, 1979.

Edwards, E.A., and Leeper, R.W.: Frostbite: an analysis of seventy-one cases, JAMA 149:1199, 1952.

Fausel, E.G., and Hemphill, J.A.: Study of the late symptoms of cases of immersion foot, Surg. Gynecol. Obstet. 81:500, 1945.

Furnas, D.W.: The cross groin flap for coverage of foot and ankle defects in children, Plast. Reconstr. Surg. 57:246, 1976.

Gage, A.A., Ishikawa, H., and Winter, P.M.: Experimental frostbite and hyperbaric oxygenation, Surgery 66:1044, 1969.

Goans, R.E.: Ultrasonic pulse echo determination of thermal injury in deep dermal burns, Med. Phys. 4:259, 1977.

Harman, J.W., and Guinn, R.P.: The recovery of skeletal muscle fibers from acute ischemia as determined by histologic and chemistry methods, Am. J. Pathol. 114:261, 1948.

Hartwell, S.W., Huger, W., Jr., and Pickrell, K.: Radiation dermatitis and radiogenic neoplasms of the hand, Ann. Surg. 160p:828, 1964.

Hauser, E.D.W.: Diseases of the foot, Philadelphia, 1939, W.B. Saunders Co.

Henshaw, R.J.: Early changes in the depth of burn, Ann. N.Y. Acad. Sci. 150:548, 1978.

Hermann, G., Schechter, D.C., Owens, J.C., and Starzl, T.E.: The problem of frostbite in civilian medical practice, Surg. Clin. North Am. 43:519, 1963.

Holm, P.C.A., and Vanggard, L.: Frostbite, Plast. Reconstr. Surg. 54:544, 1974.

Jackson, D.M.: The diagnosis of depth of burning, Br. J. Surg. 40:588, 1953.

Jackson, D.M.: Second thoughts on burn wound, J. Trauma, 9:839, 1969.

Jelenko, C. III: Chemicals that burn, J. Trauma 14:65, 1974.

Kelly, R.P., and Whitesides, R.E., Jr.: Transfibular route for fasciotomy of the leg, J. Bone Joint Surg. 49A:1022, 1967.

Knize, D.M., Weatherly-White, R.C.A., Paton, B.C., and Owens, J.D.: Prognostic factors in the management of frostbite, J. Trauma 9:749, 1969.

Lake, M.C.: The foot, Baltimore, 1938, Wm. Wood & Co.

Larkin, J.M., and Moylan, J.A.: Tetanus following a minor burn, J. Trauma 15:546, 1975.

Lewin, P.: The foot and ankle, Philadelphia, 1941, Lea & Febiger.

Lewis, T.: Observations upon the reactions of the vessels in the human skin to cold, J. Heart 15:177, 1930.

Lewis, T.: Observations on some normal and injurious effects of cold upon the skin and underlying tissues: frostbite, Br. Med. J. 2:869, 1941.

London, P.S.: The burnt foot, Br. J. Surg. 40:293, 1953.

Lyons, J.M.: Phase transitions and control of cellular metabolism at low temperatures, Cyrobiology 9:341, 1972.

Maxwell, G.P., Manson, P.N., and Hoopes, J.E.: Experience with thirteen latissimus dorsi myocutaneous free flaps, Plast. Reconstr. Surg. 64:1, 1979.

Mennell, J.M.: Foot pain, Boston, 1969, Little, Brown & Co.

Metaizeau, J.P., Gayet, O., and Prevot, J.: The use of free full thickness skin grafts in treatment of complications of burns, Prog. Pediatr. Surg. 14:209, 1981.

Miller, T.A., Switzer, W.E., Foley, W.D., and Moncrief, J.A.: Early homografting of second degree burns, Plast. Reconstr. Surg. 40:117, 1967.

Mladick, R., Georgiade, H., and Thorne, F.: Clinical evaluation of thermography in determining degree of injury, Plast. Reconstr. Surg. 38:512, 1966.

Mladick, R.A., Pickrell, K.L., Thorne, F.L., and Royer, J.R.: Ipsolateral thigh flap for total plantar resurfacing, Plast. Reconstr. Surg. 43:198, 1969.

Monk, C.J.E.: Traumatic ischaemia of the calf, J. Bone Joint Surg. 48B:150, 1966.

Moorhead, J.J.: Locating and removing foreign bodies, Am. J. Surg. 95:108, 1958.

Murbarak, S.J., and Owen, C.A.: Double incision fasciotomy of the ligament for recompression in compartment syndromes, J. Bone Joint Surg. 59A:184, 1977.

Murray, J.E., and Goldwyn, R.M.: Definitive treatment of intractable plantar ulcers, JAMA 196:311, 1966.

Norris, J.E.C.: Burns of the foot. In Jahss, M., editor: Disorders of the foot, Philadelphia, 1982, W.B. Saunders Co.

Okuboye, J.A., and Ferguson, C.C.: The use of hyperbaric oxygen in the treatment of experimental frostbite, Can. J. Surg. 11:78, 1968.

Owen, C.A.: Clinical diagnosis of acute compartment syndromes. In Mubarak, S., editor: Compartment syndromes and Volkmann's contracture, Philadelphia, 1981, W.B. Saunders Co.

Owens, J.C.: Treatment cold injuries, Postgrad. Med. 48:160, 1970.

Randolph, J.G., Leape, L.L., and Gross, R.E.: The "sprained" ankle, J. Trauma 9:972, 1969.

Roberts, W.C.: Radiographic characteristics of glass, Arch. Ind. Health 18:470, 1958.

Robson, M.C., Kucan, J.O., Piak, K.I., and Ericksson, E.: Prevention of derma ischemia after thermal trauma, Arch. Surg. 113:621, 1978.

Rudowski, W.: Burn therapy and research, Baltimore, 1976, John Hopkins University Press.

Salisbury, R.E., and Pruitt, B.A.: Burns of the upper extremity, vol. 9, Series major problems in clinical surgery, Philadelphia, 1976, W.B. Saunders Co.

Sammarco, G.J.: Soft tissue conditions in athletes feet, Clin. Sports Med. **1**:149, 1982.

Sawacki, B.E.: Reversal of capillary stasis and prevention of necrosis in burns, Ann. Surg. **180**:98, 1974.

Seddon, H.J.: Volkmann's ischaemia in the lower limb, J. Bone Joint Surg. **48B**:627, 1966.

Simeone, F.A.: Cold injury, Arch. Surg. **80**:396, 1960.

Starzl, T.E.: The problem of frostbite in civilian medical practice, Surg. Clin. North Am. **43**:519, 1963.

Tishler, J.M.: The soft tissue and bone changes in frostbite injuries, Radiology **102**:511, 1972.

Ungley, C.C.: Treatment of immersion foot by dry cooling, Lancet **1**:681, 1943.

Vanggaard, L.: Arterial venous anastomosis in temperature regulation, Acta Physiol. Scand. **76**:13A, 1969.

Vinson, H.A., and Schatzki, R.: Roentgenologic bone changes encountered in frostbite: Korea 1950-51, Radiology **63**:685, 1954.

Washburn, B.: Frostbite, N. Engl. J. Med. **266**:974, 1962.

Weatherley-White, R.C.A., Paton, B.C., and Sjostrom, B.: Observations on the treatment of frostbite, Plast. Reconstr. Surg. **36**:10, 1965.

Webster, D.R., Woolhouse, F.M., and Johnston, J.L.: Immersion foot, J. Bone Joint Surg. **24A**:785, 1942.

Whitesides, T.E., Jr.: Compartment syndrome. In Jahss, M., editor: Disorders of the foot, Philadelphia, 1982, W.B. Saunders Co.

Whitesides, T.E., Jr., Harada, H., and Marinoto, K.: Compartment syndromes and the role of fasciotomy: its parameters and technique. In American Academy of Orthopaedic Surgeons Instructional course lectures, vol. 26, St. Louis, 1977, The C.V. Mosby Co., p. 179.

21

The foot in running and dancing

The foot in running
DONALD E. BAXTER

The present interest in fitness has created new problems for the physician. The runner's enthusiasm for increased running has created biomechanical and overuse syndromes with increasing frequency. A large percentage of runner's injuries are related to a minimal structural problem in conjunction with overuse of the extremity. Overuse syndromes and problems can occur at any level of running, particularly if the runner makes an escalation of training or a major change in training character. For the physician who will deal with runner's problems, a systematic approach is necessary to sift through the multitude of possible problems.

HISTORY

Forms may be used in taking a history, thus allowing the runner to make an outline of his complaints while seated in the waiting room. A suggested format follows:
1. Chief complaint. The most severe problem should be listed first, with the duration and nature of the onset of the symptom. Lesser problems should then be listed in order of their significance.
2. Occurence of pain during runs or after runs.
3. Type of previous treatment the patient has undergone.
4. Nature of the patient's training program. Is the runner a beginner, recreational noncompetitive jogger, or a competitive runner? Has there been a recent increase in the training mileage? Has there been increased speed associated with the workouts?
5. Any recent change in shoewear. Are the shoes rotated among two or three types to avoid similar stresses? Does the patient note a specific abnormal wear pattern?
6. Use of orthotic devices. If used, have the devices been rigid or flexible orthoses; and what symptoms were changed by their use?

7. Type of surface training is carried out on. Is it hard or soft, circular or slanted?
8. Related exercises used, such as stretching and strengthening exercises. Is a systematic stretching or yoga program used? Are weights used to build up strength in a balanced manner?
9. Nutritional aspects of the runner. Are supplemental vitamins or minerals used? Is sufficient water consumed with increased training, racing, and weather conditions?

PHYSICAL EXAMINATION

The physical examination must encompass the entire lower extremity and back. This should be carried out with the patient in the standing position first, allowing him to walk and run if possible. The examination should then be continued with the patient sitting, followed by an examination with the patient in the prone and supine positions.

Standing

With the patient in the standing position, the back is observed for evidence of scoliosis, which would result in malalignment of the spine. An increase in the lumbar lordosis associated with weakened abdominal musculature should be carefully checked for. The level of the iliac wings gives one a good idea as to leg length. The patient is asked to touch the floor with his hands to give the examiner some idea as to flexibility of the hamstrings and Achilles tendons. The overall alignment of the knee is important to determine if there is any abnormality involving the patella as well as if genu varum and valgum are present. Next, the overall alignment of the foot is observed to see if both feet are in approximately the same amount of external rotation. The heel alignment gives indication not only of symmetry of the forefoot but also of increased varus or valgus configuration of the heel during running. The patient should be asked to stand on his toes to be sure that the proper

pressures rise to greater than 75 mm Hg. At times the pressure during exercise may exceed 100 mm Hg. At completion of exercise, intramuscular pressure will remain greater than 30 mm Hg for 5 minutes or longer and usually symptoms of pain and paresthesias are present. The differential diagnosis of anterior compartment syndrome or anterolateral compartment syndrome is intermittent claudication from partial femoral artery obstruction, stress fracture of the tibia or fibula, tenosynovitis or musculotendinitis (shin splints). Treatment includes resting the involved extremity giving antiinflammatory medications, and decreasing the mileage run. Most of these syndromes will subside. If they persist, a decompressive fascial release may be necessary. If the release is in the anterolateral compartment, care must be taken to decompress the superficial peroneal nerve as it penetrates the fascia. Care is taken to look for a muscle herniation at this point. If it is in the anteromedial compartment, the saphenous nerve must be released. Involvement in the deep posterior compartment is also very common in runners. Pain may be localized medially where the gastrocsoleus tapers, or it can radiate proximally or distally. Occasionally numbness in the sole of the foot is described by the runner. Results of compartment pressure measurements vary because of the nature of the problem and the difficulty in obtaining accurate measurements during exercise. Increased pressure is usually in the deep posterior compartment, but on occasion may be isolated to the posterior tibial muscle compartment.

HEEL PAIN

Most runners who complain of heel pain have plantar fasciitis or pain at the attachment of the plantar fascia and respond to appropriate rest, antiinflammatory medications, and/or longitudinal arch supports to alleviate the symptoms. An occasional patient continues to have problems despite conservative care. In a recent paper by Baxter and Thigpen (1983), it was pointed out that a motor branch to the abductor digiti quinti is located between the calcaneus and the heel spur. This particular nerve to the abductor digiti quinti is a third branch of the posterior tibial nerve (see Fig. 21-1). This particular nerve to the abductor digiti quinti passes deep to the fascia origin of the abductor hallucis muscle. Baxter and Thigpen hypothesized that some runners experience a form of compression syndrome from the abductor hallucis muscle, causing impingement on this particular nerve as it passes through and behind the fascia of the abductor hallucis muscle. This syndrome may be initiated by an episode of plantar fasciitis or by hypertrophy of the abductor hallucis muscle. As demonstrated in Figs. 21-2 and 21-3, the motor branch to the abductor digiti quinti can be compressed and/or traumatized in several areas. The first occurs at the sharp fascial edge along the superior aspect of the abductor hallucis muscle. With hypertrophy of the abductor hallucis muscle, nerve impingement may occur in this region. Also, during dorsiflexion of the toes, the abductor hallucis muscle and short flexor muscles become taut, and this too can cause both compression

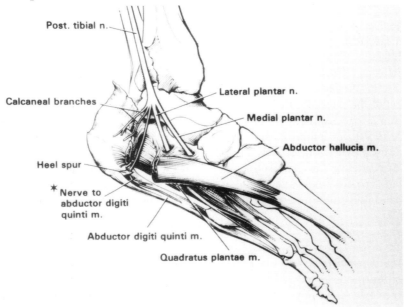

Fig. 21-2. Deep fascia of abductor hallucis muscle has been incised, exposing nerve to abductor digiti quinti. This nerve can be compressed by abductor hallucis muscle, medial tuberosity of calcaneus, or on occasion heel spur or plantar fascia. (From Baxter, D., and Thigpen, M.: Foot Ankle **5:**16, 1984. © 1984, American Orthopaedic Foot Society.)

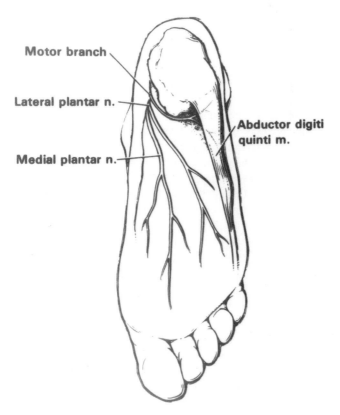

Motor branch

Lateral plantar n.

Medial plantar n.

Abductor digiti
quinti m.

Fig. 21-3. Motor branch to abductor digiti quinti muscle. (From Baxter, D., and Thigpen, M.: Foot Ankle **5:**16, 1984. © 1984, American Orthopaedic Foot Society.)

and/or tethering of the nerve during running. The last site of possible compression of the nerve is in the area of the proximal plantar fascia. Secondary to the impact of heel strike and an inflamed plantar fascia, the nerve irritation may become chronic. These patients often describe a burning pain on the medial aspect of the heel; about half note radiation of the pain into the leg.

If all attempts at conservative treatment fail in a runner with heel pain, surgery to decompress this nerve may be indicated. If surgery is performed, care should be taken to observe this particular nerve as well as the medial calcaneal branches, so that they will not be inadvertently cut, thus causing a painful neuroma and/or numbness about the heel.

PLANTAR FASCIITIS

Plantar fasciitis is a term used to describe a painful condition located about the posterior medial surface of the foot just distal to the attachment of the plantar fascia to the calcaneus. Initially, the symptoms are of gradual onset. The athlete usually carries on with training, but symptoms often become worse, being most severe after running or in the early morning. Maximum tenderness is located over the medial edge of the plan-

tar fascia just distal to the insertion of the calcaneus. There is often pain in the proximal inferior origin of the abductor hallucis muscle.

In chronic cases of plantar fasciitis, pain can actually radiate proximally into the leg, suggesting a nerve etiology of the pain. If there is burning pain into the heel or radicular pain into the leg, the nerve to the abductor digiti minimi may be compressed by an inflamed plantar fascia or hypertrophied abductor hallucis muscle.

The treatment for plantar fasciitis includes rest and application of a flexible orthosis with a ⅛-inch medial heel wedge. When symptoms improve until no pain is noted in the morning on arising, a graduated running program is begun. The orthosis is used for several months. Other treatment modalities include ice treatment, ultrasound treatment, or occasionally corticosteroid injections.

On occasion the plantar fascia can actually rupture away from the os calcis. In this case, the athlete usually gives a history of a sudden injury such as a sudden pain while running on a rigid indoor track. The pain is usually knifelike and causes significant disability for 6 to 12 weeks. When the swelling subsides in the foot, a small defect can often be palpated at the origin of the plantar fascia. Treatment for the acute form of plantar fasciitis with rupture is similar to that treatment described for chronic plantar fasciitis.

ORTHOSIS AND COMPLICATIONS OF RIGID ORTHOSES

In some runners an overuse syndrome can occur as a result of the repetitive stress of running. These people tend to have a more pronated foot than the average population, but a few may also have a cavus type foot. There are other malalignment problems such as genu varus and valgum and toeing in and toeing out that also lead to clinical problems secondary to the stress of running. Various types of orthotic devices have been used by runners and the question always arises: what if anything does an orthosis do from a biomechanical point of view? An orthosis primarily prevents hyperpronation. Cavanagh et al. (1978) selectively placed increasing thicknesses of felt along the medial border of the foot, to the eventual equivalent of 9.5 mm, and demonstrated a decrease in the degree of pronation and a decrease in the angular velocity of pronation. He further studied subjects using a force plate, and the only significant change was in the medial and lateral shear; the medial shear was decreased considerably in the subjects using the medial support. It appears that an orthosis providing a medial arch support does play a role in control of the foot by decreasing the degree as well as the rate of pronation of the foot. According to Stipe (1983), orthoses actually cause more energy consumption. It was felt that if orthoses helped correct problems with a runner's gait it could be assumed that the runner would experience an improvement in running economy as a result of wearing running orthoses. A study comparing the energy demands of running with or without orthoses was made between the responses of the subjects to running in the controlled condition (the shoes with no orthosis) and the two orthotic conditions (shoes with soft orthoses and shoes with semirigid orthoses).

The study was carried out by collecting expired air during the final 2 minutes of each run and analyzing it to determine the volume of oxygen consumed per kilogram of body weight per minute (VO_2). The study demonstrated that athletes running without orthoses required less oxygen than the athletes running with orthoses. While this situation was present at most running speeds, it was most significant during running at a pace of 7 minutes per mile or faster. The added weight of the orthoses alone could not account for the increased oxygen consumption, and it was hypothesized that the orthosis diminished the cushioning effects of the running shoe. This meant the athlete had to do more work to absorb the vertical impact of each stride.

This research suggests that an athlete does not gain running economy when he runs with orthoses in his shoes. Instead, it appears that runners who wear orthoses actually encounter an increase in the aerobic demands of running. This should not be construed as a recommendation not to wear orthoses while running a race. A decision should be made for medical reasons independent of the energetic consequences of wearing orthoses.

There are three groups of orthoses. The soft type is generally inexpensive and can be made in the office or obtained ready-made. These are the type that many runners make themselves. They use orthopaedic felt, semi-flexible cork, or leather. Many of the orthopaedic supply houses have a large selection of precut orthoses that can be used as either a temporary orthosis or a long-term orthosis to be changed intermittently.

The second type of orthoses is semiflexible. These may be made in the office but need to be fabricated by someone who understands the biomechanics of the foot and understands what function is being altered. One type may be made out of Orthoplast or Plastizote. These are heat-sensitive, semiflexible materials that become quite pliable when warm. Orthoplast is heated with warm water and Plastizote in a baking oven. Once the material is pliable it is molded onto the foot or the cast of the foot while it is attempted to hold the foot in a neutral position. Additional height of the longitudinal arch can be fabricated in layers. Once this orthosis cools, it is finished by smoothing the edges.

A third type of orthosis is a rigid orthosis that is fabricated from a positive plaster mold. A negative mold is made from the individual's foot with the foot held in the appropriate position. Once this has been done, a positive plaster cast is poured. The acrylic is poured over the positive plaster cast, and posting "bars and wedges" are added to finish the orthosis.

Indications for any orthosis are to relieve pressure from an area of the foot, to transfer pressure to a specific area, or to prevent specific motion. The main indication is in prevention of pronation in the individual with a hypermobile foot or pes planus. The use of a rigid orthosis for a high-arched, rigid, cavovarus foot is less effective, because it attempts to push the rigid foot into a different position. Selection of the orthosis is dependent on the amount of control that is needed and whether the foot is hypermobile or rigid. Rigid orthotic devices should be avoided if possible. Complications that occur with rigid orthosis include neuromas and sesamoiditis just distal to the edge of the rigid orthoses. Other problems include stress fractures of the leg as a result of inflexibility and decreased shock absorption in the foot. Cost configuration is something that must be brought into consideration. The soft orthoses are obviously the least expensive. The ideal orthosis has several characteristics. It is durable, controls motion, transfers pressure points, and is inexpensive and easy to fabricate.

SHOES

There is a multitude of shoes on the market today. More and more sophisticated shoes are being designed for training, for racing, for the heavy runner, or for the runner with a narrow foot. Good racing shoes are lightweight and should not be worn over prolonged mileage for fear of developing overuse syndromes and strains of the foot. Good training shoes have adequate compressability of the heel to cushion heel strike. They have adequate medial support to prevent hyperpronation, and they are adequately flexible to eliminate stress on the Achilles tendon from a rigid lever arm. In advising runners on buying shoes, quality control should be evaluated. Evaluation of the shoes should be carried out to assure that the sole layers are securely fastened to each other and to the upper portion of the shoe. The inner aspect of the shoes should be evaluated for protrusion and indentations. In fitting the shoe, the shoes should be fitted to the longer foot. A minimum of ¼ to ⅜ of an inch in front of the long toe should be left when measuring the length of the shoe. The calcaneus should not slip or rub excessively in the rear of the shoe. The lacing and tongue must feel comfortable on the instep to avoid irritating the superficial nerves and bony prominences.

GENERAL RULES OF TREATMENT FOR THE INJURED RUNNER

1. Change the training so that the runner runs within the limits of pain. Alter the stride length, increasing or decreasing the stride and the pace to eliminate symptoms.
2. Change to a soft, less slanted surface that has minimal curves and a surface that allows sliding, such as grass or cinders.
3. Stretching exercises are initiated if the runner's muscles are extremely tight. Stretching is done in both a linear and a rotational direction. If the runner's muscles are excessively flexible, strengthening is initiated with weights. Numerous repetitions should be done using light weights. This will increase the endurance of the muscles.
4. Ice is used for a hyperemic state in which there is swelling. Heat will often benefit the runner who has minimal swelling and where there are ischemic areas that need increased circulation.
5. Nongravity exercises are initiated using a bicycle or swimming if other treatments fail.
6. Medicines can be considered for inflammation and swelling. Aspirin can be used 3 to 4 times a day for 1 to 2 weeks. Aspirin should only be taken during periods of reduced running to avoid fluid problems, such as dehydration, that are associated with aspirin treatment. Cortisone injections should not be used in areas where tendon rupture might occur or fat necrosis might develop. It is best to avoid strong medications because of their side affects.
7. Surgery is done as a last resort, preferably after 6 to 12 months of conservative treatment. Surgical intervention includes tendon releases, bony resections for impingements, nerve releases, fascial releases, and patellar reconstruction.

Dance injuries to the foot
G. JAMES SAMMARCO

The dancer is a very special person whose feet are comparable to a concert pianist's hands. Extensive training, often beginning before the age of 10, is common, especially in girls. Classical ballet style and technique evolved from the masques and Bergamasques of the Renaissance and from fencing postures. Through the years increased strain was placed on the foot through changing styles and great leaps. In the early twentieth century the poise, balance, and symmetry that had developed into the high art form of classical technique were combined with new asymmetric individual styles and techniques of modern dance. The modern dance form requires barefoot dancing. Injuries to the foot occur whether the dancer wears a hard-toed classical ballet pointe shoe, a soft calfskin ballet shoe, a character shoe with a heel and stiff shank, or no shoe at all (McLain, 1983). Care of the entire body is an important part of training (Ambre, 1978; Kirkendall, 1983; Stonjanovic et al., 1963).

THE ARCH

In training for dance, it is important that the dancer have a well-formed arch. Although a naturally high arch is considered esthetic by dancers, it may, in fact, represent a mild to moderate cavus deformity. For the dancer who does not have a high arch, a minimum of 6 months, but more often 2 years, is necessary to develop an appropriate rotation of the hindfoot and the intrinsic and extrinsic muscle strength coordination to actively sustain the arch while performing (McLain, 1983; Sammarco, 1982).

KNUCKLING DOWN

Knuckling down occurs when the toes of the young female classical ballet dancer who is first learning to dance *sur les pointes* (on the toes) collapse within the blocked toe of the pointe shoe (Howse, 1972; Sammarco and Miller, 1982) (Fig. 21-4). A young dancer must have developed muscle strength, coordination, balance, and poise as well as the mental maturity to concentrate in a dance class for periods of up to an hour before being permitted to dance on her toes. This requires 3 years of training, and the child should be at least 11 years of age. The fault may not be observed by the teacher, since it is hidden in the pointe shoe. If the child begins to dance clumsily, this fault should be recognized and pointe dancing discontinued until strength and balance are sufficiently developed. Failure to do so predisposes the dancer to severe injury of the foot and ankle and prevents advancement in training.

SPLAYFOOT

Since the dancer stands for long periods of time in the half pointe position, i.e., on the ball of the foot, the intermetatarsal ligaments stretch, creating a splay deformity (Sammarco and Miller, 1982). This normal characteristic of the dancer's foot should not be treated surgically. In fact, over the years the flexor tendons may even sublux between the metatarsal heads. If this becomes symptomatic in dancers in their 30s and 40s, it is easily treated with a full insole molded leather arch support with a metatarsal pad. The pad may be placed in a ballet shoe.

HALLUX RIGIDUS

Dancers need the full range of motion of the hallux metatarsophalangeal joint to properly perform in all forms of dance. Hallux rigidus occurs commonly in

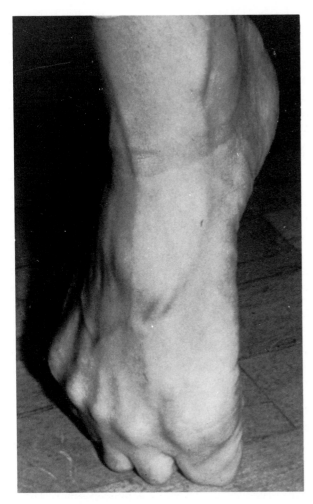

Fig. 21-4. Knuckling down is caused by dancing *sur les pointes* before young dancer has developed strength and balance. (From Sammarco, G.J., and Miller, E.H.: Foot Ankle 3:85, 1982. © 1982, American Orthopaedic Foot Society.)

male dancers. It may be accompanied by periarticular ossification of the collateral ligaments (Howse, 1983; Sammarco, 1982). Characteristically, radiographs reveal degenerative changes on the articular surfaces of the metatarsophalangeal joint. Clinically, a decreased motion of the metatarsophalangeal joint is observed. Although dancers develop this problem at an earlier age than the general population, i.e., in their 30s, the training and stage presence of the dancer, known as charisma, hide asymmetry. The dancer tends to compromise strict classical technique.

Correction of hallux rigidus in the dancer is a difficult surgical decision. Male dancers who are not required to dance *sur les pointes* will still develop metatarsalgia following an arthroplasty. Procedures that shorten the great toe, such as resection arthroplasty, allow the metatarsal pad, including the sesamoids, to migrate proximally leading to postoperative metatarsalgia. Silas-

tic arthroplasty (Howse, 1983) has been performed in unusual circumstances using a single-stem Swanson type prosthesis, but results have been inconsistent. Any procedure on the hallux may require up to 1 year for full recovery. The dancer must be counselled before surgery since a dance career tends to be short, perhaps lasting 20 years.

ACUTE AND CHRONIC PLANTAR FASCIITIS

Plantar fasciitis often occurs when the dancer returns from vacation or periods of "laying off." It is short lived and may be treated with a foam rubber arch support, physical therapy, a flexibility program, and gradually increasing the rehearsal schedule. It is important, however, that the dancer perform a flexibility program for the foot as well as the entire body everyday, whether working or not. Chronic fasciitis may be treated with a full insole molded leather arch support with a high longitudinal arch. This is placed in a ballet shoe. It is not used in a pointe shoe because of the space requirements and proprioceptive feedback needed between the foot, the shoe, and the floor. Surgical excision is not recommended.

ACUTE FLEXION INJURY

Acute flexion injury to the hallux occurs as the dancer lands from a leap. The tip of the toe is caught and a hyperflexion injury occurs, injuring the dorsal and medial capsule of the metatarsophalangeal joint of the hallux (Sammarco and Miller, 1982). This is not unlike "turf toe" seen in other athletes. Decreased motion with tenderness and pain at the metatarsophalangeal joint confirms the diagnosis. Radiographs show no fracture.

Treatment includes a compression dressing of the forefoot for 3 days followed by splinting of the first and second toes for a period of 10 days. Active range of motion is encouraged after 3 to 4 days, as tolerated.

BUNIONS

Bunions are common in dancers (Ambre, 1978; Sammarco and Miller, 1982; Tomasen, 1982; Volkov, 1975). They begin to develop at the end of the teens and occur in both male and female dancers. They are often symptomatic at the end of class, since the foot is forced into a tight shoe (Fig. 21-5). Padding with lamb's wool around the tender area is a simple and effective means of relieving pain. The dancer should chose a pointe shoe in which the box, the stiff front end of the shoe, is of proper length and stiffness. Hallux valgus and bunion can also be caused by improper dance technique, and therefore the young dancer should adhere strictly to the teacher's guidance.

Surgery for bunions that are intermittently sympto-

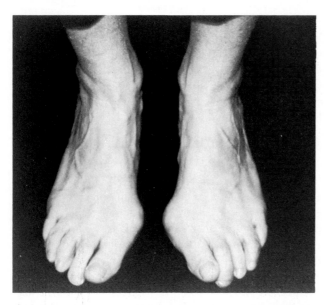

Fig. 21-5. Dancer, in fifth decade, with bunions. They are symptomatic only after leading class and relieved by elevation and comfortable shoes.

matic is not recommended, since it stiffens the hallux and often requires 1 year for recovery. Procedures that shorten the first toe may cause additional problems with pointe dancing, including poor balance and pain, and this may terminate a promising career.

HAMMERTOE

Hammertoe is common in dancers and like bunion is usually asymptomatic except toward the end of strenuous rehearsals. Appropriate lamb's wool padding in the box of a pointe shoe or around the toe of a ballet shoe will help control discomfort. The flexible deformity is best treated with foam or lamb's wool padding. If the older dancer is disabled, the severely symptomatic fixed hammertoe deformity may be treated by lengthening of the extensor tendons of that particular toe and proximal phalangeal condylectomy. Postoperatively the toe is held with a smooth Kirschner wire for a period of 4 weeks. Often such a procedure effects an apparent lengthening of the toe, and the dancer should be so advised.

METATARSALGIA
Subluxation of toe

Metatarsalgia in the young dancer can be caused by subluxation of the metatarsophalangeal joint of one of the lesser toes (Ronconi, 1983). This occurs in the second, third, or fourth toes. Diagnosis is made by holding the ball of the foot and moving the proximal phalanx up and down at the metatarsophalangeal joint to demonstrate laxity. If symptoms are disabling, surgical treat-

ment with excision of the proximal 20% of the proximal phalanx is indicated. The plantar plate of the toe should be sutured to the medial and lateral portions of the capsule over the metatarsal head so that the metatarsal pad does not migrate proximally. The toe is held in place with a smooth Kirschner wire for 4 weeks postoperatively. Dancing is permitted on the operated foot and the weight-bearing leg following removal of the wire.

Avascular necrosis of metatarsal head

Avascular necrosis of the head of the metatarsal is quite disabling in the dancer (Sammarco and Miller, 1982). Symptoms include stiffening of the metatarsophalangeal joint with pain on motion, particularly in *relevé*, i.e., rising to the demi-pointe position. Treatment includes excision of the proximal portion of the proximal phalanx, as described (Fig. 21-6). Rehabilitation requires at least 3 months of class to return to predisease level of proficiency.

Stress fracture

Stress fracture of the proximal phalanx is less common (Fig. 21-7) and may require a bone scan (see Stress Fractures) to be adequately visualized.

Sesamoiditis

Sesamoiditis occurs with a rapid onset, usually in the fibular sesamoid, and is diagnosed by pressing on the respective sesamoid with the hallux in neutral position. The hallux is then extended, and the area of tenderness moves distally as the sesamoid is pulled distally. Treatment includes appropriate padding around the tender area and antiinflammatory medication.

Interdigital neuroma

Interdigital neuroma is not uncommon in dancers and must be differentiated from subluxing toe and stress fracture of the proximal phalanx. Diagnosis is often elusive and may take several weeks with repeated examinations. Characteristic paresthesias are elicited on medial and lateral compression of the metatarsal heads as well as pressure directly over and under the nerve. If padding does not relieve the symptoms, surgical treatment is indicated. With the patient under local anesthesia, a dorsal longitudinal incision is made in the web space along with meticulous dissection to the nerve. After a few days' rest active motion is begun using the operated leg as the non-weight-bearing, "working leg," and the unoperated leg, the leg on which the dancer stands, as the leg of support.

STRESS FRACTURES

The dancer spends a great deal of time in the demi-pointe position, sometimes dancing for periods of 6

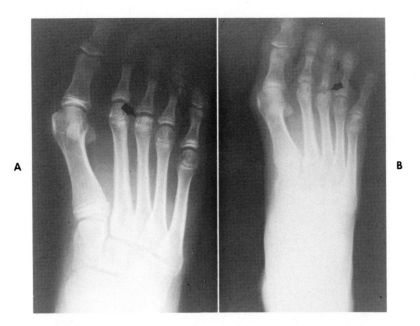

Fig. 21-6. A, Avascular necrosis of third metatarsal head is common cause of metatarsalgia. Also, note incidental finding of asymptomatic bunions. **B,** Treatment by excision of proximal portion of proximal phalanx allows return to dancing within 3 months.

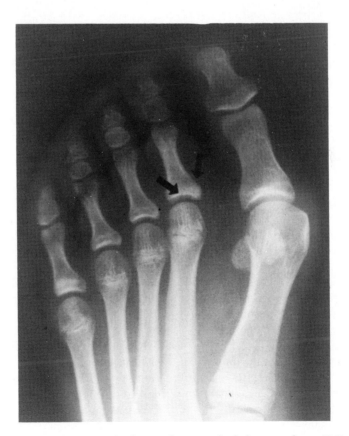

Fig. 21-7. Stress fracture (arrows) of second proximal phalanx involving 50% of articular surface of metatarsophalangeal joint. Even though onset of pain was acute, no direct trauma was involved. This was treated as a "stone bruise" for 3 weeks.

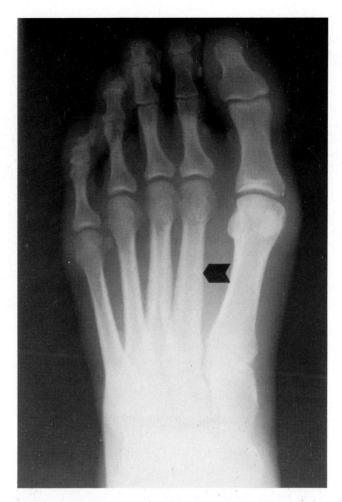

Fig. 21-8. Radiograph of young dancer's foot showing thickening of second (arrow) and third metatarsal shafts as well as lateral aspect of first metatarsal from prolonged periods spent in demi-pointe position.

hours 6 days a week. As with other high-performance athletes, the attitude of "no pain, no gain" is prevalent. The main forces within the foot pass through the dome of the talus and head of the navicular and middle cunneiform down through the second and third metatarsals (Collis and Jayson, 1972; Manter, 1946; Nikolic and Zimmerman, 1968; Pelipenko, 1973) (Fig 21-8). A secondary line of force passes laterally through the cuboid and fifth metatarsal. Stress fractures, common in dancers, tend to occur in the proximal metaphyses of the second and third metatarsals or in the tarsal bones, particularly the navicular (Fig 21-9). Less commonly a phalangeal stress fracture may occur (see Fig 21-7). This must be differentiated from other forms of metatarsalgia. These fractures may not appear on standard radiographs for several months but may be detected with bone scan (Devas, 1975; Sammarco, 1984; Wilcox et al, 1977). The dancer is often mistakenly treated for tendinitis.

Treatment includes an elastic support dressing and the use of crutches, with weight bearing, for 4 to 6 weeks, depending on the severity of symptoms. Return to a full dance schedule before healing of the fracture may cause a recurrence of symptoms. The floor on which dancing takes place must be examined to eliminate causative factors and prevent recurrence (Seals, 1983).

TRIGGER TOE

Partial rupture of the flexor hallucis longus tendon, or trigger toe, has been found in female classical ballet dancers. The injury consists of a longitudinal rent in the flexor hallucis longus tendon as it passes from beneath the sustenaculum tali through the tarsal tunnel in its own groove (Sammarco and Miller, 1979) (Fig. 21-10). The torn fibers retract on themselves, causing a fusiform swelling in the tendon at the sustenaculum tali. This swelling impinges in the tunnel as the toe is ex-

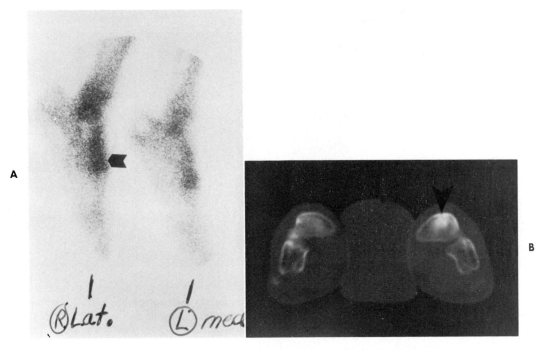

Fig. 21-9. A, Bone scan reveals increased uptake in tarsal navicular (arrow) indicating stress fracture. This was treated for 3 months as "tendinitis." **B,** Stress fracture (arrow) of tarsal navicular in same patient revealed clearly in axial CT scan.

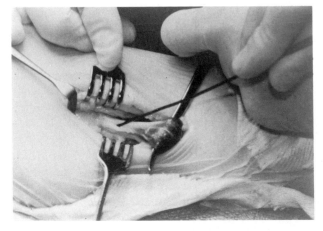

Fig. 21-10. Operative photograph of flexor hallucis longus in trigger toe. This is treated by surgical release of tunnel at posterior ankle through which flexor hallucis longus slides. Probe is inserted in rent of tendon.

tended and the dancer rises to the demi-pointe position and also when she flexes the toe during descent to the floor. It also triggers when the dancer rises to the full pointe position. It may even prevent plantar flexion of the hallux. Triggering of the tendon is palpable in the posterior medial compartment of the ankle. Treatment is sought because of ankle pain and weakness of the toe during dancing *sur les pointes.*

Surgical treatment requires a 4 cm posteromedial incision at the ankle. The flexor hallucis longus is identified and delivered through the wound. The tendon sheath is incised to the sustenaculum tali to permit unimpeded gliding of the tendon. The fusiform swelling may be skived down and the rent sutured with 5-0 running braided Dacron suture. A light compressive dressing is applied postoperatively and the dancer permitted to exercise using the operative foot as the working leg. Return to a full schedule may take several months of rehabilitation (Cobb and Sammarco, 1984).

TENDINITIS AND MYOSITIS

Clawing of the toes is often caused by muscle spasm of the leg and foot muscles following long periods of not dancing. Treatment includes antiinflammatory medication, massage, and a flexibility program daily. The dancer should perform a flexibility program whether he is employed or not. Tendinitis may occur in any of the tendons, the most common, however, being the Achilles tendon. "Dancer's tendinitis," or tendinitis of the flexor hallucis longus, may masquerade as Achilles tendinitis, but tenderness is present anterior to the Achilles tendon just above the calcaneus in the posterior medial compartment of the ankle (Hamilton, 1977). Tendinitis of the peroneus brevis and longus often gives symptoms of pain at the lateral malleolus of the ankle.

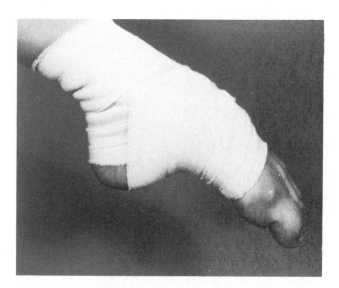

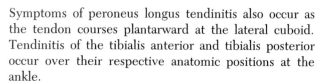

Fig. 21-11. Acute tendinitis of peroneus brevis is treated with elastic adhesive dressing until acute symptoms subside. Rehearsals and performances preclude use of such strapping because it inhibits ankle motion.

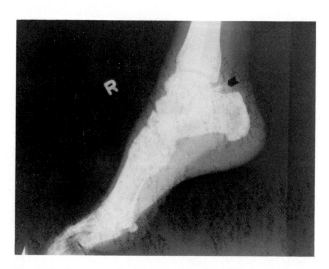

Fig. 21-12. Radiograph of dancer with os trigonum syndrome. This occurs when os trigonum (arrow) is compressed between posterior tibia and calcaneus. Bone actually increases in size because of periosteal reaction from repeated trauma.

Symptoms of peroneus longus tendinitis also occur as the tendon courses plantarward at the lateral cuboid. Tendinitis of the tibialis anterior and tibialis posterior occur over their respective anatomic positions at the ankle.

The common cause of tendinitis is overzealous or unsupervised training. Physical therapy modalities successful in treating such conditions include taping the ankle during the acute phase and the use of the foot exerciser board (Fig. 21-11), as well as instruction in a foot and ankle flexibility program (Hamilton, 1982a), and antiinflammatory medication. Chronic tendinitis may be disabling and may be associated with psychologic problems in the dancer.

Tendinitis of the flexors and extensors of the small toes is uncommon in dancers.

OS TRIGONUM SYNDROME

Posterior impingement of the os trigonum is common in dancers although rare in the general population (Hamilton, 1982; Howse, 1982; Quirk, 1982, 1983). This is because the accessory bone, present in 15% of the general population, is compressed intermittently for periods up to 6 hours a day by the dancer standing in the demi-pointe position. Often fragmentation can occur with an increase in the size of the bone as it heals (Fig. 21-12). Symptoms include pain at the posterior ankle and subtalar joint posteriorly while the dancer is standing in the demi-pointe position, on the ball of the foot.

Treatment includes a flexibility program, with atten-

tion to stretching, and antiinflammatory medication. If symptoms become disabling, surgical excision of the bony mass is indicated. However, recovery of a full range of motion may take as long as 6 months, and the dancer must be so advised.

ANTERIOR ANKLE IMPINGEMENT

Anterior ankle impingement results from osteophytes occurring on the anterior tibia and talar neck (Kleiger, 1982). If symptoms warrant, the problem is corrected by surgical excision through a small anterolateral incision.

FRACTURES

The most common fracture of the foot occurs at the fifth metatarsal neck (Sammarco and Miller, 1982). Because grossly displaced fractures may require open reduction, the period of time necessary for healing varies from 6 weeks to as long as 6 months. Open reduction is often recommended so that anatomic reduction may be achieved, thus enabling the foot to fit into a ballet pointe shoe.

Fracture of fifth metatarsal

Fracture of the fifth metatarsal styloid is uncommon in professional dancers. This avulsion fracture occurs in recreational or casual dancers and is treated by a short leg weight-bearing cast for a period of 4 weeks followed by rehabilitation. In selected cases, a compression dressing and non-weight-bearing crutch ambulation may be an alternative treatment if the dancer is not performing. Open reduction is not recommended (Jones, 1902).

Sesamoid fracture

Sesamoid fractures are of two types. One is the acute transverse fracture, which occurs following landing from a *jeté*, or jump. Symptoms include exquisite tenderness beneath the hallux and an inability to bear weight on the forefoot. A lateral radiograph of the foot confirms the diagnosis.

Treatment includes a compression dressing about the forefoot for a period of 3 weeks until symptoms subside. Following this a felt pad, ½-inch thick with relief around the area of the fractured sesamoid, is taped to the foot. During this period of convalescence, the dancer is permitted to perform a flexibility program using the injured foot as the non-weight-bearing leg.

The second, and more subtle, injury is compression fracture of the sesamoid. Symptoms may be present for periods of 18 months before diagnosis. Radiographic sesamoid views are necessary to confirm the diagnosis. Bone scan often shows a positive diagnosis at an earlier date.

Treatment includes the use of a metatarsal pad relieved under the area of the tender sesamoid for a period of 3 months. Excision of the sesamoids in the dancer is not recommended.

Dislocation

Dislocations of the toes are uncommon in the dancer and occur as a result of striking a heavy object, such as scenery. Closed reduction and appropriate splinting for 3 weeks is the recommended treatment.

SKIN AND NAILS

Dancers have heavy calluses on their feet, particularly on their toes. Modern dancers use no shoes and have thick calluses on the soles of the feet. Corns and calluses are also caused by the prolonged periods spent in a ballet pointe shoe and in the demi-pointe position in a ballet shoe. Infected soft corns are treated with cleansing and padding between the toes. Appropriate cultures should be taken before antibiotic treatment is administered. Harsh antiseptics are to be avoided. Corns are best treated with doughnut-shaped pads. During rehearsal the dancer often changes these to that part of the foot which is uncomfortable (Fig. 21-13).

Surgery to shorten or stiffen the toes to relieve calluses and allow the foot to better fit into a ballet shoe is not recommended. Convalescence may require a period of 1 year, and there is no guarantee that the dancer will return to her preoperative proficiency level.

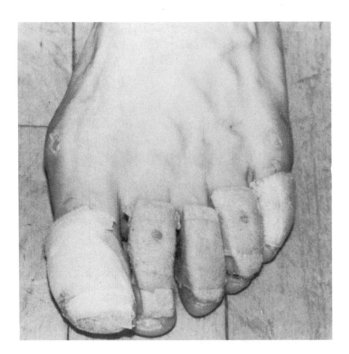

Fig. 21-13. Taping dancer's foot during rehearsal prevents soft corns from developing and alleviates pain. Tape and padding are changed from place to place during day as necessary.

Fissuring

Fissuring of the skin occurs in bare-footed modern dancers and is caused by tension at the flexion creases at the toes and metatarsal pad. The dancer applies rosin to the feet for better traction, which increases the chances of such an injury. This is best treated with gentle cleansing and a dry dressing. Prophylactic antibiotic ointment has been recommended for use while the fissure heals. This problem is minor and does not require surgery.

Common conditions of the toenails in dancers include subungual hematoma, which is usually chronic in nature and does not require draining.

Onycholysis

Onycholysis is common in ballet pointe dancers. Because of weight bearing on the tip of the toe, the nail delaminates. No treatment is indicated, since this condition is asymptomatic.

Paronychia

Paronychia is treated surgically with incision and drainage of the abscess.

Ingrown toenail

Ingrown toenail, usually on the hallux, is treated surgically by excision of the offending 20% of the nail. The germinal area of the nail should not be violated. The entire nail should not be removed, since up to one year may be required for the nail to regrow. During this time the toe is tender and difficult to fit into a shoe.

Onychomycosis

Onychomycosis is best treated with oral griseofulvin and controlled locally by clotrimazole (Lotrimin) hydrophilic oil. Excision of the toenails is not recommended, since the condition usually does not affect dancing.

REFERENCES
The foot in running

Baxter, D.E., and Thigpen, M.: Heel pain: operative results, Foot Ankle 5:16, 1984.

Cavanagh, P.R., Clarke, T., Williams, K., and Kalenak, A.: An evaluation of the effect of orthotics on force distribution and rearfoot movement during running. Presented at the American Orthopaedic Society For Sports Medicine Meeting, Lake Placid, N.Y., June 1978.

D'Ambrosia, R.D., Zelis, R.F., and Chuinard, R.G., et al: Interstitial pressure measurements in the anterior and posterior compartments in athletes with shin splints, Am. J. Sports Med., 5:127-131, 1977.

Frankel, V.H.: Fatigue fractures: biomechanical consideration, J. Bone Joint Surg. 54A: 1345, 1972.

Green, W.T.: Discrepancy in leg length of lower extremities. American Academy of Orthopedic Surgery, Instructional Course Lecture, Ann Arbor, Mich., 1951, J.W. Edwards Co.

James, S.L., Bates, B.T., and Osternig, L.R.: Injuries to runners, Am. J. Sports Med., 6:40-50, 1978.

Mann, R.A., Baxter, D.E., and Lutter, L.L.: Running symposium, Foot Ankle 1(4): 1981.

Reneman, R.S.: The anterior and the lateral compartment syndrome of the leg, The Hague, 1968, Mouton Publishers.

Slocum, D.B.: The shin splint syndrome: medical aspects and differential diagnosis, Am. J. Surg. 114:875-881, 1967.

Stipe, P.: The effects of orthotics on rearfoot movement in running, Nike Res. Newsl. 2, No. 3, 1983.

Dance injuries to the foot

Ambre, T.: Degenerative changes in the first metatarsophalangeal joint of ballet dancers, Acta Orthop. Scand. 49:317-319. 1978.

Calabrese, L., and Kirkendall, D.G.: Nutritional and medical consideration in dancers, Clin. Sports Med. 2(3):539, 1983.

Cobb, S., and Sammarco, G.J.: Flexibility program for the dancer. Clinic for the Performing Arts. Presented at the sixth Annual Dance Medicine Symposium, Cincinnati, Ohio, 1984.

Collis, W.J.M., and Jayson, M.I.V.: Measurement of pedal pressures. Am. Rheum. Dis. 31:217. 1972.

Devas, M.B.: Stress fractures, Edinburgh, 1975, Churchill Livingstone.

Hamilton, W.G.: Sprained ankles in ballet dancers. Foot Ankle 3:99, 1982a.

Hamilton, W.G.: Stenosing tenosynovitis of the flexor hallucis longus tendon and posterior impingement upon the os trigonum in ballet dancers, Foot Ankle 3:74, 1982b.

Hamilton, W.G.: Tendinitis about the ankle joint in classical ballet dancers, J. Sports Med. 5:84. 1977.

Howse, A.J.G.: Disorders of the great toe in dancers. Clin. Sports Med. 2(3):499-505, 1983.

Howse, A.J.G.: Posterior block of the ankle joint in dancers, Foot Ankle 3:8, 1982.

Howse, A.J.G.: Orthopaedists aid ballet, Clin. Orthop. Rel. Res. 89:52-63, 1972.

Jones, R.: Fractures of the fifth metatarsal bone, Liverpool Med. Surg. J. 42:103-107, 1902.

Kleiger, B.: Anterior tibiotalar impingement syndromes in dancers, Foot Ankle 3:69, 1982.

Kirkendall, D.T., and Calabrese L.: Physiological aspects of dance, Clin. Sports Med. 2:525-37, 1983.

Manter, J.T.: Distribution of compression forces in the joints of the human foot, Anat. Rec. 96:313, 1946.

McLain, D.: Personal communication, 1983.

Nikolic, V., and Zimmerman, B: Functional changes of tarsal bones of ballet dancers, Rad. Med. Fak. Zagrebu. 16:131, 1968.

Pelipenko, V.I.: Specific characteristics of the development of the foot skeleton in pupils of a choreographic school, Arkh. Anat. Gistol. Embriol. 64:46-50, June 1973.

Quirk, R.: Ballet injuries: the Australian experience, Clin. Sports Med. 2:507-14, 1983.

Quirk, R.: Talar compression syndrome in dancers, Foot Ankle. 3:65, 1982.

Ronconi, P.: Personal communication, 1983.

Sammarco, G.J.: The foot and ankle in classical ballet and modern dance. In Jahss, M., ed.: Disorders of the foot, Philadelphia, 1982, W.B. Saunders Co., pp. 1626-59.

Sammarco, G.J.: Diagnosis and treatment in dancers, Clin. Orthop. 187:165, 1984.

Sammarco, G.J., and Miller, E.H.: Partial rupture of the flexor hallucis longus in classical ballet dancers, J. Bone Joint Surg. 61A:140, 1979.

Sammarco, G.J., and Miller, E.H.: Forefoot conditions in dancers. Part 1, Foot Ankle 3:85, 1982.

Sammarco, G.J., and Miller, E.H.: Forefoot conditions in dancers. Part 2, Foot Ankle 3:93. 1982.

Seals, J.: A study of dance surfaces, Clin. Sports Med. 2:557, 1983.

Stojanovie, S., Marenie, S., and Ukropina, D.: Diseases in ballet dancers, Srp. Arh. Celok. Lek. 91:903, 1963.

Tomasen, E.: Diseases and injuries of ballet dancers, Copenhagen, 1982, Universitetsforlaget I Arhus.

Volkov, M.V.: Principles of diagnosis, treatment and prevention of occupational injuries in ballet dancers, Vestn. Khir. 114:87-90, 1975.

Wilcox, J.R., Moniot, A.L., et al.: Bone scanning in the evaluation of exercise related stress injuries, Radiology 123:699-703. 1977.

22

Congenital foot deformities

WALTER W. HUURMAN

Congenital deformities, those present at or before birth, may result from inherited (genetic) or extrinsic (environmental) influences. To understand the pathophysiology of congenital foot disorders, one must have a working knowledge of prenatal growth and foot development. Only with this background can the treatment of these disorders be competently approached.

EMBRYOLOGY

The skeletal elements of the foot are blastemic by the fifth gestational week; all are present and begin to chondrify between 5 and 6½ weeks. The cartilage anlage of each individual bone begins to ossify at a particular time in development; the pattern of ossification is quite regular. The metatarsals and distal phalanges demonstrate a periosteal collar of bone at 9 weeks, the calcaneus demonstrates a lateral perichondral area of ossification at 13 weeks, and the talus shows an enchondral center after 8 months. The tarsonavicular does not ossify until the third to fourth postnatal year.

Joints are formed with the appearance of homogeneous interzones—intermediate cell masses—beginning at the sixth gestational week. The interzones then become fissured (9½ weeks), followed by synovial tissue invasion at 11 weeks.

Differentiation of tendons begins as early as the sixth week, and by the eighth week most ligaments of the foot and ankle are differentiated as cellular condensations (Blechschmidt, 1961).

Hence we see that differentiation of the blastemas into elements arranged like those of the adult occurs between 5 and 7 weeks after conception. Individual elements of the limb appear generally in a proximal-distal sequence, and the specific time of differentiation has been determined with reasonable accuracy (Gardner et al., 1959). Knowing the time of blastemic insult in the case of a specific skeletal abnormality may guide

one to search for less obvious congenital malformations in organs differentiating at precisely the same time (Fuller and Duthie, 1974).

GROWTH AND DEVELOPMENT

Maturation begins during the fetal period and continues postnatally through adolescence. Extrinsic and intrinsic influences that are separate from the genetic code can affect growth and development of the foot at any time during these years. Because of the unique properties of the growing foot, maturation may adversely affect the developing limb by furthering a pathologic condition.

Conversely, the same phenomenon, growth, can be turned to advantage by the knowledgeable clinician to lessen or eliminate functional disability secondary to an abnormal condition. In turn, the physician must not forget the potential for reappearance of the deformity or development of a compensating iatrogenic deformity after treatment caused by the continuing effect of growth and development.

GENETICS IN THE FOOT

Congenital anomalies of the foot may be seen as part of a genetic disorder following the Mendelian rules of inheritance. As such, the foot abnormality frequently appears in association with other obvious anomalies or, on occasion, may be the only phenotypic indication of a generalized syndrome. Heritable anomalies follow either the dominant or recessive mode of transmission and may result from the influence of an autosome or the sex chromosome (Cowell and Wein, 1980).

In 1976 Zimbler and Craig presented a large series of birth defect syndromes, identifying the disorder via the abnormalities seen in the foot. Excluded from this list were foot disorders unassociated with other defects. McKusick (1975) lists several isolated anomalies (rela-

FOOT DEFORMITIES ASSOCIATED WITH OTHER PRIMARY PROBLEMS

PLANOVALGUS

Achondrogenesis (type 1)
Chromosome 18 trisomy
Chromosome 13 trisomy
Dysplasia epiphysealis hemimelica
Larsen syndrome
Marfan syndrome
Mucopolysaccharidosis IV
Multiple exostoses
Popliteal pterygium syndrome
Ehlers-Danlos syndrome
Bird-headed dwarfism
Chromosome 5P syndrome
Diaphyseal dysplasia

METATARSUS ADDUCTUS

Acrocephalosyndactyly
Smith-Lemli-Opitz syndrome
Carpenter syndrome
Cerebrohepatorenal syndrome
Clasped thumbs

EQUINOVARUS

Arthrogryposis multiplex congenita
Bird-headed dwarfism
Chromosome 18Q syndrome
Chromosome 13 trisomy
Craniocarpotarsal dystrophy
Diastrophic dwarfism
Ehler-Danlos syndrome
Larsen syndrome
Oculoauriculovertebral dysplasia
Radioulnar synostosis
Situs inversus viscerum
Stippled epiphyses

VARUS

Carpenter syndrome (acrocephalopolysyndactyly, type II)
Hypochondroplasia
Laryngeal web or atresia

CALCANEUS

Chromosome 18 trisomy
Chromosome 13 trisomy

CAVUS

Mucopolysaccharidosis
Homocystinuria
Carpal tarsal osteolysis and chronic progressive
    glomerulopathy
Phytamic acid storage disease
Urticaria, deafness and amyloidosis

POLYDACTYLY

Chondroectodermal dysplasia
Chromosome 13 trisomy
Cleft lip without cleft palate
Cleft tongue
Cyclopia
Focal dermal hypoplasia
Orofaciodigital syndrome II
Polysyndactyly
Retinal dysplasia
Stippled epiphyses

SYNDACTYLY

Acrocephalosyndactyly
Aglossia-adactyly
Ankyloblepharon
Chromosome 18P syndrome
Oligophrenia
Familial static ophthalmoplegia
Focal dermal hypoplasia
Holoprosencephalus
Hypertelorism
Laryngeal web or atresia
Lissencephaly
Meckel syndrome
Monosomy G syndrome, type II
Oculomandibulofacial syndrome
Orocraniodigital syndrome
Orofaciodigital syndrome, I and II
Popliteal web syndrome
Retinal dysplasia
Silver syndrome
Smith-Lemli-Opitz syndrome
Stippled epiphyses

From Zimbler, S., and Craig, C.: Orthop. Clin. North Am. **7:**331, 1976.

tive length of the first and second metatarsals, rotational deformity of the fifth toe, number of phalanges contained in the fifth toe) that demonstrate a dominant mode of inheritance.

Review of Zimbler and Craig's description (1976) has enabled classification of most disorders according to the mode of inheritance (see box at left). Some (e.g., Silver syndrome) have yet to show a clear genetic code but quite possibly will be classified in the future (Blechschmidt, 1961). For problems more specifically dealt with in the text, genetics are discussed under the individual disorder.

TALIPES DEFORMITIES

Talipes, derived from the Latin words *talus* ("ankle bone") and *pes* ("foot"), is a term used to describe any congenital foot anomaly. Congenital hindfoot deformities are correctly designated *talipes*, followed by a descriptive term for the morbid anatomy. A plantar-flexed hindfoot therefore is talipes equinus; if dorsiflexed, talipes calcaneus; if inverted, talipes varus; and if everted, talipes valgus.

Currently the simple contraction *talipes* is commonly used in reference to the classic clubfoot deformity. Clinically the true clubfoot presents with a triad of (1) midfoot and forefoot adductus, (2) hindfoot varus, and (3) heel equinus. Anatomically, then, *talipes equinovarus* is the appropriate descriptive term and use of simple *talipes* should probably be avoided.

Clubfoot (talipes equinovarus)

A relatively common malformation, and certainly the continuing subject of heated discussion among experts, clubfoot remains an unsolved and enigmatic congenital foot deformity. Orthopaedic literature continues to abound with articles espousing methods of treatment nearly as numerous as the number of their authors. Despite this vast experience, the etiology remains obscure, and a single best form of treatment is elusive.*

Incidence. The commonly accepted incidence in the general population is approximately 1 per 1000 births. Wynne-Davies (1964) notes the incidence as 1.24 per 1000; when broken down by sex, the male incidence is 1.62 per 1000 and the female 0.8 per 1000. This represents a distinct 2.17 to 1 predominance of male over female. There are strong hereditary factors, and if one child in a family has the deformity, the incidence among siblings rises to 2.9 per 100 or 1 in every 35 births. If the index patient is female, the incidence

---

*As Lloyd-Roberts (1964) knowingly stated: "This is an undeniably disheartening state of affairs which is in no way redeemed by the knowledge that little or no improvement has occurred since Brockman's review was published 35 years ago."

among male siblings rises to 1 in 16; however, if the index patient is male, there appears to be no significant increase in the 1 per 35 sibling incidence. Although there may be a genetic factor involved, the specific Mendelian characteristics with regard to sex linkage, dominance or recessiveness, etc., have not been worked out. It can, however, be stated with some certainty that penetrance does appear to be variable. As Cowell has pointed out, clubfeet associated with other clearly Mendelian-based syndromes (e.g., diastrophic dwarfism, Freeman-Sheldon syndrome) should not be included in genetic studies of talipes equinovarus. Currently, a multifactorial mode of inheritance seems most plausible. Nongenetic, extrinsic factors that may result in clubfoot deformity include arthrogryposis multiplex congenita, amniotic band (Streeter's) syndrome, and certain drugs taken during pregnancy (aminopterin).

Pathologic anatomy. Despite the fact that clubfoot has been recognized as a handicapping deformity since ancient times, relatively few anatomic studies have been published. Careful review of most writings reveals that dissections were usually performed on a fetus or infant who also had other significant congenital malformations.

The anatomic findings in the deformed foot of a stillborn anencephalic, myelodysplastic, or fetus with other congenital malformations potentially affecting foot development should not be used as the anatomic basis for discussion of idiopathic clubfoot. Before the excellent studies of Irani and Sherman (1963), no satisfactory series of dissections on the isolated idiopathic deformity had been reported. Although Settle (1963) confirmed the findings of Irani and Sherman later the same year, 14 of his 16 specimens had other significant deformities. Waisbrod (1973) contributed the study of eight additional idiopathic clubfeet occurring without any other significant congenital anomaly. Ippolito and Ponsetti (1980) reported their findings in five fetal clubfeet aborted between 15 and 20 weeks' gestation. At the present time these studies provide the basis for our knowledge of the pathologic anatomy.

The reason for this rather sparse information seems clear: isolated clubfoot deformity is not a cause of fetal or infant mortality, and therefore specimens are not readily available for study. Nonetheless, the idiopathic clubfeet that have been studied have had rather constant findings. A primary deformity seems to be present in the head and neck of the talus: the neck is foreshortened to absent and medially deviated, and the articular surface of the head is inclined plantarward. Other bony and soft tissue anomalies that may be present seem to be adaptive to this primary talar deformity (Fig. 22-1).

The normal talar neck has an angle of incidence with its body of 150° to 155° (Paturet, 1951; Gardner, 1956).

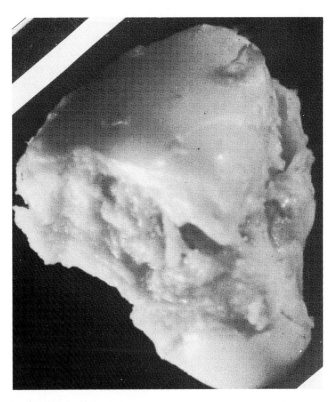

Fig. 22-1. Dorsomedial view of left talus obtained from idiopathic clubfoot in a 5-year-old child. Note shortening of neck and medial and plantar deviation of navicular articular surface.

Irani and Sherman (1963) found in their dissected specimens an angle varying between 115° and 135°. Other than adaptive changes resulting from this primary deformity, the muscles, tendons, and neurovascular and other osseous structures of the foot and leg seemed to be basically normal.

Because of the plantarward declination of the talar neck, the talar body lies more anterior in the ankle mortise than in the normal foot. The hindfoot therefore declines into equinus, and developmental contracture of both ankle and subtalar joint capsules develop accompanied by atrophy and contracture of the triceps surae muscle group (Wiley, 1959). Adaptive changes are present in the osseous structure of the talus itself. The articulations of the subtalar joint are noticeably deformed, the medial- and plantar-deviated head of the talus articulating with the anteromedial portion of the calcaneus. The posterior calcaneus is rotated laterally and held in close proximity to the fibular malleolus by a thick, strong, deformity-inducing fibulocalcaneal ligament. Settle (1963) noted that the subtalar joints were slanted medially with a single articular facet. This combination of rotation and varus of the calcaneus widens the sinus tarsi and brings the Achilles tendon insertion medial to the calcaneal midline axis. This medial dis-

placement of the Achilles tendon causes its line of pull to promote further hindfoot varus (Fried, 1959) (Fig. 22-2).

The midfoot likewise adapts to changes in the head and neck of the talus. The navicular is smaller than normal and medially "dislocated" (Brockman, 1930; Ponsetti and Smoley, 1963). This medial dislocation, however, is only apparent insofar as the navicular articulates rather properly with the medially deviated talar head, covering its articular surface (Settle, 1963; Waisbrod, 1973). It is true that the navicular is deviated medially relative to the longitudinal axis of the talar body, but this is because the anterior talus is inclined medially and plantarward. On occasion, depending on the angle of incidence of the talar neck, the navicular may be so far swung around that its medial margin articulates with the medial malleolus. The remainder of the midfoot seems to follow the talar neck and the rotated calcaneus: the cuboid is actually displaced beneath the third cuneiform and rotated toward the medial side of its normal articulation with the calcaneus. The forefoot follows the varus and adducted contour of the midfoot, completing the clinical equinovarus appearance.

If the talar deformity is severe, all adaptive changes

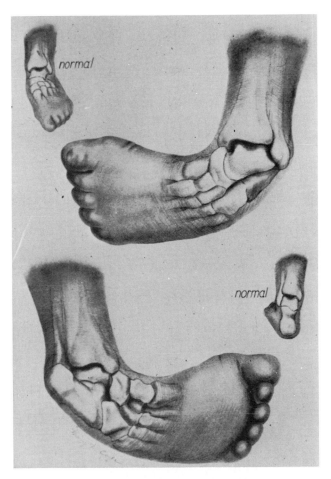

Fig. 22-2. Pathologic anatomy of clubfoot. Medially and plantar-deviated talar neck is the primary deformity; medial deviation of the navicular and hindfoot varus and equinus are adaptive. (From Settle, G.W.: J. Bone Joint Surg. **45A:**1341, 1963.)

are accentuated. The medial border of the calcaneus may be concave, the lateral column of the foot elongated, and the medial column foreshortened. With the foot swung around into equinovarus, during development the ligamentous and capsular structures on the posterior and medial side of the foot eventually become foreshortened, thickened, and quite rigid. This includes capsules of the ankle, subtalar, talonavicular, and naviculocuneiform joints. Furthermore, the deltoid and talocalcaneal interosseous ligaments become contracted and thickened. The tendinous structures (tibialis posterior, tibialis anterior, Achilles tendon), if allowed to come into opposition with deformed osseous structures, may adhere to them. This apparent abnormality of tendon insertion is adaptive and secondary to the distorted hindfoot and midfoot. On dissection, the normal insertion of these tendinous structures is always present.

When treating the idiopathic clubfoot, the physician

must constantly keep in mind the pathologic anatomy and dynamics of the growing foot. Successful treatment relies primarily on the ability of growing osseous structures to adapt and alter their shape in response to the influence of extrinsic force.

Etiology. Because the literature contains no report of an idiopathic clubfoot dissection in a fetus under 7 weeks' gestation, it has not been established whether the deformity is blastemic in origin or arises during the embryonic period. However, the presence of significantly fewer vessels in the talar neck of a fetal clubfoot, with marked disorganization of these vessels, seems to indicate that the deformity originates during the blastemic period (Waisbrod, 1973).

Bohm (1929) described four stages of normal fetal foot positioning, proceeding from a stance of equinovarus immediately after the embryonic period and progressing through gradual supination, ankle dorsiflexion, and finally, by the fourth month, pronation. A partial arrest of development during the blastemic or early embryonic stage may well be the insult that causes the deformity recognized at birth.

Radiographic evaluation. Because the osseous structures of the infant foot are small, it is nearly impossible to ascertain their true anatomic relationship by simple clinical examination. Indeed, the rather abundant heel fat pad can easily hide a great deal of hindfoot equinus. Likewise, the absence of soft tissue definition can make even a moderate amount of hindfoot varus clinically difficult to appreciate. For this reason, radiographic evaluation performed initially and intermittently during the course of treatment is necessary to adequately assess correction.

Standard radiographic views should be obtained in the anteroposterior (AP) and lateral projections. The AP view is obtained with the plantar surface flat on the film cassette in a pseudostanding position. The ankle should be slightly plantar flexed and the x-ray tube caudally directed 30°. This positioning will permit visualization of the hindfoot and allow accurate measurement of the talocalcaneal (Kite's) angle (Kite, 1930) (Fig. 22-3). The lateral view should likewise be obtained in a pseudostanding position with the ankle as neutral as possible. If the film cassette is aligned parallel with the lateral border of the foot, an oblique view of the hindfoot will result and the talus will spuriously appear to be flat topped with the fibula displaced posteriorly (Swann et al., 1969). An accurate lateral view is obtained when the hindfoot is parallel with the cassette, and in the true projection the talus is recognized as having a normal dorsally convex but anteriorly displaced articular surface.

In the AP view the longitudinal axis of the normal talus aligns well with a similar axis of the first metatar-

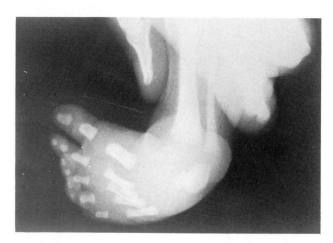

Fig. 22-3. AP view of a clubfoot in a neonate. Note reduction in Kite's angle; talus is nearly parallel with calcaneus. Neither of hindfoot structures aligns with forefoot.

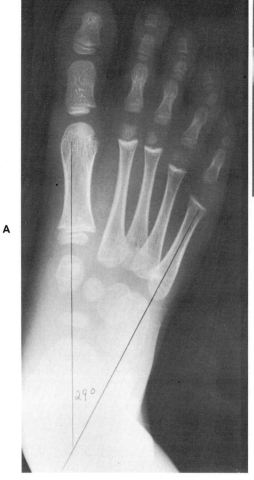

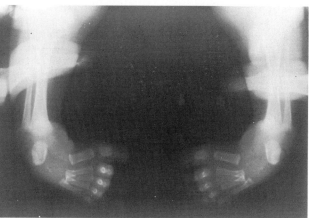

Fig. 22-4. A, Normal talocalcaneal (Kite's) angle. **B,** Bilateral clubfeet in newborn; note that neither midfoot nor forefoot align with longitudinal axes of talus and calcaneus.

sal, and the longitudinal axis of the calcaneus aligns with the fifth metatarsal. These two axes converge posteriorly, forming Kite's angle (normally 20° to 40°). With hindfoot varus the calcaneus is rotated beneath the talus, plantar flexed and, if the deformity is severe, medially bowed. This causes a decrease of Kite's angle, occasionally to 0° (Fig. 22-4). With correction of hindfoot varus, the abnormal talocalcaneal relationship reverses and the anterior calcaneus rotates laterally and the posterior calcaneal tuberosity medially, and the entire structure everts. Without a normal talo-calcaneal angle in the AP projection, the hindfoot varus has not been fully corrected.

In the lateral view the talocalcaneal angle is derived from a line drawn through the midlongitudinal axis of the ossific nucleus and a second converging line drawn along the plantar surface of the calcaneus. This angle is not static and in the normal foot will decrease with plantar flexion and increase with dorsiflexion. In the normal standing lateral projection the talocalcaneal angle measures between 35° and 50° (Heywood, 1964). A distinct overlap of the anterosuperior margin of the calcaneus on the anteroinferior margin of the talus is normally present. With clubfoot deformity and hindfoot varus, the normal lateral talocalcaneal angle is reduced, and the two structures are parallel. Furthermore, relatively little change in the angle occurs with dorsiflexion and plantar flexion. (Fig. 22-5).

Careful evaluation of the calcaneotibial relationship will demonstrate hindfoot equinus uncorrected with

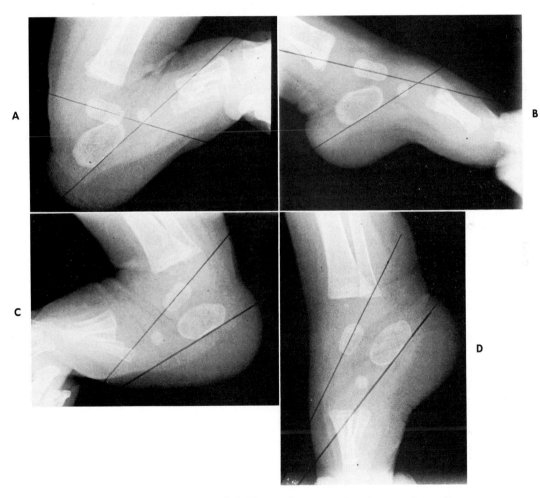

Fig. 22-5. Clubfoot in a 3-month-old child. **A** and **B,** Stress dorsiflexion–plantar flexion views of the normal foot. On stress dorsiflexion, lateral talocalcaneal angle measures 45°; on stress plantar flexion, 58°. Note overlap of the anteroinferior talus and anterosuperior calcaneus on dorsiflexion. **C** and **D,** Stress dorsiflexion–plantar flexion lateral views of opposite clubfoot. Despite stress, talocalcaneal angle is reduced and remains unchanged at 17°. On dorsiflexion, calcaneus remains in equinus and talus does not overlap anterior process of os calcis.

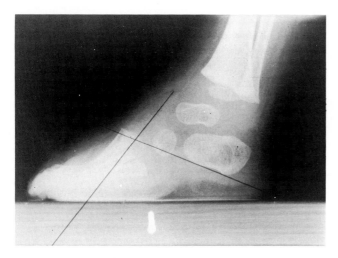

Fig. 22-6. Cavus deformity in clubfoot with foreshortened plantar soft tissues.

forced dorsiflexion. The ossific nucleus of the talus is displaced anteriorly because of the equinus deformity and, when severe, the posterior calcaneus nearly approximates the posterior malleolus.

Forefoot deformity is seen in both AP and lateral projections. On the AP view, both adduction and inversion with shortening of the medial column and lengthening of the lateral column are present. Viewed laterally, possible foreshortening of the plantar soft tissue structures may cause forefoot equinus, resulting in a cavus deformity (Fig. 22-6).

Until all the radiographic alterations have returned to normal, one cannot be satisfied that the clubfoot deformity has been corrected. Active treatment should continue until talocalcaneal parallelism is reversed in both AP and lateral views and until the stress plantarflexion–dorsiflexion radiographs demonstrate unlocking of the subtalar articulation with adequate dorsiflexion of the hindfoot. The standing lateral radiograph should present a normal plantigrade appearance with no hindfoot equinus, cavus deformity, or break of the midfoot.

Treatment. As each color has many shades and hues, so are there many degrees of clubfoot deformity. Treatment necessary to bring the foot to a plantigrade, longitudinally aligned posture depends on the degree of deformity present. Each foot must be carefully examined, both clinically and radiographically, and the treatment program must be designed to meet the demands of the deformity present.

Waisbrod (1973), in studying his eight specimens, found that the response to manual manipulation was dependent on the degree of deformity in the talar neck. In his series he was able to passively correct three feet and found, on dissection, the talar neck in each of these to have an angle in excess of 150° with the body. It is

quite likely that the apparent clubfoot that responds rapidly and readily to manipulation and casting has, in fact, little deformity in the talar neck; the initial clinical presentation may be more a postural problem. This is not to ignore these feet or to downgrade the importance of early active treatment, for the postural deformity, if persistent, can result in secondary structural change. A rather large number of clubfeet belong in the postural deformity category; and if they are treated early (from day of birth), secondary resistant changes do not have an opportunity to develop. The longer one waits before initiating treatment, the more significant and resistant are the secondary structural changes. Active treatment should begin as soon after birth as possible.

If plantar and medial inclination of the foreshortened distal talus exists to any degree, the osseous structures must be placed in an aligned position and held there during the formative years of growth and development for the foot to anatomically permit normal ambulation and normal footwear. To align the foot with the rest of extremity may require dividing secondarily shortened, thickened capsules and ligaments as well as lengthening secondarily abbreviated muscle-tendon units (Lowe and Hannon, 1973). One must always remember that the primary talar neck deformity with secondary structural change in other osseous components persists but may be altered over time by use of Wolff's law. Holding the foot in a corrected position during growth and development will create adaptive changes in the distal talus (Denham, 1967), distal calcaneus and subtalar joint, causing them to revert to near normal. However, the talus will continue to have a short neck with a somewhat flattened head, the navicular and talar body may continue to be smaller than normal, and, indeed, the entire foot and calf will probably never match the opposite member in size. If, after alignment of the foot is obtained by either serial casting or soft tissue release, the foot is not held in the corrected position for a significant period of growth and development, the neck of the talus will continue to deviate medially, the navicular and calcaneus will gradually realign with their abnormal articulations about the talar neck, and the hindfoot will drift back into varus and equinus, the forefoot into cavus and adduction.

It would therefore seem reasonable that, once alignment is obtained and reasonably stable, the foot should be held in the corrected position day and night for a moderate period of time and subsequently at night alone through at least the second period of accelerated growth and development (7 to 8 years of age). Anything less may lead to reappearance of the deformity.

Treatment at birth. The foot of a neonate with talipes equinovarus deformity is often no larger than the thumb of the treating physician. This small structure,

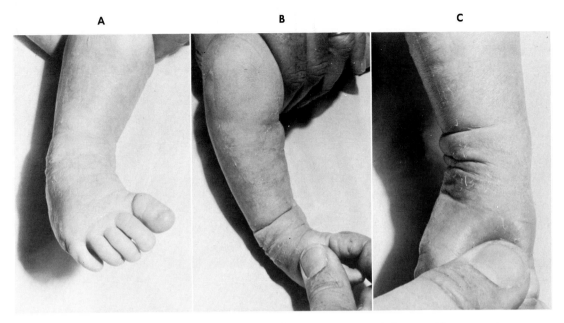

Fig. 22-7. Neonatal clubfoot deformity. **A,** Moderate equinovarus deformity. This responds to traction on medial metatarsal heads, **B,** by developing recess at lateral border of talar neck, **C,** as the navicular and forefoot are brought into alignment with tibia. It represents lateral subluxation of midfoot on medially deviated head of talus.

on careful examination, is frequently quite supple.

Longitudinal traction applied at the distal first through third metatarsals with the heel plantar flexed will result in gradual formation of a dimple over the superolateral aspect of the midfoot. This represents gradual lateral subluxation of the navicular on the medially deviated talar head as the medial column elongates with traction. The dimple or void develops at the lateral junction of the talar neck with the talar body (Fig. 22-7). Lateral subluxation of the midfoot produces normal forefoot alignment with the tibia and, if held in this position, will allow soft tissue structures of the medial column to elongate and stretch. With traction on the forefoot, the physician stretches the tightened deltoid and talocalcaneal interosseous ligaments and is able to push the posterior calcaneus into eversion and medial rotation with thumb and forefinger of the opposite hand. Forceful attempts at dorsiflexing the ankle against tightened posterior ligaments will result in a nutcracker effect (Keim and Ritchie, 1964; Dunn and Samuelson, 1974), with the contracted posterior structures acting as a hinge and the talar body within the mortise like a fulcrum. To prevent a longitudinal midfoot break with development of a rocker-bottom deformity, the physician should not attempt forceful ankle dorsiflexion.

After manipulation, the foot can be held in its realigned position by application of a corrective cast or,

as is my preference, adhesive strapping. The taping technique, a modification of the Jones method, is preferred because of the difficulty encountered in attempting to apply a corrective cast with appropriately placed pressure points on the extremely small foot of a neonate. Furthermore, taping of the newborn foot permits dynamic and passive stretching exercises during the entire time of treatment, thereby avoiding progressive joint stiffness and further muscle atrophy (Fig. 22-8).

Tape application

1. After manipulation and reduction of the clubfoot deformity and with traction applied to the distal first through third metatarsals by an assistant, apply tincture of benzoin to the foot, leg, and distal thigh in the areas to be covered by tape.

2. Place a piece of felt about 1¼ inches wide over the distal thigh with the knee flexed 90°, the free ends extending 1½ inches down the medial and lateral aspects of the leg.

3. Wrap a piece of felt of similar width about the forefoot, the free ends meeting on the lateral border of the foot.

4. At this point, or earlier, it is most helpful to follow Kite's suggestion (1930): give the baby a bottle in an attempt to promote muscle relaxation. A parent may play an active role in the treatment by assisting with this task.

5. Apply the first strip of tape, a long one, over the

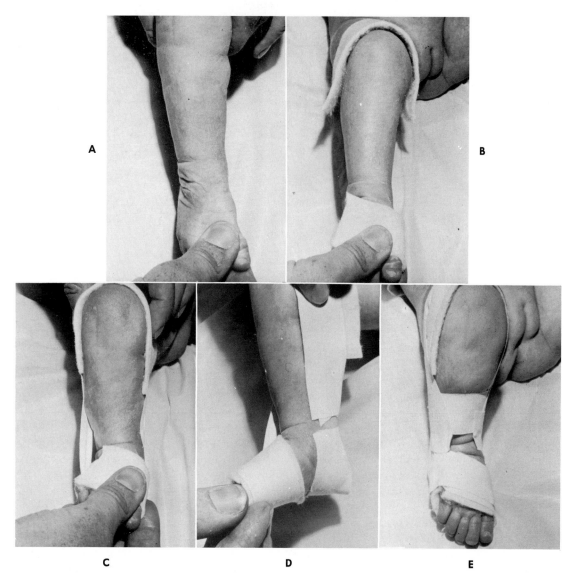

Fig. 22-8. Adhesive strapping of neonatal clubfoot. **A,** Gentle traction for several minutes applied to the medial metatarsal heads aligns foot with the leg. Note recess at lateral margin of talar neck. **B,** The areas to be covered by tape are painted with tincture of benzoin. A 1¼-inch wide strip of orthopaedic felt covers distal thigh, and a second strip surrounds forefoot. **C,** Long strip of 1-inch adhesive tape encircles foot and courses up lateral leg, over distal thigh (knee flexed) and three fourths of way down medial leg. **D,** A second long strip of tape beginning just at medial malleolus runs under calcaneus, up lateral leg, over distal thigh, and down medial leg (overlying initial tape). **E,** Two short anchoring strips encircle distal leg and foot. Foot is held in corrected position. Active and passive stretching exercises are still possible.

changes during the embryonic period. Congenital convex pes valgus is frequently seen in association with other neurologic abnormalities such as myelodysplasia, neurofibromatosis, or arthrogryposis. Because of the association of congenital convex pes valgus with congenital neurologic abnormalities, a careful search for such problems should be carried out when the deformity is encountered (Drennan and Sharrard, 1971; Lamy and Weissman, 1939; Lloyd-Roberts and Spence, 1958). As with clubfoot, very little specimen dissection has been reported.

Patterson et al. (1968) described the anatomic findings at dissection of a 6-week-old infant with congenital convex pes valgus who died of congenital heart disease; the spinal cord of the specimen was not examined. Findings in their study indicated that not until the shortened extensor tendons—including the tibialis anterior, extensor hallucis longus, extensor digitorum longus, and peronei—were serially lengthened was reduction of the talonavicular subluxation possible. Correction of hindfoot equinus was possible only after heel cord lengthening. Section of the talonavicular, subtalar, and posterior ankle capsules was carried out before tendon division but did not reduce the navicular on the talus. Moderate abnormalities in the talus and calcaneus were felt to be secondary changes and not the primary cause of the deformity. Therefore these authors contended that the primary abnormality was shortening of the muscle-tendon unit.

Drennan and Sharrard (1971) pointed out the marked association of congenital convex pex valgus with central nervous system abnormalities and presented their dissection of this deformity in a myelodysplastic child. They too felt the deformity was secondary to shortening or overpull of the dorsiflexors and everters of the foot unopposed by a weakened invertor—the tibialis posterior.

Physical findings. The problem as it presents clinically is a rigid foot with the heel in equinus and a convex sole with the head of the talus prominent on the plantar medial aspect of the tarsus. The forefoot is dorsiflexed and everted; passive correction of the deformity is not possible.

Radiographic findings. AP radiographs of the foot with the patient in a standing position demonstrate increased divergence of the talus and calcaneus. On lateral views the calcaneus is noted to be in equinus, the talus vertical, and, if ossified, the navicular dislocated onto the dorsal neck of the talus. If plantar flexion, non-weight-bearing stress projections are obtained; unlike the flexible flatfoot, the abnormal relationship between talus and the forefoot persists (Fig. 22-27). Jayakumar and Ramsey (1977) point out the essential difference between radiographic findings of the oblique or plantar-flexed talus seen in association with a flexible flatfoot and the vertical talus of congenital convex pes valgus.

Treatment. Conservative treatment, although usually unsuccessful, should be initiated as soon as possible after the patient is first seen (Becker-Anderson and Reimann, 1974). Efforts should be made at stretching the contracted anterior structures by maximally plantar flexing and inverting the forefoot, pressing the talar head dorsally, and attempting to push the navicular into a more normal relationship with the talus. Although it is not likely, serial casting after these maneuvers may result in correction of the deformity (Fig. 22-28); more likely, casting will assist in making surgical correction more successful by stretching contracted dorsal soft tissue structures (Coleman et al., 1970).

Operative treatment as advocated by Lamy and Weissman (1939) combines partial or total talectomy with lengthening of peroneal and extensor tendons as necessary (Fig. 22-29). Colton (1973) has recommended peritalar release with navicular excision as described by Stone (Fig. 22-30). Most authors agree that soft tissue procedures necessary to effect reduction include capsulotomies of the talonavicular, subtalar, and ankle joints and routine lengthening of the Achilles tendon (Coleman and Jarrett, 1966; Hark, 1950). Peroneal, anterior tibial, extensor digitorum communis, extensor hallucis longus, and posterior tibial tendons may be lengthened as necessary (Fitton and Nevelös, 1979). In addition, Eyre-Brook (1950) excised a dorsally based wedge from the navicular and placed it beneath the neck of the talus for support. He also shortened the spring ligament. Because he believed the calcaneus was not in equinus, he did not recommend posterior release. Jayakumar and Ramsey (1977) have recommended transplantation of the anterior tibial tendon into the talar neck after reduction has been obtained, thus providing dynamic support to the reduction.

I would generally recommend preoperative stretching of the anterior tendons by serial casting followed by soft tissue release of tightened talonavicular, subtalar, calcaneocuboid, and posterior ankle capsules through a Cincinnati incision (see p. 531). The Achilles tendon should be lengthened and reduction of the deformity attempted by plantar flexing the forefoot; if it is tight, dorsal tendons should be lengthened as necessary. Reduction, once obtained, should be maintained by Kirschner-wire fixation through the first metatarsal and navicular and into the neck and body of the talus. Reduction of the deformity is possible only by acutely plantar flexing the forefoot, bringing the navicular into normal relationship with the talar head. If reduction following complete capsular and extensor tendon division is still impossible, navicular excision should be carried out. A second Kirschner wire, transversely placed

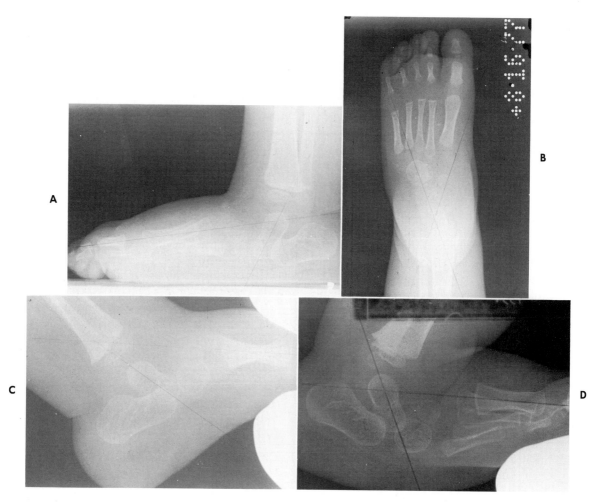

Fig. 22-27. Congenital convex pes valgus in 18-month-old child. **A** and **B,** Talar axis falls at an angle medial and plantar so that of first metatarsal. **C,** Plantar-flexion stress fails to align talus and first metatarsal. **D,** Dorsiflexion stress demonstrates persistence of hindfoot equinus. Unossified navicular is dislocated on talar neck.

Fig. 22-28. Foot of 9-year-old whose vertical talus was treated at age 2 with closed reduction and percutaneous pinning. Despite 3 months of casting, anatomic pathology recurred.

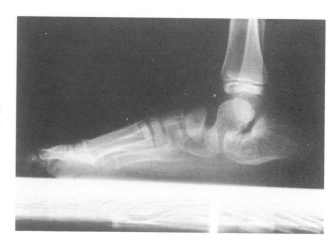

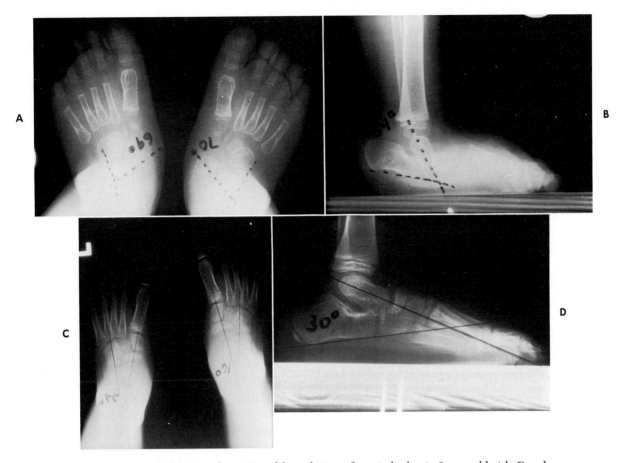

Fig. 22-29. **A** and **B,** Standing AP and lateral view of vertical talus in 3-year-old girl. **C** and **D,** Four years after open reduction accomplished by posterior capsulotomy with Achilles tendon lengthening, talonavicular capsulotomy, and peroneal and extensor tendon lengthenings followed by 4 months of casting in reduced position.

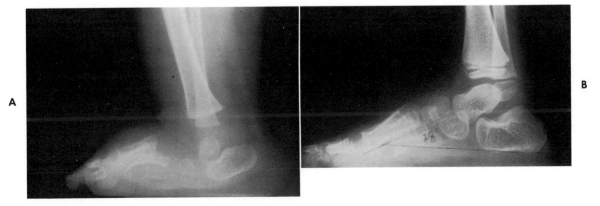

Fig. 22-30. **A,** Preoperative view of 14-month-old with vertical talus. **B,** Four years after open reduction, soft tissue release and naviculectomy. Foot is supple, plantigrade, and pain-free.

through the tuberosity of the calcaneus, is incorporated in plaster and serves as a lever to gradually bring the hindfoot out of equinus. Correction should be maintained in longleg casts for 4 to 6 months; the Kirschner wires may be removed at 3 months.

If the patient is adolescent or older, reduction of the deformity by soft tissue release and navicular excision is unlikely to be successful. By this time, foot strain and abnormal mechanics have altered other joints, and triple arthrodesis with resection of enough bone to create a plantigrade foot is the only solution. Heel cord lengthening and posterior capsulotomy may be required along with the triple arthrodesis to bring the calcaneus out of equinus.

ARTHROGRYPOSIS MULTIPLEX CONGENITA

Arthrogryposis multiplex congenita is an affliction in which multiple rigid joint deformities are evident at birth (Mead et al., 1958). Severity of both deformity and rigidity may vary from patient to patient and joint to joint. More commonly involved regions of the skeleton include the fingers, wrists, elbows, and shoulders as well as hips, knees, and feet. Not infrequently the spine is involved with a congenital-type scoliosis. Normally, the skin is smooth, muscle bulk is diminished, and fingers are rather long and slender (Sheldon, 1932). In even the mildest cases the presence of long tapered fingers may be a tip-off to the diagnosis of arthrogryposis.

Two types exist, a neuropathic form and a myopathic form (Adams et al., 1953). In many circles it is felt that the myopathic form is a type of muscular dystrophy and should be classified with the myodystrophias (Banker et al., 1957; Middleton, 1934). The etiology of arthrogryposis is generally unknown. Because many of the deformities appear to be teratologic in nature, the problem must arise sometime during the prenatal period (Drachman and Coulombre, 1962). Several causes have been proposed: intrauterine disturbances (decreased amniotic fluid, increased intrauterine pressure, mechanical compression of the fetus), inflammatory processes (rubella, viral infections, central nervous system infections) (Drachman and Banker, 1961), and environmental damage (teratogenic agents). Several attempts to work out the genetics have been made, but published series tend to be too small for any definite conclusions to be reached. At present most authorities believe heredity does not play a significant role.

Microscopic studies of arthrogrypotic specimens have shown major abnormalities in both muscle and nerve tissue. Involved muscles tend to be small, pale, and pink; some muscles are simply not present. In other areas muscle fibers may be extensively replaced by fat and connective tissue. Nervous tissue involvement in-

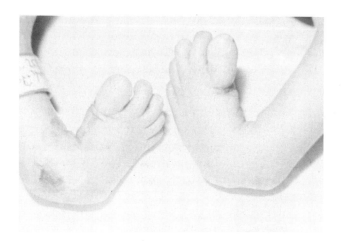

Fig. 22-31. Rigid, severe clubfeet of newborn arthrogrypotic.

cludes abnormalities of the spinal cord (i.e., a decrease or absence of anterior horn cells in the thoracic and lumbar regions). In addition, anterior roots have few fibers. Posterior roots and posterior horn cells appear to be normal (Adams et al., 1953; Drummond et al., 1974).

In arthrogryposis the foot tends to manifest the severest and most resistant of all deformities. Equinovarus is the commonest foot deformity, varying from quite mild to quite severe (Gibson and Urs, 1970). The most resistant and the most difficult to treat clubfeet are seen in arthrogryposis (Fig. 22-31). Although principles of management follow those for idiopathic clubfoot, conservative treatment often fails and the surgical approach must be extensive and radical (Drummond and Cruess, 1978).

As with the idiopathic clubfoot, treatment should begin as soon as possible after birth. Adhesive strapping in the nursery with frequent passive manipulation by nurses and parents should begin promptly. The deformity will generally not correct with longitudinal traction at the head of the first and second metatarsals, and its rigidity can be appreciated immediately.

After some foot growth and with the assumption that correction, although slow, is progressing, serial casting should begin as soon as the foot is large enough. Unlike other congenital problems, arthrogryposis does not tend to be progressive; but suspension of treatment commonly results in relapse to the initial deformity (Oh, 1976). Since the basic problem is abnormal or absent muscles and abnormal nerve structures, the goal of treatment in the arthrogrypotic clubfoot differs from that in the idiopathic condition. In arthrogryposis the goal of treatment is to change a stiff, rigid, deformed foot to one that is stiff, rigid, and plantigrade (Lloyd-Roberts and Lettin, 1970). To date, no form of treatment has been successful in obtaining or restoring any significant degree of increased mobility.

If after a period of conservative treatment it becomes obvious that full correction has not been obtained (and this is usually the case), operative intervention should proceed directly. Correction of the hindfoot is of prime importance; and if the equinus and varus can be neutralized, any residual forefoot deformity is unlikely to interfere with function. If the deformity is mild or moderate, posterior release with capsulotomy of the ankle and subtalar joints combined with segmental excision (not lengthening) of the Achilles tendon and posterior tibial tendon, accompanied by division of the posterior talofibular and deltoid ligaments, may result in a plantigrade foot. Under such circumstances the foot should be maintained in plaster in the corrected position 3 or 4 months postoperatively. It is then advisable to continue maintenance of correction in an appropriate day-night brace.

Often a moderate deformity will require a formal medial as well as posterior release. In addition to those structures released via the posterior approach, the capsules of the talonavicular, subtalar, and naviculocuneiform joints must be excised. Postoperative treatment is the same as for posterior release alone (Drummond et al., 1974). When the foot deformity is severe, soft tissue release can effect correction only by opening joints widely on the medial side of the foot. The situation has been likened to the opening of a suitcase; often there is insufficient skin and subcutaneous tissue for adequate wound closure. With such severe deformity, the "suitcase" simply closes again after removal of cast immobilization, and the deformity recurs. In this instance correction of the deformity can be obtained only by shortening skeletal elements (Menelaus, 1971).

In a young child, arthrodesis of the growing foot is inappropriate. Excision of the talus is an effective method of gaining alignment and allows skin closure without tension. In an immature, severely involved foot, talectomy results are best when the patient is between ages 1 and 5 years; the procedure can result in a plantigrade functional foot. The procedure is a demanding one and attention to detail is of prime importance.

Talectomy

A lateral curved incision following the line of the subtalar and talonavicular joints provides adequate exposure. Subcutaneous tissues should be protected and the incision carried directly to the capsules of these joints. The joints should be entered and the capsule excised; to prevent damage to the articular cartilage, an iris scissors should be used. As the dissection proceeds, the hindfoot can be manipulated into equinovarus, permitting division of the posterior and posteromedial liga-

ments. The entire talus must be excised; any remnants left behind can grow and produce a recurrent progressive deformity. After excision of the talus, a portion of the Achilles tendon should be excised. The calcaneus may then be placed in the ankle mortise; if it does not fit well, partial excision of the tip of the lateral malleolus and division of the anterior tibiofibular ligament may be necessary. The calcaneus is usually fairly stable within the ankle mortise, but a good practice is to hold the reduction with a Kirschner wire or small Steinmann pin placed up through the heel into the tibia. If excision of the talus is inadequate and the deformity is not fully corrected, the navicular may also be excised to provide further correction. One must avoid, however, excising any portion of the calcaneus, because this will have an adverse effect on the size of the foot. Postoperatively, the foot should be maintained in plaster for 3 months; the Kirschner wire can be removed at 3 to 4 weeks.

Follow-up of talectomy for arthrogryposis has generally demonstrated good results, with a plantigrade functional foot, so long as the appropriate indications for surgery were present (Tompkins et al., 1956). The procedure is indicated for badly deformed rigid equinovarus feet when additional musculoskeletal abnormalities make prolonged standing and extended ambulation unlikely. When the surgical resection is incomplete or postoperative care is inadequate, deformity will certainly recur (Fig. 22-32, A).

For the older child, triple arthrodesis is the procedure of choice. Adequate shortening of the skeletal elements to effect correction and closure of the skin without tension can be carried out during the procedure. If the triple arthrodesis does not effect complete correction, fusion of the ankle joint with appropriate resection of bone from the distal tibia may be necessary in the severely involved arthrogrypotic foot (Carmack and Hallock, 1947). Triple arthrodesis should probably not be performed when significant foot growth remains (i.e., in children under the age of 12 years).

Midtarsal wedge resection is effective in correcting cavus or forefoot equinus deformity (Fig. 22-32, B). Supramalleolar osteotomy can be used to correct hindfoot equinus in the older child, although Drummond et al (1974) believe this should be the last line of defense.

ABNORMALITIES OF TOES

Congenital abnormalities of the toes include polydactyly, syndactyly, macrodactyly, congenital hammertoe, and overlapping and underlapping toes. Congenital abnormalities of the great toe include hallux rigidus, hallux varus, and interphalangeal valgus. More than any other group of foot abnormalities, congenital toe deformities tend to be hereditary. Furthermore, some toe abnormalities are found in concert with generalized

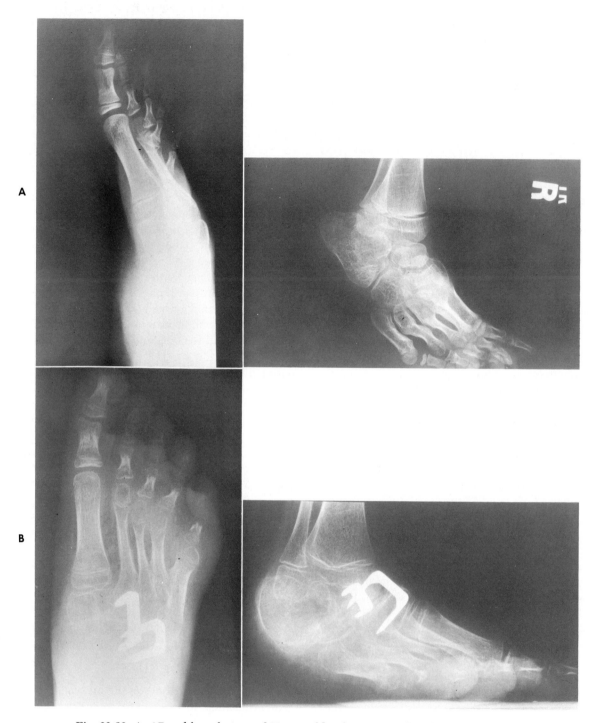

Fig. 22-32. A, AP and lateral views of 12-year-old arthrogrypotic foot that underwent talec-tomy at 15 months. **B,** Result after midtarsal dorsolateral wedge resection.

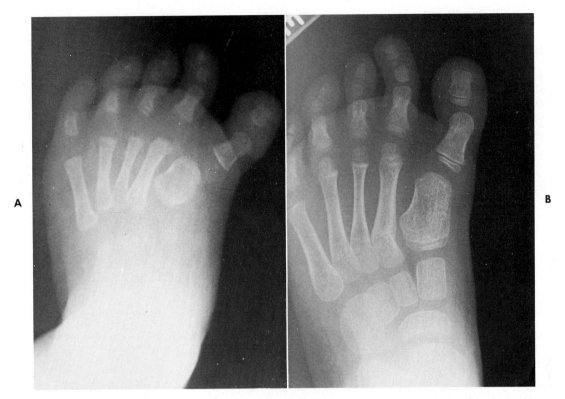

Fig. 22-33. Congenital hallux varus (atavistic first toe.) **A,** At 10 months of age; shortening of first metatarsal accompanied by medial subluxation of metatarsophalangeal joint. **B,** at 2 years and 7 months; early release of abductor hallucis. This resulted in better cosmesis and alignment.

syndromes as noted in the compilation by Zimbler and Craig (1976) (see p. 520).

Abnormalities of great toe

Congenital hallux varus. Congenital hallux varus is a rare deformity, differing from that seen as an adducted first toe accompanying metatarsus primus varus. There is no hereditary tendency for this deformity, and it is often associated with supernumerary phalanges or metatarsals; on occasion, the first metatarsal is duplicated and fused.

Clinically the deformity presents as an adduction deviation of the great toe, occasionally as much as 90° to the long axis of the foot (Fig. 22-33). Most often the deformity occurs at the metatarsophalangeal joint; however, it is sometimes seen at the interphalangeal joint. McElvenny (1941) described hallux varus in association with (1) a short thick metatarsal, (2) accessory bones or toes, (3) varus deformity of one or more of the lateral four metatarsals, and (4) a firm fibrous band along the medial aspects of the foot. This firm band, interpreted as being the abductor hallucis, has been implicated as a causative factor (Thompson, 1960).

Surgery for the condition must be tailored to meet the needs of the individual deformity. In general, sufficient skin must be retained by fashioning appropriate flaps to provide cover for the inner border of the foot. Farmer (1958) described a skin-fat flap that he uses to lengthen the short medial side of the foot, adapting the technique to the demands of the deformity. To obtain reduction, all structures along the medial side, including the metatarsophalangeal joint capsule, must be transected. To obtain correction and prevent recurrence of the deformity, the abductor hallucis must be divided. If the deformity is limited to the distal phalanx or the interphalangeal joint, symptoms may develop in adolescence and require surgical intervention. Angular deformity of the distal phalanx, either varus or valgus, can be corrected by appropriate osteotomy.

Congenital hallux rigidus. Congenital hallux rigidus is extremely rare. Its presence has been ascribed to an abnormality of the first metatarsal; elevation, excessive length, or hypermobility. More commonly the deformity appears secondary to trauma, with involvement of the first metatarsophalangeal joint or development of osteochondritis dessicans of the first metatarsal head (Kessel and Bonney, 1958). Anomalies of the first metatarsal head that cause abnormal joint surfaces can have

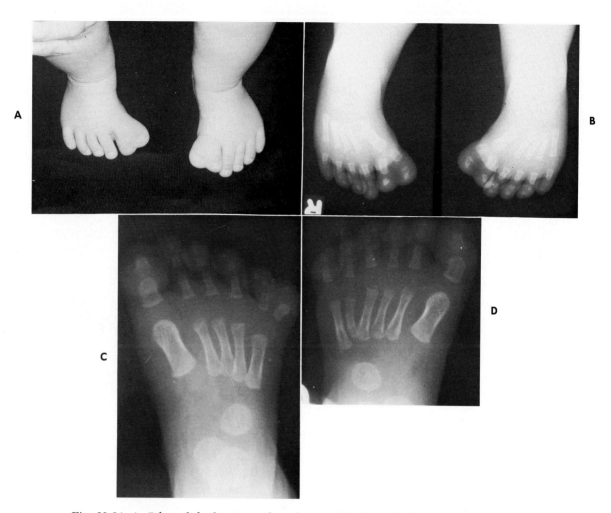

Fig. 22-34. **A,** Bilateral duplication and syndactyly of hallux. Tibialmost toe should be removed and abductor hallucis reattached to remaining proximal phalanx. If abductor hallucis is lengthened, metatarsus adductus will resolve. **B,** Radiograph of the same feet. **C,** Duplication of fifth toe; fibularmost (lateral) digit should be removed. **D,** Polydactyly with six fully developed metatarsals. If surgery is required, ray resection as well as toe amputation is necessary.

the same effect as trauma, leading to abnormal stress and degenerative joint disease. Treatment of symptomatic congenital hallux rigidus is the same as for the acquired type. Since symptoms are not usually present before adolescence, interference with future growth of the toe is not necessarily a consideration.

Abnormalities of lesser toes

Polydactyly. Often inherited as an autosomal dominant (Kirtland and Russell, 1976), polydactyly is frequently part of a generalized syndrome and may be accompanied by supernumerary fingers. If the extra digit occurs on the tibial side of the foot, it is termed *preaxial;* on the fibular side, *postaxial* (Nathan and Keniston, 1975). The literature contains many references to poly-

dactyly, but for the most part these references are made only in passing when describing the clinical characteristics of a generalized syndrome.

Recognition of the deformity in biblical times is found in 2 Samuel 21:20: "And there was again war at Goth, where there was a man of great stature who had six fingers on each hand and six toes on each foot, 24 in number; and he also was descended from the giants." Frazier (1960) noted a twelvefold increase in polydactyly among the southern black population as compared with southern whites. He described an incidence of 3.6 per 1000 live births among black children born in Baltimore.

Supernumerary toes are a clincial problem since they interfere with footwear. For this reason surgical excision is often indicated, but one must adhere to a few basic principles.* Unlike the hand, the foot does not necessitate making a decision as to which is the most rudimentary of the digits and then excising that particular one. More appropriately, the contour of the entire foot should be considered and, for the most part, the peripheral extra digit excised (Tachdjian, 1972). This is irrespective of whether it appears to be the more major digit. On the medial side of the foot, the toe closest to the tibia is usually excised; and on the lateral side, that closest to the fibula. If an abnormality of the metatarsals (bifurcation, duplication) is demonstrated radiographically, appropriate excision to obtain a normal contour of the entire foot must be considered (Fig. 22-34).

Surgical technique should be tailored to the individual case. In the usual circumstances disarticulation is carried out via a racquet-shaped incision with division and repair of ligaments and tendons as needed to prevent progressive deformity. Damage to remaining growth plates and articular cartilage must be avoided.

Muscle attachment is a more significant consideration with an accessory hallux than with other accessory toes. If the tibial hallux is excised, the abductor hallucis must be reinserted into the remaining proximal phalanx to avoid a hallux valgus deformity. Similarly, if the fibular hallux is grossly deformed and is to be excised, the adductor hallucis must be resutured into the proximal phalanx of the remaining hallux to avoid a hallux varus deformity secondary to overpull of the abductor hallucis.

Syndactyly. Like polydactyly, syndactyly is also seen in association with other congenital anomalies and syndromes. McKusick (1968) described five types of syndactyly, all transmitted as autosomal dominant traits. In the feet three types are seen:

Type I (zygodactyly): partial or complete webbing of the second and third toes; hands also involved at times.

Type II (synpolydactyly): syndactyly of the lateral two toes and polydactyly of the fifth toe in the syndactyly web.

Type III: associated with metatarsal and metacarpal fusion.

Surgical intervention for simple syndactyly of the foot is rarely indicated. The deformity is functionally insignificant and rarely becomes symptomatic. When surgery for cosmetic reasons is necessary, techniques of syndactyly release for the fingers apply as well to the toes.

The basic surgical technique involves outlining dorsal

---

*Because polydactyly frequently interferes with shoewear, excision at walking age is appropriate. At 1 year the foot and its individual structures are usually large enough to identify easily and deal with safely.

and volar skin flaps, based proximally. Flaps are incised, and this skin is used to close the cleft and reconstruct the web by suturing the flaps side to side. Opposing surfaces of the toes are then covered with free split-thickness skin grafts as required. Attempts to close flaps without using skin grafts leads to inevitable contracture and deformity.

Macrodactyly. Usually seen as a manifestation of a generalized problem (neurofibromatosis, arteriovenous fistula, hemangioma), gigantism of a toe can result in significant functional as well as cosmetic problems (Fig. 22-35). Both gait abnormalities and difficulty with footwear occur, making surgery necessary. The toe may be reduced in length by a partial or total proximal or middle phalangectomy. Circumference of a toe can be reduced by staged defatting procedures. If the third or fourth toe is involved, amputation may be acceptable. However, amputation of a gigantic second toe can result in progressive hallux valgus deformity. Tachdjian (1972) has recommended syndactyly of the second to the fourth toes if a gigantic third toe is amputated. Overgrowth of the metatarsal may be managed by epiphysiodesis at an appropriate time.

Congenital hammertoe. A rare congenital deformity, hammertoe is recognized as a flexion contracture of the proximal interphalangeal joint with or without fixed deformity of the distal interphalangeal joint. With ambulation and footwear the metatarsophalangeal joint eventually becomes hyperextended. Like syndactyly and polydactyly, hammertoe is frequently a familial problem, most often involving the middle toes. With shoe wear, callus formation over the dorsal aspect of the proximal interphalangeal joint can result in symptoms.

Because the deformity usually eventually becomes symptomatic, early treatment is indicated. In infancy, adhesive strapping combined with stretching of the contracted volar capsule of the proximal interphalangeal joint is often effective. Early surgical treatment is usually not necessary, since the deformity does not become symptomatic until early adolescence. After the foot has reached an appropriate size, correction can easily be obtained surgically by partial phalangectomy and interphalangeal fusion. If contracture of the dorsal metatarsophalangeal joint capsule has occurred, capsulotomy must also be carried out. Specifics of surgical treatment are described in Chapter 5.

Overlapping toes. Often familial, overriding is most commonly seen as the fifth toe overlapping the fourth. There is dorsiflexion of the metatarsophalangeal joint with adduction and external rotation of the digit. The condition is usually bilateral and, in about 50% of the cases, causes disabling symptoms (Cockin, 1968). Discomfort is aggravated by shoe wear and accompanying

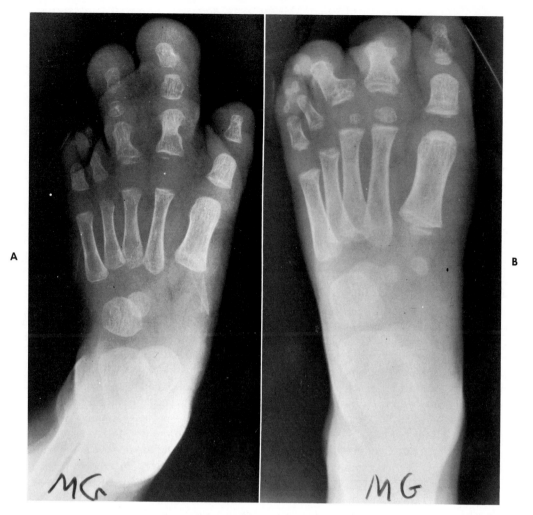

Fig. 22-35. A, Macrodactyly involving second and third toes. Digits are adult-sized at 2 years of age. **B,** Initial procedure included epiphyseodesis and soft tissue resection. Three years later interphalangeal resection and fusion with further soft tissue removal resulted in better cosmesis and shoe fit. (Courtesy Dr. Semour Zimbler, Boston, Mass.)

callus formation over the dorsal aspect of the proximal interphalangeal joint.

Because, as in hammertoe and congenital curly toe, symptoms are likely to develop later in life, early treatment may be of some benefit. In infancy, stretching the medial collateral ligament structure and dorsal medial capsule with adhesive taping into the correct position may be of some benefit. In most cases, surgical correction can be carried out without bone resection or interference with growth; therefore treatment in early childhood is possible.

Treatment. Most described procedures involve tenotomy of the extensor digitorum communis to the fifth toe as well as capsulotomy of the dorsal medial metatarsophalangeal joint.

Lapidus (1942) did the extensor tenotomy at the midtarsal level and rerouted the distal tendon stump plantarward around the medial side of the small toe, inserting the stump into the abductor digiti minimi.

I have been particularly pleased with Butler's operation (Cockin, 1968). In this procedure the entire toe is freed via a racquet incision at its base with proximal extensions dorsally and at the plantar lateral margin. After extensor tenotomy and dorsal capsulotomy the plantar capsule, if adherent, is freed from the metatarsal head. Closure of the skin is then completed with the toe in the corrected position; no postoperative cast is necessary.

Syndactylization of the fifth to the fourth toe is advocated by Scrase (1954) and Kelikian et al., (1961). A

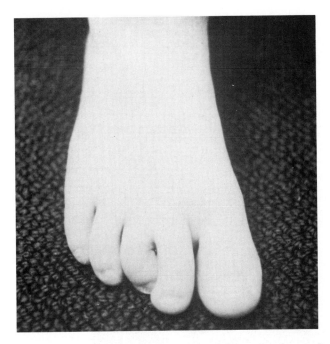

Fig. 22-36. Congenital curly toes; lateral deviation of second toe is secondary to underlapping third digit.

double-U incision between the fourth and fifth toes with excision of the intervening skin permits the syndactyly. Correction via capsulotomy and extensor digitorum tenotomy can be accompanied by removal of enough proximal phalanx to correct the deformity (Leonard and Rising, 1965).

Amputation for overlapping fifth toe generally results in pain and pressure at the head of the fifth metatarsal and therefore is not recommended. If the deformity is too severe, attempted correction without bony resection can result in vascular compromise. For this reason procedures restricted to soft tissues tend to be more applicable to children and adolescents than to adults (p. 152).

Congenital underlapping toes (congenital curly toe). Congenital underlapping toes is a common familial deformity most often seen in the lateral three toes. It presents as a combination of flexion, adduction, and internal rotation primarily at the distal interphalangeal joint (Fig. 22-36). In severe cases the proximal interphalangeal joint is also rotated and the toenail pointed laterally.

Unlike congenital overlapping toes, the congenital curly toe rarely becomes symptomatic. Early conservative treatment is not of benefit in correcting curly toe deformity.

Sweetman (1958) evaluated the long-term results of 50 cases, 21 patients treated and 29 untreated. In no patient, either treated or untreated, did the deformity

progress; 25% improved whether treated or not. Even though the deformity persisted in many cases, most patients had forgotten that it was present.

If surgery is required because of symptoms, syndactylization of the curly toe to its neighbor may be performed (Kelikian, 1965). Correction may be obtained by excising an appropriate wedge from the superolateral aspect of the distal interphalangeal joint. Sharrard (1963) recommended transfer of the extensor digitorum longus of the affected toe to the dorsolateral aspect of the extensor hood. He found that this was of benefit, particularly if the deformity was not too severe. In my hands, tenotomy of the flexor digitorum longus through an oblique incision underlying the middle phalanx, when performed in early childhood has been curative. One must take care not to cross the joint flexor crease with the incision. Postoperatively a soft dressing is sufficient.

TORSIONAL DEFORMITIES OF LOWER EXTREMITIES

In the practice of a primary care physician, perhaps the most common orthopaedic problem noted among the skeletally immature patients in the practice is some form of rotational malalignment of the lower extremities. Rarely does the problem present as a complaint of the individual but rather the result of concern on the part of parents, grandparents, or other well-meaning individuals. Diagnosis can sometimes be elusive, speculative, or unrecognized. Perhaps millions of dollars annually are spent for orthotics, braces, or other devices that are reputedly therapeutic but in fact offer no scientifically proven benefit.

The rotational deformity may obviously be either internal or external and is most often referred to as intoeing or out-toeing. If the treating physician is able to make a specific diagnosis by physical examination, then appropriate treatment or advice can be advanced on a judicious basis. The anatomic site responsible for toeing-in or toeing-out can be located anywhere between the toes and the pelvis. A torsional malalignment of foot, ankle, leg, thigh, or pelvis will result in a clinical picture most obvious at the foot. Therefore, complete appreciation of the various diagnostic possibilities, their anatomic location, and the physical findings allows one to treat appropriately, avoiding overtreatment and unnecessary expense.

Physical examination and normal parameters

Faced with a lower extremity rotational problem, physical assessment should begin with an evaluation of the individual's coordination and gait if he is ambulatory. Following a straight line of progression, the angle of gait is that subtended along the line of progression

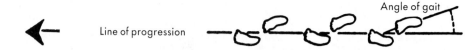

Fig. 22-37. Angle of gait when toeing-in.

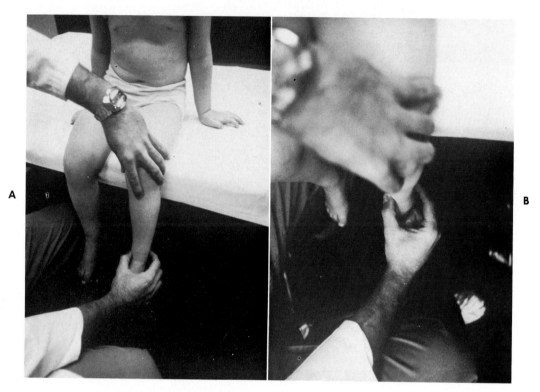

Fig. 22-38. **A,** Placement of hand for clinical measurement of tibial torsional angle. **B,** As viewed from above, normal medial malleolus is anterior to lateral by 15°.

by the foot as it strikes the floor. Under normal circumstances, the angle of gait ranges between 5° and 15° external (Fig. 22-37). While observing the individual ambulate, the examiner should note the position of the knee as related to the line of progression; this should be observed both from the front and from the back. The relationship of the foot to the knee is important in delineating the source of rotational malalignment, either above or below the knee joint.

After observing gait pattern, sequential examination of the lower limbs should be carried out. The feet should be the first specific structure examined. Starting distally allows the examiner to remain outside the patient's "space" and thereby puts the child at ease; one may then usually carry out this and the remainder of an examination with more patient cooperation. With the child supine, the plantar surface of the foot should be observed, with careful attention paid to the contour of its outer border as well as the alignment of the great toe when compared to the longitudinal axis of the first

metatarsal. The outer border of the foot should normally be straight; the great toe should continue on the long axis of the first metatarsal. The tendon of the abductor hallucis muscle should not be particularly prominent when the great toe is passively deviated toward the midline.

With the patient sitting on the edge of the examining table, the transmalleolar axis should next be evaluated. Clinically this can be accomplished by placing your index finger opposite that of the leg being examined on the lateral malleolus, the thumb on the medial malleolus. With the index finger of the other hand resting on the tibial tubercle, and using this as a guide, sight down the leg from above and determine the relationship of the transmalleolar axis to the horizontal (Fig. 22-38, A-B). Normally, the medial malleolus should be anterior to the lateral by approximately 5° at birth, progressing to 20° in adulthood (Engel and Staheli, 1974).

While the child remains in the sitting position, one may then assess the axis of the femoral neck and its

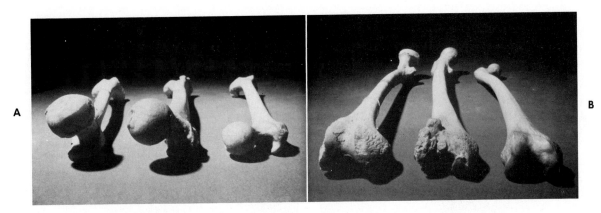

Fig. 22-39. Adult femora with varying angles of anteversion. **A,** Viewed from above; note position of greater trochanter in relation to femoral neck. **B,** Viewed from below; femoral condyles are in identical positions, femoral necks vary from 80° to 0° of anteversion. (Courtesy Shands Bone Museum, A.I. duPont Institute.)

relationship to the transcondylar axis of the femur. Since the femoral neck is in direct line with the greater trochanter (Fig. 22-39, *A-B*), rotating the extremity until the greater trochanter is palpably most lateral will allow one to determine the longitudinal axis of the neck (Fig. 22-40). The degree of femoral anteversion (relationship of the femoral neck axis to the transchondylar axis) is represented in the angle subtended by the longitudinal axis of the leg and the vertical.

Final assessment on physical examination is carried out with the patient prone. In this position, with the hip extended, the knee flexed 90°, and the ankle in a plantigrade position, one may determine the thigh-foot axis. In this position, the longitudinal axis of the foot as compared to the longitudinal axis of the thigh is normally between 0° and 10° external (Fig. 22-41). Deviation from this indicates the presence of a torsional malalignment below the knee. If the lateral border of the foot is straight, the deformity is further isolated to the area between ankle and knee.

Rotational motion of the hip is similarly assessed in this position. Total normal rotation is approximately 90°. This should consist of nearly equal internal and external rotation; in the normal individual there may be slightly more external rotation available than internal.

Using these procedures as a means of physical assessment, the examiner is able to delineate the anatomic site responsible for the rotational malalignment and approach treatment on a more scientific basis.

Treatment

Toeing-out. External rotation posturing of the lower extremities is most often physiologic. Two pathologic entities that may result in this picture include the vertical talus (see p. 548) or a neurologic disorder. If both

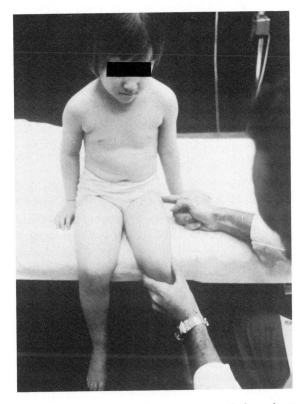

Fig. 22-40. Determination of anteversion angle by palpation of greater trochanter. Angle subtended by tibia as compared to a vertical line is equal to angle of femoral neck compared to transcondylar axis.

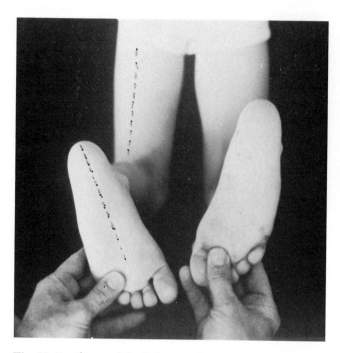

Fig. 22-41. Abnormal thigh-foot axis bilaterally, worse on left than right.

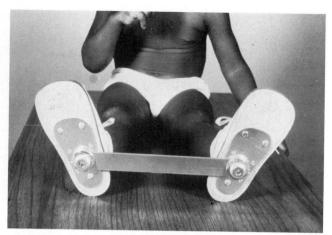

Fig. 22-42. Appropriately measured and configured Denis-Browne bar.

careful neurological assessment and examination for the presence of a vertical talus are negative, the parents may be assured that the external rotation posture of the extremity is physiologic and does not require treatment. One occasionally finds that internal rotation of the hip is limited in the infant by tight external hip rotators, perhaps because of heavy diapering or large thighs which keep the infant's hip flexed and externally rotated. External rotator stretching at the time of diaper change by internally rotating the thigh, using the flexed knee as a handle, may be of some benefit. However, it is most probable that the tight muscular and capsular structures will normally elongate as the child grows.

In the ambulatory child, external rotational posturing of the lower extremity is common before the age of 2 years. This may appear with initial ambulation as an effort on the part of the individual to provide stability in standing. This too normally resolves by 24 months of age without specific treatment (Hensinger, 1976).

Toeing-in as result of foot abnormalities. The entities of the foot responsible for internal malalignment of the foot are addressed elsewhere in this chapter (Metatarsus Adductus, Atavistic First Toe, Abductor Hallucis Tightness). Treatment of the specific foot anomaly should follow the guidelines recommended.

Tibial torsion

Torsional malalignment of the leg, either external or more commonly internal, is determined by the trans-

malleolar axis as described under Physical Examination. At birth the transmalleolar axis may be neutral, progressing to its normal 15° external by 2 to 3 years of age. The child who is seen between 6 months and 2 years of age with a complaint of toeing-in has, most commonly, persistent internal tibial torsion. It is generally felt that with growth and development a normal transmalleolar axis will develop with ambulation, and active treatment is rarely indicated. Occasionally, persistent internal torsion or deformities with a negative angle are of enough concern to warrant active intervention. If one is to treat a perceived problem that is potentially a phase of normal development, the induction of secondary iatrogenic problems must be avoided. A Denis-Browne bar no longer than the width of the individual's pelvis with the feet externally rotated no more than 45° may be applied (Fig. 22-42). More elaborate devices such as the Blount derotation brace have been used to keep the knee flexed and thereby concentrate torsional force to the ankle and leg. A bar wider than the pelvis or external rotation beyond 45° can result in secondary ligamentous laxity at the ankle or valgus deformity of the knee.

Significant external torsional deformities of the tibia are less commonly encountered. When seen, they are most frequently secondary to internal torsional deformities of the femur or malalignment of the foot as a result of neuromuscular problems. Consequently, isolated treatment of external torsional malrotation of the leg is rarely indicated.

Because of the benign nature of the problem and its probable physiologic basis, surgical approach to torsional deformities of the tibia should be performed only under rare circumstances and following a great deal of thoughtful consideration. Rotational osteotomies performed subperiosteally through a small incision in the

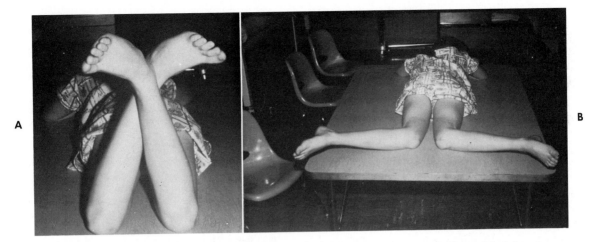

Fig. 22-43. Degree of external hip rotation available (**A**) and internal rotation possible (**B**) in presence of femoral anteversion clinically measuring 70°.

supramalleolar area may be performed without internal fixation, thus avoiding the problems associated with pins, plates, screws, etc. Maintaining corrected alignment in a long leg cast with the knee bent 90° for 6 weeks carries the least risk of complication from non-union, infection, failure of correction, etc.

Femoral anteversion

Those individuals over 2½ years of age with persistent or recently noticed toeing-in most frequently have a torsional abnormality in the proximal shaft of the femur. At birth, the longitudinal axis of the femoral neck subtends an angle of approximately 40° when compared to the transcondylar axis of the femur. During the first 2 years of life, this angle declines to 20°; further decrease to slightly over 10° in the adult occurs during the latter years of growth (MacEwen, 1976). Anterior inclination of the neck is referred to clinically as femoral anteversion. Excessive anteversion results from incomplete derotation of the upper femur as it assumes a position of extension, adduction, and internal rotation from its initial early position in the fetal limb bud. When weight-bearing, unless the acetabulum is abnormally inclined so as to receive the head of the excessively anteverted femoral neck, the extremity must internally rotate to avoid anterior subluxation. The stresses of weight-bearing, influence of growth and capsular pressures will induce remodeling, decreasing the anteversion angle. Longitudinal anteversion studies have demonstrated that an individual retains potential for remodeling until approximately 8 years of age. In children who persistently alter their gait pattern or sit in the reversed tailor position, the stresses that induce the remodeling processes are decreased. In such cases, excessive anteversion persists.

On physical examination, a significant increase in in-

ternal rotation at the hip is noted. External rotation, on the other hand, is limited to only a few degrees (Fig. 22-43, *A-B*).

It has been suggested in the past, and noted in the studies by Fabray and McEwen (1973), that bracing has little or no effect on the anteversion angle. Treatment with a Dennis Brown bar, twister cables, etc., has never shown a decrease in anteversion angle that withstood scientific scrutiny. Therefore, beyond recommending appropriate sitting habits (e.g., avoiding the reversed tailor position) the child under 8 years of age with persistent femoral anteversion and toeing-in should not be actively treated. There is no place in the treatment of this entity for prescription footwear; bracing similarly has no effect.

If, after 8 to 9 years of age, a significant cosmetic or functional deformity is present, surgical intervention may be required. Functional impairment is commonly seen in individuals who have no more than 10° of passive external rotation at the hip. It has been our policy to do a supracondylar subperiosteal derotational osteotomy without internal or external fixation. When performed as described, the risk of asymmetric or excessive derotation is minimal. Again, the complications associated with pins, plates, screws, etc., are avoided.

Technique of supracondylar femoral derotational osteotomy. Before surgery, the total amount of femoral anteversion is evaluated fluoroscopically. With the patient prone on the x-ray table, the knees are bent and the hip internally rotated until the longest image of femoral neck is present on the screen. At that point, the neck is parallel to the x-ray table; determination of the anteversion angle is possible by measuring the angle subtended by the leg against the vertical. At surgery, this degree of derotation is carried out.

1. With the patient supine on the fracture table and

the legs abducted 45°, the extremity is prepared and draped so as to allow for a medial approach to the distal femur. Using an image intensifier, the supracondylar region of the femur is identified 2.5 cm above the distal femoral physis.

2. A 4 cm longitudinal skin incision is made just anterior to the intramuscular septum, beginning just distal to the growth plate. Dissection through the subcutaneous tissue is carried out, the fascia lata is divided, and vastus medialis is retracted anteriorly.

3. The posteromedial aspect of the femoral shaft is identified and the epiphyseal vessels crossing the field are protected. A 2.5 cm longitudinal incision in the posteromedial periosteum is made, and with care the periosteum is elevated circumferentially from the femoral metaphysis at this point.

4. The femur may be divided either by predrilling the osteotomy site with a small drill bit followed by osteotomes, or with a power saw. Of great importance is maintenance of the osteotomy in a line absolutely perpendicular to the longitudinal axis of the femoral shaft.

5. Following completion of the osteotomy, the footplate of the fracture table is externally rotated, thus derotating the extremity distal to the osteotomy site. It has been unnecessary to place drains within the wound or add internal fixation devices.

6. After manipulative derotation and wound closure the extremity is placed in a longleg bilateral hip spica cast with the foot (or feet) externally rotated 90°.

Postoperatively, the patient is kept nonambulatory in the cast for a period of 6 weeks. On cast removal, hospitalization for vigorous physical therapy over a period of 4 to 6 days is necessary to regain 60° of knee motion. The patient is kept on crutch-assisted weight bearing until 90° of knee motion has been realized.

Results of this approach to the well-selected case in my hands have been universally excellent. The use of a small medial incision avoids cosmetic problems of a readily visable surgical scar. Complications of nonunion, infection, loss of position, entry into the suprapatellar pouch of the knee, or less than complete patient satisfaction have been avoided.

REFERENCES
Embryology and genetics

Blechschmidt, E.: The stages of human development before birth, Philadelphia, 1961, W.B. Saunders Co.

Cowell, H.R., and Wein, B.K.: Current concepts review: genetic aspects of club foot, J. Bone Joint Surg. 62A:1381-1384, 1980.

Fuller, D.J., and Duthie, R.B.: The timed appearance of some congenital malformations and orthopaedic abnormalities. In American Academy of Orthopaedic Surgeons instructional course lectures, vol. 23, St. Louis, 1974, the C.V. Mosby Co.

Gardner, E., Gray, D.J., and O'Rahilly, R.: The prenatal development of the skeleton and joints of the human foot, J. Bone Joint Surg. 41A:847, 1959.

McKusick, V.A.: Mendelian inheritance in man, ed. 4, Baltimore, 1975, Johns Hopkins University Press.

Zimbler, S., and Craig, C.: Foot deformities, Orthop. Clin. North Am. 7:331, 1976.

Clubfoot (talipes equinovarus)

Abrams, R.C.: Relapsed clubfoot: the early results of an evaluation of the Dillwyn Evans operation, J. Bone Joint. Surg. 51A:270, 1969.

Bohm, M.: The embryologic origin of clubfoot, J. Bone Joint Surg. 11:229, 1929.

Brockman, E.P.: Congenital clubfoot, London, 1930, John Wright & Sons, Ltd.

Cowell, H.R., and Wein, B.K.: Current concepts review: genetic aspects of club foot, J. Bone Joint Surg. 62A:1381-1384, 1980.

Crawford, A.H., Marxen, J.L., and Osterfeld, D.L.: The Cincinnati incision: a comprehensive approach for surgical procedures of the foot and ankle in childhood, J. Bone Joint Surg. 64A:1355-1358, 1982.

Denham, P.A.: Congenital talipes equinovarus, J. Bone Joint Surg. 49B:583, 1967.

Dunn, H.K., and Samuelson, K.M.: Flat topped talus: a long term report of 20 clubfeet, J. Bone Joint Surg. 56A:57, 1974.

Dwyer, F.C.: The treatment of relapsed clubfoot by insertion of a wedge into the calcaneum, J. Bone Joint Surg. 45B:67, 1963.

Evans, D.: Relapsed clubfoot, J. Bone Joint Surg. 43B:722, 1961.

Fisher, R.L., and Shaffer, S.R.: An evaluation of calcaneal osteotomy in congenital clubfoot and other disorders, Clin. Orthop. 70:141, 1970.

Fried, A.: Recurrent congenital clubfoot, J. Bone Joint Surg. 41A:424, 1959.

Gardner, E.: Osteogenesis in the human embryo and foetus. In Bourne, G., ed.: Biochemistry and physiology of bone, New York, 1956, Academic Press, Inc.

Grider, T.D., Siff, S.J., Gerson, P., and Donovan, M.M.: Arteriography in clubfoot, J. Bone Joint Surg. 64A:837-840, 1982.

Heywood, A.W.B.: The mechanics of the hindfoot in clubfoot as demonstrated radiographically, J. Bone Joint Surg. 46B:105, 1964.

Ippolito, E. and Ponseti, I.V.: Congenital clubfoot in the human fetus: a histological study, J. Bone Joint Surg. 62A:8-22, 1980.

Irani, R.N., and Sherman, M.S.: The pathological anatomy of clubfoot, J. Bone Joint Surg. 45A:45, 1963.

Johanning, K.: Exocochleatio ossis cuboidei in the treatment of pes equino varus, Acta Orthop. Scand. 27:310, 1958.

Keim, H.A., and Ritchie, G.W.: Nutcracker treatment of clubfoot, JAMA 189:613, 1964.

Kite, J.H.: The non-operative treatment of congenital clubfoot, South. Med. J. 23:337, 1930.

Lloyd-Roberts, G.C.: Congenital clubfoot, J. Bone Joint Surg. 46B:369, 1964.

Lowe, L.W., and Hannon, M.A.: Residual adduction of the forefoot in treated congenital club foot, J. Bone Joint Surg. 55B:809, 1973.

Paturet, G.: Traite d'anatomie humaine, vol. 2, Paris, 1951, Masson & Cie.

Ponseti, I.V., and Smoley, E.N.: Congenital clubfoot: the results of treatment, J. Bone Joint Surg. 45A:261, 1963.

Settle, G.W.: The anatomy of congenital clubfoot talipes equinovarus: sixteen dissected specimens, J. Bone Joint Surg. 45A:1341, 1963.

Smith, W.A., Campbell, P., and Bonnett, C.: Early posterior ankle release in treatment of congenital clubfoot, Orthop. Clin. North Am. 7:889, 1976.

Swann, M., Lloyd-Roberts, G.C., and Catterall, A.: The anatomy of uncorrected club feet, J. Bone Joint Surg. 51B:263, 1969.

Turco, V.J.: Surgical correction of the resistant clubfoot, J. Bone Joint Surg. 53A:477, 1971.

Turco, V.J.: Resistant congenital clubfoot. In American Academy of Orthopaedic Surgeons instructional course lectures, vol. 24, St. Louis, 1975, The C.V. Mosby Co.

Waisbrod, H: Congenital clubfoot: an anatomical study, J. Bone Joint Surg. **55B:**796, 1973.

Wiley, A.M.: Club foot: an anatomical and experimental study of muscle growth, J. Bone Joint Surg. **41B:**821, 1959.

Wynne-Davies, R.: Family studies and the cause of congenital club foot, J. Bone Joint Surg. **46B:**445, 1964.

Metatarsus adductus and metatarsus varus

Berman, A., and Gartland, J.J.: Metatarsal osteotomy for the correction of adduction of the fore part of the foot in children, J. Bone Joint Surg. **53A:**498, 1971.

Bleck, E.E., and Minaire, P.: Persistent medial deviation of the talar neck: a common cause of intoeing in children. Presented at the annual meeting of the American Academy of Orthopaedic Surgeons, New Orleans, 1976.

Fowler, B., Brooks, A.L., and Parrish, T.F.: The cavo-varus foot, J. Bone Joint Surg. **41A:**757, 1959.

Helbing, C.: Ueber den Metatarsus varus, Dtsh. Med. Wochenschr. **21:**1312, 1905.

Heyman, C.H., Herndon, C.H., and Strong, J.M.: Mobilization of the tarsometatarsal and intermetatarsal joints for the correction of resistant adduction of the fore part of the foot in congenital clubfoot and congenital metatarsus varus, J. Bone Joint Surg. **40A:**299, 1958.

Kendrick, R.E., Sharma, N.K., Hassler, W.E., and Herndon, C.H.: Tarsometatarsal mobilization for resistant adduction deformity of the fore part of the foot: a follow-up study, J. Bone Joint Surg. **52A:**61, 1970.

Kite, J.H.: Congenital metatarsus varus, J. Bone Joint Surg. **49A:**388, 1967.

Kite, J.H.: Congenital metatarsal varus, J. Bone Joint Surg. **32A:**500, 1950.

Lichtblau, S.: Section of the abductor hallucis tendon for correction of metatarsus varus deformity, Clin. Orthop. **110:**227, 1975.

Lincoln, C.R., Wood, K.E., and Bugg, E.I.: Metatarsus varus corrected by open wedge osteotomy of the first cuneiform bone, Orthop. Clin. North Am. **7:**795, 1976.

Lloyd-Roberts, G.C., and Clark, C.R.: Ball and socket joint in metatarsus adductus varus, J. Bone Joint Surg. **55B:**193, 1973.

McCormick, D.W., and Blount, W.P.: Metatarsus adductovarus—"skewfoot," J.A.M.A. **141:**449, 1949.

Peabody, C.W., and Muro, F.: Congenital metatarsus varus, J. Bone Joint Surg. **15:**171, 1933

Ponseti, I.V., and Becker, J.R.: Congenital metatarsus adductus: the results of treatment, J. Bone Joint Surg. **48A:**702, 1966.

Reimann, I.: Congenital metatarsus varus: on the advantages of early treatment, Acta Orthop. Scand. **46:**857, 1975.

Reimann, I., and Werner, H.H.: Congenital metatarsus varus, Clin. Orthop. **110:**223, 1975.

Specht, E.E.: Major congenital deformities and anomalies of the foot. In Inman, V.T., ed.: DuVries' surgery of the foot, ed. 3, St. Louis, 1973, The C.V. Mosby Co.

Wynne-Davies, R.: Family studies and the cause of congenital clubfoot: talipes equinovarus, talipes calcaneovalgus and metatarsus varus, J. Bone Joint Surg. **46B:**445, 1964.

Flatfeet

Bleck, E.E.: The shoeing of children—sham or science? Dev. Med. Child Neurol. **13:**188, 1971.

Bleck, E.E., and Berzins, U.E.: Conservative management of pes valgus with plantar flexed talus, flexible, Clin. Orthop. **122:**85, 1977.

Bordelon, R.L.: Hypermobile flatfoot in children, Clin. Orthop. **181:**7, 1983.

Bordelon, R.L.: Correction of hypermobile flatfoot in children by inserts, Foot Ankle **1:**143, 1980.

Chambers, E.F.S.: An operation for the correction of flexible flatfoot of adolescents, Surg. Gynecol. Obstet. **54:**77, 1946.

Harris, R.I., and Beath, T.: Hypermobile flat-foot with short tendo achillis, J. Bone Joint Surg. **30A:**116, 1948.

Helfet, A.J.: A new way of treating flat feet in children, Lancet **1:**262, 1956.

Henderson, W.H., and Campbell, J.W.: UCBL shoe insert: casting and fabrication, Tech. Rep. 53, 1967, University of California, Berkeley, Biomechanics Laboratory.

Hoke, M.: An operation for the correction of extremely relaxed flat feet, J. Bone Joint Surg. **13:**773, 1931.

Jack, E.A.: Naviculo-cuneiform fusion in the treatment of flatfoot, Am. J. Roentgenol. Radium Ther. Nucl. Med. **35B:**75, 1953.

Kidner, F.C.: The prehallux (accessory scaphoid) in its relation to flatfoot, J. Bone Joint Surg. **11:**831, 1929.

Lusted, L.B., and Keats, T.E.: Atlas of roentgenographic measurements, ed. 2, Chicago, 1967, Year Book Medical Publishers, Inc.

Miller, G.R.: Hypermobile flatfeet in children, Clin. Orthop. **122:**95, 1977.

Miller, O.L.: A plastic foot operation, J. Bone Joint Surg. **9:**84, 1927.

Rose, G.K.: Correction of the pronated foot, J. Bone Joint Surg. **44B:**642, 1962.

Semour, N.: The late results of naviculo-cuneiform fusion. J. Bone Joint Surg. **49B:**558, 1967.

Smith, S.D., Millar, E.A.: Arthrosis by means of a subtalar polyethylene peg implant for correction of hindfoot pronation in children. Clin. Orthop. **181:**15, 1983.

Templeton, A.W., McAlister, W.H., and Zim, I.D.: Standardization of terminology and evaluation of osseous relationships in congenitally abnormal feet, Am. J. Roentgenol. Radium Ther. Nucl. Med. **93:**374, 1965.

Young, C.S.: Operative treatment of pes planus, Surg. Gynecol. Obstet. **68:**1099, 1939.

Zadek, I.: The accessory tarsal scaphoid, J. Bone Joint Surg. **30A:**957, 1948.

Peroneal spastic flatfoot (tarsal coalition.)

Badgley, C.E.: Coalition of the calcaneus and navicular, Arch. Surg. **15:**75, 1927.

Conway, J.J., and Cowell, H.R.: Tarsal coalition: clinical significance and roentgenographic demonstration, Radiology **92:**799, 1969.

Cowell, H.R.: Diagnosis and management of peroneal spastic flatfoot. In American Academy of Orthopaedic Surgeons instructional course lectures, vol. 24, St. Louis, 1975, The C.V. Mosby Co.

Cowell, H.R.: Talocalcaneal coalition and new causes of peroneal spastic flatfoot, Clin. Orthop. **85:**16, 1972.

Harris, R.I.: Rigid valgus foot due to talocalcaneal bridge, J. Bone Joint Surg. **37A:**169, 1955.

Harris, R.I., and Beath, T.: Etiology of peroneal spastic flatfoot, J. Bone Joint Surg. **30B:**624, 1948.

Jayakumar, S., and Cowell, H.R.: Rigid flatfoot. Clin. Orthop. **122:**77, 1977.

Korvin, H.: Coalitio talocalcanea, Z. Orthop. Chir. **60:**105, 1934.

Leonard, M.: The inheritance of tarsal fusion and the relationship to spastic flatfoot. Presented at British Orthopaedic Research Society, 1972.

Outland, T., and Murphy, I.D.: The pathomechanics of peroneal spastic flat foot. Clin. Orthop. **16:**64, 1960.

Slomann, H.C.: On coalitio calcaneo-navicularis, J. Orthop. Surg. 3:586, 1921.

Smith, R.W. and Staple, T.W.: Computerized tomography (CT) scanning technique for the hindfoot. Clin. Orthop. **177**:34-38, 1983.

Stormont, D.M., and Peterson, H.A.: The relative incidence of tarsal coalition, Clin. Orthop. **181**:28, 1983.

Wray, J.B., and Herndon, C.H.: Hereditary transmission of congenital coalition of the calcaneus to the navicular, J. Bone Joint Surg. **45A**:365, 1963.

Congenital convex pes valgus (congenital vertical talus)

Becker-Anderson, H., and Reimann, I.: Congenital vertical talus, Acta Orthop. Scand. **45**:130, 1974.

Coleman, S.S., and Jarrett, J.: Congenital vertical talus: pathomechanics and treatment, J. Bone Joint Surg. **48A**:1026, 1966.

Coleman, S.S., Stelling, F.H., and Jarrett, J.: Pathomechanics and treatment of congenital vertical talus, Clin. Orthop. **70**:62, 1970.

Colton, C.L.: The surgical management of congenital vertical talus, J. Bone Joint Surg. **55B**:566, 1973.

Drennan, J.C., and Sharrard, W.J.: The pathological anatomy of convex pes valgus, "persian slipper foot," J. Bone Joint Surg. **53B**:455, 1971.

Eyre-Brook, A.L.: Congenital vertical talus, J. Bone Joint Surg. **49B**:618, 1950.

Fitton, J.M., and Nevelös, A.B.: The treatment of congenital vertical talus, J. Bone Joint Surg. **61B**:481, 1979.

Hark, F.W.: Rocker bottom foot due to congenital subluxation of the talus, J. Bone Joint Surg. **32A**:344, 1950.

Herndon, C.H., and Heyman, C.H.: Problems in the recognition and treatment of congenital convex pes valgus, J. Bone Joint Surg. **45A**:413, 1963.

Jayakumar, S., and Ramsey, P.: Vertical and oblique talus: a diagnostic dilemma. Scientific exhibit at the annual meeting of the American Academy of Orthopaedic Surgeons, Las Vegas, 1977.

Lamy, L., and Weissman, L.: Congenital convex pes valgus, J. Bone Joint Surg. **21**:79, 1939.

Lloyd-Roberts, G.C., and Spence, A.J.: Congenital vertical talus, J. Bone Joint Surg. **40B**:33, 1958.

Patterson, W.R., Fritz, D.A., and Smith, W.S.: The pathologic anatomy of congenital convex pes valgus, J. Bone Joint Surg. **50A**:458, 1968.

Osmond-Clarke, H.: Congenital vertical talus in infancy, J. Bone Joint Surg. **48B**:578, 1966.

Stone, K.H. (for Lloyd-Robert, G.C.): Congenital vertical talus: a new operation, Proc. R. Soc. Med. **56**:12, 1963.

Arthrogryposis multiplex congenita

Adams, R.C., Denny-Brown, D., and Pearson, C.M.: Diseases of muscle: a study in pathology, ed. 2, New York, 1953, Harper & Brothers, Hoeber Medical Division, 1953.

Banker, B.Q., Victor, M., and Adams, R.D.: Arthrogryposis multiplex congenita due to congenital muscular dystrophy, Brian **80**:319, 1957.

Carmack, J.C., and Hallock, H.: Tibiotarsal arthrodesis after astragalectomy: a report of eight cases, J. Bone Joint Surg. **29**:476, 1947.

Drachman, D.B., and Banker, B.Q.: Arthrogryposis multiplex congenita, Arch. Neurol. **5**:77, 1961.

Drachman, D.B., and Coulombre, A.J.: Experimental clubfoot and arthrogryposis multiplex congenita, Lancet **2**:523, 1962.

Drummond, D.S., and Cruess, R.L.: The management of the foot and ankle in arthrogryposis multiplex congenita, J. Bone Joint Surg. **60B**:96, 1978.

Drummond, D., Siller, T.N., and Cruess, R.L.: Management of ar-

throgryposis multiplex congenita. In American Academy of Orthopaedic Surgeons instructional course lectures, vol. 23, St. Louis, 1974, The C.V. Mosby Co.

Gibson, D.A., and Urs, N.D.K.: Arthrogryposis multiplex congenita, J. Bone Joint Surg. **52B**:483, 1970.

Lloyd-Roberts, G.C., and Lettin, A.W.F.: Arthrogryposis multiplex congenita, J. Bone Joint Surg. **52B**:494, 1970.

Mead, N.L., Lithgow, W.C., and Sweeney, H.J.: Arthrogryposis multiplex congenita, J. Bone Joint Surg. **40A**:1285, 1958.

Menelaus, M.B.: Talectomy for equinovarus deformity in arthrogryposis and spina bifida, J. Bone Joint Surg. **53B**:468, 1971.

Middleton, D.E.: Studies on prenatal lesions of skeletal muscle as a cause of congenital deformity. I. Congenital tibial kyphosis. II. Congenital high shoulder. III. Myodystrophia foetalis, Edinburgh Med. J. **41**:401, 1934.

Oh, W.H.: Arthrogryposis multiplex congenita of the lower extremities: report of two siblings, Orthop. Clin. North Am. **7**:511, 1976.

Sheldon, W.: Amyoplasia congenita, Arch. Dis. Child. **7**:117, 1932.

Tompkins, S.F., Miller, R.J., and O'Donoghue, D.H.: An evaluation of astragalectomy, South. Med. J. **49**:1128, 1956.

Talipes calcaneovalgus

Larsen, B., Reimann, I., and Becker-Anderson, H.: Congenital calcaneovalgus with special reference to its treatment and its relation to other foot deformities, Acta Orthop. Scand. **45**:145, 1974.

Wetzenstein, H.: Prognosis of pes calcaneovalgus congenita, Acta Orthop. Scand. **41**:122, 1970.

Abnormalities of toes

Cockin, J.: Butler's operation for an overriding fifth toe, J. Bone Joint Surg. **50B**:78, 1968.

Farmer, A.W.: Congenital hallux varus, Am. J. Surg. **95**:274, 1958.

Frazier, T.M.: A note on race specific congential malformation rates, Am. J. Obstet. Gynecol. **84**:184, 1960.

Kelikian, H.: Hallux valgus, allied deformities of the forefoot and metatarsalgia. Philadelphia, 1965, W.B. Saunders Co., p. 330.

Kelikian, H., Clayton, L., and Loseff, H.: Surgical syndactylia of the toes, Clin. Orthop. **19**:208, 1961.

Kessel, L., and Bonney, G.: Hallux rigidus in the adolescent, J. Bone Joint Surg. **40B**:668, 1958.

Kirtland, L.R., and Russell, R.O.: Polydactyly: report of a large kindred, South Med. J. **69**:436, 1976.

Lapidus, P.W.: Transplantation of the extensor tendon for correction of the overlapping fifth toe, J. Bone Joint Surg. **24**:555, 1942.

Leonard, M.H., and Rising, E.H.: Syndactylization to maintain correction of overlapping 5th toe, Clin. Orthop. **43**:241, 1965.

McElvenny, R.T.: Hallux varus, Q. Bull. Northwestern Univ. Med. Sch. **15**:277, 1941.

McKusick, V.A.: Mendelian inheritance in man: catalogues of autosomal dominant, autosomal recessive, and X-linked phenotypes, ed. 2, Baltimore, 1968, Johns Hopkins Press.

Nathan, P.A., and Keniston, R. C.: Crossed polydactyly: case report and review of the literature, J. Bone Joint Surg. **57A**:847, 1975.

Scrase, W.H.: The treatment of dorsal adduction deformities of the fifth toe, J. Bone Joint Surg. **36B**:146, 1954.

Sharrard, W.J.W.: The surgery of deformed toes in children, Br. J. Clin. Pract. **17**:263, 1963.

Sweetman, R.: Congenital curley toe: an investigation into the value of treatment, Lancet, **2**:398, 1958.

Tachdjian, M.O.: Pediatric orthopaedics, Philadelphia, 1972, W.B. Saunders, Co.

Thompson, S.A.: Hallux varus and metatarsus varus, Clin. Orthop. **16**:109, 1960.

Zimbler, S., Craig. C., Oh, W.H., and Iacono, V.: Exhibit presented at the annual meeting of the American Academy of Orthopaedic Surgeons, Las Vegas, 1977.

Torsional deformities of lower extremity

Engel, G.M., Staheli, L.T.: The natural history of torsion and other factors influencing gait in childhood: a study of the angle of gait, tibial torsion, knee angle, hip rotation and development of the arch in normal children, Clin. Orthop. **99:**12-17, 1974.

Fabray, G., MacEwen, G.D., and Shands, A.R., Jr.: Torsion of the femur. J. Bone Joint Surg. **55A:**1726, 1973.

Hensinger, R.F.: Rotational problems of the lower extremity. Postgrad. Med. **60:**161, 1976.

MacEwen, G.D.: Anteversion of the femur, Postgrad. Med. **60:**154, 1976.

23

Fractures and fracture-dislocations of the ankle

MICHAEL W. CHAPMAN

CRITERIA FOR TREATMENT

For best functional results in the treatment of ankle fractures, particularly those involving joints, four criteria must be filled:

1. *Dislocations and fractures should be reduced as soon a possible.* Fractures are most easily reduced early. Reduction is easier to obtain before swelling occurs and before the fracture hematoma between the fragments organizes. Furthermore, gross displacement—particularly in the ankle, subtalar, and midfoot joints—results in considerable distortion of the soft tissues and can lead to impairment of peripheral circulation, neuropraxias, and loss of skin. Early reduction minimizes these complications.

2. *All joint surfaces must be precisely reconstituted.* Nonanatomic reduction may lead to joint instability and/or joint surface incongruity, which predisposes to arthritis.

3. *Reduction of the fracture must be maintained during the period of healing.* Once anatomic reduction has been achieved, it must be held until healing of bone and ligaments sufficient to probide stability has occurred. This can be accomplished by external immobilization with a plaster cast or splints, by external fixation, or by internal fixation. External immobilization of injured joints has definite deleterious effects. The extent of these undesirable effects is largely dependent on the age of the patient; the older the patient, the more adverse the effects of long-term immobilization. In addition, holding ankle fractures anatomically by external means is difficult, and late loss of reduction in plaster is all too common.

An appreciation of the problems associated with external immobilization has prompted many surgeons, in spite of the possible risk of infection, to employ open reduction, internal fixation, and early mobilization as the treatment of choice.

4. *Motion of joints should be instituted as early as possible.* To maintain itself in a state of health, any organ or organ system must be used. Suppression of the normal functioning of the musculoskeletal system by immobilization of any of its parts is attended by numerous undesirable sequelae—including muscular atrophy, myostatic contracture, decreased joint motion, proliferation of the connective tissue in the capsular structures, internal synovial adhesions, cartilaginous degeneration, and bone atrophy. Furthermore, vascular changes occur during the period of immobilization and these often result in edema after the external support is removed. Early mobilization obviates or decreases the possible occurrence of these abnormal processes.

The most ardent protagonist for early motion after the reduction of fractures was Lucas-Championnière (1910), who based his beliefs on clinical experience. Since that time, experimental evidence has gradually appeared in the medical literature to support his contentions (Salter et al., 1980; Mitchell and Shepard, 1980).

FRACTURE CLASSIFICATION

Many classification systems for fractures and fracture-dislocations about the ankle joint exist, based for the most part, on the mechanism of injury.* Knowledge of a classification system enables the surgeon to offer better treatment through the understanding it provides of

---

*Ashhurst and Bromer, 1922; Bonnin, 1970; Kleiger, 1956; Lauge-Hansen, 1948, 1950, 1952, 1954; Mayer and Pohlidal, 1953.

Table 4. Lauge-Hansen classification of ankle fractures

Type of injury (foot position—direction of force)	Stage	Pathology
Supination—adduction	I	Transverse fracture of lateral malleolus or Torn lateral collateral ligaments
	II	Stage I plus Fracture of medial malleolus
Supination—eversion	I	Rupture (or avulsion fracture) of anterior inferior tibiofibular ligament
	II	Stage I plus Spiral or oblique fracture of lateral malleolus
	III	Stage II plus Fracture of posterior lip of tibia
	IV	Stage III plus Fracture of medial malleolus or tear of deltoid ligament
Pronation—abduction	I	Fracture of medial malleolus or tear of deltoid ligament
	II	Stage I plus Rupture of anterior and posterior ligaments of syndesmosis and fracture of posterior lip of tibia
	III	Stage II plus Oblique fracture of fibula above ankle mortise
Pronation—eversion	I	Fracture of medial malleolus or tear of deltoid ligament
	II	Stage I plus Tear of anterior inferior tibiofibular and interosseous ligament
	III	Stage II plus Tear of interosseous membrane and spiral fracture of fibula, 5 to 6 cm above plafond of tibia
	IV	Stage III plus Avulsion fracture of posterior lip of tibia

the interrelationship between the mechanism of injury and the pathologic anatomy. Occult ligamentous injury will be detected, and the optimal position of the limb in a closed reduction can be determined.

Lauge-Hansen (1948, 1950, 1952, 1954) has provided the most useful and comprehensive classification of ankle injuries; and in spite of the complex variety of ankle fractures, 98% to 99% can be fitted into his system. Most important, he emphasizes the role of the ligaments in these injuries. Students of ankle injuries are strongly advised to read the articles of Lauge-Hansen cited in the reference section.

Table 4 briefly summarizes the Lauge-Hansen classification. The Lauge-Hansen system is quite complex, however, so from a practical point of view one can look at ankle fractures in a more simplified way—as advocated by Jergesen (1959).

When assessing fractures about the ankle within a functional framework, the practitioner should consider two concepts: (1) Anatomic reduction is desirable because the restoration of normal anatomy to a weight-bearing joint is of primary importance. (2) Stability of the ankle is related to the integrity of the malleolar and syndesmosis ligaments.

The foot is securely bound to the leg by two osseous ligamentous shrouds consisting of (on the one side) the medial malleolus and the corresponding medial collateral ligament and (on the other side) the lateral malleolus and the lateral collateral ligaments. In addition, the intermalleolar space is maintained by the tibiofibular syndesmosis ligaments (Fig. 23-1). Any number of fracture and ligamentous disruption combinations can occur that may destroy the normal stability of the ankle. If we speak of the foot in relation to the leg, the basic mechanisms of injury can be thought of as (1) external rotation–eversion or abduction, (2) internal rotation–inversion or adduction, and (3) vertical loading.

Ankle injuries result from abnormal motion of the talus within the ankle mortise. Fractures of the malleoli can result from the impact of the talus on the malleoli. Fractures can also occur in tension, and the malleoli can be avulsed because of the pull exerted by the intact collateral ligaments attached to the talus.

Impact fractures tend to be spiral or oblique. Avulsion fractures tend to be at right angles to the line of pull of the ligament. Ligament failure rather than fracture may occur, so instability in any given injury can be due to a combination of fracture and ligament rup-

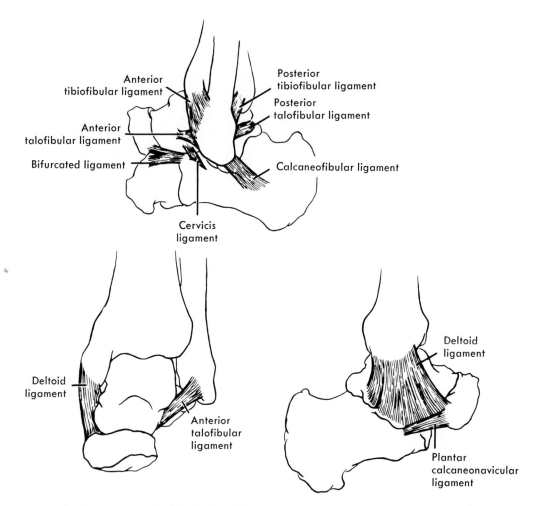

Fig. 23-1. Anatomy of ankle. (From Chapman, M.W.: Sprains of the ankle. In American Academy of Orthopaedic Surgeons Instructional course lectures, vol. 24, St. Louis, 1975, The C.V. Mosby Co.)

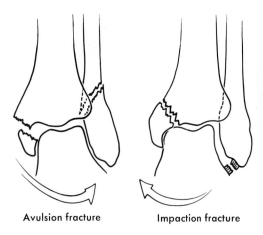

Avulsion fracture   Impaction fracture

Fig. 23-2. Mechanism of injury.

ture. Fig. 23-2 illustrates the difference between these two mechanisms.

Fig. 23-3 is four radiographs showing some of the combinations of injuries seen in external rotation–eversion and abduction-type fractures. The possible varieties of injury include the following:

1. External rotation–eversion and abduction injuries
   a. Medial side
      (1) Transverse avulsion fracture of medial malleolus
      (2) Ruptured deltoid ligament
   b. Lateral side
      (1) Spiral fracture of lateral malleolus with fracture line proceeding from distal anterior to proximal posterior (external rotation)
      (2) Spiral fracture of shaft of fibula above syndesmosis, usually associated with disruption of syndesmosis (external rotation)
      (3) Short oblique fracture of fibula in mediolateral plane below or above syndesmosis, often with

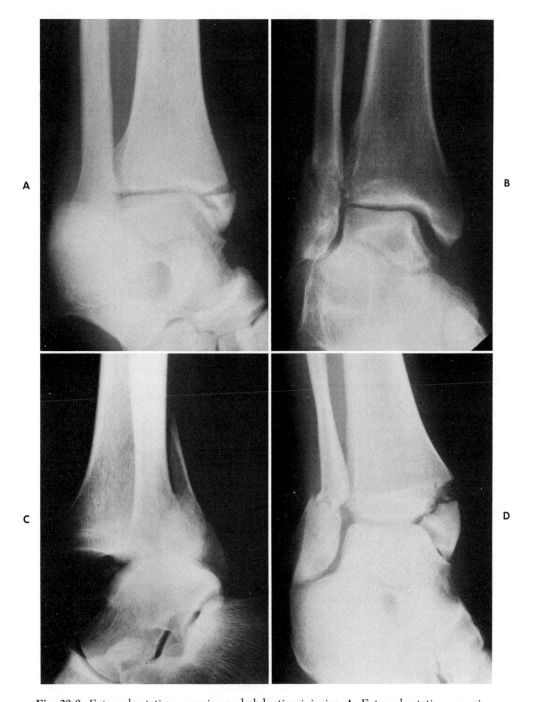

Fig. 23-3. External rotation–eversion and abduction injuries. **A,** External rotation–eversion. Transverse avulsion fracture of medial malleolus. Look for associated syndesmosis ligament ruptures and/or high proximal fracture of fibula. **B,** External rotation–eversion. Short spiral-oblique fracture of lateral malleolus with deltoid ligament rupture. **C,** External rotation–eversion. Spiral fracture of lateral malleolus with avulsion fracture of posterior malleolus. **D,** Abduction. Transverse comminuted fracture of fibula is fairly typical. Avulsion fracture of medial malleolus is usually more transverse.

small lateral butterfly fragment at fracture (abduction)
c. Syndesmosis
(1) Torn anterior tibiofibular ligament (external rotation) through complete syndesmosis rupture (more common abduction mechanism)
(2) Avulsion fracture of posterior malleolus (external rotation)

Fig. 23-4 is a radiograph of an adduction-inversion injury. The possible varieties of such an injury include the following:

2. Adduction-inversion injuries (Fig. 23-4)
a. Medial side
(1) Oblique fracture of medial malleolus extending from corner of ankle mortise proximally and medially
b. Lateral side
(1) Transverse avulsion of lateral malleolus below syndesmosis
(2) Rupture of lateral collateral ligaments
c. Syndesmosis
(1) As part of fibular fracture, torn inferior fibers rare in adduction injuries
d. Posterior malleolus
(1) With posterior medial dislocation, occasional fracture of posterior and medial malleoli

When internal fixation is being considered, the A-O system for classification of ankle fractures is very helpful (Müller, et al., 1979). The A-O system is based on the level of the fibula fracture, as the higher the fracture of the fibula, the more extensive the damage to the syndesmosis ligaments and the more likely that the ankle mortise will be unstable. I will use this system when discussing operative treatment. The three types of fractures are as follows:

Type A

Fibula	Transverse avulsion fracture below or at the level of plafond (or ligament tear)
Medial malleolus	Intact or sheared with fracture angulating upwards from corner of mortise
Posterior tibia	Usually intact, but a medial posterior fracture fragment may be present
Posterior tibia	Usually intact, but a medial posterior fracture fragment may be present
Syndesmosis	Intact
Lauge-Hansen equivalent	Supination-adduction

Type B

Fibula	Spiral fracture beginning at level of plafond and extending proximally
Medial malleolus	Intact or transverse avulsion fracture or rupture of deltoid ligament
Posterior tibia	Intact or avulsion fracture
Syndesmosis	Interosseous ligament intact; anterior and posterior inferior tibiofibular ligaments torn depending on level of fracture and severity of injury
Lauge-Hansen equivalent	Supination-eversion

Type C

Fibula	Fractured above syndesmosis
Medial malleolus	Transverse avulsion fracture or deltoid ligament tear
Posterior tibia	Avulsion fracture can occur
Syndesmosis	Always torn
Lauge-Hansen equivalent	Pronation-eversion

See Fig. 23-5 for illustration of types A, B and C.

Historically, certain ankle fractures have come to be named after the surgeon who originally described them. Before the invention of x-rays, Sir Percivall Pott (1768) described an ankle injury secondary to leaping or jumping that was a transverse fracture of the fibula, 2 to 3 inches above the distal end, associated with a tear of the deltoid ligament and lateral subluxation of the talus.

In 1819, a Frenchman named Dupuytren described a fracture similar to Pott's: a fracture of the fibula about 2½ inches proximal to its tip, accompanied by a rupture of the syndesmosis and either fracture of the medial malleolus or tear of the deltoid ligament. This fracture is a Lauge-Hansen pronation-eversion stage III.

In 1840 Maisonneuve emphasized the importance of external rotation in the etiology of ankle injuries, and his name is associated with a spiral fracture of the fibula that occurs as high as the proximal third.

An avulsion fracture of the tibial origin of the anterior inferior tibiofibular ligament, caused by abduction and external rotation, was described by Tillaux in 1872. A pull-off fracture of the fibular side can also occur.

VERTICAL COMPRESSION FRACTURES

Vertical compression fractures are typically caused by falls from a height or deceleration motor vehicle injuries. The configuration of these fractures is quite variable. The usual fracture is accompanied by hyperdorsiflexion of the ankle, producing a vertical shear fracture of the anterior tibial plafond. This injury is usually accompanied by upward impaction of the tibial plafond, compressing the metaphyseal cancellous bone. With severe compression, an explosion-type fracture occurs in which the malleoli are displaced outward as the talus drives into the central plafond of the tibia (Fig. 23-6).

Lauge-Hansen pointed out that these fractures occur in stages, with the sequence of fractures and ligament ruptures depending on the position of the foot at the

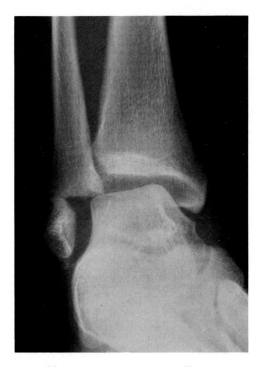

Fig. 23-4. Adduction-inversion injury. Transverse avulsion fracture of lateral malleolus below the level of syndesmosis. Talus is hinging on intact deltoid ligament.

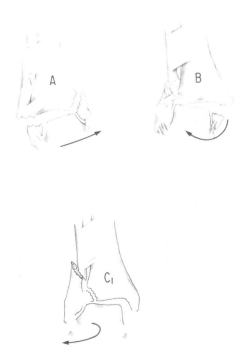

Fig. 23-5. Diagram of A-O system for classification of ankle fractures, based on level of fibular fracture. See text for details.

time of injury. These are also known as tibial plafond (French for "ceiling") fractures. When the fracture involves the metaphysis and distal shaft, it is known as a pilon (French for "rammer" or "hammer") fracture.

The A-O group classifies these into types I, II, and III, according to their severity. Type I fractures are undisplaced, Type II have joint incongruity, and Type III are comminuted with articular displacement and crushing of the cancellous bone of the metaphysis (Fig. 23-7).

Osteochondral fractures of the talus are common and must be searched for diligently in all ankle injuries. These will be discussed in Chapter 24.

Initial evaluation and emergency treatment

History. Most patients are unable to relate the exact mechanism of injury beyond the type of force involved. With a fall from a height or following a motor vehicle deceleration injury, the surgeon should look for occult impaction of the tibial plafond. The patient may describe complete dislocation of the foot on the leg with spontaneous relocation. This history, of course, would indicate a grossly unstable ankle with probable severe associated soft tissue injuries. Pedestrians hit by motor vehicles frequently have unstable adduction or abduc-

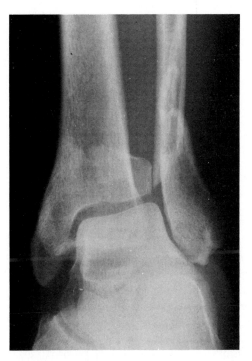

Fig. 23-6. Vertical loading–type fracture of ankle. Fibular shaft is comminuted. Tibial plafond is driven proximally, resulting in crush fracture of cancellous bone of distal tibia.

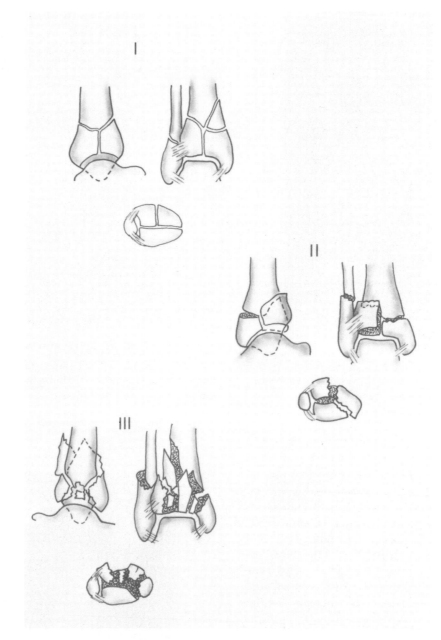

Fig. 23-7. Classification of tibial plafond fractures. *I,* Undisplaced; *II,* joint incongruity; *III,* comminuted with articular displacement and crushing of cancellous bone.

tion fractures. Weight-bearing twisting injuries are usually of the external rotation–eversion type, which makes up about 60% of all ankle fractures (Ashhurst and Bromer, 1922). Knee pain over the head of the fibula may suggest an unstable ankle with a high fibula fracture (Maisonneuve, 1840).

Physical diagnosis. Physical diagnosis is important in determining the degree of soft tissue injury, in ascertaining the presence of ligamentous injuries not evident on radiographic examination by assessing joint stability,

and in determining the neurovascular status of the foot. Radiographs will usually reveal the extent of bony injury. Careful systematic palpation to identify areas of tenderness and swelling will help localize disruptions in the structures about the ankle and the interosseous area; the full length of the fibula should also be examined.

The location of findings, plus crepitus, will usually indicate a fracture. In minor seemingly stable injuries, such as an isolated undisplaced fracture of the lateral

A   B   C

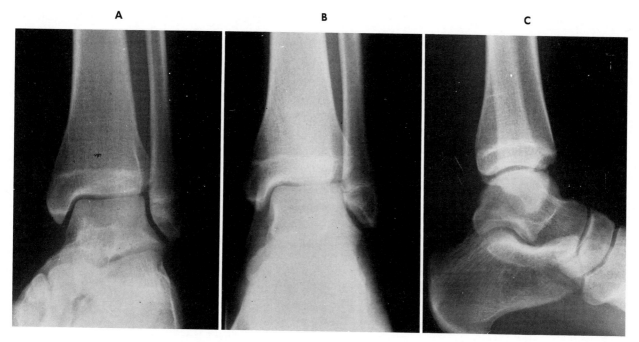

Fig. 23-8. Normal ankle in young adult. **A,** Mortise view (15° to 20° internal rotation).
B, Standard anteroposterior view. **C,** Lateral view.

malleolus, one should look carefully for evidence of deltoid and syndesmosis ligament injury. Stability of the
ankle should be gently tested in varus, valgus, and particularly external rotation. Premedication and local anesthetics may be necessary. Anterior instability of the
talus in the mortise is helpful in detecting unstable ligament injuries. Peroneal muscle spasm may hide lateral
instability. If there is a question in the examiner's
mind, examination with stress radiographs under anesthesia may be indicated. The neurovascular status of
the foot should be carefully assessed. In particular, one
should look for partial or complete common peroneal
nerve paralysis.

Radiographic findings. Anteroposterior, lateral, and
mortise views (the last, an oblique view with the foot
internally rotated 15° to 20°) should be obtained. Fractures involving the plafond may require multiple
oblique projections and biplane tomograms for full de-
lineation. After correlation of the physical examination
findings with the initial radiographic findings, further
assessment of the fracture with evaluation of the integrity of the ankle mortise and the tibiofibular syndesmosis is of paramount importance.

The integrity of the syndesmosis is best assessed on
the AP projection, as is well described by McDade
(1975) (based on Bonnin, 1970), since complete disruption, if undisplaced, will appear normal. The external

rotatory malalignment that occurs when only the anterior inferior tibiofibular ligament is torn is subtle; the
syndesmosis clear space, which represents the posterior
tibiofibular joint, does not change as the fibula rotates
outward. One must look instead at the extent of overlap
of the fibula by the anterior tibial tubercle. Comparison
views are often necessary because there is considerable
anatomic variation (Fig. 23-8).

On a good mortise view the superior articular surface
of the talus should be fully congruous with the tibial
plafond. The medial and lateral joint spaces should be
equal and comparable to the superior joint space. A line
extending distally from the posterior syndesmosis of the
tibia should pass lateral to the talus (*a-a* in Fig. 23-9).
On lateral views the talar dome should be concentric
with the tibial plafond (*b-b*).

Emergency treatment. Excessive swelling can so
compromise treatment of even minor ankle sprains that
patients should all have their lower extremities elevated
higher than their heart while undergoing initial evaluation and treatment. This usually requires that they be
placed on a gurney.

Wounds and abrasions should be cleansed and
dressed. A soft compression dressing and radiolucent
long leg splint should be applied before radiographic
examination.

Grossly distorted ankles with severe skin distortion

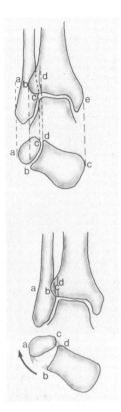

Fig. 23-9. Diagram of anteroposterior projection of ankle joint. *a*, Lateral border of lateral malleolus. *b*, Lateral border of anterior tibia. *c*, Medial border of fibula. *d*, Lateral border of posterior tibia. Rupture of anterior syndesmosis with external rotation of fibula does not affect apparent width of syndesmosis, *c-d*, or intermalleolar distance, *a-e*. However, amount of overlap of anterior tibia on fibula, distance *a-b*, and distance *b-c*, change. Distance *a-b* increases and *b-c* decreases. In most ankles, distance *b-c* is over 50% of *a-c* on anteroposterior projection. Comparison radiographs of normal ankle are very helpful.

should be reduced immediately in the emergency room to avoid skin necrosis and also to eliminate tension on the neurovascular structures.

Treatment

Soft tissue considerations. Whether treatment of these fractures is by closed or open reduction, ultimate success depends on proper assessment and management of the associated soft tissue trauma.

Abrasions should be carefully cleansed and sterily dressed. Abrasions into the dermis quickly become colonized by skin bacteria; therefore any surgery planned should be done within a few hours. After 12 to 24 hours, depending on how dirty it is, a deep abrasion may contraindicate surgery for 3 weeks or more. Ne-

glected abrasions can lead to local cellulitis with possible infection of the fracture hematoma.

Early closed reduction and elevation with a good compression dressing and splints or a cast are important to preventing edema. Ankle and foot edema can be severe, causing fracture blisters. Gross edema may contraindicate surgery and lead to loss of the initial closed reduction. Surgeons should avoid early surgery on the tensely swollen shiny-skinned "watermelon" ankle, since skin closure may be impossible and marginal wound necrosis can occur.

One should always be alert for a compartment syndrome in the leg and foot. The physical findings that should alert the clinician are tenseness in the calf, leg pain with passive stretch of the muscles, and paresis of the deep peroneal nerve.

Closed versus open treatment. Undisplaced fractures without disruption of the ankle mortise are treated with cast immobilization. Undisplaced stable fractures of the lateral malleolus and distal medial malleolus can begin immediate weight bearing in a short leg walking cast, which should be left in place for 6 weeks. Other stable injuries should be placed in a long leg cast with the knee flexed 15°. The cast must be molded to assure the maintenance of position. Weekly radiographs for at least 4 weeks are usually necessary to ensure that these fractures do not displace. Depending on the surgeon's judgment about the stability of the ankle, weight bearing can begin in either a short or a long leg cast at 4 or 6 weeks. Any fracture, whether treated closed or open, if treated in a non-weight-bearing cast, will rehabilitate more quickly and easily if given 2 weeks in a short leg walking cast before complete cast removal.

Displaced fractures or fracture-dislocations may be treated by closed reduction and cast immobilization or by open reduction and internal fixation. Open reduction and internal fixation are almost always indicated if anatomic reduction cannot be achieved. If anatomic reduction is achieved closed, it is often impossible to maintain and late displacement is frequent.

In deciding whether to accept any displacement in an ankle fracture it is important to appreciate the effects of minor displacements on the congruity of the ankle mortise. Ramsey and Hamilton (1976) showed that a 1 mm lateral shift of the talus in the mortise reduces the contact area of the ankle joint 42%. Yablon et al. (1977) showed that the talus faithfully follows the lateral malleolus. Therefore in active individuals virtually no displacement in a fracture of the lateral malleolus is acceptable. In closed treatment interposition of the periosteum or other soft tissues, particularly when the medial malleolus is fractured, can prevent good fracture apposition and thereby lead to nonunion or fibrous union.

Open reduction and internal fixation are generally indicated if ankle fractures are displaced, particularly if the talus is subluxated in the ankle mortise. Closed treatment of displaced fractures may be indicated when (1) the condition of the soft tissues contraindicates surgery, (2) the patient is nonambulatory (paraplegic), (3) the patient is elderly and sedentary, and (4) the patient has sustained multiple trauma and surgery is contraindicated.

Closed reduction

External rotation–eversion and abduction. The mechanisms of these injuries are accompanied by posterolateral subluxation or dislocation of the foot on the leg; the foot is usually externally rotated with reference to the leg. For reduction to be achieved, the foot must be brought anteriorly and medially and internally rotated on the tibia.

The malleoli are attached to the foot by the collateral ligaments; the "distal fragment" is, in reality, the foot with the attached malleoli. Hence reduction entails regaining the proper relationship of the foot to the tibia. If the deltoid ligament rather than the medial malleolus is disrupted or if the medial malleolar fragment is small, a shoulder or buttress exists medially against which the foot (talus) can be reduced. If the medial malleolar fragment is large, internal fixation of the medial malleolus may be necessary to achieve stability of the joint.

A convenient way to carry out manipulative reduction, if an assistant is available, is to flex the patient's hip and knee approximately 30° to allow the extremity to rotate externally approximately 30°. The assistant holds the limb in this position by supporting the thigh with one hand and holding the first two toes with the other hand, thereby maintaining the foot in a vertical plane. Gravity produces medial and anterior replacement of the foot; and with the foot held in a vertical position, an attitude of internal rotation of the foot relative to the leg is achieved. A cast employing the principles of three-point molding can then be applied. The knee should be flexed only 15° in the cast. Rotational control is gained through molding rather than knee flexion. These principles are embodied in the cast shown in Fig. 23-10.

Adduction-inversion mechanisms. In adduction-inversion injuries the reverse of the maneuvers described for the abduction–external rotation injury is required. There is less often a lateral buttress against which to reduce the joint, and the medial malleolar fracture line frequently runs proximally from the level of the joint.

Anterior lip fractures. It is difficult to avoid anterior subluxation in this injury when the patient is recumbent with his limb supported in the usual fashion at the foot and knee. Again the force of gravity can be used to assist the surgeon in reducing the fracture.

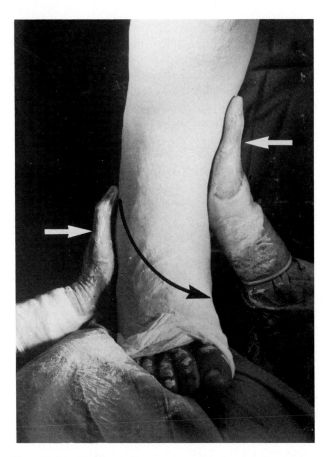

Fig. 23-10. Molding of cast to reduce external rotation-eversion type injury.

Suspend the leg over the end of the treatment table, where an assistant can carry out a posterior thrust of the foot against the leg. Or, more simply, have the patient lie prone on the table with his knee on the injured side flexed approximately 60°. An assistant supports the foot in this position, which permits the weight of the leg against the supported foot to reduce the subluxation. Reduction is maintained in this position while the surgeon applies the cast.

Vertical compression fractures. In stable impacted fractures with minimal displacement, immobilization in a neutral position with careful molding of the cast about the malleoli usually suffices. Unstable comminuted fractures present unique problems (p. 579).

Open reduction with internal fixation—indications and philosophy

Fractures of one malleolus. A fracture of one malleolus without involvement of its ligamentous component or the opposite malleolus permits using the uninjured side as a buttress to immobilize the part until healing takes place (Fig. 23-2). If only the malleolar tip is injured, simple protection from forced inversion (in the case of a lateral malleolus) or eversion (in the case of a lateral malleolus) or eversion (in the case of a medial malleolus) suffices. These are actually third-degree sprains with a small bone chip attached to the fragment.

Radiographic evidence of fracture of just one malleolus does not guarantee stability; therefore clinical evaluation of the ligamentous structures at the distal tibiofibular junction and on the opposite side of the ankle is necessary to assess the stability of the injury.

Except for avulsion fracture of the lateral malleolar tip, the most common isolated fracture of the lateral malleolus is a spiral fracture in the distal portion. Controversy exists over the indications for open reduction of these fractures. If the patient is young or middle aged, inability to achieve and hold an anatomic reduction is the indication for surgery.

What is a satisfactory reduction? Since the talus follows the lateral malleolus even in the presence of an intact deltoid ligament, small persistent displacement of the fracture can lead to talotibial incongruity. For this reason, assuming that the talus is anatomically reduced in the ankle mortise, I would accept 0.5 mm or less of shortening or widening. One millimeter or more of displacement is an indication for open reduction if the patient's age, activity level, etc., justify surgery.

Isolated fractures of the lateral malleolus per se are seldom associated with nonunion, although small avulsed fragments frequently do not unite.

Fractures of the medial malleolus, particularly those occurring below the level of the superior surface of the talus, may be asymptomatic even though they heal with fibrous union. Portis and Mendelsohn (1953) and Aufranc (1960) found little evidence to suggest that the isolated malleolar fracture, if not displaced, requires internal fixation. Fractures of the medial malleolus at the level of the plafond, however, result in complete functional loss of internal support provided by the medial collateral ligament. This fracture must be accurately reduced and internally fixed for the ankle to regain stability.

Bimalleolar fractures and fracture-dislocations. The terms bimalleolar fracture and fracture-dislocation are used to describe fractures of both malleoli, fractures of one malleolus plus complete disruption of the ligament on the opposite side, or fracture of the medial malleolus and rupture of the tibiofibular ligaments (Glick, 1964) associated with a fracture in the shaft of the fibula proximal to the tibiofibular ligament (Fig. 23-3).

Fibular fracture can occur at the proximal end of the fibula. If such a fracture is accompanied by ankle injury, one can assume that some disruption of the interosseous membrane has occurred anywhere from the distal tibiofibular syndesmosis to the level of the fibular fracture and that division of the distal tibiofibular liga-

ments has also taken place. Occasionally the injury will be manifested as a rupture of the deltoid ligament, with the line of dehiscence passing across the ankle capsule and continuing upward through the distal tibiofibular ligaments and interosseous membrane to the level of the proximal neck of the fibula. This particular combination is easy for the unwary examiner to miss, since the ankle may be relocated when the technician positions it for radiographic examination. No fracture will be seen unless a full-length radiograph of the leg, including the upper end of the fibula, is taken.

Traditional teaching in English and American orthopaedics has held that with bimalleolar fractures, the majority of which are external rotation injuries, the key to reduction and stability of the ankle mortise is the medial malleolus. Fixation of the lateral side was not believed necessary because of the intact periosteal hinge (Charnley, 1963). This is now known to be not wholly true. McDade (1975) and Yablon et al. (1977) have emphasized the key role of the lateral malleolus in determining the position of the talus in the mortise. With an intact medial osseous ligamentous bridge, subluxation of the talus in the presence of an external rotation fracture of the lateral malleolus can occur. Because the talus faithfully follows the lateral malleolus, anatomic reduction of the lateral malleolus is a must in bimalleolar fractures. Yablon et al. (1977) found that degenerative arthritis following displaced bimalleolar fractures is usually caused by incomplete reduction of the lateral malleolus with residual talar tilt.

Reduction of the lateral malleolus can be difficult. Fixation of the medial side first may lock the distal lateral malleolar fragment behind the shaft and prevent reduction. It is best to open both sides simultaneously, inspect and cleanse the joint space and fracture site(s) of debris, and reduce and then fix either the lateral side first or the medial side.

Trimalleolar fractures and fracture-dislocations. Trimalleolar fractures and fracture-dislocations include all the combinations described for bimalleolar types of fracture and dislocation plus fractures of the posterior lip of the tibia.

The fragment may vary in size and may communicate with the medial malleolar fragment; or, if it is laterally placed, it may carry the posterior tibiofibular ligament with it. If the fragment carries one fourth or more of the articular surface of the tibia with it, a high risk of posterior subluxation of the talus exists unless the fracture is internally fixed (Fig. 23-3).

Fortunately most posterior lip fragments are small and do not, in themselves, compromise the stability of the ankle (Aufranc, 1960). In ankles with a posterior fragment involving more than 25% of the articular surface, open treatment is associated with better results than closed treatment (McDaniel and Wilson, 1977).

Fractures of anterior lip of distal tibia. Fracture of the anterior lip of the distal tibia may accompany malleolar fracture as a mirror image of the posterior trimalleolar fracture-dislocation; occasionally it occurs as an isolated injury.

It is generally the result of a vertical loading injury and therefore is not usually associated with fracture of the fibular shaft or disruption of the distal tibiofibular ligaments. The anterior lip of the tibia is more often comminuted than is the posterior lip; thus internal fixation techniques may be compromised.

Open reduction and fixation are indicated when the fracture is large enough to cause talar instability (25% to 35% of the articular surface) or is a component of a comminuted fracture that is amenable to open reduction.

Occasionally a rupture of the anterior inferior tibiofibular ligament manifests itself as an avulsion fracture from the fibula or tibia. The avulsion feature from the tibia is most common and is known as a Tillaux fracture (see C-1 fracture in Fig. 23-4). If displaced, this fracture should be internally fixed with a 4.0 cancellous bone screw to stabilize the mortise.

Fractures with severe comminution and instability. It may not be possible to reduce and internally fix severely comminuted fractures of the ankle. Such injuries can be managed with external skeletal traction through the calcaneus or application of an external fixator from the tibia to the foot.

Early motion in these fractures is important to preserve ankle function and help mold the fracture surfaces. This can be achieved by performing a closed reduction with a Steinmann traction pin in the os calcis and then applying a bulky dressing or Delbet cast and placing the limb in traction on a Böhler-Braun frame. The traction will help maintain the reduction, and ankle motion can begin.

Occasionally both comminution and a complex-compound wound about the ankle create a situation in which it is impossible to employ the usual methods of malleolar fixation; yet to assure the survival of the foot and permit management of the surrounding soft tissue, stability must be achieved. In this situation the technique of driving a vertical Steinmann pin through the calcaneus and the talus into the distal tibia (Fig. 23-11) can be used to preserve the foot (Dieterlé, 1935; Childress, 1965). Because the Steinmann pin transgresses normal articular surfaces, I prefer to immobilize these fractures with an external fixator. The fixator is more versatile in that the position can be adjusted, better fixation is obtained, and conversion to a system that permits early motion is easy. A triangular frame is used with two or three pins in the tibia, one in the talus or

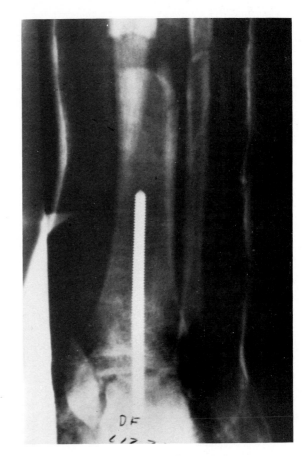

Fig. 23-11. Vertical Steinmann pin.

calcaneus, and one or two in the first metatarsal. This maintains a plantigrade foot (see Fig. 23-12).

Fractures of lateral malleolus with posterior displacement of proximal fibular fragment. Bosworth (1947), Fleming and Smith (1954), and Meyers (1957) all described bimalleolar types of fracture accompanied by displacement of the proximal fibula at the fracture site posteriorly on the tibia in a position that usually makes reduction by closed manipulation impossible. The ligamentous support of the syndesmosis apparently remains intact and holds the fibula in its dislocated position. In these types of fracture, open reduction is necessary and a posterolateral approach is appropriate (Figs. 23-13 and 23-14).

Open fractures and fracture-dislocations of ankle. The same principles of meticulous debridement, copious irrigation, and use of systemic and local bactericidal antibiotics apply to open fractures of the ankle as apply to open fractures and injuries elsewhere in the body.

Wounds in this area almost always communicate with the ankle joint. The ankle joint must be explored. Although not essential, the ankle joint capsule is usually closed primarily; if this is done, a suction tube should be left in place to permit drainage. Joint closure, as

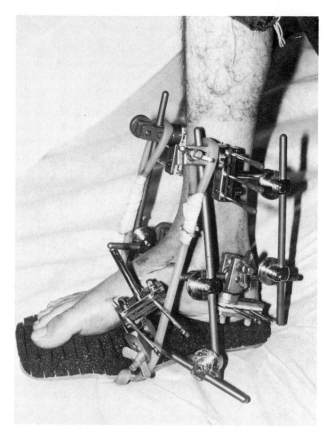

Fig. 23-12. Immobilization of severly comminuted fracture using external fixator.

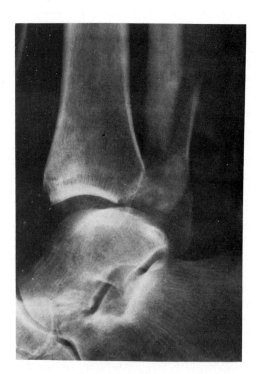

Fig. 23-13. Bosworth fracture with characteristic posterior displacement of proximal fibula.

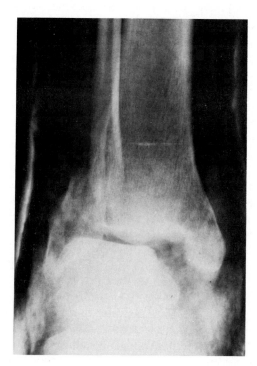

Fig. 23-14. Anteroposterior view of ankle mortise in Fig. 23-13 showing lateral subluxation of talus.

either a primary or a delayed primary procedure, is essential (Jergesen, 1959). The skin wound can be closed by primary closure, delayed primary closure, or secondary closure—depending on the degree of soft tissue damage and contamination and on the amount of elapsed time since occurrence of the injury. The safest procedure, however, is to leave the wound above the joint capsule open and carry out a delayed primary closure.

Infection is the major complication to be avoided and can be related directly to the type of wound. Gustilo and Anderson (1976) classified wounds as type I, II, or III, with type I being a wound less than 1 cm long and clean and type III having extensive soft tissue damage. In their review of open fractures Chapman and Mahoney (1977) noted that 60% of open ankle injuries had type I wounds and only 10% had type III wounds. In their series of open fractures in which immediate fixation was achieved, the infection rate in type I wounds was 2%, in type II wounds 8%, and in type III wounds 29%. This is significant insofar as it means that immediate internal fixation of ankles with type I wounds can be performed without an infection rate greater than seen in closed fractures. The risk of infection in type II and type III wounds is substantial.

In the most commonly seen open fracture-dislocation about the ankle, a transverse wound occurs at the level of the medial malleolus centered on the medial side of the leg. The foot is dislocated posterolaterally; frequently the proximal surface of the avulsed medial malleolus and the articular surface of the tibia appear in the wound. In these injuries the wound is so close to the surface of the fracture and to the joint that rigid internal fixation is necessary to protect the overlying soft tissues from pressure and recurrent tension. Since the open wound lies directly over the medial malleolus, internal fixation of the medial malleolar side can usually be accomplished with one or two screws; little if any additional dissection is necessary after the wound has been debrided and irrigated and the dislocation has been reduced.

It is unlikely that the minimal surgery required to place a medial malleolar screw will increase the risk of infection; and, in fact, the opposite may be true, since the stability achieved allows optimal treatment of the soft tissues. Again, by way of emphasis, the wounds should be closed by delayed primary closure (Fig. 23-15).

Repair of ligament ruptures. Ligamentous injuries associated with fractures are the subject of controversy in the literature and are discussed in more detail in Chapter 20.

The primary indication for repair is ligament interposition in the joint space, where exploration is necessary to achieve anatomic reduction (Coonrad and Bugg,

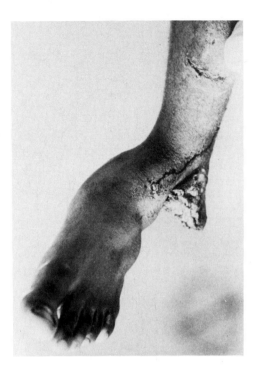

Fig. 23-15. Typical open fracture of ankle.

1954). Ruptured lateral collateral ligaments accompanying a fracture are almost always repaired. The ligaments of the tibiofibular syndesmosis usually require stabilization. Direct repair is rarely possible. Stabilization of the lateral malleolus often is sufficient; if not, a syndesmosis screw is placed. Deltoid ligament ruptures accompanying lateral fractures do not have to be repaired if joint congruity is achieved. If early mobilization, free of plaster, is planned, repair may be necessary to achieve adequate stability.

Often repair of the ligaments will be done incidental to exploration of the ankle joint on the nonfractured side to effect debridement and to look for osteochondral fractures of the talus.

Surgical technique

Early surgery is usually best for optimal results. It is best carried out on the day of injury, before edema occurs. Open reduction within 7 days of injury is little different from that achieved on the day of injury. Between 7 and 14 days, the hematoma organizes and extensive debriding of the fracture fragments is necessary to achieve reduction; anatomic reduction can usually be achieved, however. Between 14 and 21 days, callus formation, soft tissue scarring, resorption, and osteoporosis of the fractured bone ends create technical problems that compromise reduction. After 21 days, anatomic reduction is frequently impossible to achieve and closed treatment may be indicated.

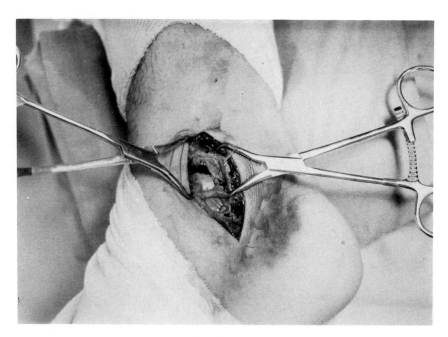

Fig. 23-16. A-O bone forceps to hold fracture.

Bivalving of the cast and surgical preparation of the skin the evening before surgery are unwise, for an accidental nick of the skin may necessitate postponement of surgery.

Unless contraindicated, a tourniquet should be employed. Unexpected comminution is often encountered, so the surgeon should have a full armamentarium of bone instruments and fixation devices available. In addition to screws, Kirschner wires, small fragment screws, small plates, malleable wire, Steinmann pins, and Rush rods or Knowles pins may be useful. One should be prepared to take an iliac bone graft in vertical compression fractures.

Medial malleolus. The skin incision should be vertical, parallel with the long axis of the tibia, and placed directly over the malleolus. Dissection is carried sharply to bone, and any undermining necessary should take place just above the periosteum. The incision must be long enough to offer good exposure without excessive retraction. It has the advantages of being extensile, being optimally located for the insertion of a screw, and avoiding significant undermining or flaps. I have never had a patient complain of a tender scar in this location. The J-shaped incision posterior or anterior and distal to the malleolus has the disadvantages of not being easily extended distally, therefore frequently compromising the exposure needed for screw insertion, and requiring undermining (which leads to an increased incidence of marginal wound slough).

1. Elevate the periosteum from the edges of the fracture line for a distance of 2 to 3 mm with a no. 15 scalpel blade used edge on. The full anterior and posterior extents of the fracture must be seen to assure accurate reduction.

2. Lightly curette and irrigate the fracture surfaces to remove all organized hematoma.

3. Explore the joint through the fracture site to detect occult chondral and osteochondral fractures of the talus and to debride and irrigate the joint as needed.

4. Anatomically reduce the fracture by grasping the malleolus transversely in a towel clip and guiding it into place with a periosteal elevator in the other hand. The reduction should be securely maintained by mechanical means while the internal fixation is inserted. The best method I have found is to use two A-O towel clip–type bone clamps or two towel clips across the fracture at its anterior and posterior borders. The towel clips are held with 4 × 8s tied through their handles (Fig. 23-16). A Bishop clamp can also be used, but I find them heavy, and they often interfere with hardware placement. The towel clip method does not interfere with hardware placement, and the clamps prevent slippage of the fracture.

5. The best fixation is obtained with two 4 mm cancellous bone screws. A pointed drill guide is used to place two 2 mm Kirschner wires from the tip of the malleolus at right angles to the plane of the fracture and as vertically as possible (Fig. 23-17, A). Each Kirschner wire is then removed and replaced with a 4 mm cancellous bone screw (Fig. 23-17, B).

Alternative fixation can be obtained with a 4.5 mm malleolar screw. The screw should enter the distal tip

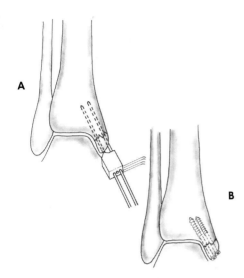

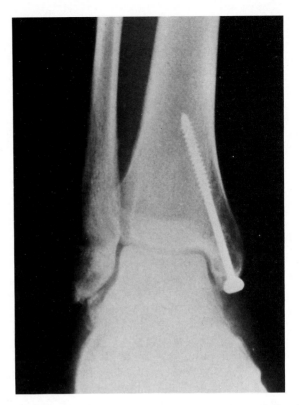

Fig. 23-17. **A,** Double fixation with two 2 mm Kirschner wires. These can be placed in the vertical or horizontal plane, depending on configuration of fracture. Pointed drill guides assure parallelism of wires. **B,** Replacement of Kirschner wires with two 4 mm cancellous screws.

Fig. 23-18. A-O malleolar screw fixing fracture of medial malleolus employing principle of lag fixation.

of the malleolus; otherwise, communication may occur and the screw head will be too prominent. The malleolar screws provided in the A-O equipment (*Arbeitsgemeinschaft für Osteosynthese,* Swiss association for study of internal fixation) are ideal although lag technique can be used with a standard bone screw (Fig. 23-18). Small or comminuted fragments not amenable to screw fixation are best fixed with two or more Kirschner wires (Fig. 23-19). I have had no experience with the Zuelzer hood plate (Zuelzer, 1958). Vertical adduction–type fractures tend to slip with a single screw. Fixation with two Kirschner wires as illustrated in Fig. 23-19 before insertion of the screw will prevent displacement.

Very small fragments may be excised, and a repair of the deltoid ligament to a drill hole in the malleolus can be effected.

Lateral malleolus. The same principles of incision and exposure described for the medial malleolus are applicable to the lateral malleolus. If syndesmosis repair is anticipated, the incision should be somewhat anterior; and if fixation of the posterior malleolus through the same incision is planned, the incision should be placed somewhat posterior.

The configuration of the fracture determines the type of fixation to be employed. Ideal fixation provides interfragmentary compression and rotational control. Oblique and spiral fractures whose lengths are greater than one and one half times the diameter of the bone at the level of the fracture are best fixed with interfragmentary lag screws.

Neutralization of the forces across the fracture should

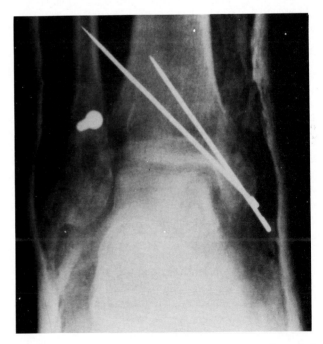

Fig. 23-19. Kirschner wire fixation of comminuted medial malleolar fracture. Note that one wire was left excessively long.

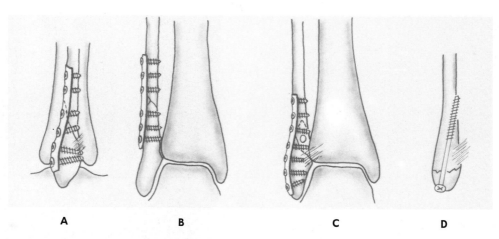

Fig. 23-20. A, Lateral views showing posterior plate applied with spiral fracture just above syndesmosis. Note interfragmentary lag screw through plate. **B,** Lateral plate for fracture of fibular shaft. **C,** Lateral plate used as buttress plus anteroposterior lag screw for fixation of oblique fracture at syndesmosis. **D,** Single malleolar screw used to fix transverse avulsion-type fracture below syndesmosis.

always be accomplished. A one-third tubular plate applied to the lateral border of the fibula is sufficient. Ideally, five cortexes of fixation above and below the fracture should be obtained. If a lateral plate is used and the fracture is at the syndesmosis, only unicortical screws will be possible in the distal fragment, and the plate will serve as a buttress.

This configuration of an anteroposterior interfragmentary screw and lateral plate provides biplanar fixation. The plate can be placed anteriorly or posteriorly, and the interfragmentary lag screw can then be placed through the plate. This is technically more difficult, however. Often the interfragmentary lag screw must be placed through a separate anterior stab wound.

For the interfragmentary screw, I prefer to use a 3.5 mm cortical screw with overdrilling of the near cortex. If comminution is a problem, then a 4.0 mm cancellous screw can be used. The best plate is a one-third tubular bent to fit the malleolus and fixed with 3.5 or 4.0 mm screws. Fig. 23-20 shows a suggested configuration of fixation for various fractures of the lateral malleolus and fibula. Fig. 23-21 is a radiograph of similar fixation for a fracture of the shaft of the fibula. The empty screw holes were not filled because of comminution.

I no longer use interfragmentary fixation with Rush rods or Steinmann pins, as they offer poor rotational control, and in oblique fractures shortening may occur.

The A-O tension-band wire technique is useful for transverse fractures at or below the syndesmosis and comminuted fractures (Fig. 23-22).

Posterior malleolus. Injuries to the posterior malleolus are usually posterolateral and are best fixed through a posterolateral approach with the patient prone. The

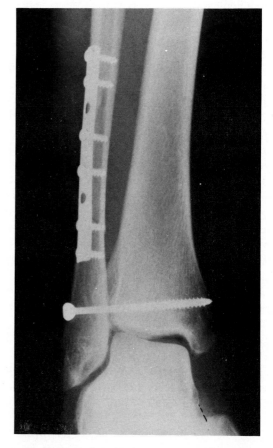

Fig. 23-21. Plate fixation of fracture of fibula.

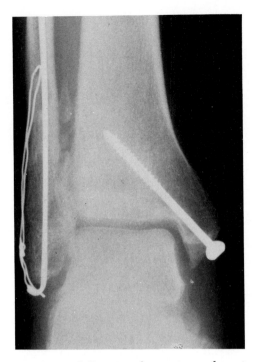

Fig. 23-22. Intramedullary Kirschner wires and tension band figure-eight wire used to fix fracture of lateral malleolus.

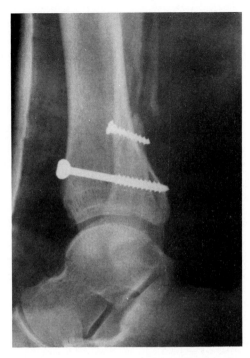

Fig. 23-23. Fracture of posterior malleolus fixed with interfragmentary malleolar screw placed through anterior stab wound. Before comminution there is a small defect in articular surface of tibial plafond.

lateral and medial malleoli can easily be repaired with the patient prone. Preoperative radiographs should be carefully assessed. Occasionally a posterior malleolar fracture is an extension of a medial malleolar fracture and should be approached medially.

Because of limited exposure, posterior malleolar fractures can be difficult to internally fix. Since the intraarticular component of the fracture cannot be seen when reduced, the entire extraarticular portion of the fracture should be visualized to ensure the accuracy of reduction. Fixation with two Kirschner wires while the malleolus is held in place ensures that reduction will not be lost during screw placement. To guarantee optimal closure of the intraarticular component, the screw should be at right angles to the fracture and just above the tibial plafond.

If the screw cannot easily be placed from posterior to anterior, it can be placed from anterior to posterior through a small stab wound (Fig. 23-23).

Syndesmosis separations. Syndesmosis separations that are unstable should be stabilized. Occasionally stabilization of an associated fibular fracture provides adequate stability, and fixation across the syndesmosis can be avoided. With fibular fractures above a syndesmosis separation, some surgeons elect to treat only the syndesmosis separation. This is acceptable; but great care must be exercised to avoid residual external rotational

deformity of the distal fragment and avoid overtightening the syndesmosis screw, which can produce a valgus malposition of the lateral malleolus. Proximal migration of the lateral malleolus should be avoided by making certain that shortening at the fracture site has not occurred. It is usually best to stabilize the fibula first and then the syndesmosis. I always plate the fibula.

When transfixing the syndesmosis, the surgeon should take care to ensure that the fibula is reduced posteriorly into the tibial sulcus. Fixation is obtained with a screw (Fig. 23-24). Fully threaded screws are best, as they avoid overreduction of the syndesmosis. The syndesmosis must be properly reduced when the screws are inserted, however. A malleolar screw can also be used, but with the lag effect possible, one must avoid overtightening the syndesmosis. The screw is best inserted at right angles to the distal tibiofibular joint, passing from the posterolateral border of the fibula anteromedially into the tibia.

These screws must be removed at 6 weeks in most patients before unprotected weight bearing is allowed, because the dynamic function of the fibula (McMaster and Scranton, 1975; Scranton et al., 1976) may lead to screw fracture.

Tibial pilon (plafond) fractures. A comminuted fracture of the ankle is usually caused by vertical loading that produces compression of the cancellous bone above

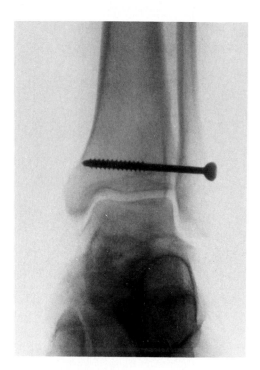

Fig. 23-24. Syndesmosis rupture fixed with malleolar screw.

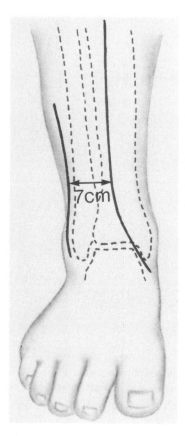

Fig. 23-25. Preferred incisions for operating on comminuted fractures of distal tibia and fibula. Lateral incision is over mid-lateral border of fibula. Avoid injury to superficial peroneal nerve. Tibia is approached anteriorly. Incision swings medially as one proceeds distally. Seven centimeters should separate the two incisions.

the tibial plafond. An unstable fracture of the distal shafts of the tibia and fibula may be associated. See Fig. 23-7. Because the degree of comminution and the poor condition of the soft tissues make internal fixation impossible, closed treatment may be indicated. The surgeon must weigh the goals of surgery against such risks as increased soft tissue trauma from multiple or larger incisions and the ill effects of prolonged surgery. Some advocate restoration of the joint surfaces and treatment of the remainder of the fracture with a cast. This is the worst of all possible choices, however, as one has taken th risk of surgery, not achieved sufficient stability for early motion, and subjected an intraarticular fracture to surgery and prolonged immobilization.

In this fracture the best results will be achieved with restoration of the normal anatomy, stabilization, and early motion to restore joint physiology.

Müller et al. (1979) advocate total reconstruction of comminuted fractures with multiple fixation devices, including large buttress plates, to stabilize the shaft component and permit early mobilization in the absence of external fixation. This type of reconstruction is usually possible only with A-O type of equipment. The procedures are difficult and should be undertaken only by surgeons who are intimately familiar with the method and do more than an occasional fracture of this type. To avoid the complications of wound sloughing and infection, the surgeon's soft tissue technique must be atraumatic and meticulous.

The preferable skin incisions are depicted in Fig. 23-25. The anterior incision exploits the interval between the anterior tibial tendon and extensor hallucis longus. Flaps are developed at the level of the periosteum. The periosteum must be left attached to the anterior fragment, which can easily be opened like a book to reveal the central comminution of posterior fragments.

Although not as versatile as the direct anterior approach, the transfibular approach can be used when the fibula is fractured and the syndesmosis ruptured (Wiggins, 1975). Bone graft is usually required, and most commonly I remove it through a small window in the proximal tibia. Iliac crest bone can also be used.

The steps in reconstructing a comminuted pilon fracture of the tibia with an associated fracture of the fibula are as follows.

1. The fibula is brought out to length and internally fixed with a plate and screws. This restores normal length to the tibia fracture and reveals the extent of communication and crush of cancellous bone (Fig. 23-26).

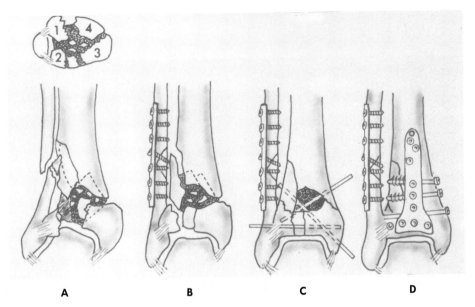

Fig. 23-26. Steps in reconstruction of typical pilon fracture.

2. The tibia fracture is exposed and reduced. Typically the plafond is in four pieces with some central comminution, as depicted in Fig. 23-26, *A*. Because of interlocking, often all four major fragments must be reduced and temporarily fixed with Kirschner wires or screws (Fig. 23-26, *C*). The goal is to reassemble the fracture into a main distal and proximal fragment, which can then be brought together. The talus can be used as a template against which the tibia is reconstructed. Before the plate and screws are applied, defects are filled with bone graft.

3. The Kirschner wires are then replaced with screws and a buttress plate. In Fig. 23-26, *D*, the use of an anterior spoon plate is depicted. A T-plate or medial cloverleaf plate can also be used, depending on the configuration of the fracture. An example of the complex reconstruction often required is shown in Fig. 23-27.

The wounds are then closed. Tension must be avoided. If necessary a deep layer can be closed, the skin left open, and a delayed closure carried out.

Postoperative care. In the immediate postoperative period the most frequent problem is swelling, which can be controlled by bed rest and elevation. I do not use casts postoperatively, as the fractures are stable after fixation. In the vast majority of cases, a shortleg Robert Jones dressing with splints can be used. If a cast is used, it should be routinely univalved anteriorly and spread.

Fractures that are unstable after fixation usually require a long leg non-weight-bearing cast for 6 weeks followed by 2 weeks in a short leg walking cast.

Stable fractures can be treated according to the need for early joint mobilization and the surgeon's confidence in his repair.

In their series of patients in whom a stable situation was produced at the time of internal fixation, Burwell and Charnley (1965) described a minor modification of the usual postoperative care for internal fixation of ankle fractures. In the early postoperative period, the injured limb was removed from the protective plaster cast for active non-weight-bearing exercise and a long leg cast was replaced by a short leg plaster cast. The authors reported an early recovery of maximum range of motion in patients thus treated.

In most cases I keep the Robert Jones dressing in place for 1 week. I then apply a brace or bivalved short leg cast and begin supervised dorsiflexion and plantar flexion exercises. To avoid an equinus contracture, a splint must be in place when the patient is not exercising. This can be removed when the patient can actively dorsiflex within 5° of the normal side. Unprotected weight bearing is delayed until 8 weeks and in pilon fractures until 12 weeks or longer if required for union.

EPIPHYSEAL INJURIES OF ANKLE IN CHILDREN

Ankle fractures are less common in children than adults. The ligaments are stronger than the physeal plates, so ligament tears are uncommon and epiphyseal injuries are more common. The physeal plates are zones of weakness that produce fracture patterns different from those seen in adults. Growth disturbances from fractures about the ankle are common, and there

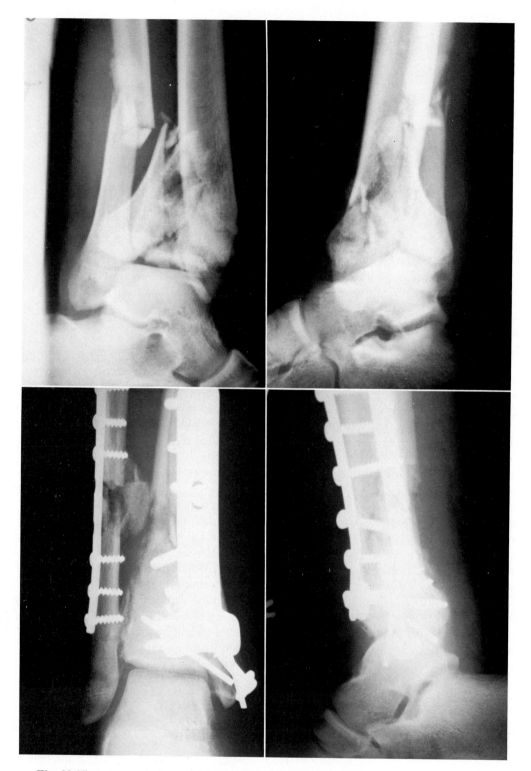

Fig. 23-27. Anteroposterior and lateral radiograph of fixation of comminuted pilon fracture.

is a tendency to underestimate the severity of the injury.

Diagnosis requires a high degree of suspicion. Radiographs are essential, and comparison views are very helpful. Stress radiography may be necessary to reveal an occult epiphyseal slip.

Fibula

A Salter-Harris (S-H) type I slip of the lateral malleolus is the most common injury. Reduction is rarely necessary, as most of these are avulsion injuries that are minimally displaced. Treatment with a shortleg walking cast for 3 to 4 weeks suffices.

Tibia

Eversion–external rotation injuries tend to produce S-H type II displaced fractures of the tibial epiphysis with a greenstick fracture of the fibula above the syndesmosis. The ankle mortise is undisturbed. Closed reduction and cast immobilization for 3 to 6 weeks is adequate treatment. Because the perichondral ring is disrupted, weight bearing is not advisable. Damage to the lateral side of the tibial epiphysis can occur with these injuries. Follow-up yearly radiographs until maturity are advisable. Type I injuries of this epiphysis can occur but are rare. Treatment is as just outlined.

Fractures of the medial malleolus are usually S-H type III or IV injuries. Growth disturbance caused by these injuries is common. Open reduction and Kirschner wire fixation parallel to the physeal line are usually advisable.

TILLAUX FRACTURE

In early adolescence, the medial portion of the tibial epiphysis begins to close. An external rotation force may avulse the anterior lateral portion of the epiphysis, producing an S-H type III injury. The ankle is usually rotationally unstable. Although these can often be treated with closed reduction and a long leg cast, open reduction and Kirschner wire fixation is indicated if anatomic position cannot be achieved by closed reduction.

TRIPLANE FRACTURE

Triplane fracture is a complex fracture of the distal tibial epiphysis that resembles an S-H type IV injury in the coronal plane medially, an S-H type II injury in the coronal plane laterally, and an S-H type III injury in the sagittal plane laterally (Fig. 23-28). Diagnosis is often difficult. Tomograms and CT scans are often helpful. Anatomic reduction is essential. This can usually be achieved closed, but open reduction may be required.

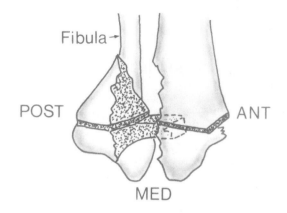

Fig. 23-28. Triplane fracture.

COMPARTMENT SYNDROME

Compartment syndrome of the leg or foot occurs where increased pressure within the fascial compartments compromises the circulation and function of the nerves and muscles in the compartment(s). The most common causes in the foot and leg are increased compartment content (from bleeding and/or edema) and externally applied pressure (from a tight cast). Decreased compartment volume (from closure of the fascia too tightly or from traction) can also be causal. Foot surgeons must be aware of this problem, because the leg is the most common site of compartment syndrome.

The symptoms and signs of compartment syndrome are as follows:

1. Pain out of proportion to clinical situation
2. Pain with passive stretch of the muscles in the involved compartment
3. Tenseness of the compartment
4. Hypesthesia and decreased sensation

Adjunctive diagnostic techniques are tissue pressure measurements and nerve function tests. Depending on the patient and the measuring technique used, normal is usually less than 10 mm Hg. Over 30 mm Hg is definitely abnormal (fasciotomy may be indicated), and fasciotomy is nearly always indicated if the pressure is over 50 mm Hg.

In the leg, all four compartments usually require decompression. This can be accomplished by the single-incision parafibular technique described by Matsen (1980).

In the foot, decompression of all compartments can be achieved through a single incision on the non-weight-bearing surface of the medial arch.

REFERENCES AND SUGGESTED READINGS
Criteria for treatment

Akeson, W.H.: An experimental study of joint stiffness, J. Bone Joint Surg. **43A**:1022, 1961.

Clark, D.D., and Weckesser, E.C.: The influence of triamcinolone acetonide on joint stiffness in the rat, J. Bone Joint Surg. **53A**:1409, 1971.

Collins, D.H., and McElligott, T.F.: Sulphate ($^{35}SO_4$) uptake by chondrocytes in relation to histological changes in osteoarthritic human articular cartilage, Ann. Rheum. Dis. **19**:318, 1960.

Davenport, H.K., and Ranson, S.W.: Contraction resulting from tenotomy, Arch. Surg. **21**:995, 1930.

Dziewiatkowski, D.D., Benesch, R.E., and Benesch, R.: On the possible utilization of sulfate sulfur by the suckling rat for the synthesis of chondroitin sulfate as indicated by the use of radioactive sulfur, J. Biol. Chem. **178**:931, 1949.

Ely, L.W., and Mensor, M.C.: Studies on the immobilization of the normal joints, Surg. Gynecol. Obstet. **57**:212, 1933.

Evans, E.B., Eggers, G.W.N., Butler, J.K., and Blumel, J.: Experimental immobilization and remobilization of rat knee joints, J. Bone Joint Surg. **42A**:737, 1960.

Frankshteyn, S.I.: Experimental studies on mechanism of development of contractures due to immobilization in casts, Khirurgiia **8**:44, 1944.

Frugone, J.E., Thomsen, P., and Luco, J.V.: Changes in weight of muscles of arthritic and immobilized arthritic joints, Proc. Soc. Exp. Biol. Med. **61**:31, 1946.

Gasser, H.S.: Contractures of skeletal muscle, Physiol. Rev. **10**:35, 1930.

Hall, M.C.: Cartilage changes after experimental immobilization of the knee joint of the young rat, J. Bone Joint Surg. **45A**:36, 1963.

Harrison, M.H.M., Schajowicz, F., and Trueta, J.: Osteoarthritis of the hip: a study of the nature and evolution of the disease, J. Bone Joint Surg. **35B**:598, 1953.

Lucas-Championniére, J.: Précis du traitement des fractures par le massage et la mobilisation, Paris, 1910, G. Steinheil.

McLean, F.C., and Urist, M.R.: Bone: An introduction to the physiology of skeletal tissue, Chicago, 1955, University of Chicago Press.

Menzel, A.: Ueber die Erkrankung der Gelenke bei dauernder Ruhe derselben: eine experimentelle Studie, Arch. Klin, Chir. **12**:990, 1871.

Müller, W.: Experimentelle Untersuchungen über die Wirkung langdauernder Immobilisierung auf die Gelenke, Z. Orthop. Chir. **44**:478, 1924.

Peacock, E.E., Jr.: Some biochemical and biophysical aspects of joint stiffness: role of collagen synthesis as opposed to altered molecular bonding, Ann. Surg. **164**:1, 1966.

Ranson, S.W., and Sams, C.F.: A study of muscle in contracture: the permanent shortening of muscles caused by tenotomy and tetanus toxin, J. Neurol. Psychopathol. **8**:304, 1923.

Salter, R.B., and Field, P.: The effects of continuous compression on living articular cartilage: an experimental investigation, J. Bone Joint Surg. **42A**:31, 1960.

Scaglietti, O., and Casuccio, C.: Studio sperimentale degli effetti della immobilizzazione su articolazioni normali, Chir. Organi Mov. **20**:469, 1936.

Sokoloff, L., and Jay, G.E., Jr.: Natural history of degenerative joint disease in the small laboratory animals. 4. Degenerative joint disease in the laboratory rat, Arch. Pathol. **62**:140, 1956.

Solandt, D.Y., and Magladery, J.W.: A comparison of effects of upper and lower motor neuron lesions on skeletal muscle, J. Neurophysiol. **5**:373, 1942.

Thaxter, T.H., Mann, R.A., and Anderson C.E.: Degeneration of immobilized knee joints in rats: Histological and autoradiographic study, J. Bone Joint Surg. **47A**:567, 1965.

Trias, A.: Effect of persistent pressure on the articular cartilage, J. Bone Joint Surg. **43B**:376, 1961.

Thomsen, P., and Luco, J.V.: Changes of weight and neuromuscular transmission in muscles of immobilized joints, J. Neurophysiol. **7**:245, 1944.

Tschmarke, G.: Experimentelle Untersuchungen über die Rolle des Muskeltonus in der Gelenkchirurgie. 3. Mitteilung: Fixationskontrakturen und die Beeinflussung ihrer Entwicklung, Arch. Klin. Chir. **164**:785, 1931.

Fractures and fracture-dislocations of ankle joint

Ashhurst, A.P.C., and Bromer, R.S.: Classification and mechanism of fracture of the leg bones involving the ankle. Based on a study of three hundred cases from the Episcopal Hospital, Arch. Surg. **4**:51, 1922.

Aufranc, O.E.: Trimalleolar tracture dislocation, J.A.M.A. **174**:2221, 1960.

Bonnin, J.G.: Injuries to the ankle, Darien, Conn. Hafner Publ. Co., 1970.

Bosworth, D.M.: Fracture-dislocation of the ankle with fixed displacement of the fibula behind the tibia, J. Bone Joint Surg. **29**:130, 1947.

Burwell, H.N., and Charnley, A.D.: The treatment of displaced fractures at the ankle by rigid internal fixation and early joint movement, J. Bone Joint Surg. **47B**:634, 1965.

Chapman, M.W., and Mahoney, M.: The place of immediate internal fixation in the management of open fracture, Abbott Soc. Bull. **8**:85, May, 1976.

Charnley, J. The closed treatment of common fractures, Baltimore, 1963, The Williams & Wilkins Co.

Childress, H.M.: Vertical transarticular-pin fixation for unstable ankle fractures, J. Bone Joint Surg. **47A**:1323, 1965.

Coonrad, R.W., and Bugg, E.I.: Trapping of the posterior tibial tendon and interposition of soft tissue in severe fractures about the ankle joint, J. Bone Joint Surg. **36A**:744, 1954.

Cooperman, D.R., Seigel, P.G., and Laros, G.S.: Tibial fractures involving the ankle in children, J. Bone Joint Surg. **60A**:140-146, 1978.

Dieterlé, J.: The use of Kirschner wire in maintaining reduction of fracture-dislocations of the ankle joint: a report of two cases, J. Bone Joint Surg. **17**:990, 1935.

Dupuytren, G.: Of fractures of the lower extremity and luxations of the foot. In Medical Classics **IV**:151-172, 1939.

Fleming, J.L., and Smith H.O.: Fracture-dislocation of the ankle with the fibula fixed behind the tibia, J. Bone Joint Surg. **36A**:556, 1954.

Glick, B.W.: The ankle fracture with inferior tibiofibular joint disruption, Surg. Gynecol. Obstet. **118**:549, 1964.

Gustilo, R.B., and Anderson, J.T.: Prevention of infection in the treatment of one thousand and twenty-five open fractures of long bones, J. Bone Joint Surg. **58A**:453, 1976.

Jergesen, F.: Open reduction of fractures and dislocations of the ankle, Am. J. Surg. **98**:136, 1959.

Kleiger, B.: The mechanism of ankle injuries, J. Bone Joint Surg. **38A**:59, 1956.

Lauge-Hansen, N.: Fractures of the ankle: analytic historic survey as the basis of new experimental, roentgenologic and clinical investigations, Arch. Surg. **56**:259, 1948.

Lauge-Hansen, N.: Fractures of the ankle. II. Combined experimental-surgical and experimental-roentgenologic investigations, Arch. Surg. **60**:957, 1950.

Lauge-Hansen, N.: Fractures of the ankle. IV. Clinical use of genetic roentgen diagnosis and genetic reduction, Arch. Surg. **64**:488, 1952.

Lauge-Hansen, N.: Fractures of the ankle. III. Genetic roentgenologic diagnosis of fracture of the ankle, Am. J. Roentgenol. Radium Ther. Nucl. Med. **71**:456, 1954.

Maisonneuve, J.G.: Recherches sur la fracture du perone, Arch. Gen. Med. **7**:165, 433, 1840.

Matsen, F.A., III: Compartmental Syndromes, New York, 1980, Grune & Stratton, Inc.

Mayer, V., and Pohlidal, S.: Ankle mortise injuries, Surg. Gynecol. Obstet. **96:**99, 1953.

McDade, W.C.: Treatment of ankle fractures. In Instructional Course Lectures, American Academy of Orthopaedic Surgeons, vol. 24, St. Louis, 1975. The C.V. Mosby Co.

McDaniel, W.J., and Wilson, F.C.: Trimalleolar fractures of the ankle. And end result study, Clin. Orthop. **122:**37, 1977.

McMaster, J.H., and Scranton, P.E.: Tibiofibular synostosis: a cause of ankle disability, Clin. Orthop. **111:**172, 1975.

Meyers, M.H.: Fracture about the ankle joint with fixed displacement of the proximal fragment of the fibula behind the tibia, J. Bone Joint Surg. **39A:**441, 1957.

Mitchell, N., and Shepard, N.: Healing of articular cartilage in intra-articular fractures in rabbits, J. Bone Joint Surg. **62A:**628-634, 1980.

Müller, M.E., Allgower, M., and Willenegger, H.: Manual external fixation, New York, 1979, Springer-Verlag New York, Inc.

Portis, R.B., and Mendelsohn, H.A.: Conservative management of fractures of the ankle involving the medial malleolus, JAMA **151:**102, 1953.

Pott, P.: Some few general remarks on fractures and dislocations, London, 1768, Hawes, Clarke, Collins.

Ramsey, P.L., and Hamilton, W.: Changes in tibiotalar area of contact caused by lateral talar shift, J. Bone Joint Surg. **58A:**356-357, 1976.

Salter, R.B., and Harris, W.R.: Injuries involving the epiphyseal plate, J. Bone Joint Surg. **45A:**587, 1963.

Salter, R.B., Semmonds, D.F., and Malcolm, B.W., et al.: The biological effect of continuous passive motion on the healing of full-thickness defects in articular cartilage, J. Bone Joint Surg. **62A:**1232-1251, 1980.

Scranton, P.E., McMaster, J.H., and Kelly, E.: Dynamic fibular function, a new concept, Clin. Orthop. **118:**76, 1976.

Wiggins, H.E.: Pronation-dorsiflexion fractures with involvement of distal tibial metaphysis—case studies. In Instructional Course Lectures, American Academy of Orthopaedic Surgeons, vol. 24, St. Louis, 1975, The C.V. Mosby Co.

Yablon, I.G., Heller, F.G., and Shouse, L.: The key role of the lateral malleolus in displaced fractures of the ankle, J. Bone Joint Surg. **59A:**169, 1977.

Zuelzer, W.A.: Use of hookplate for fixation of ununited medial tibial malleolus, JAMA **167:**828, 1958.

24

Fractures and dislocations of the foot

JESSE C. DeLEE

Introduction

Fractures and dislocations of the foot are among the most common injuries in the musculoskeletal system. Historically these injuries have been considered minor and their treatment often relegated to a secondary position. Hillegass[7] reports that of every 300 men working in heavy industry, 15 working days per month are lost as the result of foot problems, 65% of which are the result of trauma. The disability resulting from these injuries and their frequency warrant more close attention in their diagnosis and management.[8] The following general comments on the diagnosis and management of fractures and dislocations of the foot are meant to establish the basic principles. More detailed remarks are presented for each particular injury.

CLINICAL DIAGNOSIS

In evaluating patients with trauma to the foot, it is essential to obtain a thorough history. One must determine the general state of health with regard to such diseases as gout, diabetes, and circulatory problems before the initiation of treatment.[4] A detailed history of the mechanism by which the injury occurred will direct the examiner in his physical and radiographic examination.[4] In addition, it will provide a clue to the degree of soft tissue injury associated with the fracture.

Once the history is taken, the physical examination must be carried out systematically. Klenerman[9] emphasizes that while forefoot injuries are easily diagnosed,

Editor's note: Because of the extensive list of references in this chapter, they are numbered and filed after each section for the reader's convenience.

midfoot and hindfoot injuries often times go undetected. Because of the high incidence of multiple fractures in the injured foot,[4] careful palpation for points of tenderness is performed to detect any area of occult injury.[3,14] The importance of evaluating the circulatory status of the foot cannot be overemphasized. It is important to compare the arterial pulsations of the involved foot with the normal foot, particularly in the elderly patient in whom absent pulsations may not be secondary to the fracture but to preexisting vascular disease.

In displaced fractures and dislocations, evaluation of the overlying skin for signs of ischemia is important so that early reduction can be performed to prevent skin sloughing. Evaluation of the range of motion of the ankle, subtalar, midtarsal, and metatarsophalangeal joints is carried out within the limits of pain as part of a routine examination. A careful motor examination of intrinsic and extrinsic muscles is recorded both before and after treatment. The sensory examination is essential to detect loss secondary to the injury and such preexisting conditions as a diabetic neuropathy, which could produce a Charcot joint in the injured foot.

RADIOGRAPHIC DIAGNOSIS

Only after a careful history and physical examination are radiographs considered. The standard views used in evaluating the foot are the anteroposterior, lateral, and oblique views. The lateral view of the foot is helpful in evaluating fractures of the calcaneus and neck and body of the talus in addition to evaluating the midtarsal bones. Metatarsal overlap limits the usefulness of the lateral view in evaluation of the metatarsals and phalanges. The oblique view is particularly useful in evaluating the calcaneocuboid joint and in overcoming the metatarsal overlap noted on the lateral view. Additional radiographs, such as the anteroposterior view of the ankle are useful in evaluating the articular surface of the talus and the lateral aspect of the calcaneus. Axial views of the heel, special views of the subtalar joint, polytomography, and arthrography are also indicated in certain instances. The use of the computed tomography scan in evaluating fractures and dislocations in the foot will be extended as experience with its use increases.

TREATMENT

The prime objectives in the treatment of fractures and dislocations of the foot are: (1) avoiding stiffness and loss of mobility; (2) preventing bony prominences, which may result in pressure phenomena from the use of a shoe; and (3) restoring the articular surfaces. The goal of treatment of fractures and dislocations of the foot is a flexible plantigrade foot with good bony alignment.

Once the diagnosis is certain, dislocations and fractures of the foot should be reduced as soon as possible. The reduction is easier to obtain before swelling occurs and before the hematoma between the fracture fragments organizes. Additionally, gross displacement of dislocations and fractures of the foot can result in localized pressure on the skin with vascular compromise and skin loss. Immediate reduction of the displacement can limit these complications.

It is important to remember that a perfect anatomic result does *not* necessarily ensure that mobility will be maintained. In fact, McKeever[12] emphasizes that all too often a perfect radiograph is seen, but the foot is so stiff that the patient cannot walk without pain. However, Klenerman[9] emphasizes the importance of restoring the foot to its normal shape even in cases in which joint mobility cannot be achieved. He stresses the importance of maintaining the relative lengths of the medial (talonaviculocuneiform) and lateral (calcaneocuboid) columns of the foot, and of avoiding any abnormal prominence on the plantar aspect of the foot.

Chapman[1] emphasizes the importance of anatomic restoration of joint surface within the foot and advocates open reduction and internal fixation where applicable to restore joint continuity. In addition, Klenerman[9] stresses that mobility of joints of the foot, so essential in normal function, is not likely to be regained if joint surfaces remain notably incongruous. He also emphasizes that although a period of immobilization may be beneficial to soft tissue healing, it can lead to stiffness of joints, even those which are not involved in the injury, because of hemorrhage and extravasation about the adjacent joints.

Because of the close relationship of subtalar with midtarsal motion, limitation of motion of either of these joint complexes will secondarily limit the motion in the other.[2,10] Therefore isolated injuries to midtarsal or subtalar joints must be actively mobilized to prevent secondary limitation of the linked joint.[2,10]

Giannestras and Sammarco[5] emphasize that, since the foot is a weight-bearing structure, the preservation of soft tissue is as important as the reduction of the fracture. They note that patients experience a great deal of difficulty attempting to walk on scarred soft tissue, even if the bones of the foot are anatomically reduced.[5] Heck[6] also stresses the concept that fractures and dislocations of the foot are not solved simply by restoration of the continuity of a bone or joint complex, but rather by the simultaneous treatment and rehabilitation of the soft tissues. He emphasizes that the response to treatment of injuries to soft parts of the foot adjacent to a fracture is dependent on their early recognition and proper management. If for any reason one does not obtain supple soft tissues about the fracture, the final result will be impaired function of the foot and toes.

Lapidus and Guidotti[11] strongly emphasize the need for early mobilization in injuries of the foot. They note that the only two indications for immobilization of a fracture or dislocation are: (1) to maintain the reduction of the fragments, and (2) to eliminate motion between fragments to prevent nonunion. They note that immobilization of a badly injured foot for 6 weeks or longer (the time usually required for bony union) will almost invariably produce fibrous ankylosis of the small joints of the foot, with resultant muscular atrophy and limitation of joint motion.

Chapman[1] stresses that if immobilization can be accomplished by internal fixation, earlier institution of joint motion is possible and should be encouraged. However, if cast immobilization is required, leaving the toes free so that motion at the metatarsophalangeal joints can be encouraged will help decrease edema and stimulate muscle function in the calf and foot. In addition, I have found that by leaving the toes exposed in a cast and using them to pick up small objects, swelling can be decreased and earlier mobility stimulated.

In cases in which stability of the fracture or dislocation allow early weight bearing, Hillegass[7] reports that such early weight bearing decreases the period of disability following injury. He believes it prevents the development of osteoporosis, decreases swelling by early muscle contraction, and permits slight motion in the small joints of the foot (even in a cast), which helps to prevent stiffness. Mullen and Gamber[13] also noted the importance of early mobilization and weight bearing to prevent long-term disability. Chapman[1] emphasizes that immobilization of the foot in a non-weight-bearing mode is accompanied by muscular atrophy, myostatic

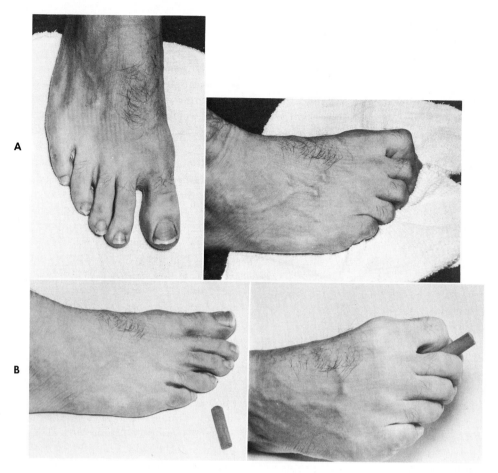

Fig. 24-1. Foot exercises used to institute early muscle contraction and range of motion. **A,** Using toes to bunch up a towel. Exercise can also be done in a cast if toes are left free. **B,** Picking up small objects with toes helps stimulate intrinsic muscle function.

contracture, decreased joint motion, proliferation of connective tissue and capsular structures, internal synovial adhesions, and cartilaginous degeneration. Early mobilization obviates or decreases the possible occurrence of these abnormal processes.[1] In situations in which postoperative immobilization is indicated *without* weight bearing, consideration can be given to bivalving the short leg cast and instituting early motion *without* weight bearing. Once motion is restored, immobilization can be continued until union occurs. The stability of the fracture or dislocation must be considered before this method is recommended.

If weight bearing needs to be delayed, Omer and Pomerantz[14] suggest using a patellar tendon–bearing plaster cast or brace to relieve weight bearing but to allow mobilization. Evaluation of stability, determined at the time of reduction, and cast immobilization will help decide if early weight bearing, with its known benefits, can be instituted.

Following the period of fracture immobilization, an

intensive rehabilitation program, specialized for the foot, should be instituted to ensure restoration of joint function and muscle strength. I have found an Unna boot or Gelocast to gently support the foot and yet allow progressive motion of the joints for the first week after cast removal, helps prevent swelling. Exercises with the foot, including bunching a towel with the toes (Fig. 24-1, *A*) and picking up small objects with the toes (Fig. 24-1, *B*), help to institute muscle contraction and range of motion to the foot and ankle. McKeever[12] points out that many injuries to the foot result in crushing, stretching, or tearing of the soft tissues in addition to the fractures. This produces hemorrhage, which extravasates through the soft tissue and infiltrates the tissue interstices. The result is dense intraarticular and extraarticular adhesions and fibrosis, all of which severely limit the normal flexibility of the foot. In addition, this can be accompanied by demineralization of bone and can result in Sudeck's atrophy or reflex sympathetic dystrophy in the limb. It is McKeever's

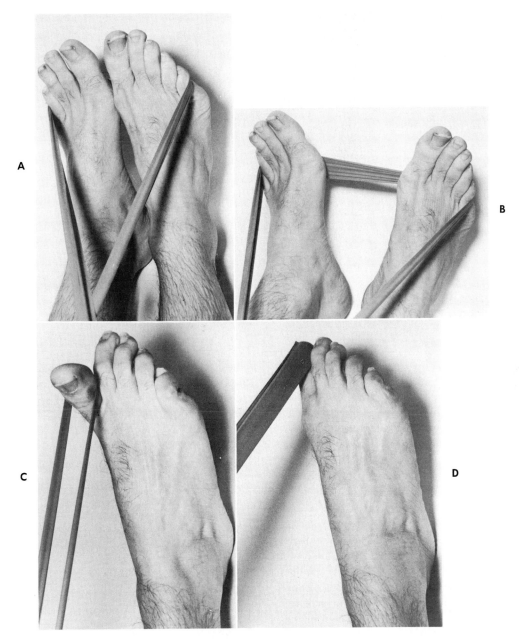

Fig. 24-2. Elastic bandage can be used to supply gentle resistance for early strengthening and motion exercises. This can be used for ankle dorsiflexion–plantar flexion (**A**), and inversion-eversion (**B**), and metatarsophalangeal motion (even in a cast) of foot (**C** and **D**).

opinion[12] that prolonged immobilization of a foot distended with blood is a common precursor to this disabling syndrome. Discussion of the diagnosis and treatment of reflex sympathetic dystrophy is beyond the scope of this chapter; however, by early motion, elevation, and early weight bearing, it can often be prevented.[12]

Lapidus and Guidotti[11] recommend early mobilization combined with swimming-pool walking exercises for treatment of fractures of the ankle or tarsal bones.

These swimming-pool walking exercises are performed on a daily basis. Walking is started in the deepest part of the pool so that the buoyancy of the patient's body in the water results in a weightless state. The patient is instructed to walk as though he were walking on normal ground. Although Lapidus and Guidotti recommend the treatment of some fractures of the foot *initially* in this manner, if the fractures are unstable and require immobilization, I have found this method very useful following a period of immobilization. Although a

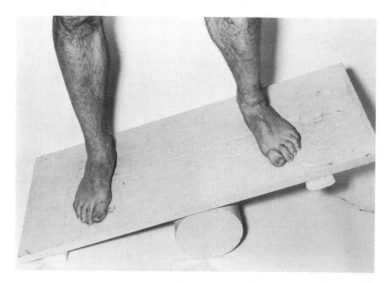

Fig. 24-3. Use of a "Bongo Board" to help retrain the foot in proprioception. Balancing on board using cylinders of increasing diameter facilitates progression of proprioceptive development.

whirlpool used for soaking before instituting range of motion exercises is helpful in improving range of motion, it does not allow actual weight bearing with support of the water as swimming-pool walking does.

I have found the use of an elastic bandage for gentle resisted dorsiflexion–plantar flexion, inversion-eversion, and abduction-adduction, helpful early in restoring both joint motion and muscle power (Fig. 24-2). Later, strengthening exercises, including resisted ankle plantar flexion–dorsiflexion, and inversion-eversion are added as pain permits. Proprioceptive exercises are instituted when strength allows painless ambulation. A simple means of proprioceptive training is the use of a board placed on a cylinder ("Bongo Board"), which helps in two-dimensional retraining (Fig. 24-3). Eventually placing the board on one half of a round ball will introduce three-dimensional tilt for proprioception education.

Stretching exercises for the Achilles tendon and gentle stretching of the subtalar, midtarsal, and metatarsophalaneal joints is also indicated. The metatarsophalangeal joints can be actively assisted in their range of motion, again, using an elastic bandage (Fig. 24-2, C and D). If swelling occurs during this period of rehabilitation consideration is given to a compression dressing such as a Jobst compression stocking or Ace wrap. Contrast baths alternating heat and cold are used later if recurrent swelling becomes a permanent problem.

After rehabilitation is complete, the use of a longitudinal arch support, particularly for midtarsal injuries, and a protective liner in the shoe made of a material such as Plastizote to relieve the plantar aspect of the foot help to restore the weight-bearing function of the foot. Special shoe alterations and appliances are mentioned later under each specific injury.

REFERENCES

1. Chapman, M.W.: Fractures and dislocations of the ankle and foot. In Mann, R.A., editor: DuVries' surgery of the foot, ed. 4, St. Louis, 1978, The C.V. Mosby Co.
2. Close, J.R., Inman, V.T., Poor, P.M., and Todd, F.N.: The function of the subtalar joint, Clin. Orthop. **50**:159-179, 1967.
3. Coker, T.P., Jr., and Arnold, J.A.: Spots injuries to the foot and ankle. In Jahss, M.H., editor: Disorders of the foot, vol. 2, Philadelphia, 1982, W.B. Saunders Co.
4. Garcia, A., and Parkes, J.C.: Fractures of the foot. In Giannestras, N.J., editor: Foot disorders: medical and surgical management, ed. 2, Philadelphia, 1973, Lea & Febiger.
5. Giannestras, N.J., and Sammarco, G.J.: Fractures and dislocations in the foot. In Rockwood, C.A., Jr., and Green D.P., editors: Fractures, vol. 2, Philadelphia, 1975, J.B. Lippincott Co.
6. Heck, C.V.: Fractures of the bones of the foot (except the talus), Surg. Clin. North Am., **45**:103-177, 1965.
7. Hillegass, R.C.: Injuries to the midfoot: a major cause of industrial morbidity. In Bateman, J.E., editor: Foot science, Philadelphia, 1976, W.B. Saunders Co.
8. Johnson, V.S.: Treatment of fractures of the forefoot in industry. In Bateman, J.E., editor: Foot science, Philadelphia, 1976, W.B. Saunders Co.
9. Klenerman, L.: The foot and its disorders, ed. 2, London, 1982, Blackwell Scientific Publications.
10. Lapidus, P.W.: Mechanical anatomy of the tarsal joints, Clin. Orthop. **30**:20, 1963.
11. Lapidus, P.W., and Guidotti, F.P.: Immediate mobilization and swimming pool exercises in some fractures of foot and ankle bones, Clin. Orthop. **56**:197-206, 1968.
12. McKeever, F.M.: Fractures of the tarsal and metatarsal bones, Surg. Gynecol. Obstet. **90**:735-745, 1950.

13. Mullen, J.P., and Gamber, H.H.: Management of severe open foot injuries, J. Bone Joint Surg. **54A**:1574, 1972.

14. Omer, G.E., and Pomerantz, G.M.: Principles of management of acute injuries of the foot, J. Bone Joint Surg. **51A**:813-814, 1969.

Fractures of the calcaneus

The calcaneus is the most commonly fractured of all the tarsal bones,[89,167] constituting 60% of all major tarsal injuries.[27] Of all patients with calcaneus fractures, 10% have associated fractures of the spine,[52,96,157] and 26% have other associated extremity injuries.[52,99,157] About 7% of these fractures are bilateral, and less than 2% are open.[107]

The economic importance of these fractures is apparent in that, although they represent only 2% of all fractures, 90% occur in men between 41 and 45 years of age.* They occur most often in middle-aged industrial workers.† The economic impact becomes even more apparent when one considers that 20% of patients may be incapacitated for up to 3 years following fracture, and many are still partially incapacitated as long as 5 years after the fracture.[130]

Conn[30] in 1926 termed calcaneus fractures "serious and disabling injuries in which the end results are incredibly bad," and Mercer[122] called calcaneus fractures the most disabling of all injuries. The pessimism surrounding these fractures was echoed by Cotton and Henderson,[33] and by Bankart, who termed the results of treatment of crush fractures of the calcaneus "rotten."[9]

Although some aspects of the treatment of calcaneus fractures are well accepted, a standard method of treatment is not agreed on by most authors.[163] The first written report of a closed treatment was by Bailey[8] in 1880, while Morestein[127] in 1902 first reported open reduction and internal fixation of calcaneus fractures. Since these very early reports, the emphasis on treatment has vacillated between open and closed methods. There is no current concensus of opinion regarding the treatment of all calcaneus fractures. Additionally, the direct comparison of various treatment modalities is difficult for several reasons:

1. Different authors have used different methods of classification of calcaneal fractures, making comparison difficult.[199]
2. There are no true prospective studies available comparing the various treatment modalities.
3. Methods of postfracture evaluation have varied greatly, making comparison of results difficult.[144]

*References 46, 78, 107, 121, 128, 134, 138, 162, 190-192, and 195.
†References 1, 17, 162, 190-192, and 195

The purpose of this section is to present the logic and theory for each method of treatment and to combine in my "Author's Preferred Method," the points of each method of treatment that I have found most useful.

ANATOMY

The calcaneus transmits the weight of the body to the ground and forms a strong lever for the muscles of the calf.[3] The calcaneus consists of an internal structure of cancellous bone surrounded by an outer shell of cortical bone.[11,129] This cortical shell is very thin except at the posterior tubercle, and the enclosed pattern of cancellous bone reflects the static and dynamic strains to which the calcaneus is exposed.[73] Traction trabeculae radiate from the inferior cortex of the calcaneus, while compression trabeculae converge to support the posterior and anterior articular facets. Soeur and Remy[173] have termed this condensation of bone trabeculae beneath the anterior and posterior facets *the thalamic portion of the calcaneus.* According to Letournel,[105] however, Destot termed the posterior articular surface of the calcaneus *the thalamus.*[105]

The so-called neutral triangle with its sparseness of trabeculae is located just beneath the crucial angle of Gissane (Fig. 24-4). According to Hardy,[73] the neutral triangle is where blood vessels reach the medullary cavity of the calcaneus and therefore is a common site for the early manifestations of blood-borne infection.

The calcaneus has six distinct surfaces: superior, inferior, lateral, medial, posterior, and anterior.[160]

Superior surface

The superior surface of the calcaneus can be conveniently divided into three parts: posterior, middle, and anterior[160,195] (Fig. 24-5).

The posterior third of the superior surface is completely nonarticular. It is perforated by multiple vascular foramina.[160] This posterior nonarticular portion of the calcaneus joins with the middle surface and marks the highest portion of the bone, "the posterior peak."[194]

The middle one third of the superior surface consists of the large posterior facet of the calcaneus. The articular surface of the posterior facet is convex along the longitudinal axis of the cancaneus.[160]

The anterior one third of the superior surface consists of the sinus tarsi, the sulcus calcanei, and the articular surfaces of the anterior and middle facets. The anterior and middle facets form a concavity that corresponds to the convexity of the talar head.[160] The anterior articular surface is supported by the beak of the os calcis, and the middle surface is supported by the sustentaculum tali.[160,194] Variations occur in the contour and degree of separations of these two articular sur-

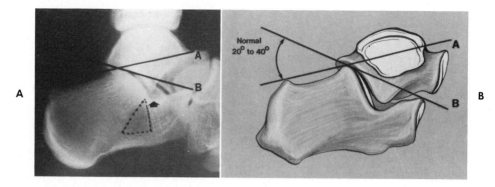

Fig. 24-4. A, "Neutral triangle" (dotted lines) beneath crucial angle of Gissane (arrow). Note sparcity of trabeculae in neutral triangle. **B,** Bohler's tuberosity joint angle. Line *A*, from highest point on posterior articular surface to most superior part of calcaneal tuberosity. Line *B*, from highest point on anterior process of calcaneus to highest part of posterior articular surface. Intervening angle (arrow) is Bohler's tuberosity joint angle (20 to 40 degrees).

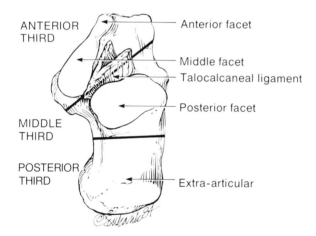

Fig. 24-5. Superior surface of calcaneus is divided into thirds. Posterior one third is extraarticular, middle one third contains posterior facet, and anterior one third contains articular surface of middle and anterior facets.

faces. The anterior and middle facets can either be separate or confluent.[160]

The tarsal canal separates the middle and posterior articular facets. This canal is narrow and is oriented obliquely forward, laterally, and inferiorly.[160] The intraosseous talocalcaneal ligament inserts in the floor of the canal, and it serves to separate the posterior facet from the anterior and middle facets[58] (Fig. 24-5). Although the anterior, middle, and posterior talocalcaneal articular facets have separate synovial cavities and are curved in opposite directions, they function as a single reciprocal unit.[73]

Inferior surface

The inferior surface of the calcaneus is triangular with the base located posteriorly and the apex anteriorly.[160] The inferior surface is composed of a medial and a lateral tuberosity, with the medial tuberosity being the main weight-bearing structure.[160] The medial tuberosity gives origin to the abductor hallucis muscle, and the lateral tuberosity gives origin to the abductor digit minimi. According to Sarrafian,[160] 36% of os calci have a heel spur, which is a shelflike anterior bony projection originating from the medial tuberosity.

Lateral surface

The lateral surface of the body of the calcaneus is flat and contains a shallow groove for the peroneal tendons.[160] A separate groove for the peroneus longus tendon is present on the lateral aspect of the os calcis in 85% of specimens,[160] while a definite groove for the peroneus brevis tendon is present in only about 3% of specimens.

Medial surface

The configuration of the medial calcaneal surface is determined mainly by the sustentaculum tali, a large triangular projection with a posterior base and an anterior apex.[160] Its superior surface represents the middle articular facet of the calcaneus, and its inferior surface is curved into a groove for the flexor hallucis longus tendon and provides attachment for the fibrous tunnel for this tendon.[160] Additionally, the tibiocalcaneal component of the deltoid ligament and the superomedial calcaneonavicular ligament insert on the upper border of its medial surface.

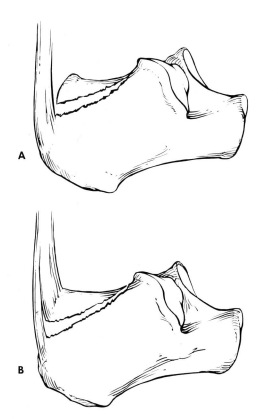

Fig. 24-6. A, According to Sarafian,[160] upper surface of posterior surface is free from attachment of Achilles tendon. B, According to Lowy,[87] however, there is great variability at point of insertion of the Achilles tendon. As indicated here, the Achilles tendon can insert very proximally on calcaneus.

Posterior surface

The posterior surface of the calcaneus is also triangular in shape with the apex superior and the base inferior. The overall contour of this surface is convex.[160] Sarrafian[160] stresses that the lower border of this posterior surface serves as the insertion for the Achilles tendon, while the upper portion of the posterior surface is free from tendinous insertion (Fig. 24-6).

Anterior surface

The anterior surface of the calcaneus is entirely articular.[160] It is saddle shaped, convex transversely, and concave vertically. It serves as the articulation between the calcaneus and cuboid.

Tuberosity joint angle

Bohler[17] in 1931 described the tuberosity joint angle, or "salient" angle, which is noted on the lateral radiographic projection (see Fig. 24-4). This angle is formed by the intersection of two lines: (1) a line from the highest point on the posterior articular surface to the most superior point of the calcaneal tuberosity (a) (see Fig. 24-4, A), and (2) a line from the highest point on the anterior process of the calcaneus to the highest part of the posterior articular surface (b) (see Fig. 24-4, B) Bohler[17] considered the normal angle to be between 30° and 35°, while Palmer[137] reported the angle can vary from 10° to 40°. Stephenson[174] also reports a great deal of variation in the tuberosity joint angle in the normal foot, ranging from 25° to 40° with an average of 35°.[174] The angles in the right and left calcanei of the same individual are equal.[17]

In severe fractures of the os calcis, this angle becomes smaller, straight, or even reversed.[134] The angle can therefore be taken as a relative measure of the degree of compression and deformity in calcaneus fractures.[150,160] According to Bohler[17] the displacement evidenced by change in the angle is maintained by the muscle pull of the gastrocnemius.

While Stephenson[174] stresses that the tuberosity joint angle is a measure of the height of the posterior facet, McLaughlin[110] pointed out that reduction or reversal of the tuberosity joint angle simply measures the degree of proximal displacement of the tuberosity and can therefore be decreased in both intraarticular and extraarticular fractures of the calcaneus (Fig. 24-7). Rosendahl-Jensen[154] also stresses that the angle is simply an expression of the form of the calcaneus and that it gives no information on the position of the surfaces of the subtalar joint or of the location of the bone in relationship to the other bones of the tarsus.

The tuberosity joint angle therefore can be an expression both of posterior facet involvement in an intraarticular fracture and of simple proximal displacement of the tuberosity of the calcaneus in fractures that are entirely extraarticular[24,28,110,154,174] (Fig. 24-7). This must be kept in mind when considering its value in evaluation of fractures of the calcaneus.

Crucial angle of Gissane

A thick and strong cortical strut exists within the calcaneus and extends from the front of the bone to the posterior margin of the posterior subtalar facet. This strut is angled, and the angle supports the lateral process of the talus.[48] This angle was termed "The Crucial Angle" by Gissane in 1947 (see Fig. 24-4, A).[48,60] According to Stephenson,[174] the crucial angle also shows a great deal of individual variation, ranging from 120° to 145° with an average of 130° in the normal, uninjured foot. Again, the angle in the two normal feet of an individual should be approximately equal.[147] The densities on the lateral radiograph that make up the crucial angle consist of the subchondral bone of the posterior facet and the subchondral bone of the anterior

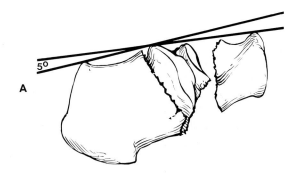

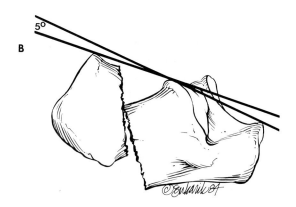

Fig. 24-7. A, Intraarticular fracture with decrease in Bohler's tuberosity joint angle. **B,** Extraarticular fracture with decrease in Bohler's tuberosity joint angle.

and middle facets. The angle therefore gives some indication of the relationship of the posterior, anterior, and middle facets.

When axial compression forces are applied, the lateral process of the talus acts as a bursting wedge, pointing directly into the crucial angle in the floor of the calcaneal sulcus.[58,73] This produces the primary fracture line in calcaneal fractures, which extends from the crucial angle to the inferior surface of the calcaneus (See Figs. 24-30, *A* and 24-31, *A*).[47] Secondary fracture lines may also emanate from the crucial angle.[47,174]

CLASSIFICATION

Attempts to classify fractures of the calcaneus have been made by many authors.[17,31,47,75,157] However, no single classification system has been completely satisfactory, largely because of the implications of a statement by Cotton and Wilson[34] in 1908 that it was not possible to classify "the fracture in a nut subjected to the stresses of a nutcracker." Horn[79] too emphasized that any classification system is limited by the tremendous number of variations possible in fracture patterns.

For practical purposes, fractures of the calcaneus are usually divided into two general groups: intraarticular and extraarticular fractures.[69] Essex-Lopresti strongly emphasized the importance of simplifying these classification systems by dividing calcaneus fractures generally into those that involve the subtalar joint and those that did not.[48] This simple classification is based on the fact that the extraarticular calcaneus fracture tends to have a very good prognosis, while the prognosis of intraarticular fracture is much less predictable and satisfactory.[48]

Extraarticular fractures of the calcaneus are less common, composing from 25% to 35% of all calcaneus fractures.* Intraarticular fractures make up from 70% to 75% of all calcaneus fractures.[17,48,107,199] Within the intraarticular fracture group, Essex-Lopresti identified two distinct fracture patterns: tongue and joint depression.[48] Essex-Lopresti further divided extraarticular fractures into tuberosity fractures and fractures involving the calcaneocuboid joint. Essex-Lopresti stressed the importance of long-term disability of associated subluxation of the talar head at the talonavicular joint in comminuted calcaneus fractures and of involvement of the calcaneocuboid joint.

Rowe et al.[157] presented a classification modified from the system presented by Watson-Jones.[188] They divided fractures of the calcaneus into five types (Fig. 24-8). The first three types are separate from the last two in that they do not involve the subtalar joint. These extraarticular fractures are easier to treat and have a uniformly better prognosis than fractures in which the subtalar joint is involved.[48,134]

In this section I will use a classification system (Table 4) based primarily on that of Rowe et at.[157] (Fig. 24-8) for extraarticular fractures and on that of Essex-Lopresti[48] (Table 5) for intraarticular fractures. The discussion of the various fracture types will follow this classification system. I have considered sustentaculum tali fractures as intraarticular fractures because the sustentaculum contains the middle subtalar facet on its superior surface. Also, although anterior process fractures are considered extraarticular, they can involve the subtalar or calcaneocuboid joints, in which instance the prognosis is less favorable.

MECHANISM OF INJURY

In addition to having distinctly different prognoses, extraarticular and intraarticular fractures of the os calcis are the result of different mechanisms of injury.

Cave stressed that many extraarticular fractures result from twisting injuries that avulse fragments of bone, such as the avulsion fracture of the Achilles tendon insertion that results from a violent contraction of

---

*References 17, 48, 98, 99, 107, and 199.

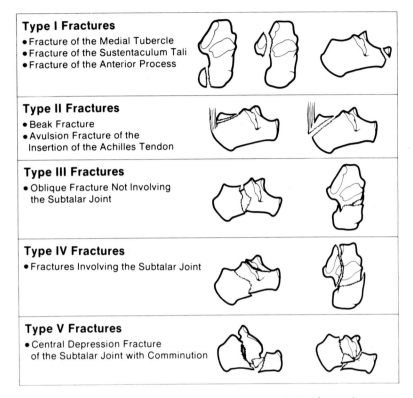

Type I Fractures
- Fracture of the Medial Tubercle
- Fracture of the Sustentaculum Tali
- Fracture of the Anterior Process

Type II Fractures
- Beak Fracture
- Avulsion Fracture of the Insertion of the Achilles Tendon

Type III Fractures
- Oblique Fracture Not Involving the Subtalar Joint

Type IV Fractures
- Fractures Involving the Subtalar Joint

Type V Fractures
- Central Depression Fracture of the Subtalar Joint with Comminution

Fig. 24-8. Classification of calcaneal fractures by Rowe et al. (Redrawn from Rowe, C.R., Sakellarides, H.T., Freeman, P.A., and Sorbie, C.: JAMA **184**:920-923, 1963.)

Table 4. Author's classification of calcaneus fractures.

I. *Extra articular fractures*
   A. Anterior process fracture (This can occasionally be intraarticular; in which case the results may be poor.)
   B. Tuberosity fracture: beak and avulsion fractures
   C. Medial or lateral process fracture
   D. Fracture of the body without involvement of the subtalar joint
II. *Intraarticular fractures*
   A. Sustentaculum tali fracture
   B. Tongue fracture
   C. Joint depression fracture
   D. Comminuted fracture
III. *Stress fractures*

Table 5. Classification of Essex-Lopresti

I. *Fractures not involving the subtalar joint*
   A. Tuberosity fractures
      1. Beak type
      2. Avulsion of the medial border
      3. Vertical fracture
      4. Horizontal fracture
   B. Fractures involving only the calcaneocuboid joint
      1. Parrot-nose type
      2. Various types
II. *Fractures involving the subtalar joint*
   A. Without displacement
   B. With displacement
      1. Tongue-type of displacement
      2. Central lateral depression of the joint
      3. Sustentaculum tali fracture
      4. Comminution from below (including severe tongue and joint depression types)
      5. From behind and forward with dislocation of the subtalar joint

the gastrocnemius-soleus muscle group (see Fig. 24-24) or the avulsion of the anterior process of the calcaneus caused by inversion of the foot.[27] Dodson[45] also emphasizes that twisting injuries of the foot produce the relatively minor extraarticular fractures. A direct blow can also result in fracture of the medial tubercle or an extraarticular fracture of the body of the calcaneus without displacement.[45]

On the other hand, intraarticular fractures are most commonly the result of a fall from a height, with the patient's weight concentrated on the heels on landing.* Dodson[45] stresses that any patient who falls over 2 feet should be suspected of having a calcaneus fracture.

Although intraarticular calcaneus fractures are usually secondary to a fall from a height in civilian life, in war they usually result from a force inflicted from below, such as an exploding land mine beneath a military vehicle.[70] These war fractures are usually even more comminuted than those caused by falls and are often open with extensive soft tissue damage.[70]

It is important to emphasize that every degree of severity of fracture can result from a fall, depending on the distance fallen, the quality of the bone in the calcaneus, the firmness of the surface on which the patient lands, and the position of the foot and leg when the foot strikes the ground.[72,129,140] It is the various combinations of bone quality, height of fall, and foot position that produce the varying degrees of comminution and fracture patterns, which make classification of these fractures so difficult.[72] Also, Barnard[11] correctly emphasizes that such a fall with the patient landing on a hard surface dissipates force to the ankle joint, skin, fibrous tissue, bone, and soft tissue structures about the ankle, midfoot, and forefoot. Therefore the actual fracture of the calcaneus and resulting damage to the subtalar joint is only a small part of the overall injury. The severity of the soft tissue injury associated with these fractures must be kept in mind when treatment and results are considered. Finally, because the usual mechanism is a fall from a height, these fractures are bilateral in up to 9% of patients.[98,99,134,140,178]

Since a fall from a height is the most common cause of these fractures, associated injuries in general are quite frequent.[48,76,99,157,162] Rowe et al.[157] noted associated injuries in 26% of all patients with calcaneus fractures, while associated injuries were reported in 60% of the patients reported by Lance et al.[98,99] and in nearly 70% of those reported by Slatis et al.[141] These injuries include compression fractures of the lumbar spine, which have been reported in 3% to 12% of cases,[48,76,99,157,162] and associated lower extremity fractures, which can occur in up to 10% of patients.[199]

---

*References 45, 50, 75, 107, 129, 177, and 189.

Cotton and Henderson[33] noted that such falls result in vertical compression of the calcaneus, which then expands laterally, pushing bone out beneath the fibula. The body of the calcaneus is therefore reduced in height and spread out laterally so that a considerable mass of bone piles up beneath the lateral malleolus and may impinge on it later.[71] King stresses that the area beneath the posterior facet has a paucity of trabeculae, and therefore a downward force on the fixed os calcis, such as occurs in a fall, can result in impaction of the outer two thirds of the posterior facet into the os calcis.[93]

Palmer[137] produced a very clear explanation of the mechanism of calcaneal fracture secondary to a fall. According to him, the tuberosity calcanei is forced upward by the impact when it strikes the ground, while the articular portion of the calcaneus is driven downward by the talus, resulting in a vertical shearing fracture.[14] (Fig. 24-9). If the foot is in a marked varus position when it strikes the ground, an extraarticular fracture of the medial tubercle can result. However, if the foot is in valgus on impact, a lateral shearing fracture will result. In most cases, this lateral shearing fracture is not restricted to the tubercle. Instead, the line of fracture starts on the medial side and runs laterally and upward, entering the posterior facet of the talocalcaneal joint and splitting it into two fragments[137] (Fig. 24-9, A). This fracture line may continue anteriorly to involve the calcaneocuboid joint also. The large fragment produced by this lateral shearing force is separated from the medial undisplaced portion of the calcaneus. Within this large lateral fragment, a secondary fracture of the compression type can occur, with the articular surface and underlying bone being driven down into the spongy bone of the calcaneus. The degree of compression of this articular surface corresponds to the maximal displacement at the time of the accident (Fig. 24-9, B). When the compression force is removed, the lateral fracture recoils downward, forming a step-off in the joint space (Fig. 24-9, C).[137] This secondary compression fracture of the lateral component can consist of the articular surface of the lateral one half of the posterior talocalcaneal joint, or the fragment can extend posteriorly to include the upper part of the tuberosity. The latter is the so-called tongue-type fracture mentioned by Essex-Lopresti.[48]

RADIOGRAPHIC EVALUATION

Proper radiographic visualization is essential in evaluation and treatment of calcaneal fractures. For any classification system to be accurate, excellent radiographic visualization of all components of the fracture is essential.[2,102,134,163] Most authors believe that any patient with a calcaneal fracture should be evaluated by a

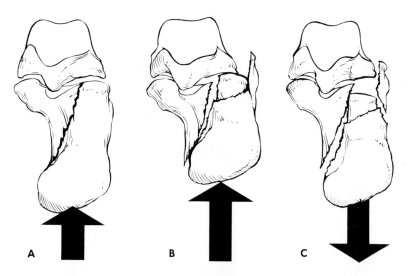

Fig. 24-9. Mechanism of fracture of calcaneus according to Palmer. **A,** Fracture line begins medially and runs laterally to exit into posterior facet. **B,** Articular surface is maximally displaced at time of injury. **C,** When compression force is removed, lateral surface recoils downward, forming step-off in articular surface of posterior facet. (Redrawn from Palmer, I.: J. Bone Joint Surg. **30A:**2-8, 1948.)

minimum of three radiographic views: an anteroposterior view of the foot (the so-called dorsoplantar view), a lateral view, and an axial view.* Additionally, an anteroposterior view of the ankle may be helpful.[178]

Because fractures of the calcaneus may be bilateral, it may be advisable to take radiographs of both feet.[58] Also, Hazlett recommends taking radiographs of the uninjured foot to establish a baseline for Bohler's angle and to detect any congenital anamolies that may confuse the appearance of the contralateral fractured calcaneus.[74] Additionally, Horn,[79] Hermann,[76] and O'Connell et al.[134] all recommend routinely taking lumbar spine radiographs in patients with calcaneal fractures, whether or not they have back complaints, in an effort to detect mild compression fractures of the lumbar and lower thoracic vertebra, which may otherwise go unnoted.

Standard radiographic views

The anteroposterior view of the midfoot (Fig. 24-10) is taken with the foot flat on the cassette and the central ray directed vertically downward, centered over the calcaneocuboid joint. This view demonstrates the extent of involvement and degree of displacement of fractures into the calcaneocuboid joint.[2,103,178] Since Vestad[184] reports that 23% of calcaneal fractures involve the calcaneocuboid joint, this view is essential in evaluation. In addition, medial subluxation of the talus at the talonavicular joint can occur in severe fractures,

and is well demonstrated on this anteroposterior view of the midfoot.[79,133,177] Finally, the amount of lateral spread of the lateral calcaneal surface is clearly visualized on the anteroposterior view.[79]

The lateral view (Fig. 24-11) is useful in detecting the amount of vertical displacement of the tuberosity of the calcaneus as it is reflected in Bohler's tuberosity joint angle.[2,178] In addition, it may or may not demonstrate involvement of the posterior facet of the subtalar joint and/or the calcaneocuboid joint.[2]

The axial view (Fig. 24-12) clearly demonstrates the medial concave and lateral convex surfaces of the body of the calcaneus.[2,178] Also, the articular margin of the posterior facet located on the lateral side of the foot and the sustentaculum tali and medial subtalar facet joint located on the medial side of the foot are clearly seen in this view.[2] Widening of the body of the calcaneus is also demonstrated on the axial view.[114,115] According to McReynolds[114,115] the axial view demonstrates the most significant deformity in calcaneal fractures, that being the marked depression and overriding of the superior medial fragment. It clearly demonstrates the main fracture line, which begins in the medial cortex of the calcaneus and inclines upward and outward into the posterior facet joint.

Essex-Lopresti[48] cautioned that interpretation of the axial view can be difficult. He stressed that the appearance of the subtalar joint on the axial view will depend on the angle at which the central ray strikes it. Often the subtalar joint is not shown at all on this view. The main change in appearance obtained by altering the an-

---

*References 45, 74, 76, 105, 167, and 184.

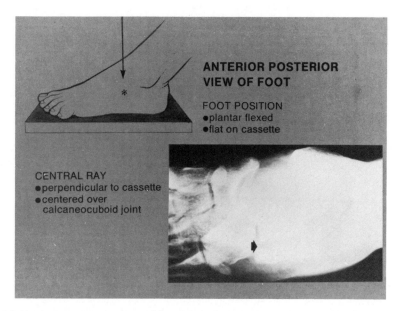

Fig. 24-10. Anteroposterior view of foot. Note fracture into calcaneocuboid joint (arrow).

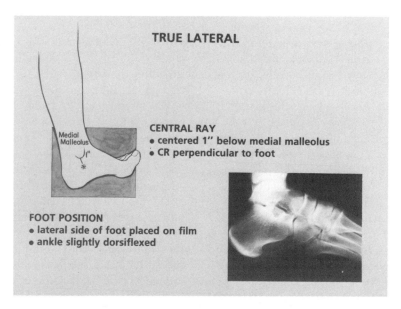

Fig. 24-11. Lateral view of foot.

gle at which the tube is directed is lengthening or foreshortening of the body of the calcaneus. Unless the central x-ray strikes the subtalar joint tangentially, its outline will not show up against the mass of spongy bone anterior to it. Furthermore, Essex-Lopresti pointed out that if the joint is simply displaced downwards and forwards, i.e. in the line of the central ray, no deformity will be present. Finally, Stephenson[174] emphasizes the importance of the axial view being taken with the radiographic tube tangential to the posterior facet in order to delineate any step-off in the posterior facet joint.

An anteroposterior view of the ankle has been recommended by few authors,[103,114,178] because it demonstrates piling up of bone from the lateral cortex of the calcaneus beneath the fibular malleolus. Additionally, it will detect associated ankle injuries.[178]

In addition to the standard views described here,

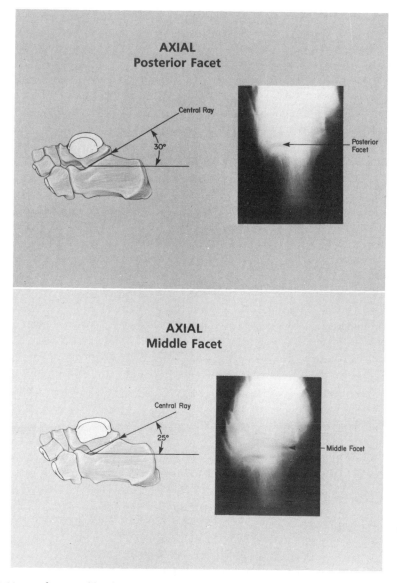

Fig. 24-12. Axial view of heel. Variation in angle of central ray is necessary for visualization of medial and posterior facets.

special views that demonstrate the subtalar joint in detail may be essential to correctly classify these fractures and to demonstrate joint congruity, particularly in intraarticular calcaneal fractures.[4,21,123,179,184]

Radiographic evaluation of subtalar joint

Anthonsen's view. Anthonsen[4] described a radiographic view in which the central ray is directed at a point just below the medial malleolus with the dorsiflexed foot in the lateral position on the film. The tube is tilted 25° caudally and 30° dorsoventrally (Fig. 24-13).[183,187] According to Anthosen, this view is particularly useful in visualizing the posterior and middle facets of the subtalar joint.[4,178] Schottstaedt,[163] Soeur

and Remy,[173] and Warrick and Bremner[187] strongly recommended the use of Anthosen's view. However, according to Isherwood[83] it is often difficult to produce these two Roentgen tube tilts simultaneously. Although foot position can be adjusted to counter this problem, Isherwood believes double-angulation of the tube combined with foot positioning makes it difficult to reproduce the view. He therefore suggested three additional oblique views for evaluating the subtalar joint: oblique lateral, medial oblique axial, and lateral oblique axial.

Oblique lateral view (oblique dorsoplantar). The inner border of the foot is placed on the film and the sole inclined 45° to the film. The tube is centered 1 inch below and 1 inch anterior to the lateral malleolus. This

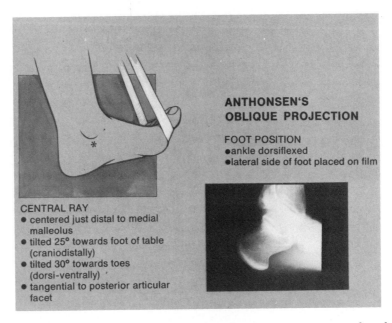

Fig. 24-13. Anthosen's view of calcaneus. This view demonstrates posterior and medial facets of subtalar joint.

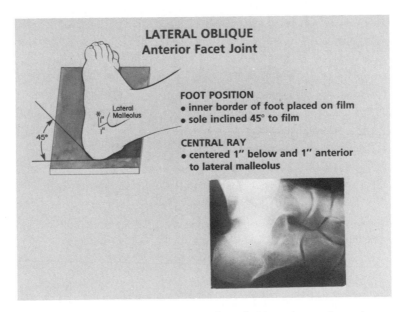

Fig. 24-14. Oblique dorsoplantar view (oblique lateral). Note clarity of anterior process and calcaneocuboid joint.

view clearly demonstrates the anterior process of the calcaneus and the calcaneocuboid joint (Fig. 24-14).[178]

Medial oblique axial view. The foot is dorsiflexed and inverted, this position being maintained by a broad bandage held by the seated patient. The knee is rotated 60° and the foot rests on a 30° wedge. The tube is directed axially and tilted 10° towards the head, being centered 1 inch below and 1 inch anterior to the lateral malleolus (Fig. 24-15). This projection gives an "end-on" view of the tarsal canal, as noted in Anthonsen's view, and has the added advantages of (1) placing the sustentaculum close to the film for bone detail, and (2) being more easily reproduced by having a flexed angulation of the tube. The medial oblique axial view

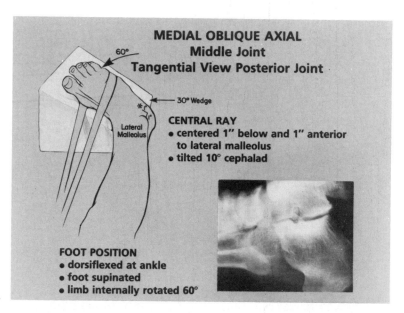

Fig. 24-15. Medial oblique axial view. Note clarity of medial and posterior facets of subtalar joint.

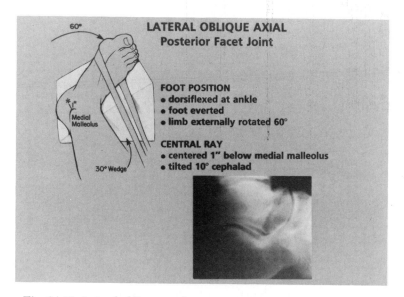

Fig. 24-16. Lateral oblique axial view. Posterior facet is seen in profile.

is used to demonstrate the medial joint and also to give a tangential view of the convexity of the posterior joint.

Lateral oblique axial view. The foot is dorsiflexed and inverted, the position again being maintained by asymmetric pull on a broad bandage. The knee is laterally rotated 60° and the foot rested on a 30° wedge. The tube is directed axially, tilted 10° towards the head, and centered 1 inch below the medial malleolus (Fig. 24-16). The tube direction and tilt are therefore fixed for both the medial and lateral oblique axial views. The lateral oblique axial view is excellent to demonstrate the posterior facet joint in profile.

Broden's projections. McReynolds[114,115] strongly suggested the use of Broden's projections I and II to evaluate the posterior subtalar facet[21] (Fig. 24-17). These views are based on the theory that the best examination of the posterior facet joint is performed by two projections in planes perpendicular to each other and at 45° to the long axis of the foot. Using these two

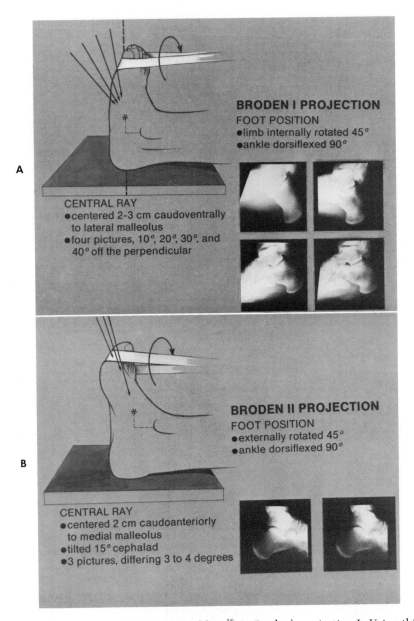

CENTRAL RAY
● centered 2-3 cm caudoventrally to lateral malleolus
● four pictures, 10°, 20°, 30°, and 40° off the perpendicular

BRODEN I PROJECTION
FOOT POSITION
● limb internally rotated 45°
● ankle dorsiflexed 90°

CENTRAL RAY
● centered 2 cm caudoanteriorly to medial malleolus
● tilted 15° cephalad
● 3 pictures, differing 3 to 4 degrees

BRODEN II PROJECTION
FOOT POSITION
● externally rotated 45°
● ankle dorsiflexed 90°

Fig. 24-17. Broden's radiographic views of foot.[18] **A,** Broden's projection I. Using this view, one can see entire posterior facet from front to back. **B,** Broden's projection II. This view demonstrates dorsoplantar compression at joint surface and sinus tarsi.

projections, McReynolds believed that one can see the entire posterior facet from front to back.

Broden's projection I. The patient is supine. The leg and foot are rotated inward 45° with the ankle joint at a right angle. The central ray is directed at a point 2 to 3 cm caudoventrally to the lateral malleolus. Four exposures are taken with the tube angled at 40°, 30°, 20°, and 10° respectively towards the head. The picture taken with the tube angled at 40° demonstrates the anterior part of the talocalcaneal joint, and the exposure

with the tube angled at 10° demonstrates the posterior aspect. Exposures with the tube angled at 30° or 20° may demonstrate the articulation between the sustentaculum tali and the talus (Fig. 24-17, A).[21]

Broden's projection II. The patient is supine. The foot and leg are turned 45° outwards with the ankle joint held at 90°. The central ray is directed at a point 2 cm caudal anteriorly to the medial malleolus with the tube angled 15° towards the head. Three exposures with a difference of 3° or 4° are then made (Fig. 24-17,

B). According to Broden, this view is useful to demonstrate the height of the articular cartilage and also to demonstrate dorsoplantar compression at the joint surface. Additionally, the sinus tarsi is distinctly visible.[21]

Conventional tomography and computed tomography

Letouronel[105] suggests that horizontal tomography may be useful to further delineate subtalar joint fractures. However, Soeur and Remy[173] did not find tomography particularly useful in evaluating these fractures. I have found polytomography to be useful in evaluating the subtalar joint in patients who cannot position their foot for the special views just described. Polytomes are more applicable to the evaluation of calcaneal fractures than tomograms, because they represent thinner cuts through the area of interest.

Recently, computed tomography (CT) has been introduced as a helpful aid in evaluating fractures of the calcaneus.[171,172] According to Smith and Staple,[172] CT scan evaluation of the hindfoot is useful, particularly in healed calcaneal fractures with residual pain and in tarsal coalition. They were particularly impressed with the fact that the CT scan would often demonstrate complete dislocation of the peroneal tendons following calcaneal fracture.

Smith and Naple also demonstrated that CT scanning is useful in evaluating the subtalar joint for fractures.[172] Although they believe that the hindfoot examination should be done with the patient fully weight bearing, the diameter of the gantry opening of most CT scanners precludes the standing position. They therefore devised a plantigrade position of the foot for scanning of the hindfoot. The feet are placed solidly on a table extension, requiring ankle plantar flexion of about 20°. The table extension is then raised to an angle of about 10° to reduce the effort required by the patient to hold the foot in a plantar-flexed position. The gantry is then tilted 5° cranially. Thus the central ray is within 5° of a line perpendicular to the plantar aspect of the foot. The posterior subtalar joint is clearly visualized using this technique. The advantages of CT scanning include better visualization of the subtalar joint, and patients in plaster casts can be scanned without removal of the plaster and with more comfort. I have no experience using CT scanning in evaluating acute calcaneus fractures.

TREATMENT: GENERAL PRINCIPLES

The variety of approaches to the treatment of calcaneal fractures presented in the literature is evidence of the frustration associated with managing this fracture. Standardization of treatment is nearly impossible, because the damage sustained by the os calcis varies within such great limits as to present difficult problems in management.[70,103] Little disagreement surrounds the treatment of extraarticular fractures, with good results reported in the majority of cases.[43,48,99,157] It is the management of displaced intraarticular fractures (involving the subtalar joint) where the majority of controversy exists.* As emphasized by Dart and Graham,[38] most authors champion a particular technique, but fracture patterns vary so greatly that recommending a single technique for treatment is as irrational as would be treating all fractures of the femur, regardless of location or type, in one particular way. Additionally, comparison of one method of treatment with another is very difficult, because so many variables are present that statistical significance becomes doubtful.[38]

The goal of treatment is solid union with normal motion in the talocalcaneal, calcaneonavicular, and calcaneocuboid joints.[80] All fractures of the calcaneus should be managed as severe injuries and consideration given to hospital admission and elevation to avoid edema and discourage the spread of the fracture hematoma.[38] Pumping motion of the toes and early range of motion to the foot help prevent the development of stiffness and induration that often are the overriding disabilities.[125] Horn[79] recommends restoration of the articular congruity, correction of widening of the calcaneus beneath the lateral malleolus, restoration of the height from the malleoli and the plantar surface of the heel pad, and early range of motion to restore function. Other authors, however, are not concerned about reduction but instead encourage early activity and exercise in an effort to restore function to the foot.[12,138,158] When dealing with the fractured calcaneus, one must remember this controversy regarding the necessity of fracture reduction in the overall scheme of calcaneus fracture management. I strongly endorse the recommendations of Miller,[125] who stresses that any treatment method *must* include early pumping action of the toes and early range of ankle, subtalar, and midfoot motion to prevent stiffness and induration.

One must remember that severe fractures may be less disabling than some of the more minor fractures, because a severe fracture can damage the subtalar joint to the degree that it becomes virtually ankylosed.[72] In such cases there may be little pain even when the deformity is severe.[72]

Finally, the ideal method for managing fractures of the calcaneus that involve the subtalar joint has not been discovered.[9] One must remember, however, that the degree of accuracy of anatomic restoration of calcaneal contour may not parallel the excellence of the functional result in many cases.[120]

---

*References 9, 17, 34, 43, 48, 74, 76, 99, 112-115, 120, 137, 142, 146, 157, 174, 178, 191, and 196.

Extraarticular fractures

Extraarticular fractures (fractures *not* involving the subtalar joint) seem to do well with nearly any form of treatment.[28,52,53,69,76] Unfortunately, however, these extraarticular fractures constitute only about 25% of all calcaneal fractures.[25,28,52,99]

Allan[3] reports that extraarticular fractures rarely produce disability. Essex-Lopresti[48] found that 92% of patients with extraarticular fractures were back to full work in under 6 months and that 93% had no or only trivial symptoms. Additionally, extraarticular fractures treated by exercise alone had slightly better results than those treated in plaster.[48] Rosendahl-Jensen[154] reported bad results in only 5.6% of all extraarticular fractures. Pridie[146] also reports that early motion and freedom from weight bearing produce good results in extraarticular fractures and that the patients generally return to their preinjury occupations. Extraarticular fractures then, as a group, tend toward a favorable long-term prognosis and, unless substantially displaced, can be treated in a conservative fashion. The various types of extraarticular fractures will be considered in the sections that follow.

FRACTURES OF ANTERIOR PROCESS OF CALCANEUS

Fracture of the anterior process of the calcaneus is classified as an avulsion type fracture of the calcaneus by Rowe et al.[40,157] Although historically this fracture has been considered an unusual injury, recent authors report that it is more common than previously appreciated.[18,57,81,143] This is secondary to the fact that in the past this fracture was often misdiagnosed as a sprain of the ankle. The true incidence of anterior process fracture is difficult to determine, because the injury is often missed. Reports of the frequency have varied from 3% to 23% of fractures of the calcaneus.[84,154,157]

Anatomy

Anatomically, this portion of the calcaneus has been variously named the anterior lip,[18] the anterior process,[29] the anterior superior portion,[36] the anterior superior process,[106] the promontory,[143] and the anterior end of the calcaneus.[188] Whichever term is preferred, this anterior process forms a saddle-shaped promontory that varies in length and breadth.[40,143] It can be completely absent, or it can overhang the adjacent proximal superior portion of the cuboid with an appearance similar to a parrot's beak.[85] The anterior process of the calcaneus is not seen radiographically in patients under the age of about 10 years.[40,85] and there is no physis in the area to cause confusion with the fracture. Rarely, however, an accessory ossicle, the calcaneus secundaris, occurs at this site, and it may be confused with a fracture.[40,81,94,181,197]

Fractures of the anterior process of the calcaneus have previously been classified as nonarticular calcaneal fractures, referring to their lack of involvement of the subtalar joint.[40,154,157] However, the saddle-shaped promontory of the anterior process articulates inferiorly with the cuboid.[39,40,49,81,85] Additionally, when the anterior process is well developed, its medial surface may consist of a cartilaginous articular surface that articulates with the slightly flattened facet on the inferior portion of the neck of the talus and hence may be involved in the subtalar joint.[85] Therefore when the fracture includes a large portion of the anterior process, both the subtalar and calcaneocuboid joints may be involved (Fig. 24-18). The significance of articular involvement of the calcaneocuboid joint has been previously noted only in relation to the uncommon compression fracture of the cuboid.[81] However, irrespective of its size, this process articulates over its entire distal surface with the cuboid, and therefore when it is fractured the calcaneocuboid joint is usually involved.[85,143] Although it is conceivable that a small cortical avulsion from the *lateral* cortex of the anterior process could be extraarticular, it is more likely that most of these fractures are indeed intraarticular, involving the calcaneocuboid and often the anterior talocalcaneal joints. Indeed, Jahss believes that occasional poor results seen with this fracture are related to intraarticular involvement of the fractures.[85] Because of the variation in size of the anterior process and the size and/or presence of the variable anterior talocalcaneal facet, the size of the fracture fragment may determine the presence or absence of articular involvement.

Several ligaments have points of attachment along the calcaneal promontory. Most important of these is the strong bifurcate ligament.[85] It originates from the lateral aspect of the anterior calcaneal process. The calcaneonavicular portion inserts distally into the adjacent navicular and the calcaneocuboid portion distally into the cuboid.[85] Additionally, a small portion of the extensor digitorum brevis muscle may originate from this bony prominence.[40] The dorsal calcaneocuboid ligament connects the calcaneus and cuboid superiorly. Jahss and Kay[85] clearly delineated the presence of the anterior interosseous talocalcaneal ligament, which arises in the sinus tarsi from the posterior surface of the base of the anterior calcaneal process and extends dorsally to insert into the inferolateral margin of the neck of the talus. He theorizes that the anterior interosseous ligament acts as a stabilizing point of fixation, while the calcaneocuboid ligament avulses the anterior process fragment with flexion and inversion of the foot.

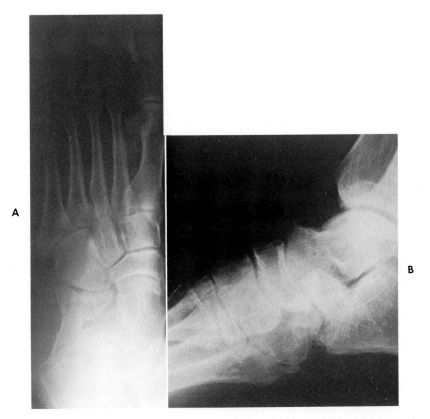

Fig. 24-18. A, Displaced fracture of anterior process of calcaneus with involvement of articular surface of calcaneocuboid joint. Because of size of fracture, anterior subtalar joint is also involved. **B,** Degenerative arthritis in calcaneocuboid, subtalar, and talonavicular joints following symptomatic treatment.

Mechanism of injury

Three mechanisms of injury have been reported to cause fracture of the anterior process of the calcaneus.[40]

1. Inversion and plantar flexion is the mechanism favored by most authors.* This mechanism is felt to result in avulsion of the anterior process by the bifurcate ligament. Because this is the same mechanism that produces the more common sprain of the anterior talofibular ligament of the ankle, the two entities are often confused with each other. This has resulted in the fracture being referred to as the "fracture sprain"[18] (Fig. 24-19, A). Experimental studies on the production of these fractures confirm that the process may be fractured with forced flexion combined with inversion.[85] However, occasionally this mechanism may produce isolated rupture of the calcaneocuboid ligament.[7] Jahss and Kay were unable to determine experimentally whether the anterior interosseous ligament and/or the calcaneocuboid ligament were responsible for isolated

*References 7, 29, 40, 57, 64, and 143.

fractures of the anterior calcaneal process.[85] They concluded, however, that since both are tight in inversion and plantar flexion, either or both may be responsible for the avulsion.[85]

2. Dachtler[36] described this fracture in association with a handcar injury in which the patient was struck just above the ankle posteriorly, resulting in a violent dorsiflexion injury to the foot. In this mechanism, the anterior process is forced downward into equinus against the cuboid, producing an impaction force that fractures the promontory[18,49,64] (Fig. 24-19, B).

3. Finally, forceful abduction of the forefoot with a fixed hindfoot can result in a compression fracture of the anterior process of the calcaneus.[81] King[92] reported three cases of such a compression fracture in which the mechanism appeared to be sudden abduction of the forefoot. Jaekle[84] also reported a similar fracture caused by a crushing injury. Hunt[81] emphasizes the importance of separating this type of fracture from the avulsion type because of the increased injury and more common displacement of the anterior process fracture

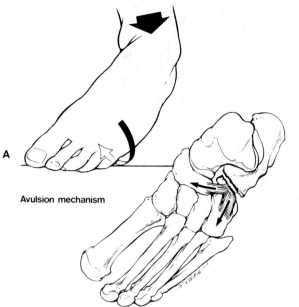

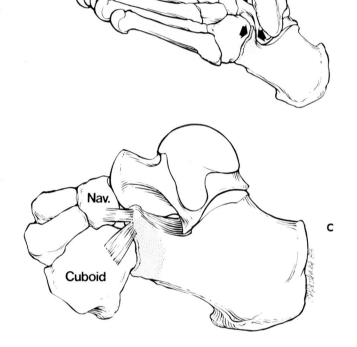

Fig. 24-19. A, Inversion and plantar flexion result in avulsion of anterior process by bifurcate ligament. This is the same mechanism that produces a sprain of anterior talofibular ligament, hence the term *sprain fracture*.[2] **B,** Anterior process is forced inward against cuboid, producing impaction force that fractures anterior process. **C,** Abduction and supination of forefoot forces cuboid against inferior aspect of calcaneus. This portion of anterior process is compressed and posteriorly displaced.[12]

by this mechanism.[81] He stresses that this results in severe derangement of the calcaneocuboid joint.[81] Gellman emphasizes that this mechanism may also result in damage to adjacent structures, particularly the cuboid articular surface. He theorizes this may have contributed to the severe peroneal spasticity King noted in his patients[57] (Fig. 24-19, *C*).

Diagnosis

History. The history of a "cracking sensation" at the time of the injury is common.[7] The patient may complain of pain, but it often is not severe enough to be disabling.[18] The pain is located on the outer aspect of the midportion of the foot. In the non-weight-bearing position this pain is minimal,[64] and a considerable increase in pain occurs with weight bearing.[7,18,49,57] This often leads patients to ignore the fracture and contributes to the large number of misdiagnoses and late diagnoses reported in the literature.[7,18,57]

Clinical diagnosis. Clinical examination of the foot reveals localized tenderness and swelling in a small, well-defined area 3 to 4 cm anterior and slightly below the lateral malleolus[7,40] (Fig. 24-20). This corresponds to an area on the dorsal surface of the calcaneocuboid joint.[18,57] The location of tenderness and swelling should immediately suggest a differential diagnosis that includes injury to the lateral malleolus, the lateral ligaments of the ankle joint, and the base of the fifth metatarsal. *Careful* location of the point of maximal tenderness helps differentiate these entities.[7,18,40,64] Additionally, supination of the entire foot at the *ankle* does not reproduce pain as it does in lateral ligamentous injury of the ankle.[7] Manipulation of the foot into inversion and adduction does increase the pain and spasm.[7,18,40]

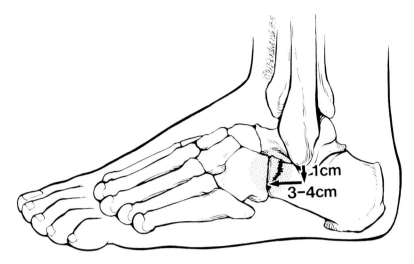

Fig. 24-20. Anterior process is located slightly below and 3 to 4 cm anterior to lateral malleolus. Point tenderness in this area suggests anterior process fracture.

This entity must be suspected when a patient with a history of trauma has marked peroneal spasm following a suspected ankle injury.[35,92]

Radiographic diagnosis. The fracture cannot usually be seen on routine anteroposterior radiographs of the foot and only occasionally is it visible on the lateral view.* Although superoinferior views of the foot have been recommended to detect this fracture,[36] most authors agree that this area is best seen on an oblique projection of the foot in which the adjacent bones do not overlap.[49,106,197] These oblique views must be taken at several different angles to separate the shadow of the anterior process from that of the front and undersurface of the talus.[57] Bachman et al.[6A] suggest these radiographs be taken with a central beam directed 15 to 20 degrees superior and posterior to the midfoot. This projects the anterior process over the neck of the talus enough that the fracture can be easily visualized[40] (Fig. 24-21, *A* and *B*). Gellman[57] suggests a caudal and dorsal direction of the central ray so that it passes 15° to 25° cranially and 10° to 15° ventrally. However, the precise angles must be adjusted individually to meet the variations in the size and shape of the anterior calcaneal process in different patients.[7]

In spite of these special views, tomograms may be necessary to demonstrate the anterior process fracture and particularly to determine whether or not an anterior talocalcaneal facet is present and involved in the fracture.[32,35] Conway and Cowell[32] have demonstrated the value of lateral tomography of the talocalcaneal

joint to evaluate this anterior facet. Polytomography may also be useful to evaluate involvement of the calcaneocuboid joint. Finally, Jahss has suggested that subtalar arthrography combined with oblique radiographs may be important in evaluating the anterior talocalcaneal joint.[85]

When evaluating the radiographs it is important to distinguish between an acute fracture of the anterior process (Fig. 24-22, *B*), a nonunion of this fracture (Fig. 24-22, *C*), and an accessory ossicle, the calcaneus secundarius, which when present is located near the anterior process of the calcaneus[197] (Fig. 24-22, *A*). The calcaneus secundarius, however, is usually round or ovoid in shape with its cortex sheathing the bony density.[18,143] The smooth edges and rounded appearance of this anomaly help to differentiate it from an acute fracture or a nonunion[18] (see Fig. 24-22, *A*). Although some authors have mentioned the possibility of confusing this fracture with an nonunited epiphysis,[143] Piat reports no such secondary epiphyseal center at this location, thereby excluding the possibility of an united epiphysis confusing the diagnosis.[143] In the acute fracture, the fragment is usually triangular in shape[40] and the fracture surfaces are irregular (Fig. 24-22, *B*). A nonunion is also triangular in shape, but the fracture surfaces are sclerotic (Fig. 24-22, *C*).

To adequately outline a plan of treatment, the oblique views and/or tomograms must be *carefully* studied to determine (1) the size of the fracture fragment, (2) the degree of displacement, and (3) the presence of subtalar and calcaneocuboid joint involvement.

---

*References 18, 36, 40, 57, 143, and 197.

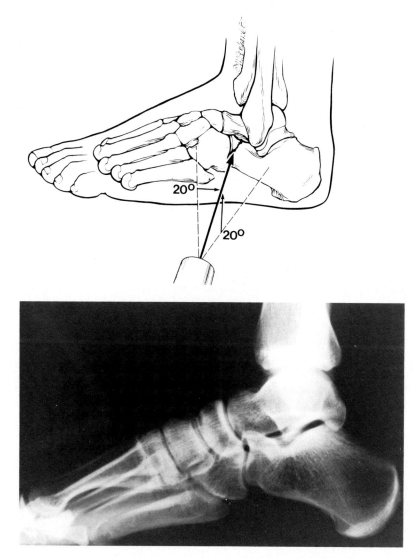

Fig. 24-21. Oblique view obtained by angling central beam 20° cephalad and 20° posterior projects anterior process over neck of talus, allowing excellent visualization.[8]

Treatment

A great deal of controvery surrounds the treatment of fractures of the anterior process of the calcaneus. Most authors report the majority of these fractures unite in 2 to 3 months whether rigid or semirigid immobilization is used.[36,39,57,85,154] Gellman recommends a simple below-the-knee cast for severe cases and believes that an elastic bandage is sufficient for the less severe injuries.[57] He does not permit weight bearing for 4 weeks.[57] Backman et al.[7] recommend elastic bandage immobilization for 2 to 3 weeks unless the injury is severe, in which case a cast is applied. Bradford and Larsen also recommend either an elastic bandage or a short leg plaster boot, depending on the degree of associated injury.[18] Likewise, Green recommends immo-

bilizing the foot with either an adhesive strapping or a plaster in the neutral position, with weight bearing only after 2 weeks.[64]

Debold and Stimson emphasize that maintaining function of the subtalar joint is more important that anatomic repositioning of the fracture.[39] They stress that prolonged immobilization and associated edema may lead to stiffness and weakness of the subtalar and other small joints of the foot.

Jahss also stresses that, although rigid immobilization gives more comfort, in his experience a cast has been associated with Sudeck's atrophy and extremely disabling stiffness of the entire foot and ankle.[85] He therefore recommends the use of an Unna boot as treatment for these fractures.

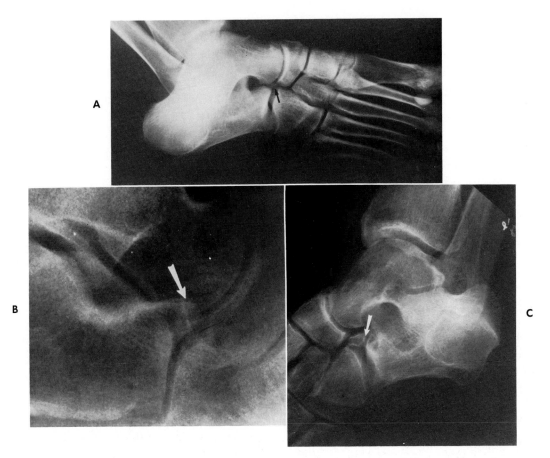

Fig. 24-22. A, Os calcaneus secondarius, an accessory ossicle. Note ovoid shape and irregular edges (arrow). **B,** Fracture of anterior process of calcaneus. Note triangular shape and irregular edges of fracture surface (arrow). **C,** Nonunion of anterior process of calcaneus. Sclerotic margins and triangular shape help differentiate it from os calcaneus secondarius. (**B** and **C** From Degan, T.F., Morrey, B.F., and Braun, D.P.: J. Bone Joint Surg. **64A:**518-524, 1982.)

Although these fractures usually heal with 4 to 6 weeks of immobilization by either simple adhesive strapping or a plaster cast,[106] Degan et al. emphasize that they may not be completely asymptomatic after this period of immobilization.[40] In fact, 28% of their patients required *more* than 1 year to become asymptomatic or to realize the final extent of recovery from this injury. Based on this experience, they recommend up to 1 year of nonoperative treatment before any surgical treatment is considered.[40]

The question of whether or not *immediate* surgical intervention in the form of excision would shorten the convalescence has often been raised.[18,85] Because most of these fractures heal without sequelae, both Jahss and Kay[85] and Bradford and Larsen[18] feel that such aggressive treatment is open to criticism. However, excision

of the neglected fracture fragment that has progressed to nonunion with continuous pain and disability has been reported to be successful.[40,49,197] Finder et al.[49] Degan et al.[40] and Jahss and Kay[85] caution against performing such an excision before adequate time for recovery has elapsed. Excision of the nonunion may not result in permanent symptomatic relief, and recovery after the excision may be prolonged.[40,49]

Likewise, the place of open reduction and internal fixation of *displaced* fractures of the anterior process of the calcaneus is not clear. Rowe et al.[157] report open reduction in two patients in whom the fracture fragments were large enough, and Watson-Jones[88] notes that operative intervention may be indicated when large fragments of the anterior process of the calcaneus are separated and tilted. Hunt[81] reported a displaced fracture of the anterior process of the calcaneus secondary to an abduction force in which a good result was obtained following open reduction and internal fixation. It must be remembered that in this case the fracture fragment was quite large and was associated with midtarsal subluxation. Open reduction in this situation not only restores the articular surface of the calcaneocuboid joint but also reduces and stabilizes the subluxation of the midtarsal joint.

Although Jahss and Kay[85] mention open reduction and internal fixation of larger fragments to correct a step-off on the articular surface of the calcaneocuboid joint, they caution against this procedure because of the good results reported from conservative treatment of most of these fractures. However, Gould, in discussing this article,[85] recommends that large fragments be treated by immediate surgical intervention. The determination is made whether the fracture should be firmly fixed and motion immediately initiated or the fragment should be excised. He emphasizes that which ever approach is used, *immediate* postoperative motion is essential. He stresses that restoration of subtalar and midtarsal motion is as critical as restoration of joint surface alignment.[85]

Finally, in patients who have not had relief of symptoms following excision of the calcaneal fragment, Bradford and Larsen mention triple arthrodesis as a final attempt to relieve their pain.[18]

Results

The prognosis following fracture of the anterior process of the calcaneus is quite good, particularly if the fragment is *small* and minimally displaced. The large majority of these fractures unite without sequalae in 2 to 3 months.[36,39,85] Degan et al. report satisfactory results with no limitation of activity following conservative treatment of these fractures.[40] However, they stress that the time for recovery averages 10 months, and at follow-up less than half of their patients were completely pain free. The main factor associated with long-term disability and poor results is delay in diagnosis and treatment.[18,40,106] Although Jackie and Clark[84] report that involvement of the calcaneocuboid joint is unimportant and disability from this involvement practically nil, Hunt and Gould stress the importance of restoring the articular surface of the calcaneocuboid joint.[81,85] The size of the fragment also affects results because the larger fragments have more involvement of the calcaneocuboid articular surface.[81]

Although they noted no loss of motion of the subtalar or Chopart's joint following excision of the fragment, Degan et al. did report occasional ossification in the area of excision at follow-up.[40] They report that recovery is often prolonged following excision and that in patients who received no early treatment (22 to 24 months after fracture), an unsatisfactory result was obtained after fragment excision.[40]

AUTHOR'S PREFERRED METHOD OF TREATMENT

I consider it extremely important to completely evaluate this fracture radiographically *before* deciding on the method of treatment. Oblique radiographs and even polytomes may be required to distinguish the size of the fracture fragment, the degree of displacement, and the presence or absence of anterior subtalar and calcaneocuboid joint involvement.

In patients with acute fractures of the anterior process of the calcaneus, treatment is based on the size of the fracture fragment, the associated soft tissue injury, and the degree of displacement. For small, nondisplaced fragments, in which involvement of the calcaneocuboid joint is minimal, immobilization in a soft tissue compression dressing with non-weight bearing is initiated. If there is marked associated soft tissue swelling, a short period of immobilization in a posterior splint is used. An Unna boot is applied when swelling has decreased. As soon as comfort allows, motion of the subtalar and Chopart's joint are initiated under the direction of a physical therapist. Additionally, toe flexion exercises are instituted in an effort to help decrease edema in the foot. The *main* goal is to restore motion in these two joints. Weight bearing is usually delayed for 2 to 4 weeks, based on the associated pain. The patients are informed that recovery may take 3 to 4 months following this seemingly minor injury.

Cast immobilization for 4 weeks is used when soft tissue injury is severe. Because of the inability to institute early motion with this method, I seldom use this approach.

In patients with a large, displaced fracture fragment involving a major portion of the calcaneocuboid and/or anterior subtalar joint, consideration is given to open reduction and internal fixation or excision, depending on fragment size. I prefer a longitudinal incision over the calcaneocuboid joint and parallel to the sole of the foot. In my experience this incision, which is parallel to the sural nerve fibers, results in less neuroma formation and fewer tender surgical incisions. It is important to stress that if either one of these methods are selected, the patient *must* initiate immediate range of motion so that subtalar and Chopart's joint motion is not lost.

Excision of fracture fragments that represent a painful nonunion is withheld until at least 1 year after injury in an effort to allow complete recovery before surgical intervention.

TUBEROSITY FRACTURE: BEAK AND AVULSION FRACTURES

Anatomy

Beak and avulsion fractures of the calcaneus, which involve the posterosuperior aspect of the calcaneus, are well recognized.[34,147,187] These fractures do not involve the subtalar joint unless the posterior fragment is unusually large.[164] Essex-Lopresti,[48] Bohler,[17] and Rothberg[156] reported this injury to be extremely rare. Rowe et al.[157] and Lyngstadaas[109] report that it makes up 3% of calcaneus fractures.

The classification of fractures of the posterosuperior aspect of the calcaneus is based on involvement of the insertion of the Achilles tendon into the calcaneus.[108,109] Watson-Jones[188] and Bohler[17] have termed those fractures that do *not* involve the Achilles tendon insertion *beak fractures* (Fig. 24-23, *A*). They termed those fractures that do involve the Achilles tendon insertion *avulsion fractures*[17,188] (Fig. 24-23, *B*). This avulsed fragment can vary in size from a small sliver of bone located beneath the Achilles tendon to a large mass consisting of the entire posterior tuberosity of the calcaneus.[134]

The posterior surface of the calcaneus has three distinct areas or subdivisions.[108] Most inferior on the posterior surface is a roughened area for the fibrofatty tissue of the heel pad. The middle surface, into which the Achilles tendon is inserted, joins the upper surface, which is smooth and is related to a bursa that lies deep to the Achilles tendon.[108] The Achilles tendon is separated from the proximal one half of the posterior surface of the calcaneus by this bursa.[147] Fractures related to this bursa only are the so-called beak fractures, whereas those extending into the middle portion of the posterior surface involve the Achilles tendon insertion (Fig. 24-23).

The Achilles tendon attachment is *usually* positioned in the middle one third, but in 5% of patients it is located in the upper one third, of the posterior surface.[73,79] Both Korn[96] and Lowy[108] demonstrated that the point of insertion of the Achilles tendon may cover a variable portion of the posterior aspect of the calcaneus.

Additionally, Sutro[175] has demonstrated degenerative changes at the point of insertion of the calcaneal tendon in persons over the age of 50. These changes, when present in an already high insertion, may produce the appearance of a "beak" type fracture radiographically when, in fact, the entire insertion of the tendo Achilles has been avulsed.[175] Finally, Protheroe[147] casts doubt on the exact differentiation between "beak" and "avulsion" fractures on an anatomic basis. In two of the patients he reported, he found that the Achilles tendon

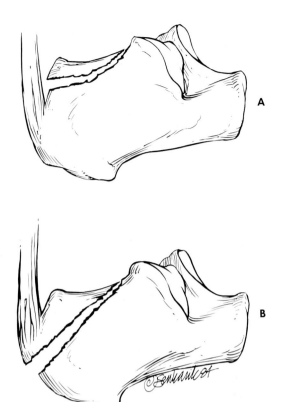

Fig. 24-23. Beak (**A**) and avulsion (**B**) fractures of calcaneus.

was adherent to the *entire* posterior aspect of the calcaneus and hence inserted more proximally into the posterior surface of the calcaneus than has been classically described. One of these fractures was radiographically identical to a beak fracture, but at surgery was found to be a true avulsion.

Because of the variability in location of the insertion of the Achilles tendon and the changes pointed out by Sutro[175] associated with aging, the only way to accurately differentiate beak and avulsion fractures is by clinical examination or surgical exploration, *not* by radiography.[147] Lowy[108] cautions that if the clinical diagnosis is in doubt, it is a good idea to explore the heel, because failure to gain accurate reduction of the fracture (and hence Achilles tendon continuity) will produce substantial disability.

Mechanism of injury

According to Watson-Jones[188] and Bohler[17] beak fractures are caused by direct trauma to the posterior surface of the calcaneus, while avulsion fractures are secondary to a violent contraction on the Achilles tendon.[188] Parkes,[139] Korn,[96] and O'Connell et al.[134] also attribute avulsion fractures to violent pull by the Achilles tendon with the foot in a fixed position. According to Lyngstadaas[109] and Rothberg,[159] the most common mechanism is a fall, which causes the patient to strike his heel on a hard surface with the triceps surae tensed. Garcia and Parkes[54] believe when a patient lands with the knee in full extension and the ankle in plantar flexion after a jump, it produces tension in the Achilles tendon that avulses the insertion.

Clinical diagnosis

Patients give a history of a fall on the foot and of feeling a "pop" in the heel or a direct blow to the heel with sudden pain.[108,139] They complain of pain in the heel and in avulsion fractures, walk with a flatfooted, antalgic gait.[108,139] In addition to pain in the heel and calf, there is commonly weakness of plantar flexion.[108,147] Clinically the heel is grossly swollen and, after the first 12 to 24 hours, may have ecchymosis and bullous formation in the area of the tuberosity.[44,50,106,147,156]

In avulsion fractures with displacement there may be a palpable hollow between the calcaneus and the avulsed fragment that contains the Achilles tendon insertion.[147,156] Also, in avulsion fractures one can demonstrate a loss of function of the Achilles tendon by absence of plantar flexion with calf compression. Lowy[108] emphasizes the diagnosis of an avulsion fracture is based on the clinical examination and *not* on radiographs. As mentioned earlier, the variability of insertion of the Achilles tendon is responsible for avulsion fractures appearing radiographically as beak fractures. Careful *clinical* examination is essential to distinguish these two injuries and permit correct treatment selection.

Radiographic diagnosis

Radiographically, both beak and avulsion fractures are best seen on a lateral view of the foot and ankle, which demonstrates a fracture involving the posterosuperior aspect of the tuberosity of the calcaneus.[9,114,139,147] Although beak fractures usually involve *less* than the upper one-half of the tuberosity of the calcaneus, while "avulsion" fractures *never* involve less than one-half of the tuberosity, the clinical examination is the *key* to distinguishing these two injuries. Classically both of these fractures demonstrate separation at the fracture site with only minor comminution.[147] Displacement is the key to fracture evaluation, as either beak or avulsion fractures which are displaced may require reduction.

Treatment

Treatment recommendatiaons are based on *clinically* distinguishing between avulsion and beak fractures. It is essential to determine whether the fracture fragment contains the Achilles tendon insertion.

Beak fractures. Garcia and Parkes[54] recommend that nondisplaced beak fractures be treated by immobilization of the foot in the neutral position or slight plantar flexion for a period of 6 weeks without weight bearing.[54] In displaced beak fractures (those that do not contain the Achilles tendon insertion), Schottstaedt[164] and Sisk[167] recommend closed reduction and immobilization in a plantar-flexion cast for 6 weeks. Heck[75] reports that the surgeon can reposition a displaced beak fracture by applying direct pressure to the fragment with his or her thumb while the foot is in plantar flexion. Following reduction, Heck recommends a short leg cast for 6 weeks. If displaced beak fractures are not treated by closed reduction, the closeness of the skin overlying the displaced fracture fragment can produce skin necrosis.[147]

Avulsion fractures. Schottstaedt[163,164] and Slatis et al.[168] treated nondisplaced avulsion fractures of the calcaneus in a non-weight-bearing cast in equinus position for 6 weeks, followed by non-weight bearing for an additional 2 weeks.[163,164,168]

The most important effect of displaced avulsion fractures of the calcaneus is impairment of heel cord function.[147] The greater the displacement of the avulsed fracture, the greater the functional loss and the more need for accurate reduction. There is general agreement that displaced avulsion fractures have to be repositioned,[75,157] and the need for accurate reduction of the avulsed fracture is stressed by most authors.[108] Closed reduction by direct pressure over the displaced fragment with the foot in plantar flexion has been recommended.[44,96] Following closed reduction, Key and Conwell[90] recommended immobilization in a long leg cast with the knee bent and the foot plantar flexed. Other authors recommend open reduction and internal fixation in all patients in whom the avulsion fracture is displaced.[146,167]

Parkes[139] and Lowy[108] recommend open reduction and internal fixation with a screw, followed by a cast with the foot in the equinus position for 6 weeks. The displaced fragment containing the Achilles tendon insertion can be fixed with a screw either from above and through the fragment or from below, through the calcaneus, and into the fragment[108] (Fig. 24-24). Schottstaedt[163,164] recommended open reduction using a medial or lateral incision that parallels the Achillles tendon. He stressed that timing of surgery depends on the degree of swelling present.[163,164]

The choice of open versus closed methods of reduction of avulsion fractures must take the patient and the displacement into consideration. According to McLaughlin,[110] if the insertion of the Achilles tendon is merely tilted upward direct pressure over the fragment and casting in plantar flexion produces a good result.

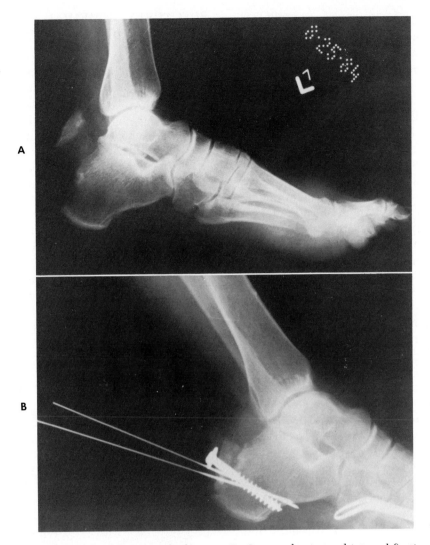

Fig. 24-24. A, Avulsion fracture of calcaneus. **B,** Open reduction and internal fixation using A-O 4 mm cancellous screw.

However, if the fracture is tilted *and* rotated with displacement, he believes that open reduction and internal fixation are necessary.[110] In elderly patients with impaired function or decreased demands who have slightly displaced avulsion fractures, treatment by soft dressing immobilization and physical therapy will produce a good result.[147] However, younger patients with displacement of an avulsion fracture must have open reduction and internal fixation if normal function is to be expected.[147]

Prognosis

According to Key and Conwell[90] and Parkes,[139] the prognosis for both fracture union and function are excellent when avulsion and beak fractures are reduced. Heck[75] and O'Connell et al.[134] report excellent results

unless the fracture involves the posterior subtalar joint, which rarely occurs unless the fragment is large.

The complications of persistent displacement of avulsion fractures include weak plantar flexion and difficulty climbing stairs.[147] Finally, skin slough over persistently displaced beak fractures has been reported.[147]

AUTHOR'S PREFERRED METHOD
OF TREATMENT

In my opinion, the most important aspect in evaluating these patients is to *clinically* distinguish between beak and avulsion fractures. Weakness of ankle plantar flexion and loss of passive plantar flexion on squeezing the calf are signs I rely on to determine whether the fracture fragment contains the insertion of the Achilles tendon. If these tests are inconclusive in a young patient who has a displaced fracture, I explore the fracture. If the Achilles tendon is attached to the fracture fragment, I perform internal fixation of the fracture.

Beak fractures. In beak fractures in which the displacement is minimal, i.e., if the fracture fragment does not pose any threat to the overlying skin, I use a short leg walking cast for 4 to 6 weeks. I allow early weight bearing *only* if the clinical examination confirms that the fracture is truly of the beak variety and that the insertion of the Achilles tendon is intact. If continuity of the tendon is not certain, non-weight bearing is selected because of the potential for Achilles tendon activity to produce displacement of the fracture.

In displaced fractures in which the overlying skin seems to be at risk, I perform a closed reduction. With the knee bent and the ankle in plantar flexion, I apply direct pressure to the displaced fragment. If the reduction is successful, I use a short leg cast in plantar flexion for 6 weeks followed by progressive weight bearing. Early active motion to the metatarsophalangeal joints is encouraged. If the fracture is markedly displaced and cannot be reduced by closed methods, open reduction via an incision lateral to the Achilles tendon is recommended. Care is taken to avoid injury to the sural nerve when this approach is used. I prefer A-O cancellous screws for fixation. If stable fixation is obtained postoperatively, no immobilization is used and early motion of all foot joints is instituted. Progressive weight bearing is allowed at 4 to 6 weeks postoperatively.

Avulsion fractures. I believe that avulsion fractures of the calcaneus that are displaced to any degree must be reduced unless the patient is elderly and very inactive. The clinical examination is used to confirm the discontinuity of the Achilles tendon mechanism.

I prefer open reduction unless the local skin conditions are unacceptable. I use an incision lateral to the Achilles tendon. Once the reduction is obtained, fixation using either 6.5 mm or 4.0 mm A-O cancellous screws, depending on the fracture fragment size, is performed. Following open reduction and internal fixation, I place the foot in an equinus short leg cast for 4 weeks, followed by a short leg walking cast with the foot in the neutral position for 2 weeks. Progressive weight-bearing and intensive range-of-motion exercises out of plaster are then instituted.

Finally, I emphasize the importance of careful evaluation of the lateral radiograph to make certain that neither beak nor avulsion fractures communicate with the posterior subtalar joint because of the adverse affect on long-term prognosis. If such communication is noted, accurate open reduction, stable internal fixation, and immediate range of motion is my choice of treatment.

FRACTURES OF MEDIAL AND LATERAL PROCESSES OF CALCANEUS
Anatomy

The medial process serves as the origin of the abductor hallucis and the medial portion of the flexor hallucis brevis and plantar fascia. The lateral process serves as the origin of the abductor digit minimi. Fractures of the medial or lateral process of the tuberosity of the calcaneus are uncommon injuries,[45,54] the medial tubercle being the most frequently fractured. These fractures are rarely significantly displaced[110] (Fig. 24-25).

Mechanism of injury

These fractures occur when an abduction or adduction force is exerted on the heel as it strikes the ground in eversion, which produces a fracture of the medial process, or inversion, which causes a fracture of the lateral process.[45,54] A less common mechanism occurs when the medial aspect of the heel receives a glancing blow from below while the foot is held in a valgus position.[52,110]

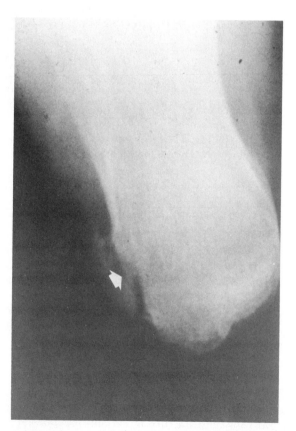

Fig. 24-25. Fracture of medial process of tuberosity of calcaneus.

Clinical diagnosis

Patients give a history of having fallen or jumped from a height, landing directly on the heel. The heel is thickened and swollen, and ecchymosis will appear within the first 24 hours.[110] In medial process fractures, the posteromedial sulcus of the heel is flattened, and the entire hindfoot may be tender.[110]

Tenderness may be localized to the posteromedial or posterolateral surface of the heel depending on the location of the fracture.[54] Additionally, there may be tenderness on the plantar aspect of the heel.[54] Range of motion to the ankle, midfoot, and forefoot joints is usually within normal limits.[54]

Radiographic diagnosis

Radiographically the diagnosis is confirmed on the axial view of the calcaneus or a posteroanterior view of the foot[54,84,110] (Fig. 24-25).

Treatment

McLaughlin[110] recommended simple immobilization of these fractures in a walking cast until union occurs. Bohler[17] also recommends a short leg cast for 6 weeks with immediate weight bearing.

Garcia and Parkes[54] recommend elevation in a pressure dressing. Ice is applied and early range of motion instituted. In displaced fractures, they recommend reduction by molding the heel and applying a well-padded plaster around it.[54] As swelling usually decreases in 7 to 10 days, a cast change may be necessary. The cast is removed after 4 weeks, and the patient is begun on range of motion and kept non-weight bearing for an additional 4 weeks. Schottstaedt[163] and Kalish[89] recommended a plaster cast for 5 to 6 weeks for undisplaced fractures of the tuberosities. Because displaced fractures can produce widening of the heel, they believe consideration should be given to reduction by manipulation using the pressure of the heel of the hand or a compression clamp followed by a short leg cast for 4 to 8 weeks.[89,163]

Dodson[45] also bases treatment recommendations on fracture displacement. He recommends elevation and compression followed by non-weight bearing and range of motion in nondisplaced fractures. If the fracture is displaced, he too recommends reduction by compression and application of a well fitted non-weight-bearing cast, which is worn for 8 weeks. Schofield[162] also recommends closed reduction following injection of the fracture site with an anesthetic.

Jaekle and Clark[84] report that fractures consisting of a longitudinal split with slight medial-to-lateral separation produce minimal disability. However, if the medial or lateral tuberosity has any degree of proximal displacement, a painful heel will result unless it is reduced. McLaughlin[110] mentioned shoe modifications if malunion results in a painful prominence.

Prognosis

Persistent tenderness in the heel, managed by shoe modification or padding, is the main long-term problem that has been reported.[58,110] Nonunion of the displaced fragment, requiring excision, has also been mentioned.[54]

Author's preferred method of treatment

In nondisplaced fractures and those with only minimal separation of the fracture surfaces, I use a compression dressing with ice and elevation. Range of motion exercises of the ankle, subtalar, midtarsal, and metatarsophalangeal joints are instituted immediately. Once pain and swelling have subsided, a well-molded short leg walking cast is worn for 3 to 4 weeks. A shoe with a well-padded heel is then recommended.

In fractures with proximal displacement and/or marked mediolateral separation, I attempt closed reduction by applying mediolateral compression on the heel using the heels of my hands. If this method is not successful in reducing the separation, compression with a Bohler clamp is used if the patient's local skin circulation is not compromised and the fracture is significantly displaced. After reduction of a displaced fracture, a well-padded short leg non-walking cast is applied with mediolateral molding about the heel to maintain the reduction. The patient is kept non-weight bearing for 4 weeks. Weight bearing for an additional 2 weeks in a walking cast is then recommended.

If closed reduction is not successful, I treat these patients in the same manner as if the fracture were nondisplaced. This is because I have not seen long-term disability significant enough to warrant open reduction and internal fixation.

FRACTURE OF BODY OF CALCANEUS NOT INVOLVING SUBTALAR JOINT
Anatomy

Of fractures of the body of the calcaneus, 20% do not involve the subtalar joint.[54,157,187] The only criterion for a fracture to be included in this group is a lack of involvement of the subtalar and calcaneocuboid joints. The fracture line usually extends from the posteromedial to the anterolateral aspect of the calcaneus, lying behind the subtalar joint.[28] Even though the subtalar joint is not involved in the fracture, displacement of the fracture can occur in a proximal direction, resulting in reduction of the tuberosity joint angle, or in a

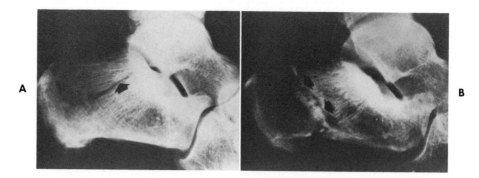

Fig. 24-26. **A,** Extraarticular fracture of body of calcaneus; undisplaced. **B,** Extraarticular fracture of body of calcaneus with proximal displacement of tuberosity and reduction in Bohler's tuberosity joint angle.

mediolateral direction, producing widening of the heel.[158,164]

Mechanism of injury

The same mechanism that produces intraarticular fractures of the calcaneus can result in a fracture of the calcaneal tuberosity *without* involvement of the subtalar joint.[28] According to Chapman, the most common mechanism is that of landing on the heel after a fall or sustaining a severe blow from below while standing.[28] Additionally, Garcia and Parkes[54] emphasize that a fall from a height with the heel in the neutral or valgus position produces this extraarticular fracture. Since the fall is usually not from a great height, there is often little comminution or displacement of this type of fracture.[139]

Clinical diagnosis

The signs and symptoms of this fracture are similar to those of an intraarticular fracture. The patient usually gives a history of a fall from a height with sudden severe pain and the inability to bear weight.[54] Swelling and ecchymosis of the heel are present shortly after the injury.[54,139] In addition to generalized pain and swelling about the heel, there is tenderness to pressure on both the medial and lateral aspects of the heel.[45,54] If the fracture is displaced in a proximodistal direction, plantar-flexion weakness may be present. Motion of the ankle and subtalar joint are usually painful.

Radiographic diagnosis

Garcia and Parkes[54] emphasize that, although this fracture is best seen on the lateral view of the foot, it is extremely important to obtain other views to make certain there is no involvement of the subtalar joint.[45,139] They recommend the axial view to rule out subtalar involvement.[54] On the lateral view, Bohler's

tuberosity joint angle can be determined and compared to the uninjured side (Fig. 24-26).

Treatment

Controversy exists as to the best way to treat these fractures.[47] However, because fractures without subtalar involvement usually have good results, most authors recommend minimal treatment.[45,54,157,163,164] Garcia and Parkes[54] and Dodson[45] recommend ice, elevation, a compression dressing, and institution of early range of dorsiflexion–plantar flexion, inversion-eversion, and toe motion for fractures without displacement. They recommend that patients be kept non-weight bearing for 12 weeks to prevent displacement of the fracture. Rowe et al.[157] recommend immobilization in a short leg cast if the fracture is nondisplaced. Geckeler[56] recommended early protected weight bearing in an equinus cast for nondisplaced fractures. Early weight bearing is believed to prevent loss of muscle tone and disuse changes in the joints of the foot.[56]

Rowe et al.[157] recommend closed reduction of displaced fractures. Schottstaedt[163,164] recommends reduction by traction and immobilization in a cast molded with mediolateral compression if the heel is widened.[163] Wilson[193] also recommends the use of a Bohler compression clamp followed by a short leg cast in fractures with marked mediolateral displacement (Fig. 24-27).

According to Garica and Parkes[54] and McReynolds,[114] if the fracture exits posterior to the articular surface of the posterior facet and is displaced proximally, it should be reduced with a percutaneous Kirschner wire to pull the fragment down. Once reduction has been obtained in this manner, the traction wire is incorporated into a long cast with the knee bent at 45° to relax the Achilles tendon. Dodson[45] also recommends insertion of a percutaneous Steinmann pin into the main fragment to act as a lever to permit reduction of the fracture. This

placed and rotated downward at its outer margin. Aitken believed that the medial one half of the posterior facet in these fractures is usually not displaced. Displacement of the lateral half, however, resulted in a markedly irregular joint surface.

Essex-Lopresti[48] emphasized that the pattern of the fracture is remarkably constant. According to him, the biomechanics of this fracture involve vertical loading of the calcaneus by the talus at the crucial angle of Gissane.[48] The posterior subtalar joint is forced into eversion, with the lateral process of the talus being driven into the crucial angle. This produces a primary fracture line extending in the lateral cortex from the crucial angle to the plantar calcaneal surface (Figs. 24-30, A and 24-31, A). If the force is expended at this point, it results in a nondisplaced intraarticular fracture. However, if the force continues, a secondary fracture line is produced. The secondary fracture line extends from the crucial angle of Gissane posteriorly. The secondary fracture line produces two distinct types of displacement, tongue type and joint depression (Figs. 24-30, B and 24-31, B). In the first, the tongue type, the secondary fracture line runs straight back from the crucial an-

gle to the posterior border of the tuberosity. The anterior end of this large fracture fragment consists of the outer one half of the subtalar articular surface and the upper border of the body (see Fig. 24-30, B). As the force continues, the front end of the tongue is driven further down. While the tuberosity is still in contact with the ground, it is forced upwards and backwards. This results in the anterior end of the tongue being depressed *inside* the lateral wall of the body (see Fig. 24-30, C). An axial radiograph taken of this stage of the displacement demonstrates a step-off between the inner and outer components of the subtalar joint.

In the second, or joint depression, type the secondary fracture line runs across the calcaneal body to just *behind* the posterior facet of the subtalar joint. The lateral fragment consists of a well-defined unbroken piece of bone carrying the articular cartilage of the lateral half to two thirds of the posterior subtalar joint (see Fig. 24-30, B). When the fracturing force continues, the lateral one-half joint fragment is depressed into the spongy bone of the calcaneus *inside* the lateral wall, which is driven outwards. An axial radiograph of the calcaneus taken at this stage demonstrates the shearing

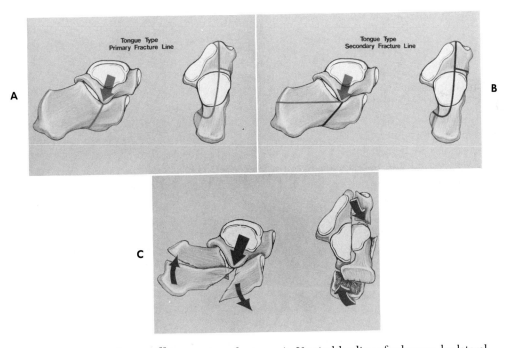

Fig. 24-30. Essex-Lopresti[36] tongue-type fracture. **A,** Vertical loading of calcaneus by lateral process of talus produces primary fracture line from crucial angle of Gissane to plantar calcaneal surface. **B,** Secondary fracture line runs back to exit at posterior border of calcaneal tuberosity. Resulting tongue-shaped fragment contains outer one half of posterior facet and upper border of body of calcaneus. **C,** With further progression of force, anterior end of tongue is depressed inside lateral wall of body, and tuberosity is displaced proximally. (Courtesy B.D. Burdeaux, M.D., Houston, Tex.)

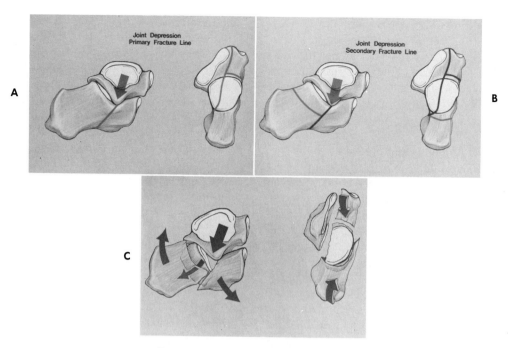

Fig. 24-31. Essex-Lopresti[36] joint depression type fracture. **A,** Vertical loading by lateral process of talus produces primary fracture line from crucial angle of Gissane to plantar calcaneal surface. **B,** Secondary fracture line runs across calcaneal body to exit *just* behind posterior facet. Lateral fragment contains lateral one half to two thirds of posterior facet and contains little soft tissue attachment. **C,** With further progression of force, lateral one half joint fragment is depressed into spongy bone of calcaneus inside lateral wall. Primary fracture line opens up, displacing tuberosity proximally with loss of tuberosity joint angle.

fracture of the sustentaculum tali with displacement and bulging of the lateral wall. With further progression of the force, in addition to the inferior and posterior displacement of this articular fragment, the primary fracture line produced by the lateral process of the talus can open up, resulting in the tuberosity of the calcaneus being forced superiorly with the loss of the tuberosity joint angle and spreading of the primary fracture line (Fig. 24-31, *C*).

Palmer believed that this shearing fracture was the primary force in calcaneal fractures.[137]

Soeur and Remy's classification[173] is similar to that of Essex-Lopresti,[48] with their "semi-lunar fracture" resembling the joint depression, and the "comet-shaped group" resembling the tongue fracture.

Essex-Lopresti emphasized that there is always a step-off with this displacement varying from 3 to 10 mm, between the outer and inner fragments of the posterior subtalar joint. At the moment of maximal compression, the medial (sustentacular) one half of the posterior facet is depressed down to the level of the outer one half. However, on release of the compression force, soft tissue resilience of the foot causes the sus-

tentacular one half to be drawn up by its intact attachments to the talus. The outer half of the facet, buried inside the lateral wall, no longer has any attachments to the talus and therefore remains depressed. The height of the step-off is therefore a measure of the recoil that has occurred.

In cases in which the force is even greater, gross comminution of the remainder of the body of the calcaneus occurs, resulting in a severely comminuted fracture that does not fit in either the tongue-type or joint depression classification. These have been termed *comminuted fractures*.[89] According to Stephenson,[174] this mechanism produces a traumatic flatfoot deformity that has four components: (1) spread of the lateral wall; (2) depression of part of the posterior facet; (3) avulsion of the superomedial border of the calcaneus, which may include a portion of the posterior facet; and (4) shortening, which is a result of muscle forces crossing the bone. According to King,[93] 95% of fractures of the calcaneus involving depression of the posterior facet can be classified into either the tongue or joint depression type as described by Essex-Lopresti.

McReynolds[114] on the other hand, believed that the

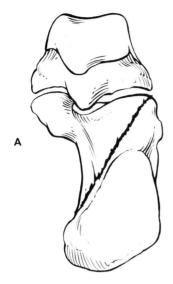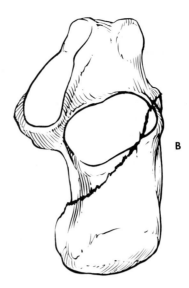

Fig. 24-32. A, According to McReynolds,[93] main fracture line begins in medial cortex and extends upward, outward, and anterior, to exit in posterior facet. **B,** Fracture line exits more laterally in the posterior facet than reported by Essex-Lopresti.[36] This fracture line produces a large superomedial fragment, reduction of which McReynolds believes is crucial.

oblique fracture originating in the medial cortex and extending upward, outward, and anteriorly to exit in some portion of the articular surface of the posterior facet is the primary fracture line. McReynolds emphasized that the point at which the oblique fracture line enters the posterior facet varies but that it is far more lateral than had been assumed by Essex-Lopresti. For this reason, the superomedial fragment often contains the sustentaculum tali and much more of the articular surface than the lateral fragment (Fig. 24-32). There is medial displacement, overriding, and rotation of the superomedial fragment in 90% of both tongue-type and joint depression fractures. McReynolds found this to be the most constant significant deformity in these fractures.[93] He based his treatment on the restoration of the position of this large superomedial fragment.

In this section, I will use the Essex-Lopresti classification of intraarticular fractures of the calcaneus.

Clinical and radiographic diagnosis

Clinical diagnosis. The patient often gives a history of having fallen from a height.[90,110] Indeed, according to Bohler,[17] the history of a vertical fall on the heel from a height of more than 5 meters should suggest a calcaneus fracture. There is rapid swelling with severe pain in the heel.[84,114] According to McReynolds, the pain is secondary to marked bleeding from the cancellous bone and to the fact that the heel is tightly enveloped in fascia, which prevents extravasation of the blood into the adjacent subcutaneous tissues.[114] Later,

there is discoloration about the medial and lateral sides of the heel.[114] Occasionally the hemorrhage and discoloration may extend up the calf some distance away from the heel.[114] If treatment is delayed, severe swelling and bleb formation in the skin over the medial and lateral aspects of the heel develops.

Objectively, there is tenderness and ecchymosis in the tissues surrounding the calcaneus.[54] Clinically the normal contour of the hindfoot is distorted.[54] The arch may also be flattened and the distance from the heel to the lateral malleolus shortened compared to the normal foot. According to Key and Conwell, the longitudinal arch of the foot is flattened by upward displacement of the tuberosity and sagging of the inner border of the foot, and the malleoli are lowered because of the upward displacement of the tuberosity.[90] Point tenderness is limited to the os calcis.[84] Subtalar motion is limited and painful, while ankle motion is painless.[54,84,90] One can usually palpate excess bone behind and below the external malleolus secondary to the bulge of the lateral calcaneal wall.[90] Upward and forward displacement of the tuberosity of the callcaneus in severely comminuted fractures tends to relax the Achilles tendon and decrease plantar-flexion power, the so-called Hoffa's sign.[90,139] Inability to bear weight, broadening and swelling of the heel, and a hematoma that extends anteriorly towards the sole all help, according to Bohler,[17] to distinguish calcaneal fractures from fractures of the ankle.

If the mechanism of injury is a fall, one must look

for associated compression fractures of the lumbar spine.[27,54] Parkes emphasizes the importance of palpation of both the spine and the ankle to detect the tenderness that suggests these commonly associated fractures.[139]

Radiographic diagnosis. A complete radiographic evaluation is essential in all patients with a history of a fall from a height and heel pain. Routine radiographs used to evaluate intraarticular fractures of the calcaneus include an anteroposterior, a true lateral, and an axial view. Anthonsen's view, Broden's projections I and II, the oblique dorsoplantar view, the medial oblique axial view, and the lateral oblique axial view can then be used to delineate the degree of involvement of the subtalar joint. A complete description of these special radiographic views and their interpretation is found on pp. 605-609.

Radiographs of the lumbar spine are mandatory in patients who suffer a significant fall and all patients who complain of back pain and who have spine tenderness on physical examination.

Treatment

A review of the current literature reveals no universally accepted method for the treatment of intraarticular fractures of the calcaneus. According to Cave,[27] severely comminuted intraarticular fractures treated by expert fracture surgeons result in acceptable functional and economic results in no more than 50% of cases, no matter whether treatment is by manipulation and plaster fixation, wire traction, or open reduction.[27] He stresses that the surgeon *must* avoid overtreating the fracture while neglecting the remainder of the foot.[27]

Deyerle[42] reports that patients treated by open reduction and internal fixation or by immediate arthrodesis have no better results than those treated conservatively.[42] Thoren[179] stated that, while in fractures with severe displacement open reduction may give a better result, in similar cases early physical therapy can give sufficient results to warrant use of this method instead of open treatment.

In addition to conflicting reports regarding the best means of treatment of those fractures, there is difficulty in comparing the different reports in the literature, because most evaluations depend on the patients' own concept of their results, an interpretation that is not always reliable.[67] Additionally, authors have used different objective evaluation systems in reporting their results.

At present there is no one method suitable for the treatment of all of these fractures. There are five basic methods of treatment of intraarticular fractures of the calcaneus: (1) closed treatment without reduction, (2) closed reduction with and without immobilization, (3) open reduction and internal fixation with and without bone grafting, (4) primary subtalar or triple arthrodesis, and (5) excision. Each of these methods will be discussed here, with the strengths and weaknesses of each emphasized in an effort to help the reader select the treatment modality most useful in each particular situation.

CLOSED TREATMENT WITHOUT REDUCTION

Closed treatment of calcaneus fractures *without* an attempt at reduction has been advocated by many authors.* In 1946 Roberts and Sayle Creer emphasized the value of conservative treatment without reduction.[152] Trickey[180] emphasized that this is *not* treatment by neglect and that the method must be learned and carefully supervised. Bankart,[9] Thoren,[179] and Essex-Lopresti[48] reported good results with early motion and non-weight bearing. They reported no loss of position with this method of treatment as long as early weight bearing is avoided.

McLaughlin[111] considered the physician treating a calcaneus fracture to be on the horns of a dilemma. By using early motion without reduction, he or she accepted deformity to maintain motion. On the other hand, by attempting a reduction, the physician accepted the stiffness inherent in the immobilization that is necessary to maintain the reduction.[111] McLaughlin preferred early motion without reduction for the following reasons: (1) immobilization is not necessary for union, (2) these fractures will heal with or without treatment, (3) immobilization of these fractures invariably produces a stiffened foot, and (4) such a stiff foot is usually painful.

Since os calcis fractures will not be displaced by early active motion of the foot and ankle, and because nonunion of the calcaneus is practically unheard of, Cave believed that early motion and partial weight bearing could be allowed without harm using crutches and a well-fitted shoe soon after injury.[27] Early range of motion to the foot and toes helps maintain muscle tone and improve the circulatory status of the extremity.[27]

According to Lance et al.,[98] stability of calcaneus fractures is secondary to bony impaction at the time of injury, and therefore immobilization is not necessary. Their treatment consists of compression, early range of motion and non-weight bearing for 12 weeks. They emphasized that early weight bearing can result in a further loss of Bohler's angle.[99]

The disadvantage of this form of treatment is that the deformity present at the time of injury must be compatible with good function.[98] If it is, good results can

---

*References 10, 11, 13, 15, 45, 52, 55, 95, 130, 131, 134, 166, and 179.

be obtained with early range of motion. Lance et al.[98] report that fractures treated by compression dressing and early motion produced 55% satisfactory results, while operative treatment produced only 48% satisfactory results with a significant 17% complication rate. They set forth the following criteria for closed treatment: (1) proper weight-bearing alignment of the hindfoot, (2) freedom of the peroneal tendons from impingement from the lateral bulge; (3) a congruent relationship between the posterior facets of the talus and calcaneus, and (4) an elderly patient. If patients meet these criteria, 99% returned to their preinjury level of activity.

Lapidus and Guidotti[100] also emphasize the importance of avoiding long-term immobilization. They believe any attempt at reduction using either a compression clamp or skeletal traction will require prolonged immobilization of 6 to 8 weeks to maintain the alignment. This results in fibrous ankylosis of the subtalar joint *and* the other joints of the foot. A stiff, painful foot results. They therefore recommend the use of swimming pool exercises, using the buoyancy of the body in the water to unweight the injured limb. The patient initially begins in the deep water and progressively moves to shallower water as pain allows. Their patients returned to work in 3 to 5 months. Lapidus and Guidotti[100] believe that early range of motion helps to mold the articular surfaces of the involved joints and to decrease swelling. On the other hand, Hazlett[74] believes that early range of motion does little to restore the irregular joint surfaces when the incongruity is marked.

Barnard[10,11,13] recommends elevation, ice packs, movement of the foot and ankle 5 minutes of every hour, and avoidance of weight bearing for 6 weeks. The first shoe used by the patient has the heel elevated to produce 45° of ankle equinus. The heel is gradually decreased in height over the next 6 weeks until the foot is flat. If the patient cannot cooperate with this method of treatment, Barnard[11] recommends a walking cast with a sponge rubber pad about the heel with the foot in equinus position after the swelling has decreased. The height of the cast heel is decreased until the foot is in the normal position, usually after about 6 weeks.

Parkes[138,140] also advocates early motion and nonweight bearing without reduction in the treatment of these fractures. The patient is admitted to the hospital, and a compression dressing is applied from the foot to the knee. Ice bags are applied to the heel and the foot is elevated. After 24 hours, the patient is encouraged to move the foot and ankle in all directions. These exercises are performed once every waking hour. The whirlpool can be used to help the patient perform these exercises. After 3 to 5 days, when the pain begins to subside, the compression dressing is replaced by an elastic stocking. The patient is allowed to dangle his legs briefly over the side of the bed several times a day for 1 to 2 days and is then allowed up on crutches *without* weight bearing on the fractured heel. When not ambulatory on the crutches, the foot is kept elevated. The patient is then fitted with a walking Oxford shoe with a well-molded heel and built-in arch. The patient slowly increases the amount of pressure he applies to the foot. Between 4 to 8 weeks after injury, most patients can bear full weight, and many return to work after 6 to 12 weeks. Parkes emphasizes that if pain from arthritis or peroneal tenosynovitis develop following this mode of treatment, they are treated as necessary later. He emphasizes that it may take up to 2 years to get an optimal result.[139] He recommends this treatment particularly for surgeons who have no experience in treating the fractures of the calcaneus, as it offers an acceptable result in most patients.

Salama et al.[158] recommend early immediate elevation, ice, and early range of motion. Exercises are instituted within 24 hours. Resisted plantar flexion is emphasized to overcome the weakness of the gastrocnemius, which is secondary to the shortened triceps surae resulting from proximal fracture displacement. They begin partial weight bearing at 4 to 6 weeks after fracture and are continued on partial weightbearing for an additional 4 to 6 weeks. Using this method of treatment, they report satisfactory results in 82% of cases.[158]

When treating these fractures by early motion without reduction, Vestad emphasizes the importance of avoiding cast immobilization.[184] Gage and Premer[52] report that the results using plaster immobilization without reduction are less satisfactory than early range of motion without immobilization. Dick[43] recognized the problem of stiffness in the foot following calcaneus fractures and recommended that a cast not be used postoperatively. Lindsay and Dewar[107] found that in conservatively treated patients, those whose fractures were manipulated had poorer results than those treated by early motion without reduction.

In reviewing the literature, good results are reported in a variety of fractures treated in this manner. The common theory is that early motion without immobilization avoids a stiff, painful foot, which is often produced when cast immobilization is used. However, the criteria for which patients should be treated in this fashion are not clear. Vestad[184] recommends this method of treatment in patients over 50 years of age and those with severely displaced fractures. Kalish[89] recommends this method for diabetics and patients with peripheral vascular disease because of the high incidence of complication in these patients following other forms of treatment. On the other hand, Burghele and Serban[24] report that since a valgus heel, flatfoot deformity, and painful arthrosis may occur following this method of treatment, reduction should be considered in patients who have severe flatfoot deformity and a valgus heel. Finally, Harris[70] reports that even severely comminuted fractures of the calcaneus resulting from war injuries, with marked displacement and soft tissue injury, often do fairly well after this treatment in spite of the marked deformity.

CLOSED REDUCTION
Closed reduction with immobilization

Since early motion without reduction necessitates that the surgeon accept the displacement initially present, reduction and maintenance of the reduction is a method of treatment recommended by some. Indeed, although McLaughlin preferred early motion without reduction as the main form of treatment, he gave three indications for reduction of calcaneus fractures: (1) if the tuberosity of the calcaneus is displaced proximally, it should be transfixed with a pin and pulled down to restore gastrocsoleus length; (2) in the grossly widened calcaneus fractures in which the lateral fragment is jammed up beneath the fibula, it should be reduced by compression either manually or using a clamp; (3) occasionally, if the displaced posterior articular facet is driven into the calcaneus without comminution, reduction is indicated.[6,59,110,111]

The goals of closed reduction and fixation include: (1) restoration of Bohler's angle, (2) restoration of the normal width of the calcaneus, and (3) attempt to restore the congruity of the subtalar joint. Cotton and Wilson in 1908[34] emphasized the importance of decreasing the width of the heel following calcaneus fractures to prevent the lateral buildup of callus beneath the distal end of the fibula. Calcaneal width was reduced by pounding on the lateral surface of the calcaneus with a mallet, after which the foot was placed in plaster. However, Carothers and Lyons[26] found that when long-term immobilization was used following Cotton's reduction, lateral motion of the foot was entirely missing. The patients complained of the inability to walk on uneven terrain. They therefore modified Cotton's technique by removing the cast at the tenth postreduction day and instituting early motion while denying weight bearing for 8 weeks. They found that subtalar motion was restored relatively quickly. They report that this method resulted in a painless heel with good subtalar motion.

Wilson[194] also modified Cotton's technique for comminuted fractures. While one assistant maintains pull on the leg and another exerts countertraction on the dorsum of the foot and the back of the heel, the lateral spread of the heel is reduced by a direct blow over a broomstick placed beneath the lateral malleolus. This results in decreased width of the calcaneus and restoration of the proximal displacement of the tuberosity. If the reduction is acceptable, the foot is placed in a short leg cast with sponge rubber padding placed beneath the medial and lateral malleoli. The foot is in moderate plantar flexion, and pressure is applied to the heel to maintain alignment and the decreased width. After 10 days the cast is removed and early motion is begun. The patient is kept non-weight bearing for 8 weeks and wears a stiff-soled shoe.

Bohler's method. Bohler[17] in 1931 recommended closed reduction with traction. His goal was to correct the axial deviation, flattening, and shortening of the calcaneus. Reduction is performed after 6 to 10 days to allow the swelling in the foot to subside. With the patient under anesthesia, the fracture is disimpacted by placing the sole of the foot over a wooden wedge and forcing it into plantar flexion. The foot is then prepped, and two pins are inserted, one through the tibia four fingerbreadths above the ankle joint and a second, parallel to the first, through the posterior upper corner of the tuberosity of the calcaneus. Both of these pins are then connected to wire stirrups. Using these pins and stirrups, traction is applied first in the longitudinal axis of the leg to reduce the tuberosity joint angle and then in the axis of the body of the calcaneus to reduce shortening. Next, a screw vice is used to apply pressure medially and laterally beneath the malleoli to reduce the lateral spread. The reduction is then checked radiographically. An unpadded cast is applied from the toes to the popliteal fossa with the traction still in place. When the plaster hardens, the fracture alignment is maintained by the pins. The pins remain in for 3 to 5 weeks, at which time a walking plaster and stirrup are applied. When the fracture is healed, a Blucher-type shoe with a custom arch support is prescribed, and gradual weight bearing is permitted.

Aitken[2] used a modification of Bohler's pin traction and Cotton's reduction methods for calcaneus fractures. He recommended immediate reduction to prevent further swelling and hematoma formation, because he believed delaying reduction allows clot organization, which can prevent reduction. He placed the foot medial side down on padding, and placed a rolled-up towel over the lateral aspect of the calcaneus. The towel was then struck with a hammer. This corrected the lateral spread of the calcaneus. If it failed, a Bohler clamp was applied to reduce the residual displacement. If there was upper displacement of the tuberosity, it was grasped by tongs and a crutch was placed in the arch of the foot, just distal to the calcaneocuboid joint. The tongs were pulled down and the crutch was forced into the arch. This resulted in restoration of the arch and reduction of tuberosity displacement. If this method resulted in reduction, the foot was casted with pads placed beneath the medial and lateral malleoli. The cast was changed as swelling dictated, but the patient remained casted for 10 weeks. Following this, the foot was placed in a stiff-soled shoe.

Olson[135] also modified Bohler's technique by using two turnbuckles to connect the pins in the tibia and os calcis. The turnbuckles are used to manipulate the fracture and maintain the reduction. According to Olson, the turnbuckles make fracture reduction and maintenance easier than casting.

Leonard[103] notes that since there are no fibrous structures passing between the adjacent articular surfaces of the posterior subtalar joint (which are necessary for traction to reduce depressed articular fragments), the logic behind Bohler's traction method is questionable. Allan[3] and Burghele and Serban[24] also report failure of reduction of the displaced posterior facet with Bohler's method. Schofield[162] reported good results with this technique and emphasizes the importance of restoring the normal weight-bearing alignment of the foot. However, Conn[31] reported that, although alignment of the foot may be improved by traction methods, subtalar motion is often limited. He[31] recommended triple arthrodesis after reduction by Bohler's technique because of the stiffness present after traction treatment and casting. Gossett[62] reports that reduction by traction followed by early mobilization helps to decrease the incidence of stiff foot. However, according to Aitken, although the subtalar joint is often stiff after cast removal, it usually loosens up with ambulation, and 75% of patients treated in this manner return to gainful employment.[2]

Harris[70] found that while traction by Bohler's method would correct the gross alignment of the foot, it had no effect on restoring articular surface alignment. He therefore recommended fusion in conjunction with this reduction. Traction and heel compression were used to reduce the fracture. The traction pins were incorporated into a cast. If fracture reduction was not acceptable, fusion was carried out 10 days following reduction. According to Lindsay and Dewar,[107] reduction of calcaneus fractures is achieved in only 30% of patients when pin traction is used. Additionally, they report an 11% incidence of pin tract infection when pins are used for reduction. Lance and Carey[99] report that three fourths of the patients treated by pin traction have unsatisfactory results, the group with the highest failure rate. They therefore suggest that pin traction be removed from the armamentarium of the surgeon treating calcaneus fractures.

Hermann's method. Hermann in 1937 reported a modification of Bohler's method of treatment.[76] After being administered a general or spinal anesthetic, the patient is turned on the side opposite the fracture and a sandbag is placed under the medial aspect of the heel. A rolled towel is placed beneath the lateral malleolus, and a wooden or rubber hammer is used to deliver a blow to the piled-up bone beneath the lateral malleolus. The blows are repeated until the normal depression beneath the lateral malleolus is restored. The heel is then molded by hand, and the subtalar motion is tested. Hermann believes that the lateral submalleolar bone block has not been sufficiently removed unless subtalar motion is restored at this point. After the lateral spread is reduced, tongs are used to grasp the upper posterior part of the calcaneus, and traction is applied. Countertraction is applied from a crutch placed in the arch of the foot just distal to the calcaneocuboid joint. This maneuver is done to overcome the posterior vertical pull of the calf muscles and the inferior horizontal pull of the intrinsic muscles of the foot. The tongs are then removed. A small roll of felt is placed obliquely beneath the medial and lateral malleoli, and a plaster of paris cast is applied with the foot in slight inversion and extreme plantar flexion. The cast is removed after 2 weeks and the submalleolar pads replaced. The foot is placed at a right angle and a new cast applied. New cast and pads are applied up to 10 or 12 weeks postfracture to maintain constant pressure beneath the malleoli. The patient is then fitted with a brace, and weight bearing is begun. Hermann reported 73% good results using this method of treatment. However, Giannestras and Sammarco[58] reported that the end results of Hermann's method are no better than the nonreduction methods mentioned earlier. McReynolds emphasized that Hermann's method can be expected to do little more than change the tuberosity joint angle and is not likely to reduce the displaced posterior facet.[112]

Modified Hermann's method. Giannestras recommended the use of a modified Hermann method for selected displaced tongue-type fractures.[54,58] The patient is placed on a fracture table while under general anesthesia. A heavy, threaded Kirschner wire is inserted through the calcaneal tuberosity close to the superior cortex of the fragment. The knee is flexed 80° over a knee support on the fracture table, thereby relaxing the gastrosoleus muscle. Traction is exerted on the calcaneus through a Kirschner bow that incorporates the threaded pin while countertraction is applied at the knee. Traction is continued until the articular fragment is disimpacted and separated. According to Giannestras, the posterior articular fragment can be distracted from its bed by exerting sufficient traction on the intraosseous talocalcaneal ligament.[54] When traction is released, the fragment will then settle into its original bed without any residual displacement. This traction force re-establishes the tuberosity joint angle of the calcaneus. The heel is palpated to be certain that the mediolateral spread of the calcaneus has been reduced. In an acceptable reduction, a finger can be placed between each of the malleoli and the lateral or medial cortices of the calcaneus. If the normal width has not been restored by the traction, a compressive force is applied with a Bohler's clamp.

A radiograph is taken to see whether the tuberosity joint angle has been re-established and the tongue fragment returned to its normal position. A long leg cast is applied with molding about the heel and a roll of sheet wadding placed beneath the malleoli. The Kirschner wires are incorporated into the cast. At the end of 3 weeks the cast and Kirschner wires are removed and a new, well-molded long leg cast is applied for 3 more weeks. When the cast is removed the patient is begun on an exercise program to encourage range of motion. No weight bearing is permitted until there is radiographic evidence of union.

Essex-Lopresti's method. Essex-Lopresti[48] credited William Gissane with introducing the method of closed reduction of intraarticular fractures of the calcaneus by means of a specially designed stainless steel spike introduced into the calcaneus and incorporated into a plaster cast.

According to Essex-Lopresti,[48] although both open and closed reduction using the spike for fixation can achieve good reduction, they suffer from the disadvantage that postoperative fixation in plaster is necessary. Some of the feet were quite stiff after such immobilization. For these reasons, he introduced a small shoe-shaped plaster slipper designed to hold the spike after reduction and yet to enable ankle, subtalar, and midtarsal joint movement to begin the day after operation. He found the shoe-shaped plaster sufficient to hold the reduction in spite of early motion. This technique incorporates all the features of treatment necessary for a good result: exact reduction, minimal trauma, and immediate exercise of the joints to prevent stiffness.[48]

Essex-Lopresti[48] clearly distinguished between two types of displaced intraarticular calcaneal fractures, the tongue and joint depression types. He recommended closed reduction with a Gissane spike for the tongue-type fracture and open reduction using the Gissane spike to maintain reduction of the joint depression type.

For the tongue-type fracture, the patient is anesthetized and placed in the prone position on the operating table. An incision is made over the displaced tuberosity of the calcaneus *lateral* to the insertion of the achilles tendon. A Gissane spike or heavy (3/16-inch) Steinmann pin is introduced into the tongue fragment in the axis

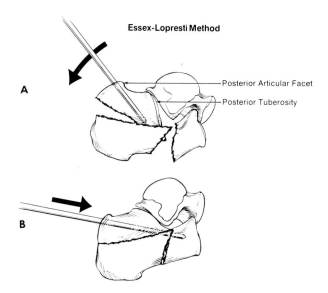

Fig. 24-33. Essex-Lopresti's method of reduction. **A,** In tongue-type fracture, Gissane spike or Steinmann pin is inserted into calcaneal tuberosity, lateral to Achilles tendon, being careful not to cross fracture site. Pin is then used to manipulate tongue fragment into position. **B,** After radiographs confirm reduction of the fracture, the pin is driven into anterior end of calcaneus to maintain reduction.

of the calcaneus, angling slightly towards its lateral wall (Fig. 24-33). Roentgenographs are taken in the axial and lateral planes to determine the position of the pin. It must be in the tongue fragment but should not cross the fracture line. The knee is flexed to a right angle, with the forefoot in one hand and the handle of the spike in the other. The reduction is effected by lifting the knee just clear of the table. According to Essex-Lopresti, the fragment can be felt to click loose during this maneuver, and the handle of the spike will move upwards as the tongue fragment rotates. The weight of the leg and thigh as it is lifted off the table, exerts a sufficient force to pull the sustentacular fragment into alignment with the body of the os calcis. The displaced fragments are now lying in their correct relationship, and the depressed tongue fragment is once again clear of the bulged-out lateral wall. The heels of the surgeon's hands are then used to press the medial and lateral walls together and line up the tuberosity and sustentaculum tali. While the reduction is held by an assistant, a slipper cast is applied that incorporates the spike. The patient is kept on bed rest for 10 days.[48] The spike and plaster are removed in tongue fractures at the end of 4 weeks. Essex-Lopresti then recommended a protective below knee plaster for 4 additional weeks. The patient is kept non-weight bearing for a total of 8 to 10 weeks, at which time radiographs indicate union. Weight bearing and walking exercises are then instituted.

According to Pozo et al.[144] early range of motion provides the most effective treatment for soft tissue and also contributes to molding of a congruous subtalar joint. Deyerle[42] also believes that early range of motion to the foot helps prevent the peroneal tendons from becoming tethered to the lateral calcaneus.

Roberts and Sayle Creer[152] and Bertelsen and Hasner[15] reported shorter periods of incapacitation after treatment by early range of motion than after reduction and casting. Finally, Rosendahl[155] recommends early exercise to maintain subtalar motion, because restoration of subtalar motion paralleled good results in his patients. Most important, however, *no* authors have shown that early motion results in further displacement of calcaneal fractures.

Most authors prefer to delay weight bearing for 6 to 12 weeks to allow fracture healing and to prevent further fracture displacement. According to Rosendahl,[155] early weight bearing often produces poorer results because of secondary compression and fracture displacement, which result in an increased valgus deformity of the heel. Even though Rockwood[153] recommends early weight bearing, he carefully places the heel of the cast so that all weight is borne *anterior* to the calcaneus to prevent weight transfer across the calcaneus and secondary fracture displacement. Additionally, he emphasizes the importance of restoring motion *before* casting and early weightbearing.

Overall, most authors agree that no matter what form of treatment is selected in these fractures, early motion to alleviate soft tissue swelling and restore subtalar motion is the *cornerstone* of treatment. Early, unprotected weight bearing with or without plaster fixation can lead to secondary displacement and is not generally recommended.

Damage to soft tissues and fat pad of heel

The complex structure of the heel pad, which is necessary for painless weight bearing, has been expertly described by Blechschmidt.[16] Essex-Lopresti,[48] Miller and Lichtblau,[126] and Schottstaedt[163] have all emphasized the importance of damage to the soft tissue of the heel pad in affecting long-term prognosis.

According to Miller, the columns of fat in the heel pad normally create a hydraulic effect that cushion the heel during weight bearing.[125] If this hydraulic action is lost, no salvage procedure, including arthrodesis, will relieve this cause of pain.[126] Harris[71] stressed that the weight-bearing function of the heel pad can be compromised by the impact of the acute injury or by long-term localized pressure from the bony prominences of a malunion. Either of these can result in a painful heel. Barnhard[12] and Lance et al.[99] emphasize that plantar pain resulting from damage to the fibrofatty elements

in the heel pad is a disaster and is not helped by any surgical treatment.

Although damage to the fibrofatty elements of the heel pad is a prognostic factor that is beyond the control of the surgeon, he must recognize this as a postinjury cause of pain that, at present, has no surgical treatment.

Age

Essex-Lopresti[48] introduced the concept of a relationship between the age of the patient and results following calcaneus fractures. He believed that patients over the age of 50 had lost some of the mobility of their subtalar joint. Since their feet had an age-related stiffness, better results were to be obtained by conservative treatment consisting of early exercise therapy. For these reasons, he suggested that patients over the age of 50 did better with closed treatment consisting of early exercise, while patients under the age of 50 were better treated by open reduction. In spite of his recommendations, Gaul and Greenburg,[55] Pennal and Yadav,[142] and Lindsay and Dewar[107] could find no relationship between patient age and long-term results.

Associated injury

Gaul and Greenberg[55] emphasize that associated fractures, particularly those involving the ipsilateral lower extremity, have a strongly adverse affect on the outcome of fractures of the calcaneus. This is likely because of constraints on treatment of the calcaneal fracture that ipsilateral injuries impose on the physician. Indeed, Vestad[184] stresses that *systemic* injury in itself does not have any effect on the long-term result after these fractures.

Involvement of midtarsal joints

Involvement of the calcaneocuboid and/or talonavicular joints by communication with the original fracture or subluxation secondary to original displacement of the calcaneal fracture can result in pain in the midfoot following calcaneal fracture.

Conn[31] warned of prolonged disability following involvement of the calcaneocuboid joint in calcaneal fractures. Heck[75] also reported that involvement of the calcaneocuboid joint by the calcaneal fracture can result in pain in this joint. If pain in the calcaneocuboid joint persists after the primary fracture has healed and shoe modifications are not helpful, arthrodesis of the calcaneocuboid joint may be indicated.

Talonavicular joint subluxation secondary to a calcaneal fracture healing in a position of displacement has been reported and can be symptomatic.[90] If incongruity and/or posttraumatic arthritis of the midtarsal joints can be identified at a specific cause of pain following calcaneus fracture, consideration should be given to arthrodesis, either alone or in combination with subtalar fusion.[75]

COMPLICATIONS FOLLOWING CALCANEAL FRACTURES

Most authors have emphasized that results after calcaneus fractures can continue to improve for a long time. According to Gage and Premer,[52] a long period of slow improvement may last up to 2 years. Essex-Lopresti reported continued improvement over a 3- to 6-year period, while Lindsay and Dewar[107] report that results can improve up to 10 years following fracture. Therefore one must wait at least 18 to 24 months before assigning a disability and relating that disability to a specific complication of the fracture.

Complications following calcaneal fracture are mainly related to malunion, stiffness, and soft tissue injury, because nonunion of calcaneus fractures is extremely rare.[14,111] According to McLaughlin,[111] most of the complications following calcaneus fractures are contained in a clinical syndrome characterized by a gait abnormality resulting from a stiff and painful foot. Pain is the predominant feature of this syndrome, and there appears to be a tendency to attribute this symptom to mechanical disorders in the subtalar joint.[111] This presumption is strengthened by radiographic evidence of gross distortion of the joint by the fracture. The origin of pain following subtalar fractures, however, is debatable.[86] Indeed, McLaughlin taught that the *greater* the involvement of the talocalcaneal joint, the more likely it is for an eventual spontaneous fibrous ankylosis to occur, which should eliminate pain in the area.

It is essential that the examiner delineate the exact cause of pain following a calcaneal fracture so that treatment can be directed appropriately. Pain following a calcaneal fracture can arise from the subtalar joint,[53] the midtarsal joint,[30] the ankle,[107] the malleoli,[82,111] and the soft tissues of the heel pad.[124] However, difficulty in determining the exact cause of heel pain following calcaneal fractures led Sallick and Blum[159] to recommend complete sensory denervation of the heel for persistent pain following fractures of the calcaneus.

Heel pain

Heel pain following calcaneal fracture is usually located in one of three anatomic areas: laterally, over the point of the heel, and medially. According to O'Connell et al.[134] lateral heel pain is first, medial heel pain is second, and pain over the point of the heel is third in frequency of occurrence.

Lateral heel pain. Lateral heel pain is usually caused by an abnormality in the subtalar joint, peroneal teno-

synovitis, fibular abutment, or calcaneocuboid joint involvement.

Subtalar joint pain. Key and Conwell[90] and Reich[149] believed that pain from subtalar arthritis is the leading cause of disability after calcaneus fracture. On the other hand, Bankart[9] believed undue importance had been placed on subtalar arthritis as a source of pain following calcaneal fracture.

According to Johansson et al.[87] and Thomas,[176] pain secondary to subtalar arthritis is usually located on the lateral and plantar aspects of the foot, is increased with walking or stressing the subtalar joint, and is relieved by the injection of lidocaine (Xylocaine) into the joint.[87] Garcia and Parkes[54] emphasize that pain on inversion or eversion of the foot that is referred to the area of the sinus tarsi suggests subtalar arthritis. If these clinical signs are present, the authors recommend injecting the joint with a local anesthetic. If the pain is relieved, subtalar fusion may be indicated. If the injection does not relieve the symptoms, the leg can be immobilized in a short leg cast. If immobilization relieves the pain, it is another sign that arthrodesis may relieve the patient's pain. Dodson[45] recommends injection of the subtalar joint with steroids in an effort to *treat* subtalar arthritis. If this fails, arthrodesis is indicated.

If subtalar arthritis is believed to be the cause of the pain, Bankart,[9] Rosendahl-Jensen,[154] Sisk,[167] and McLaughlin[110] recommend subtalar arthrodesis. Isolated subtalar arthrodesis is adequate treatment for subtalar arthritis *if* subtalar injection has completely relieved the patient's pain, indicating that the calcaneocuboid and talonavicular joints are not involved in producing the pain. If these joints are involved, triple arthrodesis should be performed. Subtalar arthrodesis in these situations usually produces better results if done within 1 year of fracture rather than waiting for a prolonged time.[87]

McReynolds[115] stressed that while arthrodesis for malunited fractures may stop subtalar pain, it will do nothing for the widening, shortening, and valgus deformity of the calcaneus, which result in a broad flatfoot and can be a problem in shoe fitting. Kalamachi and Evans[88] report a technique of subtalar arthrodesis through a posterior approach in which a graft is taken from the lateral heel in patients with old calcalcaneus fractures. By taking the graft from the calcaneus, the width of the heel is decreased, the valgus of the heel is corrected, and the peroneal tendons are decompressed.

Deyerle,[42] on the other hand, believes that stiffness and the inability to control the foot on uneven ground are more frequent causes of disability than subtalar pain from arthritis. Indeed, Slatis et al.[169] report a decreased range of motion of the subtalar joint in 74% of all patients following calcaneal fracture and in 89% of those with a depressed intraarticular fracture. Lance et al.[98] report that the loss of one half of subtalar motion resulted in unsatisfactory function in 75% of their patients. However, Letournel[105] reports that a normal life and sports participation are possible with a subtalar joint that has one half of normal motion. Indeed, patients who retain one fourth of the normal range of motion functioned better than patients who underwent arthrodesis. However, Pozo et al.[144] report that neither the degree of stiffness of the subtalar joint nor the radiographic evidence of degenerative joint disease corresponded well with the patient's symptoms.

Peroneal tendinitis and fibular abutment. When the lateral cortex of the calcaneus bursts in severely comminuted fractures, fragments may be displaced in a mediolateral plane and come to lie below the tip of the lateral malleolus. If they unite in this position, they produce a lateral bony prominence posterior and inferior to the lower end of the fibula.[114] The resulting permanent bony prominence can impinge the peroneal tendons against the fibula, entrap them in callus, force them anteriorly, and occasionally actually result in abutment against the tip of the fibula.[115,170] Magnuson[82] in 1923 was the first to recognize this lateral piling up of bone beneath the external malleolus, and he recommended removing the mass to create a trough for the peroneal tendons. Key and Conwell[90] report that excess bone behind and beneath the external malleolus is the second most common cause of heel pain following calcaneal fracture.

McLaughlin[110] and Barnard[10-13] reported that crowding of the peroneal tendons under the lateral malleolus often produces peroneal tenosynovitis and spasm, resulting in a valgus forefoot and a painful spastic flatfoot. According to Parvin and Ford,[141] peroneal tendinitis should be suspected if there is pain below the tip of the malleolus aggravated by supination and pronation. To treat this problem, McLaughlin's recommended treatment of this[111] was a longitudinal incision of the peroneal tendon sheaths, leaving intact the retinaculum to prevent subluxation of the tendons from their fibular groove. Also, Lindsay and Dewar[107] caution that pain beneath the tip of the lateral malleolus may also be secondary to injury to the lateral ligaments of the ankle at the time of the original fracture.

Fitzgerald and Coventry[51] report that antalgic gait, limited subtalar motion, and point tenderness over the peroneal tendons at the inferior peroneal retinaculum are the physical findings suggestive of peroneal tenosynovitis. The diagnosis is further substantiated if the pain is relieved by injection of 1 to 2 ml of local anesthetic into the tendon sheath. Peroneal tenography,

performed by the intrasynovial injection of Hypaque into the common peroneal tendon sheath proximal to the ankle will reveal a complete or partial block at the level of the inferior retinaculum.[51] Conservative treatment by the injection of steroids may relieve the symptoms. However, if steroid injection fails, excision of the bony prominence beneath the peroneal tendon sheath[51] or release of the tendon sheath may be helpful.[54]

Deyerle reports that peroneal dysfunction can also result from the tethering of the peroneal tendons as they course behind the malleolus in the region of the fracture.[51] In some patients, spreading of os calcis can actually push the peroneal tendons out of the tunnel behind the fibula, and they can become dislocated *anterior* to the fibula. Patients with dislocated peroneal tendons have inability to resist inversion and complain of instability and lack of control of the foot.[66,77] According to Deyerle, this condition is greatly improved by excising the excess bone in the region of the old healed fracture and rerouting the peroneal tendons beneath the fibula. He also emphasizes the importance of a peroneal synoviogram in the diagnosis and treatment of peroneal tenosynovitis to determine if the tendon sheath is only obstructed or actually dislocated anteriorly.

In addition to peroneal tenosynovitis and spasm, Isbister[82] reports "abutment" of the tip of the fibula against the displaced lateral wall of the calcaneus as a cause of pain.[75] Although Magnuson and Cotton recommended excision of the displaced lateral calcaneal bone, Isbister[82] believes that resection of the tip of the fibula is a simpler procedure. He recommends resection of 1 cm of the tip of the fibula subperiosteally. Interestingly, he reports that this procedure will relieve symptoms wheth   they are secondary to impingement, compressio   of the peroneal tendons, or direct bony abutment. Ie reports success following this method of treatment in 80% of patients treated.

Both Deyerle[42] and Isbister[82] emphasize the importance of prevention in lateral peroneal tenosynovitis and fibular abutment. They recommend primary fracture treatment, which tends to narrow the width of the heel immediately behind the fibula and tends to lengthen the os calcis.[42,82] Deyerle[42] also emphasizes the importance of regular vigorous contractions of the peroneal tendons in any form of treatment to prevent them from becoming tethered at the site of the lateral wall of the calcaneus.

On the other hand, Reich[148] believed that disability after the calcaneus fracture was secondary to degenerative joint disease of the subtalar joint, not impingement of the peroneal tendons. Because of difficulty in delineating whether subtalar arthritis or peroneal tenosynovitis or "abutment" are responsible for lateral pain after calcaneus fractures, Mann[116] prefers to decompress the peroneal tendons at the time of subtalar fusion. The lateral calcaneal cortex beneath the peroneal tendons is removed intact. The cancellous bone beneath the lateral cortex is removed and used for grafting the subtalar joint. This decreases the width of the calcaneus. The intact cortex is then reinserted into the defect to decrease the potential for scarring between the exposed cancellous bone and the peroneal tendons.

Calcaneocuboid arthritis. Key and Conwell[90] believed that traumatic arthritis of the calcaneocuboid joint is the third most common cause of pain following calcaneal fracture. McLaughlin[110] too reports that derangement of the calcaneocuboid joint can be a significant source of pain. The pain may be caused by actual involvement of the calcaneocuboid joint by the original fracture[110] or by stiffness or malposition of the joint resulting from a malunion of the calcaneus. Selective injection of the calcaneocuboid joint, which relieves the patient's pain, suggests that isolated calcaneocuboid fusion is indicated. If the injection relieves only part of the patient's pain, fusion of the calcaneocuboid and/or talonavicular joints in conjunction with subtalar arthrodesis should be considered.

Pain over point of heel

Bony prominence. A recognized cause of heel pain following calcaneus fractures is the plantar heel spur. Barnard,[11] Dodson,[45] Reich,[150] and Key and Conwell[90] all mentioned pain on the plantar surface of the calcaneus following a fracture. Bony projections secondary to persistent plantar displacement of fracture fragments or to exuberant callus formation on the plantar aspect of the calcaneus can produce localized tender areas or painful callosities.[45,134,163] According to McLaughlin,[111] this tenderness results from the concentration of pressure on the plantar aspect of the fracture deformity, particularly when the calcaneal arch is reversed. Garcia and Parkes[54] recommend initial treatment by local injection. However, such injections usually fail, and excision of the bone fragment may be required.[54] Although Garcia and Parkes,[54] Key and Conwell,[90] Barnard,[11] and Dotson[45] mentioned resection of the bony prominence of these malunions, McLaughlin[111] warned that such prominences should be surgically approached only with great caution. He emphasized that postoperative fibrosis in the area of bone excision may produce as much discomfort on weight bearing as did the original lesion, even if the skin incision is kept well away from the weight-bearing area. He preferred to place soft rubber heels and foam rubber "doughnuts" inside the shoe in a position to protect the tender area from pressure.

Finally, McReynolds[114] and Key and Conwell[90] mentioned pain on the plantar aspect of the foot resulting from malunion. This pain, located over the posterior end of an angulated fracture of the calcaneus just anterior to the tuberosity, occurs with weight bearing. If this pain is severe, they recommended excising the plantar fragment and using it as a bone graft in an opening wedge osteotomy of the calcaneus just anterior to the tuberosity. This is done to restore the normal contour of the plantar surface of the calcaneus. No results of this technique were reported.

Heel pad damage. In addition to exostoses, exuberant callus, and plantar prominence secondary to malunion, many authors mention damage to the heel pad itself as contributing to heel pain. According to Barnard,[11,12] Dodson,[45] and Pozo et al.,[144] pain on the *plantar* surface of the heel with weight bearing is not pathognomonic of subtalar joint problems. Instead, this pain may arise from rupture of the fibrous septae and the fat-filled compartments in the soft tissue over the plantar aspect of the calcaneus. This results in loss of the hydraulic buffer that protects the heel with weight bearing. Additionally, according to Barnard, long-term immobilization predisposes to fibrosis of these tissues,[12] which further compromises their hydraulic function.

O'Connell et al.[134] note that pain over the heel that is reproduced with minimal pressure is usually related to disruption of the fibrofatty elements of the heel pad and to secondary scar formation. In their review of calcaneus fractures, Lance et al.[98] found that loss, atrophy, or fibrosis of the heel pad is associated with an unsatisfactory result in every case. Obviously, if damage to the heel pad is present in addition to a plantar spur, simple excision of the spur will not result in relief of pain.

I have found xeroradiographs very useful in demonstrating loss of thickness of the heel pad following calcaneus fracture and use them frequently in evaluating heel pain after calcaneus fracture. If there is loss of heel pad function, Dodson[45] recommends treatment simply with a heel cushion or an orthosis in the shoe.

Medial heel pain

Ankle joint and flexor tenosynovitis. According to Barnard[10,11] and O'Connell et al.,[134] the second most common site of pain following calcaneus fractures is beneath the medial malleolus. This pain is not caused by subtalar arthritis.[134] Although it may be secondary to spreading of the calcaneus, both Barnard[10,11] and O'Connell, et al.[134] suggest it is most likely caused by damage to the ankle joint itself and the flexor tendons that pass beneath the medial malleolus. O'Connell et al.[134] believe that this damage is compounded by immobilization, which results in further stiffness and arthrofibrosis of the ankle. These authors recommend active early mobilization of the ankle joint and the medial flexor tendons to prevent arthrofibrosis of the ankle

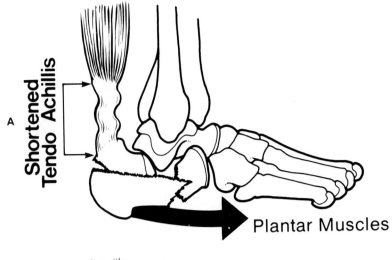

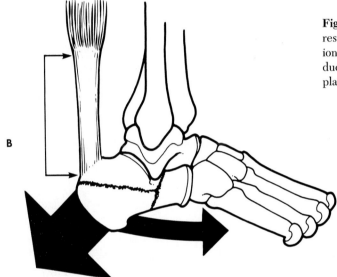

Fig. 24-36. A, Upward displacement of calcaneal tuberosity results in shortening of Achilles tendon and weak plantar flexion. It also results in loss of longitudinal arch of foot. **B,** Reduction of fracture restores Achilles tendon length and hence plantar-flexion power. Longitudinal arch is also restored.

and posttraumatic tenosynovitis of the flexor tendons.[10,11,134]

Nerve entrapment. Guillen-Garcia et al.[65] note that the tarsal tunnel is bordered on its medial side by the os calcis and report tarsal tunnel syndrome following fractures of the calcaneus, particularly when the medial wall is displaced into the tunnel. They report a 10% incidence of tarsal tunnel syndrome following these fractures. The patients complain of medial heel pain and paresthesias in the distribution of the posterior tibial nerve. The pain is frequently worse at night or with walking or standing. According to these authors, the diagnosis is based on the clinical picture but can be assisted by a trial injection of a local anesthetic into the tarsal tunnel. They report that only 28% of patients require operative decompression of the posterior tibial nerve and its branches but that when decompression is performed, the results are excellent.

Finally, Hall and Pennal reported six patients with sural nerve injury secondary to the surgical exposure of the calcaneus.[67] These patients complained of an ache and pain in the lateral aspect of the heel. In my experience, pain from iatrogenic cutaneous nerve damage is extremely recalcitrant to treatment.

Weakness of plantar flexion

McLaughlin[110] and Barnard[12] mentioned that malunion of the calcaneus with upward displacement of the tuberosity usually results in effective lengthening of the Achilles tendon and reduction in calf power. The resulting disability is marked weakness and reduction in the ability to plantar flex the foot (Fig. 24-36). McLaughlin[111] believed when there is severe upward displacement of the calcaneal tuberosity, primary treatment of the fracture should include measures to return the tuberosity to its normal level and to hold the calf muscles at normal length until the fracture unites. In this way, weakness of plantar flexion can be prevented.

Initially, patients whose fractures have *healed* with the tuberosity displaced superiorly walk with a flat-footed gait and are unable to take off from or stand on their toes. According to McLaughlin, however, compensatory shortening of the calf muscles eventually results in a satisfactory gait.[110] Surgical shortening of the Achilles tendon is not recommended in these patients.[12,110]

Fixed flatfoot

According to McLaughlin, upward displacement of the posterior half of the os calcis also results in elimination of the longitudinal arch of the foot[111] (see Fig 24-36, *A*). The normal plantar arch of the hindfoot is reduced, eliminated, or reversed. If the upward displacement of the tuberosity is sufficient to reverse the plantar arch of the os calcis, it should be corrected.[111] Only by reducing the displacement can flatfoot deformity be minimized and painful weight bearing at the apex of a rocker-bottom heel be prevented.[111]

Stiffness of forefoot and toes

Barnard,[11,12] O'Connell et al.,[134] and Pozo et al.[144] mention stiffness and pain in the forepart of the foot and toes, areas not involved in the fracture, as significant causes of disability. These authors relate this stiffness and pain to initial injury to the ankle and midtarsal joints that is complicated by the long periods of immobilization and disuse so often used to treat calcaneus fractures. According to Barnard, fibroblastic adhesions and thickening of the capsular elements around the midtarsal joints are responsible for this stiffness. Indeed, Pozo et al.[144] report that, in addition to the fact that 80% of their patients had less than 50% of normal subtalar motion, 20% had at least a 50% restriction of ankle motion and 15% had at least a 50% reduction of midtarsal motion. I have also seen stiffness of the metatarsophalangeal joints after calcaneus fractures. According to Pozo et al.,[144] the combined stiffness of these joints produced a stiff foot and an unsatisfactory outcome. According to McLaughlin,[111] a stiff midfoot can produce a shuffling gait, because attempts to push off with the forefoot are accompanied by midtarsal pain. Once this condition is established, high shoes with a well-fitted arch support rigid enough to relieve the midtarsal joints from the strain of ambulation may help decrease symptoms.

These reports of stiffness of the forefoot further emphasize the importance of early motion to the ankle, subtalar, midtarsal, and metatarsophalangeal joints in an effort to produce a mobile foot following calcaneus fracture.

Reflex sympathetic dystrophy

Reflex sympathetic dystrophy following fracture of the calcaneus has been reported.[110,111] Severe, burning pain associated with shiny, cold, and discolored skin around the heel should suggest this diagnosis. Early motion, progressive weight bearing, and early use of the foot will prevent development of reflex sympathetic dystrophy. Indeed, Rockwood[145] notes that with his method of early motion and weight bearing, reflex dystrophy has not been noted.

The treatment of established reflex sympathetic dystrophy is beyond the scope of this text.

Infection

Infection following open reduction of intraarticular calcaneus fractures has been mentioned by many authors. The magnitude of the original injury, the precarious nature of the blood supply about the heel, and the gross swelling usually present in these fractures all predispose to infection following open reduction.[111] Letournel[105] reported a 10% incidence of skin necrosis following open reduction, with nearly one half of these patients developing severe infection. Debridement followed by closure over suction drains was recommended to treat the infection. However, in all patients in whom an infection developed, the subtalar joint remained stiff and a fair or poor result was recorded.

AUTHOR'S PREFERRED METHODS OF TREATMENT

As the review of the modes of treatment recommended for intraarticular fractures of the calcaneus reveals, many factors are believed to affect results. However, it is my opinion that *early active* range of motion of the subtalar, ankle, midtarsal, and metatarsophalangeal joints is the *key* to the successful treatment of these fractures and *must* be stressed, no matter which treatment method is selected.

Nondisplaced intraarticular fractures

I treat all nondisplaced intraarticular fractures by the application of a compression dressing and elevation with ice. Pain medication adequate to control the patient's discomfort is essential. Active range of motion of all joints in the foot, emphasizing the subtalar joint, is encouraged.

I believe the responsibility of prescribing and supervising range of motion exercise is the physician's *not* the physical therapist's. In my experience, subtalar motion is poorly understood by patients, and explanation by the physician is essential for patient understanding and cooperation.

Once swelling has subsided and the patient has demonstrated the ability to actively move the subtalar, ankle, midtarsal, and metatarsophalangeal joints, he is discharged on crutches. He is kept non-weight bearing on crutches for 4 to 6 weeks in well-fitting support hose. Partial weight bearing in a well-fitted shoe is then instituted. Weight bearing is progressed within the tolerance of pain. Range of motion exercises are continued until fracture union and painless weight bearing are achieved.

Alternatively, once motion has been restored, a short leg "drop foot" cast with a weight-bearing heel placed anterior to the anterior border of the tibia can be applied (see p. 636). Weight bearing is progressed, and the cast is removed in 4 to 6 weeks. This treatment scheme is useful in patients who cannot manage non-weight bearing for 4 to 6 weeks.

Displaced intraarticular fractures

I treat displaced intraarticular fractures initially with a sterile prep of the foot, application of a compression dressing, elevation with ice, and early motion of the ankle, subtalar, midtarsal, and metatarsophalangeal joints. I instruct the patients in each of these motions myself, particularly motion of the subtalar joint. Routine radiographs consisting of anteroposterior, lateral, and axial views are obtained. Specialized views, including Anthonsen's and Broden's projections I and II (see p. 605) are obtained as necessary to demonstrate the posterior facet of the subtalar joint. Recently I have begun using CT scans to further evaluate the fracture. I then attempt to classify the fracture as a tongue, joint depression, or comminuted type, using the terminology of Essex-Lopresti.

Tongue-type fractures

I prefer to treat tongue-type intraarticular fractures by the method of Essex-Lopresti. The patient is placed in the prone position under acceptable anesthesia. A ⅛-inch smooth Steinmann pin is inserted into the calcaneal tuberosity just lateral to the Achilles tendon. The pin is directed into the long axis of the calcaneus, aiming slightly lateral, toward the calcaneocuboid joint. Care is taken not to cross the fracture site. Axial and lateral radiographs are taken to confirm pin position.

The knee is then flexed 90° and lifted off the table with one hand on the Steinmann pin and the other supporting the dorsum of the foot. A click is usually heard as the reduction occurs. Occasionally, a shaking motion is necessary to free the tilted tongue fragment from inside the lateral cortex of the calcaneus. After this reduction maneuver is performed, lateral and axial radiographs are taken to evaluate the accuracy of the posterior facet reduction. If the fracture is reduced, the Steinmann pin is driven across the fracture into the anterior process of the calcaneus. A slipper cast is then applied incorporating the pin, as recommended by Essex-Lopresti. This allows the patient to continue with ankle and subtalar motion while the reduction is maintained. The pin is removed at 4 to 6 weeks, the foot is placed in a "drop foot" cast, and weight bearing is begun. The degree of plantar flexion is decreased at serial cast changes. The cast is discontinued at 8 to 10 weeks.

If the fracture is not reduced, particularly in the young, active patient, the pin is removed, the patient is placed in the supine position, and the heel is reprepped. Through a lateral incision as described by Stephenson,[137] the fracture fragment is elevated and fixed to the medial aspect of the calcaneus using small A-O cancellous screws. The wound is closed, a soft tissue dressing is applied, and the patient is begun on early range of motion exercises of the subtalar joint. Weight bearing is not allowed for 8 to 10 weeks. I stress the importance of careful evaluation of the skin in the area of the heel before open reduction. Excessive swelling, abrasions, or bleb formation constitutes a contraindication to open reduction.

In patients with diabetes mellitus, arteriosclerotic vascular disease, or other types of circulatory compromise in the lower extremity and in the debilitated patient, I do not use percutaneous pin fixation or open reduction. Tongue-type fractures in these patients are treated by early motion and "drop foot" casting (see p. 636).

Joint depression and comminuted fractures

Although open reduction and internal fixation of the joint depression type fracture is ideal, in my experience subtalar stiffness results, and the risk of infection and loss of reduction are substantial, even with an anatomic reduction. For these reasons, I prefer closed reduction combined with early motion in treating these fractures. I use open reduction of joint depression fractures only in the young patient who has severe joint depression but *little* comminution, a combination that is quite uncommon.

My goal in treating the comminuted calcaneus fracture is to attempt to restore the *external* morphology of the calcaneus. This consists of restoring the normal width of the heel, correcting mediolateral displacement, and correcting superior migration of the posterior tuberosity. I have found that early motion after closed reduction of these displacements gives the best results.

Patients with joint depression and comminuted fractures are treated initially with sterile prep, compression dressing, elevation with ice, and early motion of the ankle, subtalar, midtarsal, and metatarsophalangeal joints.

Careful radiographic evaluation of the *external morphology* of the calcaneus is then undertaken. The lateral view of the foot demonstrates the degree of superior migration of the tuberosity of the calcaneus. If such superior migration is marked, i.e., Bohler's angle is neutral or reversed, two problems can occur: (1) relative shortening of the Achilles tendon, which produces weak plantar flexion and a poor gait; and (2) a bony prominence at the site of the primary fracture line on the *plantar* aspect of the foot, resulting in a rocker-bottom foot (see Fig. 24-36).

The axial view demonstrates calcaneal widening, varus-valgus angulation, and mediolateral displacement of the tuberosity of the calcaneus. In my opinion, closed reduction should be instituted to correct all of these displacements.

Superior displacement of the tuberosity

Superior displacement of the tuberosity can usually be reduced by simply plantar flexing the foot. However, if this is successful, it requires casting to maintain the reduction, and casting prevents early motion. Therefore I use a ⅛-inch Steinmann pin inserted into the tuberosity of the calcaneus and driven across the fracture site into the anterior calcaneus to hold the reduction. If the anterior process is comminuted and does not provide adequate fixation, the pin is driven across the calcaneocuboid joint into the cuboid to stabilize its position. Once again, a slipper cast is applied to allow early range of motion of the ankle and subtalar joints. Further management follows Essex-Lopresti's method of treating tongue-type fractures (see p. 634).

Mediolateral spread, displacement, or angulation

Mediolateral spread of the calcaneus is reduced by placing the heels of the surgeon's palms beneath the malleoli to compress the calcaneus and restore its width. The patient is placed in the prone position and the knee is flexed 90°. The heel is grasped between the heels of the surgeon's palms. The thigh is lifted off the table and the heel "shaken" to disimpact the fracture. The heel is then compressed. If more compression is required, a Bohler's clamp can be used.

If there is significant mediolateral displacement or varus-valgus angulation of the tuberosity of the calcaneus (resulting in an abnormal weight-bearing alignment of the hindfoot), these displacements are reduced by applying varus or valgus stress to the tuberosity of the calcaneus. The reduction is confirmed radiographically. This compression and molding decompresses the lateral heel and peroneal tendons and also places the heel parallel to the floor for weight bearing.

If the mediolateral displacement or varus-valgus angulation recurs after closed reduction, a Steinmann pin can be inserted into the tuberosity fragment and driven across the fracture, thereby stabilizing it into the anterior process of the calcaneus in a reduced position. The foot is then placed in a slipper cast incorporating the pin, and early motion of the ankle and subtalar joints is instituted. The pin is removed at 4 to 6 weeks, the foot is placed in a "drop foot" cast, and weight bearing is instituted with a heel placed anterior to the tibia. The cast is removed at 8 to 10 weeks, and the foot is placed in a sturdy boot, the heel of which is progressively decreased in height.

If the closed reduction is stable, it does not require a pin for maintenance of the reduction. The patient is kept on bed rest with the foot elevated in a compression dressing with ice packs. Adequate pain medication is prescribed. Intensive ankle, subtalar, midtarsal, and metatarsophalangeal joint motion are instituted. Once the swelling has subsided and motion has been restored, usually at 7 to 10 days, a "drop foot" cast is applied. This is a short leg cast applied with the patient seated and the leg hanging off the bed. The foot assumes a *slight* equinus position under the force of gravity only. (This is *not* a full equinus cast.) A walking heel is then applied to the cast *anterior* to the anterior border of the tibia. A heel is placed so that body weight is transmitted through the walking heel, up through the metatarsals, across the navicular and talus, and up the tibia, thereby bypassing the calcaneus and preventing further displacement. When the cast is dry, the patient begins to toe touch and increases weight bearing as tolerated. In my experience, early cast-protected weight bearing promotes muscle contraction and stimulates venous return, which results in less swelling in the foot after treatment. The cast is removed at 6 to 8 weeks, and the patient is fitted with a tight lace-up boot or cowboy boot with an elevated heel. The heel is slowly decreased in height over the next 3 to 4 months.

It is important to emphasize to the patient that continued improvement in function will occur for 18 to 24 months following the fracture. Only after this time has passed is consideration given to reconstructive surgery, such as arthrodesis. Additionally, careful evaluation to determine the exact cause of postfracture disability is essential before *any* surgical treatment is instituted. I am particularly careful to evaluate heel pad damage, usually with xeroradiography, because in my experience this damage precludes a good result from any surgical treatment.

STRESS FRACTURES OF CALCANEUS

A stress or fatigue fracture is defined as a break in the continuity of normal bone caused by repeated subthreshold stresses or as a break in the continuity of abnormal bone caused by repeated normal stresses.[38,100,101] The os calcis is the tarsal bone most commonly affected with stress fractures.[37] D'Ambrosia and Drez[37] suggest that gait variations play a role in the anatomic predisposition to stress fractures in certain tarsal bones.

According to Leabhart,[101] the first stress fractures were reported by Brehithaupt in 1855 in the painful feet of soldiers. Scheller[161] reported 590 stress fractures, of which 4 involved the calcaneus. Hullinger[80] in 1944 reported 53 stress fractures of the calcaneus in Army recruits. Van DeMark and McCarthy[183] also noted that stress fractures of the calcaneus were a frequent cause of painful heels in soldiers. Finally, Leabhart in 1959 reported 134 stress fractures of the calcaneus in soldiers, stating that this fracture occurred in 0.45% of new recruits. Nearly three fourths of the patients in Leabhart's series had bilateral fractures, and less than 10% had been physically active before enlistment in the service. He found no relationship between abnormal foot structure and the incidence of calcaneal stress fractures.

Clinical diagnosis

Calcaneal stress fractures have been misdiagnosed as tenosynovitis, tendinitis, arthritis, rheumatic fever, cellulitis with lymphagitis, and neurosis.[101] The clinical examination is essential in preventing such misdiagnoses.

The key to the diagnosis of stress fracture of the calcaneus is a high index of suspicion.[37] Stress fractures usually occur in long-distance runners and Army recruits. Patients complain of painful swelling of the heel, which occurs within the first 7 to 10 days of increased training.[101] They do not give a specific history of trauma. According to Leabhart,[101] edema in the area of the precalcaneal bursa, anterior to the Achilles tendon, is highly suggestive of a stress fracture. Tenderness over the posterosuperior aspect of the calcaneus in the area of the stress fracture is diagnostic.[101] According to Leabhart, stretching the heel cord by dorsiflexion of the foot does not substantially increase the pain. Although the edema subsides with rest, the tenderness usually persists until the fracture is healed.[101] Pain on mediolateral compression of the calcaneus and a positive radiograph at 3 weeks confirm an os calcis stress fracture.[37]

Radiographic diagnosis

The radiographs are negative until 10 to 14 days after the onset of symptoms, at which time a definite line or density is usually seen in the postersuperior aspect of the calcaneus, perpendicular to the trabecular stress lines.[37,101] The fracture line increases in density up to 6 weeks after the beginning of symptoms, then the density gradually resolves.[101] The radiographic differential diagnosis of a stress fracture of the calcaneus includes osteogenic sarcoma, osteomyelitis, and osteoid osteoma.

Radionuclide bone scanning will substantiate the diagnosis as early as 2 to 8 days from the onset of symptoms.[145] Because it takes 2 to 3 weeks before radiographic changes are manifested, a positive bone scan permits early treatment, which can forestall the development of the full clinical and radiographic syndrome of a stress fracture.[145] Prather et al.[145] found that patients with negative bone scans never developed subsequent radiographic changes in the bone but there was a 24% incidence of false positive bone scans. According to D'Ambrosia and Drez,[37] a false positive bone scan is the result of accelerated bone remodeling in these highly active individuals. Standard radiographs, on the other hand, have a false negative rate of 71% when performed early in the clinical syndrome.[144]

Treatment

According to D'Ambrosia and Drez,[37] treatment is symptomatic, with symptoms resolving in 2 to 3 weeks.[37] Leabhart[101] found that weight bearing on crutches with a ½ inch sponge rubber heel insert decreases the symptoms. He reports that attempts to return patients to stressful ambulatory status before 8 weeks usually resulted in recurrence of symptoms. Importantly, he reports that no calcaneal stress fracture underwent displacement.

AUTHOR'S PREFERRED METHOD OF TREATMENT

My experience with stress fractures has been mainly with long-distance runners. These patients present with a gradual onset of pain in the heel. The symptoms must be distinguished from plantar fasciitis and Achilles tendinitis. Differentiating Achilles tendinitis and plantar fasciitis is most easily done on the basis of the specific area of point tenderness. If there is still confusion, a bone scan will help to distinguish these entities.

I treat patients with calcaneal stress fractures by limitation of the inciting activity until the symptoms subside. Contrast baths using heat followed by ice help decrease the symptoms. Once the symptoms have subsided, a heel pad and possibly an arch support in the running shoe are useful in preventing recurrence. Resumption of the activity that caused the stress fracture is usually not possible before 4 to 6 weeks. If activity is resumed earlier, the symptoms usually recur. I have not seen a stress fracture of the calcaneus undergo displacement.

DISLOCATION OF CALCANEUS

Dislocation of the cancaneus at the subtalar and calcaneocuboid joints is a rare injury, with only eight cases reported in the recent literature.[25,68,185] According to Hamilton,[68] the mechanism of injury is a great force against the lower leg that causes the leg to be displaced backwards against a fixed heel. Twisting injuries have also been implicated in causing this dislocation.[25] The calcaneus usually dislocates laterally[25,68,185] however, an inferior dislocation has also been reported.[185]

Treatment in all but one of the cases reported in the literature has been by closed reduction followed by cast immobilization in a short leg cast[25,68,185] for 6 to 9 weeks.[68]

In a single case reported by Viswanath and Shephard,[185] closed reduction of a lateral dislocation of the calcaneus was unsuccessful. Open reduction was performed through a lateral approach but was unstable and required a Kirschner wire across the calcaneocuboid joint for stability. At followup, this patient had a persistent limp and slight varus deformity of the heel. However, most reports in the literature indicate that these patients recover a useful foot without significant disability.[68,185]

None of the cases in the literature had intraarticular fractures associated with this dislocation. Such fractures could render the reduction unstable and require internal fixation. These fractures can also lead to more severe long-term subtalar and midfoot stiffness and disability.

REFERENCES

1. Aaron, D.A.R.: Intra-articular fractures in the calcaneus, J. Bone Joint Surg. **56B:**567, 1974.
2. Aitken, A.P.: Fractures of the Os-Calcis: treatment by closed reduction, Clin. Orthop. **30:**67-75, 1963.
3. Allan, J.H.: The open reduction of fractures of the os calcis, Ann. Surg. **141:**890-900, 1955.
4. Anthonsen, W.: An oblique projection for roentgen examination of the talo-calcanean joint, particularly regarding intra-articular fracture of the calcaneus, Acta Radiol. **24:**306-310, 1943.
5. Arnesen, A.: Fracture of the os calcis and its treatment. Acta Chir. Scand. [Suppl.] **234:**2-70, 1958.
6. Arnesen, A.: Treatment of fracture of the os calcis with traction and manipulation, Acta Chir. Scand. **132:**566-573, 1966.
7. Backman, S., and Johnson, S.R.: Torsion of the foot causing fracture of the anterior calcaneal process, Acta. Chir. Scand. **105:**460-466, 1953.
8. Bailey, F.A.: Proc. Oregon Med. **7:**68, 1880.
9. Bankart A.S.B.: Fractures of the os calcis, Lancet **2:**175, 1942.
10. Barnard, L.: Non-operative treatment of fractures of the calcaneus, J. Bone Joint Surg. **45A:**865-867, 1963.
11. Barnard, L.: Non-operative treatment of fractures of the calcaneus, Instr. Course Lect. **28:**249-251, 1973.
12. Barnard, L., and Odegard, J.K.: Conservative approach in the treatment of fractures of the calcaneus, J. Bone Joint Surg. **37A:**1231-1236, 1955.
13. Barnard L., and Odegard, J.K.: Conservative approach in the

treatment of fractures of the calcaneus, J. Bone Joint Surg. **52A:**1689, 1970.
14. Bellenger, M., Vander Elst, E., and Lorthior, J.: Les fractures du calcaneum: leur traitement des sequelles, Acta Orthop. Belg. **17:**59-167, 1951.
15. Bertelsen, A., and Hasner, E.: Primary results of treatment of fracture of the os calcis by "Foot-free walking bandage" and early movement, Acta Orthop. Scand. **21:**140-154, 1951.
16. Blechschmidt, E.: The structure of the calcaneal padding, Foot Ankle **2:**260-283, 1982.
17. Bohler, L.: Diagnosis, pathology, and treatment of fractures of the os calcis, J. Bone Joint Surg. **13:**75-89, 1931.
18. Bradford, C.H., and Larsen, I.: Sprain-fractures of the anterior lip of the os calcis, N. Engl. J. Med. **244:**970-972, 1951.
19. Brattstrom, H.: Primary arthrodesis in severe fractures of calcaneum, Nord. Med. **50:**1510-1511, 1953.
20. Brindley, H.H.: Fractures of the os calcis: a review of 107 fractures in 95 patients, South. Med. J. **59:**843-847, 1966.
21. Broden, B.: Roentgen examination of the subtaloid joint in fractures of the calcaneus, Acta Radiol. **31:**85-91, 1949.
22. Brown, J.E.: Early ambulation of os calcis fractures, Clin. Orthop. **63:**252, 1963.
23. Burdeaux, B.D.: Reduction of calcaneal fractures by the McReynolds medial approach technique and its experimental basis, Clin. Orthop. **177:**87-103, 1983.
24. Burghele, N., and Serban, N.: Reappraisal of the treatment of fractures of the calcaneus involving the subtalar joint, Ital. J. Orthop. Traumatol. **2:**273-279, 1976.
25. Carey, E.J., Lance, E.M., and Wade, P.A.: Extra-articular fractures of the os calcis, J. Trauma. **5:**362-372, 1965.
26. Carothers, R.G., and Lyons, J.F.: Early mobilization in treatment of os calcis fractures, Am. J. Surg. **83:**279-280, 1952.
27. Cave, E.F.: Fractures of the os calcis: the problem in general, Clin. Orthop. **30:**64-66, 1963.
28. Chapman, M.W.: Fractures and fracture-dislocations of the ankle and foot. In Mann, R.A., editor: DuVries' surgery of the foot, ed. 4, St. Louis, 1978, The C.V. Mosby Co.
29. Christopher, F.: Fracture of the anterior process of the calcaneus, J. Bone Joint Surg. **13:**877-879, 1931.
30. Conn, H.R.: Fractures of the os calcis: diagnosis and treatment, Radiology **6:**228, 1926.
31. Conn, H.R.: The treatment of fractures of the os calcis, J. Bone Joint Surg. **17:**392-405, 1935.
32. Conway, J.J., and Cowell, H.R.: Tarsal coalition: clinical significance and roentgenographic demonstration, Radiology **92:**799-811, 1969.
33. Cotton, F.J., and Henderson, F.F.: Results of fracture of the os calcis, Am. J. Orthop. Surg. **14:**290-298, 1916.
34. Cotton, F.J., and Wilson, L.T.: Fractures of the os calcis, Boston Med. Surg. J. **159:**559-565, 1908.
35. Cowell, H.R.: Talocalcaneal coalition and new causes of peroneal spastic flatfoot, Clin. Orthop. **85:**16-22, 1972.
36. Dachtler, H.W.: Fractures of the anterior superior portion of the os calcis due to indirect violence, Am. J. Roentgenol. **25:**629-631, 1931.
37. D'Ambrosia, R.D., and Drez, D.J.: Prevention and treatment of running injuries, Thorofare, New Jersey, 1982, Charles B. Slack, Inc., pp. 25-31.
38. Dart, D.E., and Graham, W.P.: The treatment of fractured calcaneum, J. Trauma, **6:**362-367, 1966.
39. DeBold, C., Jr., and Stimson, B.B.: Treatment of injuries involving the subtalar joint, Am. J. Surg. **93:**604-608, 1958.
40. Degan, T.J., Morrey, B.F., and Braun, D.P.: Surgical excision for anterior-process fractures of the calcaneus, J. Bone Joint Surg. **64A:**519-524, 1982.

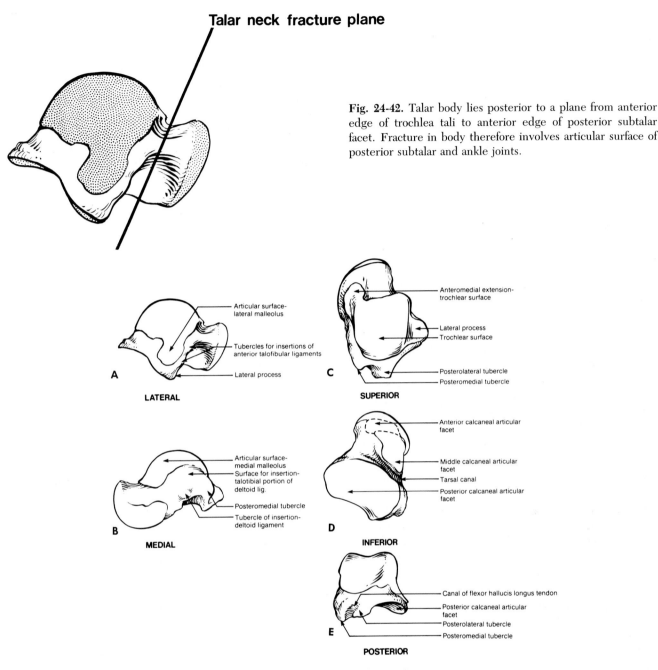

Talar neck fracture plane

Fig. 24-42. Talar body lies posterior to a plane from anterior edge of trochlea tali to anterior edge of posterior subtalar facet. Fracture in body therefore involves articular surface of posterior subtalar and ankle joints.

Fig. 24-43. Five surfaces of talar body. **A,** Lateral. **B,** Medial. **C,** Superior. **D,** Inferior. **E,** Posterior.

Neck

The neck of the talus has four surfaces: the superior, lateral, medial, and inferior. The superior surface of the neck is limited posteriorly by the anterior border of the trochlea tali and anteriorly by the articular surface of the talar head. The talotibial capsule inserts along this superior surface, just proximal to the insertion of the capsule of the talonavicular joint. The lateral surface of the neck provides an insertion of the medial aspect of the inferior extensor retinaculum.[124] The inferior surface of the neck forms the roof of the sinus tarsi and sinus canal (Fig. 24-39). The medial surface provides an area for insertion of the talonavicular ligaments.[124]

Body

The body of the talus is arbitrarily divided into five surfaces: the lateral, medial, superior, inferior, and posterior (Fig. 24-43).

The lateral surface of the body of the talus consists of a large articular surface, the facies malleolaris lateralis[124] (Fig. 24-43, A). The lateral talocalcaneal ligament inserts at the apex of the lateral process. Along the anterior border of the trigonal articular surface of the lateral surface are two tubercles for insertion of the anterior talofibular ligament. Along the posteroinferior border of the lateral malleolar surface lies a groove for attachment of the posterior talofibular ligament.

The medial surface presents two areas: the superior and inferior (Fig. 24-43, B). The superior portion is occupied by the articular facet, or facies malleolaris medialis.[124] This articular surface is shaped like a comma, with a long axis oriented anteroposteriorly. The inferior portion is nonarticular and consists in its anterior half of a depressed surface perforated by numerous vascular foramina. Under the tail of the superior surface, the posterior half of the inferior surface consists of a large oval area that provides insertion for the deep component of the deltoid ligament.[124]

The superior surface of the body is shaped like a pulley, with the groove of the pulley near the medial border (Fig. 24-43, C). The transverse diameter of the superior surface is greater anteriorly than posteriorly.[124]

The inferior surface consists of the facies articularis calcanea posterior[124] (Fig. 24-43, D). This articular surface is quadrilateral in shape and is concave in the long axis while being flat transversely. It articulates with the posterior facet of the calcaneus.

The posterior surface consists of posterolateral and posteromedial tubercles that flank the sulcus for the flexor hallucis longus tendon[124] (Fig. 24-43, E). The posterolateral tubercle is larger and more prominent than the posteromedial tubercle. This posterolateral tubercle contributes an inferior articular surface that is in continuity with the posterolateral aspect of the posterior calcaneal surface of the talus. An accessory bone, the os trigonum, may be found in connection with the posterolateral tubercle.[124]

OPEN FRACTURES OF TALUS

Because of the nature of trauma that results in fractures of the talus, these injuries often result in open wounds.* The wounds are often of the bursting type, and the wound margins are often ischemic.[25,36] In open fractures and fracture-dislocations, antibiotic coverage is begun immediately on the patient's arrival. An antibiotic providing both gram-positive and gram-negative coverage is recommended.[46,104] One must consider these antibiotics therapeutic and not prophlylactic, as such wounds are known to be contaminated at the time of injury.[104] The choice of antibiotic is changed only

*References 3, 8, 40, 43, 64, 86, and 106.

after cultures taken in the emergency room and the operating room reveal microbial sensitivities that demand such a change. Immunization against tetanus by the use of tetanus toxoid and/or human immune globulin must be considered in light of the patient's history.[46]

Giannestras and Sammarco[46] recommend an attempt to reduce the open fracture-dislocation in the emergency room and the application of a simple sterile dressing. When the patient is taken to the operating room, the wound is completely debrided, including skin edges and all necrotic tissue, and irrigation is performed. Once a complete debridement is performed, these authors recommend a change of instruments to perform the open reduction and internal fixation. The skin is left open following the open reduction, and a plaster splint is applied to the leg. At 48 to 72 hours the patient is brought back to the operating room for wound examination and possible closure. Giannestras and Sammarco emphasize that if the wound cannot be closed at that time, surrounding ligamentous, capsular, and other soft tissues should be used to cover the joint. The wound is reexamined in another 48 hours. If the wound still cannot be closed, plastic surgery consultation is obtained for skin grafting, muscle pedicle flap, or a free flap to obtain joint closure.

AUTHOR'S PREFERRED METHOD OF TREATMENT

In open fracture-dislocations of the talus, the basic principles of management of open fractures must be *strictly* followed. Cultures are obtained in the emergency room immediately on arrival. I prefer not to attempt reduction, as this may result in further contamination of the ankle and subtalar joints if done before a complete soft tissue debridement is performed. A sterile dressing is applied to the open wound after a povidone-iodine (Betadine) prep is performed. The patient is taken *immediately* to the operating room for debridement and reduction of the fracture-dislocation. Any delay at this point in treatment will result in significant soft tissue necrosis caused by the persistent dislocation.

I prefer a cephalosporin as the initial antibiotic, which is begun immediately on arrival in the emergency room, after the initial wound culture is taken. This antibiotic is continued until culture and sensitivity reports from the cultures taken in the emergency room or operating room dictate a change in antibiotic coverage. Antibiotics are continued for 48 to 72 hours, depending on the degree of initial contamination. The patient's tetanus immunization history is evaluated, and tetanus toxoid and/or immune globulin given is indicated.

The patient is brought to the operating room immediately and undergoes a routine 10-minute surgical prep. Following draping, the edges of the open wound are debrided, and a second set of cultures is taken. The area from which the body of the talus has been subluxated or dislocated is thoroughly debrided. Any tissue with a suggestion of necrosis is sharply excised. Following extensive debridement of all tissue of questionable viability, a thorough irrigation is performed. I prefer to use a series of irrigating solutions that includes povidone-iodine solution diluted with normal saline, followed by a triple antibiotic solution containing colistin sulfate (polymixin), neomycin, and bacitracin, and finally normal saline. Following the debridement and an extensive irrigation, a sterile dressing is applied. The limb is then reprepped and redraped and new surgical instrumentation is opened.

The particular talar fracture is then dealt with as indicated in the coresponding sections of this chapter. Once reduction and internal fixation have been performed, the wound is left open and the extremity placed in a short leg splint. The patient is returned to the operating room in 48 to 72 hours. At this time the wound over the joint and the talus are closed, if the wound is clean. If there is insufficient soft tissue or skin for closure or if the wound does not appear clean, a second debridement of necrotic tissue is performed, and the wound is again left open. The wound is reexamined 48 hours later and the decision is made to use skin grafting, local muscle pedicle grafting, or a distant free flap to obtain coverage. It is my opinion that coverage of this wound within the first 5 to 7 days is essential (providing the wound is clean) to prevent the long-term sequelae of talar osteomyelitis.[36]

FRACTURES OF HEAD OF TALUS

Fractures of the head of the talus are rare injuries, being less common than fractures of the talar neck or body.[13,25] Coltart[25] reports that 5% and Pennal[106] that 10% of all fractures and dislocations of the talus involve the talar head. The disability arising from these fractures can be severe.[13] Contusion and fibrillation of the articular cartilage of the talonavicular joint, which is associated with these fractures, may result in severe arthritis and pain on weight bearing, and may later require talonavicular fusion.[126]

Fractures of the head of the talus are of two varieties. The first is compression fractures of the head of the talus, as described by Pennal,[106] Schrock,[126] and Boyd and Knight.[13] These injuries represent simple impaction of the talar head and are often associated with compression fractures of the tarsal scaphoid.[13] The second variety is fractures of the talar head in the longitudinal or oblique plane, both of which result in two or more major fragments of the head of the talus.[126]

Mechanism of injury

Two mechanisms of injury producing talar head fractures have been proposed. According to Pennal,[106] the compression-type fracture results from a longitudinal compression force that acts on the foot when it is in some degree of plantar flexion. Coltart[25] reports that the force of impaction is transmitted along the longitudinal axis of the foot through the metatarsals and navicular to compress the talar head. This force usually produces a fracture in the medial portion of the talar head.[106] Coltart[25] suggests that, because of the association of talar head fractures with midtarsal joint dislocations, abduction and adduction may be important in addition to longitudinal compression in producing these injuries.

On the other hand, Garcia and Parkes[43] believe that this injury is caused by a fall on the completely extended (dorsiflexed) foot. In this mechanism, the talar head is presumably compressed against the anterior edge of the tibia by the force transmitted from the forepart of the foot to the navicular.[43]

Clinical diagnosis

The patient gives a history of a fall or motor vehicle accident in which the foot is plantar flexed at the time of impact. He complains of pain over the dorsal aspect of the foot in the region of the talonavicular joint.[40,43,46] There is usually point tenderness and swelling over the head of the talus. If the diagnosis is delayed, ecchymosis may be present.[43,46] Attempted dorsiflexion and plantar flexion of the midtarsal joint will reproduce the pain.[43,46] Additionally, inversion and eversion of the hindfoot will produce pain in the talonavicular area.[43] Ankle motion, if performed *without* stress at the midtarsal level, is not painful. Careful palpation of the calcaneocuboid and the subtalar joints for tenderness will detect an associated midtarsal subluxation that has spontaneously reduced, a finding which is important in planning treatment.

Radiographic examination

Fractures of the head of the talus may be demonstrated on the anteroposterior, lateral, and oblique radiographs of the foot. Careful evaluation of the outline of the talar head and neck on the *lateral* radiograph may be particularly helpful in making the diagnosis and determining displacement.[40] Although the fractures of the talar head are often comminuted, they are seldom displaced, because the fragments are held in place by the strong intertarsal ligaments of the foot.[43,46]

If routine radiographs do not give a clear indication of fracture location and size, particularly in the longitudinal or oblique (nonimpaction-type) fractures, polytomography may be useful. It is important to radiographically differentiate between a single displaced fracture fragment and a comminuted fracture for treatment purposes. Careful evaluation of the films, particularly for associated injury of the scaphoid and the calcaneocuboid joint, is important.

Treatment

Nondisplaced fractures. Dunn et al.[40] recommended that nondisplaced fractures be treated in a short leg cast with partial weight bearing allowed for a minimum of 3 weeks. Boyd and Knight[13] also recommended that compression fractures of the head of the talus be immobilized in a non-weight-bearing cast for 3 to 4 weeks, followed by a walking cast until union has occurred. They suggested that, if there is a tendency to flattening of the longitudinal arch of the foot, an arch support should be used after the walking cast is removed. Giannestras and Sammarco[46] recommended that a Whitman-type steel arch support be fitted in the shoe for a period of 3 months following cast removal in an effort to decrease the stress on the talonavicular joint. Pennal[106] noted that these fractures are usually located in the medial portion of the head, and that although there may be several fracture lines, significant displacement is not common. He recommended that these nondisplaced fractures be treated by mobilization in a walking cast for 4 to 6 weeks.

Displaced fractures. In cases in which the fracture of the talar head is displaced, resulting in disruption of the talonavicular joint, Pennal suggests fragment excision.[106] According to Schrock[126] a displaced fragment of the talar head may be excised *only* if more than one half of the talar head remains intact. On the other hand, Dunn et al.[40] recommend that displaced fractures of the talar head be treated by open reduction and internal fixation if the fracture fragments are large enough *and* if closed reduction is unsuccessful. Following open reduction, they recommend partial weight bearing in a short leg cast until healing occurs.

Boyd and Knight[13] report that distortion of the talonavicular joint following this injury is significant and may result in traumatic arthritis, which will necessitate midtarsal arthrodesis for pain relief. Schrock[126] also reports that the associated contusion and fibrillation of the articular cartilage may result in traumatic arthritis, requiring talonavicular fusion. Garcia and Parkes[43] state that although the prognosis is generally good, chondromalacia of the head of the talus or osteoarthritis of the talonavicular joint may develop, requiring arthrodesis of this articulation. However, before fusion, they recommend a steroid injection on one or two occasions in an effort to postpone arthrodesis.[43] Although Dunn et al.[40] prefer triple arthrodesis when there is isolated talonavicular arthritis, Garcia and Parkes[43] believe isolated talonavicular fusion is the most conservative approach. Should this fail, a triple arthrodesis can be performed.

AUTHOR'S PREFERRED METHOD OF TREATMENT

I emphasize the importance of careful palpation to detect associated occult injury to the calcaneocuboid or subtalar joints. Careful radiographic examination of these areas for associated fractures is essential. If on clinical examination there is tenderness over the calcaneocuboid joint, one must consider that the talar head fracture has been associated with a midtarsal subluxation or dislocation that has spontaneously reduced. Stress radiographs are helpful in determining the degree of this subluxation or dislocation. If injury to these joints occurs, treatment is altered as indicated on p. 782.

Isolated talar head fractures of the impaction type that are comminuted but nondisplaced are treated in a short leg non-weight-bearing cast for 3 weeks. This is followed by a weight-bearing cast for an additional 3 to 5 weeks, depending on the degree of comminution. The cast is well molded in the longitudinal arch. Cast immobilization is discontinued when union is present. The toes are left free in the cast to encourage early active range of motion to the metatarsophalangeal joint. After cast immobilization, the shoe is fitted with a firm longitudinal arch support.

For those fractures in which there is a displaced fracture involving the talonavicular joint, I prefer open reduction and internal fixation or fragment excision, depending on the size of the fragments. I prefer not to excise a fragment of the talar head if the remaining head of the talus makes up less than one half of the articular surface. Open reduction and internal fixation using Kirschner wires or A-O small screws for the single large displaced fragment has been successful in my hands. Following open reduction, if fracture fixation is stable, the patient is begun on an early range of motion program while still in the hospital. Once motion has been restored to the midtarsal and subtalar joints, a short leg cast is worn until union occurs. After union, a longitudinal arch support is recommended.

If the fracture fragments are excised, the foot is immobilized in a short leg walking cast for 3 weeks followed by a rigorous range of motion exercise program. Once motion has been restored, a longitudinal arch support is recommended.

For patients who develop traumatic arthritis of the talonavicular joint following these fractures, I prefer isolated talonavicular arthrodesis. Before this arthrodesis is performed, I inject local anesthetic into the talonavicular joint under fluoroscopic control as a diagnostic test. The patient is then allowed to be up and walking about. If the injection produces pain relief, an isolated talonavicular fusion is performed. If the pain persists, sequential injection of the talonavicular, calcaneocuboid, and subtalar joints is performed to see which of these joints is responsible for the pain. Arthrodesis of one, two, or all three of the joints is performed based on the results of injection. Isolated arthrodeses of small joints in the foot have produced good results in my patients when this type of preoperative evaluation has been performed.

If the calcaneocuboid joint has been subluxed but not dislocated, the talar head fracture is managed as described previously, but weight bearing is delayed for 3 weeks to allow healing of the calcaneocuboid joint capsule. If there has been frank dislocation, consideration is given to percutaneous pinning of the calcaneocuboid joint. Such pins can be inserted under radiographic control and then cut off and bent beneath the skin, to be removed later. In these patients, weight bearing is delayed for 4 to 6 weeks, at which time the pins are removed.

FRACTURES OF NECK OF TALUS

Fractures and fracture-dislocations of the neck of the talus make up 50% of all major injuries to the talus.* The significance of these injuries is the result of the frequency and severity of the complications and long-term disability they produce.[107]

Coltart[25] credits Fabricius of Hilden with the first account of an injury to the talus in 1608. Sir Astley Cooper[26,106] first described the natural history of dislocation of the talus in 1818. Sir James Syme[141] in 1848 reported that of 13 patients admitted to the Royal Infirmary of Edinburgh with compound fracture-dislocation of the talus, only 2 survived. Therefore he recommended below-the-knee amputation for these injuries, a procedure that still produced a mortality of 25% in his era. Stealy[139] in 1909 reviewed the literature to that date and noted a 50% mortality following open fracture-dislocation of the talus.

Anderson[2] in 1919 while serving as consultant surgeon to the Royal Flying Corps, collected 18 cases of fracture-dislocation of the talus resulting from airplane crashes and coined the term *aviator's astragalus* for this injury because of its occurrence in "belly landings" of small aircraft.[90] Coltart[25] in 1952, in an excellent and detailed review, described 228 injuries of the talus which he collected from the Royal Air Force.

Hawkins[53] in 1970 suggested a classification of vertical fractures of the neck of the talus. This classification is based on the radiographic appearance at the time of

---

*References 25, 53, 62, 106, 115, and 140.

injury and divides these fractures into three groups (groups I, II, and III). Hawkins noted that vertical fractures of the neck of the talus frequently enter a portion of the talar body; in these injuries, the fracture line involves the trochlea *and* the articular surface of the posterior facet of the subtalar joint. He included these fractures with fractures that only involved the talar neck in his classification. In my experience, those fractures which involve the body have an increased incidence of degenerative arthritis of both the ankle and the subtalar joint, and also an increased incidence of aseptic necrosis. Indeed, Mindel et al.[86] reported that the incidence of satisfactory results in fractures of the talar *neck* with dislocation was 64% compared with the 29% satisfactory results in fractures of the talar *body* with dislocation. Schrock[99] also reports the level of fracture in the talus is of significance in predicting viability of the body. Because of this difference in prognosis, I have chosen to separate fractures of the talar neck and body in this chapter.

In Hawkins[53] group I injuries the vertical fracture in the neck of the talus is undisplaced (Fig. 24-44, A). The body of the talus maintains its normal relationship in both the ankle and subtalar joints. In group I injuries only one of the three main sources of blood supply to the talus is interrupted: those vessels which enter the foramina on the dorsal and lateral aspect of the neck of the talus and progress proximally into the body.

In group II injuries (Fig. 24-44, B), the vertical fracture of the neck of the talus is displaced, and the subtalar joint is either subluxed or dislocated. The associated subtalar dislocation may occur medially, secondary to an inversion force, or laterally if secondary to an eversion force. According to Penny and Davis,[107] medial dislocation is more frequent. If the subtalar dislocation is complete, the injuries are frequently open because of the thin subcutaneous layer of tissue at the level of the ankle joint. The relationship of the talus in the ankle joint is normal, and the head of the talus retains its normal relationship with the navicular and the anterior facet of the subtalar joint. In group II injuries, at least two of the three sources of blood supply to the talus are interrupted: the blood supply proceeding proximally from the talar neck (as in group I) and that entering vascular foramina located inferiorly in the roof of the sinus tarsi and tarsal canal. The third main source of blood supply, that entering vascular foramina on the medial surface of the talar body, may also be injured.

In group III injuries, the vertical fracture of the neck of the talus is displaced and the body of the talus is dislocated from *both* the ankle and the subtalar joints (Fig. 24-44, C). The body of the talus is often extruded posteriorly and medially to be located between the posterior surface of the tibia and the

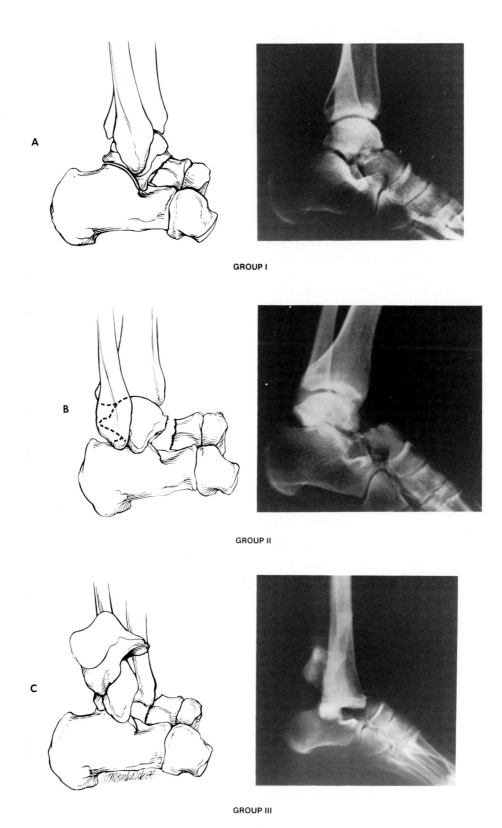

GROUP I

GROUP II

GROUP III

Fig. 24-44. For legend see opposite page.

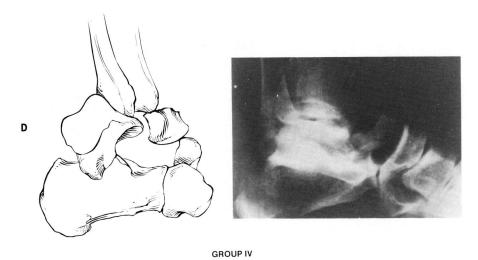

GROUP IV

Fig. 24-44. A, Group I[52]: Nondisplaced fracture of talar neck. Subtalar joint alignment is anatomic. **B,** Group II[52]: Displaced fracture of talar neck with associated subluxation or dislocation of subtalar joint. **C,** Group III[52]: Displaced fracture of neck of talus with talar body dislocated from both subtalar *and* ankle joints. **D,** Group IV[12,17]: Displaced fracture of talar neck associated with dislocation of body from ankle or subtalar joint and with additional dislocation or subluxation of head of talus from talonavicular joint. (Reprinted with permission from Canale, S.T., and Kelly, F.B., Jr.: J. Bone Joint Surg. **60A:**143-156, 1978.)

Achilles tendon. The head of the talus maintains its normal relationship with the navicular. All three of the main sources of blood supply to the body of the talus are damaged in group III injuries. The foot adopts a position of slight eversion and lateral dislocation.[107] More than one half of group III fracture-dislocations are open injuries, and in the closed injuries the overlying skin and occasionally the neurovascular bundle are in jeopardy.[98] Pantazopoulos et al.[102] presented an unusual group III fracture-dislocation of the talus in which there was a fracture of the neck of the talus with complete dislocation of the body that was difficult to detect. The body was displaced and rotated 180° on its transverse axis, so that it was lying upside down in the ankle joint.

Canale and Kelly[17] added a fourth type of dislocation, group IV, in which there is a fracture of the talar neck associated with dislocation of the body from the ankle or subtalar joint *and* dislocation or subluxation of the head of the talus from the talonavicular joint. In this injury, damage to the vascularity of *both* the body (as in group III injuries), and the head and neck fragments are possible[74] (Fig. 24-44, *D*). Boyd and Knight[13] have also reported a fracture of the neck of the talus with dislocation of the head. Pantazopoulos et al.[103] reported a variation of a group IV injury in which there was a dislocation of the head of the talus while the body of the talus remained reduced.

Shelton and Pedowitz[129] believe that the main shortcoming of Hawkins' classification is the failure to emphasize slight subluxation as opposed to frank dislocation of the subtalar and tibiotalar joints. They emphasize the possibility of momentary subluxation or dislocation of these joints that spontaneously reduces *before* radiographic studies. This can only be diagnosed on stress films.[129] Such spontaneously reduced fracture-dislocations may appear to be group I injuries but instead may be group II or III injuries with their attendant increased morbidity.

This discussion of fractures in the neck of the talus includes coronal fractures through the neck. Saggital fractures that exit through the talonavicular joint and therefore involve the head of the talus are not included in this section.

Anatomy

The neck of the talus represents the weakest portion of that bone, located where the sulcus of the talus reduces its thickness considerably. The fracture line usually begins dorsally in the talar sulcus and exits inferiorly along the line of insertion of the interosseous talocalcaneal ligament (Fig. 24-45, *A*). Fractures that occur more posteriorly and involve both the articular surface of the talocrural and posterior facet of the subtalar joint (Fig. 24-45, *B*) are discussed under Fracture-Dislocations of Body of Talus (See p. 683).

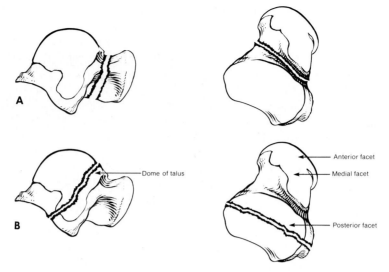

Fig. 24-45. A, Fracture of talar neck exits inferiorly between middle and posterior subtalar facets of talus. **B,** Fracture of talar body involves both ankle joint and articular surface of posterior subtalar facet.

Mechanism of injury

Fractures of the talar neck are most common in motor vehicle accidents, airplane crashes, and falls from heights.* Anderson[2] identified the mechanism as a hyperdorsiflexion force exerted on the sole of the foot by the rudder bar of an aircraft on impact, hence the term *aviator's astragalus.* Penny and Davis[107] emphasize that a hyperdorsiflexion injury produced by the clutch or brake pedal of an automobile reproduces this mechanism of the aviator's astragalus. The same mechanism occurs in a fall if the forepart of the foot strikes the rung of a ladder or some other object on the ground.[107] Pennal[106] reports that although the mechanism of talar neck fracture is usually a force from below, the opposite force, in which a weight falls on the dorsum of the foot, can produce a talar neck fracture.

With a dorsiflexion injury, the posterior capsular ligaments of the *subtalar* joint are the first structures to rupture. The neck of the talus then impacts against the anterior edge of the distal tibia, and a fracture line develops through the neck and enters the nonarticular portion of the subtalar joint between the middle and posterior facets.[107] Jensenius[59] likens the anterior margin of the tibia to a wedge driven into the dorsal aspect of the neck of the talus (and occasionally into the anterior part of the trochlea), resulting in a fracture with an angle opening to the dorsum.[59] If the force ceases at this point, a nondisplaced fracture of the talar neck (group I) occurs. With continuation of the dorsiflexion force, the calcaneus and remainder of the foot, includ-

ing the head of the talus, subluxate or dislocate anteriorly. At this point, if there is an inversion component to the force, the foot may subluxate or dislocate medially, while a concomitant eversion force results in lateral dislocation of the foot.[107] If the dorsiflexion force subsides at this point, the body of the talus tips into equinus (being dislocated at the subtalar joint), and the fracture surface of the talar neck rides on the upper surface of the os calcis (group II).[106,107] If the dorsiflexion force continues, however, rupture of the posterior capsular ligaments of the *ankle*, the strong posterior talofibular ligament, and the superficial and posterior portions of the deltoid ligament occurs.[26,106,107] The body of the talus is then forced backward out of the ankle mortise. It follows the curve of the posterior facet of the os calcis, rotating so that the undersurface of the talus faces downward and outward, while the neck of the talus points upward and outward.[106,107] The body of the talus comes to lie in the interval between the posterior aspect of the medial malleolus and the anterior aspect of the Achilles tendon. The posterior tibial neurovascular structures may escape injury by this mechanism as they lie anterior to and are protected by the flexor hallucis longus tendon.[107]

According to Penny and Davis,[107] in group III fractures the talus pivots around the remaining intact fibers of the deltoid ligament. This produces a kinking of the deltoid ligament that may obstruct the only remaining vascular pathway to the body of the talus. According to Pennal,[106] if there is a fracture of the medial malleolus, the attachment of the deltoid ligament to the talus is protected. He stresses the importance of this anatomi-

---

*References 7, 17, 41, 43, 53, 62, 64, 103, and 126.

ation using two A-O compression screws or one A-O compression screw and a Kirschner wire to prevent rotatory displacement is recommended.

Shelton and Pedowitz[129] also recommend closed reduction. If closed reduction is not satisfactory or is unstable, they recommend open reduction and internal fixation using a medial approach with osteotomy of the medial malleolus. They take particular care to avoid damage to the arterial branches to the talus located in the deltoid ligament. Once an anatomic reduction of the talar neck is obtained, stabilization with interfragmentary compression screws is performed. If there is a defect at the fracture site, they recommend cancellous bone grafting from the distal tibial metaphysis.

Hawkins[52] reports anatomic closed reduction was obtained in 40% of his group II patients. Even with adequate closed reduction, aseptic necrosis occurred in 40% of these injuries.[52] When closed reduction was not successful, open reduction through an anteromedial arthrotomy provided good visualization of the medial and superior aspects of the talar neck fracture. He suggests drilling two Steinmann pins from the navicular and head of the talus through the fracture site and into the body of the talus to secure fixation and maintain reduction.

Trillat et al.[143] recommend a unique method of treatment that combines closed reduction under fluoroscopic control and fixation with a lag screw inserted from the *posterior* tubercle of the talus to stablize group II fractures. Lahaut[69] first used this posterior approach to insert a tibial graft through the posterior tubercle to stabilize a talar fracture. Lemaire and Bustin[73] recommend this technique in both group II and III fractures. Group II fractures are first reduced by manipulation under fluoroscopic control. Anatomic alignment is obtained and maintained by plantar flexion of the foot. In the group III fractures, open reduction is necessary. Once reduction is obtained, the posterior tubercle of the talus is approached through a posterolateral incision adjacent to the Achilles tendon. A Kirschner wire is introduced under fluoroscopic control from the posterior tubercle, along the longitudinal axis of the talus, perpendicular to the fracture line.[73] An A-O cancellous screw is then inserted parallel to the Kirschner wire. Despite the fact that good fixation was obtained, the authors did not use early range of motion. Instead, they immobilized the foot and ankle for 4 to 6 weeks following surgery. The advantages of this approach in group II injuries are (1) it avoids immobilization in the equinus position, (2) it shortens the time to union, and (3) it allows immediate mobilization if stable fracture fixation is achieved.[73] The authors emphasize that fixation achieved by means of Kirschner wires or a screw introduced from the *anterior* fragment into the body of the talus *rarely*

achieves firm fixation with compression in the appropriate plane. The authors agree with Trillat et al.[143] that this technique is superior to closed reduction or to open reduction and fixation using an anterior approach for Group II injuries. Also, the posterolateral approach may preserve some of the blood supply to the body of the talus which enters anteromedially. However, the method does not prevent osteonecrosis.[73]

Group III injuries

Closed. In Hawkins' group III fractures, the talar body is displaced both from the ankle and subtalar joints. The talar body usually rests posteriorly and medially, rotating around the deep fibers of the deltoid ligament.[52] The blood supply to the body of the talus is completely disrupted, with the possible exception of that through the deltoid ligament.[52] The Committee on Trauma of the American Orthopaedic Foot Society in 1983 recommended early *anatomic* reduction to decompress the remaining deltoid ligament vessels, to allow the maximum surface area for revascularization across the talar neck fracture, and to ensure an anatomic reduction of the subtalar joint.[32] Although McKeever,[80,81] and Boyd and Knight[13] suggest early subtalar fusion in these patients with a talus devoid of soft tissue may hasten revascularization of the talus, this has not been shown to accelerate revascularization.[52]

Nearly 50% of group III injuries are open[98]; however, if the injury is not open, the displaced body usually puts extreme tension on the overlying skin, which can result in necrosis unless prompt reduction is instituted.

Although closed reduction is recommended by most authors, it is usually not successful.[40,98,106,129] Pennal[106] and Shelton and Pedowitz[129] recommend *immediate* closed reduction unless there is an open wound that demands debridement. This reduction is performed under general or spinal anesthesia, as muscle relaxation is essential. A large Kirschner wire or Steinmann pin is inserted transversely through the calcaneus. The calcaneus is plantar flexed and everted, and the joint distracted using this pin as a handle. Pressure is then applied from behind the body of the talus to force it forward into the mortise. Coltart[25] reports that Armstrong used a Steinmann pin inserted into the talar body to control the body while manipulating it into the mortise of the ankle joint. The subtalar dislocation, which is usually medial, is then reduced by applying traction to the forefoot and lateral pressure on the calcaneus with the ankle in equinus. A long leg, bent-knee cast is applied with the foot in eversion and equinus. Routine postreduction radiographs are carefully reviewed to detect a varus angulation of the talar neck fracture which will lead to delayed or malunion. If this occurs, immediate open reduction is recommended.

If closed reduction fails, Shelton and Pedowitz[129] recommend open reduction through a medial approach, sparing the deltoid ligament. The talar neck fracture is anatomically reduced and fixed internally with an interfragmentary compression screw. A short leg non-weight-bearing cast in neutral position is recommended for 3 months, or until fracture union is present radiographically. Weight bearing is delayed until fracture healing is complete, usually in 12 weeks.

Pennal,[106] Penny and Davis,[107] and Giannestras and Sammarco[46] recommend a *posteromedial* approach for open reduction. They cite the following advantages for the posteromedial approach: (1) it is centered directly over the fractured body, which allows direct visualization of the neurovascular structures; and (2) it is easily extended to allow osteotomy of the medial malleolus, which protects the medial talar vascular supply.[107] Lemaire and Bustin[73] also recommended the posteromedial approach, because it allows fixation of an associated malleolar fracture and also permits insertion of a screw from posterior to anterior for fixation of the talar neck fracture.

Deyerle and Burkhardt[37] emphasize the importance of osteotomy of the medial malleolus for better exposure in group III injuries. They believe that this technique completely protects the remnants of the deltoid ligament and its associated vascular supply to the talus. Using this method for early anatomic reduction, they report aseptic necrosis in only 10% of group III injuries. Indeed, Hawkins[52] notes that revascularization of the necrotic talus begins medially and progresses laterally, suggesting that vessels persist in the deltoid ligament that supply the talar body. Dunn et al.[40] recommend a lateral approach to avoid further damage to these important medial arteries to the talar body.

Open. Open group III injuries produce a particular challenge to the orthopaedist, as the decision of whether or not to retain the contaminated body of the talus must be made. Removal of the talar body, particularly when it is open and devoid of soft tissue attachment has been suggested by some authors.[12,47] Gibson and Inkster[47] reported that although partial talectomy was unsatisfactory, complete talectomy may indeed produce a satisfactory result. However, Miller and Baker,[84] and Boyd and Knight[13] caution against talectomy because of poor results, i.e., shortening, pain with weight bearing, instability, and lack of endurance. They suggest if talectomy is necessary, it should be considered temporary, and that tibiocalcaneal fusion should be performed later. Bohler[10] and Coltart[25] recommend the talar body not be discarded, as its removal causes severe and lasting disability. Winkler[149] also recommends against talectomy, because an ankle without a talus is invariably painful and disabled, and such patients are frequently incapable of any type of weight bearing.

Penny and Davis[107] believe the best solution in the working man is to discard the body of the talus, wait for primary wound healing, and then proceed with an early Blair[8] fusion. In those patients in whom it is preferable to retain the body of the talus, they prefer primary rigid internal fixation using an A-O cancellous screw. This allows easier management of associated soft tissue injury without the problems associated with casting.

Percy[108] recommends that the completely dislocated talar body be cleansed and replaced, because the bony stock it provides may be needed later for reconstruction. Indeed, Sneed[135] reported a case in which the talus was completely dislocated and replaced, and revascularization proceeded with a good functional result. O'Brien[98,99] emphasizes that in the open dislocation, the talus should not be discarded unless infection or late presentation prevent its salvage. In these instances, the talus is removed and tibiocalcaneal fusion is performed at a later date.

Although it provides stability, tibiotalar fusion is difficult to obtain, results in some loss of heel height with difficulty fitting shoes, and allows no tibiopedal motion.[8,13,34,90] As a result, Blair introduced a modified tibiotalar fusion for these injuries. In patients with fractures of the neck or body, neither the head nor distal part of the neck of the talus are involved; therefore the anterior and middle calcaneal articular facets of the talus remain intact. In a Blair fusion, a sliding bone graft anteriorly from the tibia is inserted into the remaining neck of the talus (see Fig. 24-52). This does not shorten the limb, and it maintains some subtalar motion through the retained anterior and medial subtalar facets; thus late progressive deformity does not occur. Morris et al.[91] and Dennis and Tullos[34] have reported excellent results using the Blair modified tibiotalar arthrodesis. Poor results were noted only if a pseudarthrosis developed.[34] In an open injury, initial wound debridement and secondary closure are performed, with the Blair fusion performed later when the wounds are healed. A more complete discussion of the Blair fusion can be found under Prognosis and Complications.

Group IV injuries. Group IV fractures, in which there is a fracture of the talar neck and subluxation or dislocation of the talar body and a dislocation of the head of the talus have rarely been reported in the literature.[12,17,103] Shelton and Pedowitz[129] advise anatomic reduction and temporary fixation of the talonavicular joint. Boyd and Knight[13] and Canale and Kelly[17] report that open reduction, with or without internal fixation, is necessary in the management of these injuries.

In this group of patients aseptic necrosis of both the talar body and head fragments is possible.[74]

Prognosis and complications

The prognosis in fractures of the neck of the talus is directly related to Hawkins' classification of the fractures. Lorentzen et al.[77] report that 46% of their group I patients had complications, including aseptic necrosis, osteoarthritis, and painful subtalar joints. Despite union without aseptic necrosis, Penny and Davis[107] note 50% of patients with group I fractures have unsatisfactory results. Group II injuries have even a less favorable prognosis. Penny and Davis[107] report aseptic necrosis in 20% and Hawkins[52] in 42% of patients with group II injuries. Although union occurred in all fractures, persistent subtalar joint symptoms in spite of an anatomic reduction were noted. Also, delayed union occurs in up to 15% of group II fractures.[110] In group III fractures, aseptic necrosis varies between 90% and 100%,[52,107] and nonunion occurs in 10% of patients.[52,107] Group IV injuries have been too infrequently reported to give an accurate accounting of the prognosis.

The complications most frequently noted following fractures of the neck of the talus include: (1) skin necrosis, (2) osteomyelitis, (3) delayed union or nonunion, (4) malunion, (5) traumatic arthritis, and (6) avascular necrosis of the talus. Although it is rarely mentioned, Dunn et al.[40] report that injury to the posterior tibial nerve and artery can occur, particularly if the body is dislocated. According to McKeever,[81] the treatment of these complications is primarily prophylactic and depends on prompt and accurate reduction at the time of initial treatment. He emphasizes that once the complications occur, any treatment must be considered salvage.

Early complications

Skin necrosis. The lack of excess subcutaneous tissue and skin over the dorsum of the foot predisposes the skin in this area to pressure necrosis from underlying displaced talar fractures.[81] Indeed, Gillquist et al.[81] report that postoperative skin necrosis occurs in the majority of patients. Although skin necrosis was common in their series, Gillquist et al.[48] did not find a relationship between soft tissue loss, infection, and the functional end results. They did note, however, that osteomyelitis changes the prognosis substantially.

If skin necrosis occurs, McKeever[81] recommends excision of the gangrenous skin and closure of the area of skin loss with a flap of skin and subcutaneous tissues. Garcia and Parkes[43] and Giannestras and Sammarco[46] have also emphasized the importance of early debridement and coverage of the necrotic skin areas in an attempt to prevent any superficial infection from contaminating the joint and the talar body. Septic arthritis or

talar osteomyelitis, which may complicate skin necrosis, are catastrophic.[48]

Osteomyelitis. If the fractured talus is contaminated and osteomyelitis develops, it is very recalcitrant to treatment.[81] According to Dunn et al.,[40] McKeever,[81] and O'Brien,[98] established osteomyelitis of the talus can only be eliminated by excision of the talus. Because of the disability that results from talar excision, tibiocalcaneal or Blair fusion is indicated later.* Gillquist et al.[48] report uniformly poor results if infection occurs after these injuries. For these reasons, most authors recommend thorough debridement, delayed closure, and prophylactic antibiotic coverage to prevent this sequela.

Late complications

Delayed union and nonunion. Although delayed union is not uncommon,[77] definite nonunion is unusual after talar neck fractures. The severity of disruption of talar blood supply, particularly in group II and III injuries, the lack of thick periosteum on the talar neck, and the small fracture area available for repair (See Fig. 24-46, *B*) are responsible for delayed union in these fractures. If weight bearing is not restricted until union is evident radiographically, the nonunion rate will be unacceptably high. Peterson et al.[109] believe that delayed union is present when no healing is radiographically evident within 6 months. This occurred in slightly over 10% of their patients, none of whom went on to develop a nonunion. Miller[85] reports no cases of nonunion in his patients. Mindell et al.[86] noted delayed union in over 10% of their cases and report it associated with an increased incidence of poor results.

Lorentzen et al.[77] noted nonunion in less than 5% of fractures, but report that all were symptomatic. Avascular necrosis was a contributory factor in only one case.

Hawkins[53] reports nonunions only in group III fractures and found that all had associated aseptic necrosis. Direct bone grafting of an established nonunion can be considered if union is not present 12 months after fracture.[17,66] Talectomy as a salvage procedure for nonunion is suggested only if there is a lack of talar neck bone stock.

Malunion. Malunion results from accepting a poor reduction or loss of an acceptable reduction. Persistent displacement at a talar neck fracture is likely to result in incongruity and degenerative arthritis in the ankle, subtalar, and/or midtarsal joints (see Fig. 24-46). McKeever[80,81] warns against loss of reduction during the first few weeks of cast immobilization as swelling subsides and the foot becomes less secure in the cast. To prevent displacement and malunion, he stresses the

---

*References 8, 13, 17, 25, 40, and 149.

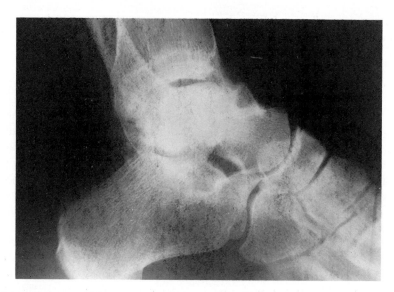

Fig. 24-49. Malunion of fracture at junction of talar body and talar neck prevents normal ankle dorsiflexion.

importance of open reduction or closed manipulative reduction secured by internal fixation.

Canale and Kelly[17] have stressed the frequency of malunion following talar neck fractures. They note that malunions can occur in the dorsal or varus position.[17] A dorsal malunion (one in the lateral plane) results in pain and restricted dorsiflexion of the ankle (Fig. 24-49). Dunn et al.[40] mention a dorsal exostosis of the talar neck as a complication of these fractures. They are not certain whether this is secondary to injury to the anterior capsule of the ankle, to callus formation at the fracture site, or to malunion. They mention that removal of the exostosis has restored dorsiflexion in some cases.

Varus malunion of the talar neck produces varus positioning of the forefoot.[17] This causes excessive weight bearing on the lateral side of the foot with plantar callus formation and pain. Also, almost one half of the patients reported by Canale and Kelly[17] with varus malunion developed degenerative arthritis of the subtalar joint, which required surgical treatment.

Traumatic arthritis of subtalar and talocrural joints. Fractures of the neck of the talus, even when not complicated by aseptic necrosis, are associated with subtalar arthrofibrosis and arthritis secondary to the original injury and the immobilization that is necessary until union occurs.[32,81]

Lorentzen et al.[77] stress that the most important complication of fractures of the neck of the talus is not aseptic necrosis, but osteoarthrosis, particularly of the subtalar joint. One third of their patients with talar neck fractures developed talotibial osteoarthritis, and over half developed subtalar osteoarthrosis. Addition-

ally, 24% of their patients had *both* talotibial and subtalar osteoarthrosis. While the incidence of talotibial osteoarthritis increased from group I to III, the incidence of subtalar osteoarthritis was essentially the same in the two groups.

Dunn et al.[40] report that restricted ankle and subtalar motion were responsible for a poor result in over half of their patients. They believe that restricted ankle dorsiflexion is caused by prolonged immobilization in equinus and recommended that this position be avoided. They believe that loss of subtalar motion is secondary to the damage to the articular surfaces at the time of the subtalar dislocation in group II and III injuries.

Canale and Kelly[17] used decreased range of motion in the involved joint associated with radiographic evidence of arthritic changes as the definition for traumatic arthritis. Using this definition, almost half of their patients with talar neck fractures had traumatic arthritis in the subtalar joint. Importantly, one third of the patients who developed subtalar arthritis had malunion of their fractures. In the remainder, the etiology of the arthritis was believed to be the amount of initial disruption of the subtalar joint or possibly aseptic necrosis of the inferior aspect of the body.[17]

Lemaire and Bustin[73] also note loss of subtalar motion and osteophyte formation in both the tibiotalar and subtalar joints, even following anatomic reduction and stable internal fixation of group II and III fractures. However, these patients were not managed with early motion. McKeever[81] suggests the arthrofibrosis can be minimized by promoting venous drainage with elevation of the foot and by beginning early range of motion

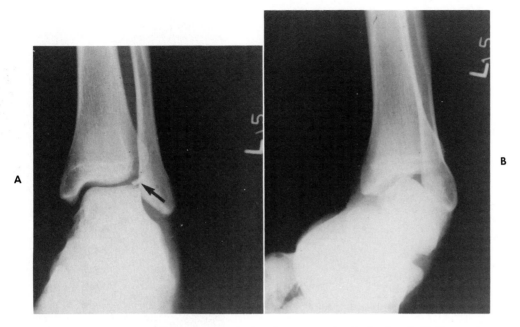

Fig. 24-55. A, Transchondral fracture of talar dome, completely displaced. **B,** Stress view shows associated lateral ligament disruption.

which suggests a vascular insult as the cause. Kappis[60] in 1922 was the first to use the term *osteochondritis dissecans* as applied to the ankle joint, while Rendu[119] in 1932 first reported a case of intraarticular fracture of the talus. Defects in the talar dome have, since these original descriptions, been reported under a confusing terminology.[95] Lesions with identical radiographic characteristics have been classified by some as fractures and by others as osteochondritis dissecans.[4,5] The most recent concept is that the lesion termed *osteochondritis dissecans of the talus* is not caused by idiopathic aseptic necrosis but instead by an injury.[4,100,116] Ray and Coughlin[116] report that the condition is caused by trauma, but stress that the trauma can be in the form of a single recognized episode, or more importantly, repeated minor unnoticed episodes. Such injuries result in a localized decrease in vascularity, leading to avascular separation of a loose fragment of cartilage and subchondral bone.[116]

Roden et al.[120] report that almost all such lesions that occur on the *lateral* aspect of the talus (Fig. 24-55) are secondary to trauma, rarely heal spontaneously, and are frequently the source of continued symptoms. On the other hand, they found that the majority of lesions on the *medial* aspect of the talus (Fig. 24-56) are not secondary to a *recognizable* episode of trauma, produce fewer symptoms, and frequently heal spontaneously. Canale and Belding[16] also noted that there were differences between the medial and lateral lesions: the lat-

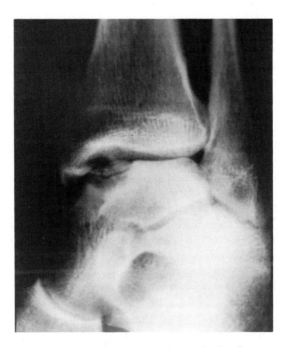

Fig. 24-56. Stage III lesion of medial talar dome.

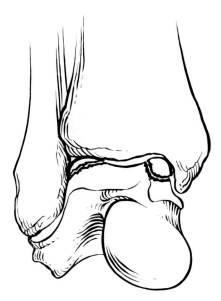

Fig. 24-57. Medial lesions are often cup shaped, while lateral lesions are waferlike or flakelike. (Redrawn from Canale, S.T., and Belding, R.H.: J. Bone Joint Surg. **62A:**97-102, 1980.)

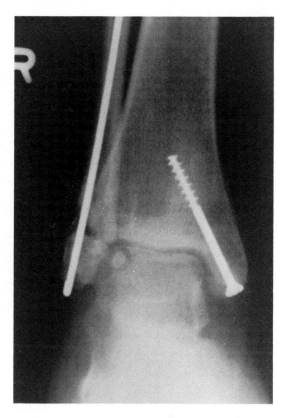

Fig. 24-58. Bimalleolar fracture of ankle treated by open reduction and internal fixation. Note lesion in lateral dome of talus, which was not detected at time of open reduction.

eral lesions seem to be traumatic in origin, while the medial lesions appear to be either traumatic or atraumatic. Additionally, the lateral lesions are wafer-shaped while the medial lesions are cup-shaped (Fig. 24-57), and the lateral lesions are more frequently associated with persistent symptoms and degenerative changes. They were unable to state, however, that the lateral lesion was a transchondral or dome fracture and that the medial lesion represented a true osteochondritis dissecans. Indeed, Berndt and Harty[4] in 1959 demonstrated that both the medial and lateral talar dome lesions of osteochondritis dissecans were transchondral or osteochondral fractures secondary to trauma. O'Donoghue[100] is also of the opinion that the majority of cases of so-called osteochondritis dissecans are in fact osteochondral or chondral fractures that arise from avulsion or shearing fractures or from direct compression.

Marks[78] in 1952 reported a case in which progression of a simple flake fracture of the talus to definite osteochondritis dissecans occurred. Alexander and Lichtman,[1] in an effort to combine the concepts of transchondral fracture and osteochondritis dissecans, reported that the lesion referred to in the literature as osteochondritis dissecans in reality represents a "compression lesion" of the articular surface of the talus, and that these lesions may progress to the actual loose body formation and fragment separation. They also noted that the diagnosis of a transchondral fracture of the talar dome is often delayed because initial radiographs are negative or because the injury seems so trivial that radiographs are not even taken.[1] Also, Shelton

and Pedowitz[129] note that these fractures are commonly associated with more obvious injuries to the malleoli and/or the adjacent ligaments, which tend to obscure their detection (Fig. 24-58).

In 1959 Berndt and Harty[4] classified lesions of the dome of the talus into four stages, as follows: stage I, a small area of compression of subchondral bone; stage II, a partially detached osteochondral fragment; stage III, a completely detached osteochondral fragment which remains in the talar crater; and stage IV, displaced osteochondral fragment (Fig. 24-59). Alexander and Lichtman[1] believe the lesion termed *osteochondritis dissecans*, particularly those in which a history of trauma is indefinite, actually represent a Berndt and Harty stage I compression lesion, which is painless at the onset because no ligaments are torn. It is with further weight bearing that this lesion progresses to a stage II or III lesion.

In spite of confusion regarding the terminology of fracture versus the concept of osteochondritis dissecans, for the purpose of discussion in this chapter, these lesions are considered as one. The fact that treatment recommendations and prognosis are not depen-

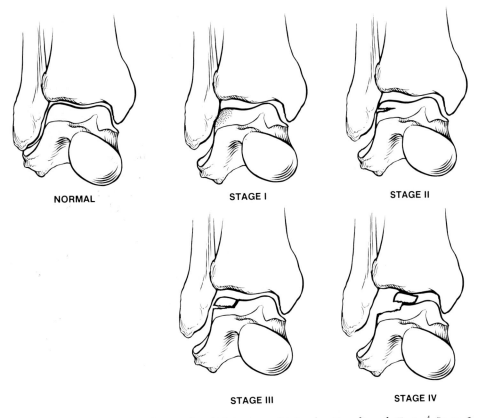

NORMAL **STAGE I** **STAGE II**

STAGE III **STAGE IV**

Fig. 24-59. Classification of osteochondral lesions of talus by Berndt and Harty.[4] Stage I, Small area of compressed subchondral bone. Stage II, Partially detached fragment. Stage III, Completely detached fragment remaining in talar crater. Stage IV, Fragment loose in joint.

dent on the etiology justifies the discussion of these entities under one heading.

Anatomy. The dome is that part of the talus which articulates with the lower articular surface of the tibia and fibula.[92] A secure fit of the dome of the talus into the ankle mortise, particularly in dorsiflexion, predisposes it to the shearing forces necessary to produce transchondral fractures. Inversion or eversion of the foot and ankle, which are necessary to produce these fractures, may produce associated injuries of the medial or lateral collateral ligaments of the ankle[84] (see Fig. 24-55).

Berndt and Harty[4] found that 43% of these lesions are in the lateral aspect of the talus, while 57% are located on the medial aspect of the dome of the talus. Canale and Belding[16] found an almost equal distribution of medial and lateral lesions. Those lesions on the medial aspect of the dome of the talus are usually located in the posterior third, while lesions in the lateral portion are most commonly located in the middle third of the talus.[4,16,28]

Pathology. Berndt and Harty[4] believe that once an osteochondral fracture occurs, whether it be on the me-

dial or lateral dome, it can heal like other fractures, but *only* if it is reduced *and* immobilized until union occurs. They emphasize that in stage I, II, and III fractures, the blood supply of the compressed or avulsed fragment has been cut off at the fracture line. The process of healing can occur only by the ingrowth of capillaries from the adjacent talus *across* the fracture line. The fracture fragment is avascular until a new blood supply arrives from the adjacent talus. These authors emphasize that if immobilization of the fracture in stages I, II, and III is incomplete or of too short a duration, resultant motion at the fracture line will shear off ingrowing capillaries and prevent the reparative process. Also, unless stage I and II lesions are immobilized, continued weight bearing may rupture the remaining attachment of the fragment and convert it to a detached stage III or completely displaced stage IV lesion.[4]

The gross appearance of the dome of the talus will depend on the stage of the lesion, varying from the appearance of normal cartilage with slight softening and discoloration over the lesion to an actual defect in the articular surface of the affected bone in situations in which there is a displaced osteocartilaginous loose body.[116] In the stage I lesion,[28] no damage may be evident on superficial examination of the talar dome; the injury may be caused entirely by a compression force resulting in microscopic injury to the bony trabeculae supporting the articular cartilage. The overlying articular cartilage does not become necrotic initially, since it obtains the majority of its nutrition from the synovial fluid.

Once the fragment becomes displaced, its bed becomes covered with a fibrous coating of host tissue as a new reparative process begins. Once the fragment is removed, the defect can become filled with fibrous connective tissue that restores the original shape of the talus and is of sufficient firmness to act as a satisfactory replacement for the missing bone.[4]

Mechanism of injury. Although reports of lesions of the talar dome without a history of trauma are present in the literature, there is overwhelming agreement that the majority of these injuries are posttraumatic in nature.[121] Lindholm et al.[75] found that trauma, such as a fall from a height or a twisting injury during a sporting activity, was the main cause of these lesions. Vaughan and Stapleton[145] stressed that, even though trauma is a major factor, at least some patients have an underlying predisposition to the lesion, possibly a local area of decreased vascular supply to the subchondral bone, which might produce a necrotic area with minimal injury.

Current literature suggests that osteochondral fractures of the talus are caused by inversion injuries.[28,78] O'Farrell and Costello[101] suggest that if the foot is plantar flexed during inversion, a medial lesion results from compression of the medial talar dome by the tibia. On the other hand, if the foot is dorsiflexed, a lateral talar lesion results from shearing forces produced by striking the fibula.

The most detailed investigation into the mechanism of these injuries was that reported by Berndt and Harty.[4] They found that with strong inversion of the dorsiflexed foot, a lesion of the lateral border of the talar dome resulted. This fracture was located at the middle or anterior half of the lateral border of the talus. With ankle dorsiflexion, the wider anterior half of the talus fits tightly into the ankle mortise. Inversion then impacts the lateral dome against the articular surface of the fibula. It is for this reason that the injury may be accompanied by tearing of the lateral ankle ligaments.[78,95] On the other hand, when the foot is in plantar flexion, the narrow posterior half of the talar dome occupies the mortise, and forceful inversion accompanied by medial rotation of the tibia on a fixed foot results in posteromedial talar impaction.

Rosenberg[22] emphasizes a clinical correlation with the mechanism of injury. He notes that the lateral lesion is easily recognized as an acute fracture, because it is elevated by the levering effect of the articular facet of the fibula. On the other hand, the medial lesion occurs as a result of impaction against the medial malleolus and is rarely displaced. These medial injuries become demonstrable radiographically only when absorption of bone has occurred at the impaction fracture site.

Finally, Mukherjee and Young[92] report an unusual fracture of the *anterior* dome of the talus, the mechanism of which they ascribe to plantar flexion and vertical compression, whereby the anterior edge of the lower articular surface of the tibia fractures the anterior aspect of the dome of the talus.

Clinical diagnosis. The diagnosis of osteochondral fracture of the talus is often missed in the early stages, because many of these patients are originally treated as though they had sprains, the fracture being overlooked.[1,95] Also, Alexander and Lichtman[1] reported that 28% of these patients have associated fractures, usually of the malleoli (Fig. 24-58). In these situations, the clinical examination may divert one's attention from the possibility of an injury to the dome of the talus.

Canale and Belding[16] found that the majority of patients, and all patients with lateral lesions, had a history of trauma to the ankle.[1,75,116,122] Other authors have also found a history of trauma in most patients although in some instances it seems insignificant.[116] In most series, patients are predominantly athletic males in the second and third decades of life.[129]

Berndt and Harty[4] stress that there are no symptoms pathognomonic of a transchondral fracture. In fact, Roden et al.[120] stressed that lesions of the lateral talar dome are more frequently associated with definite symptoms, while medial dome lesions usually have minimal symptoms. The symptoms vary depending on the stage of the injury, i.e., acute or chronic.[28,101,116] Acute fractures are often misdiagnosed as sprains, while patients with chronic injuries are misdiagnosed as arthritic. The symptoms of acute transchondral fracture are those of an inversion sprain, i.e., pain and tenderness in the torn lateral collateral ligaments, swelling of the ankle, ecchymosis, and limited motion.[4,101] However, stage I lesions may be almost painless because of the absence of sensory fibers in the compressed articular cartilage and a lack of associated ligamentous change.[1,28] In the chronic injury the symptoms depend to a large degree on the amount of healing of the associated torn ligaments and on the size and displacement of the fracture fragment. The symptoms suggest arthritis and include freedom of pain when the joint is at rest, but crepitus, stiffness, swelling, and limited motion after exercise.[4,101,116] Tenderness, crepitation, recurrent swelling, clicking, or symptoms of "a weak ankle" all should suggest the possibility of a fracture of the dome of the talus.[30,95,151] In stage IV lesions, locking occurs in addition to the symptoms of osteoarthritis.[4]

The physical findings in acute injury include swelling and tenderness.[92] The location of point tenderness can often determine the location of the lesion in the talar dome. In midlateral lesions, tenderness is usually located between the talus and tibiofibular syndesmosis,[97,116,129] while in posteromedial lesions tenderness is usually present behind the medial malleolus.[129] Marks[78] noted that there was swelling beneath the lateral malleolus and tenderness over the whole insertion of the lateral collateral ligament of the ankle, most marked over the attachment of the anterior and middle fasciculi to the talus and calcaneus respectively.

Flexion and extension of the ankle are normal, but there is marked limitation of inversion by pain, and of eversion by swelling, in acute injuries.[78,97]

Limitation of motion, locking, instability (secondary to associated ligamentous injury or to a loose body), and a palpable loose body may be present in cases of long-standing injury.[116]

Radiographic examination. Although the clinical history of an inversion sprain should suggest the diagnosis of an osteochondral fracture of the talus, radiographs are mandatory to establish the diagnosis. It is important to emphasize that when only the articular cartilage is damaged, i.e., in a stage I injury, the fracture may not be noted radiographically. The medial lesion in particular is commonly the result of impaction against the medial malleolus and is rarely displaced, and therefore it may become demonstrable radiographically only when absorption of bone and/or sclerosis has occurred at the fracture site. Indeed, Shelton and Pedowitz,[129] Alexander and Lichtman,[1] and Vaughan and Stapleton[145] stress the importance of repeat radiographic examination in certain patients in an effort to prevent a delay in diagnosis, which often leads to chronic disability. If pain about the ankle persists following an injury (despite normal initial films), these authors recommend repeating the radiographs as they may detect a stage II or III lesion that has developed from an undetected stage I injury.

Roden et al.[120] stressed that anteroposterior and lateral radiographs of the ankle are not adequate for diagnosis. Berndt and Harty[4] recommend a minimum of three views of the ankle, anteroposterior, oblique (10° of medial rotation), and lateral, all centered over the joint line and taken with the foot in the neutral position. The anteroposterior view usually demonstrates the medial margin of the dome of the talus clearly, but the lateral border of the talar dome is obscured by the lateral malleolus, which is superimposed over the lateral talar dome.[28,95] The oblique view with 10° of medial rota-

tion of the limb demonstrates the talofibular joint and gives a clear view of the lateral border of the talar dome.

Newberg[95] and Yvars[151] stress that even anteroposterior, lateral, and oblique views may not demonstrate the lesion. They therefore recommend taking the internal oblique radiographs of the ankle in neutral, plantar flexion, and dorsiflexion. In addition, Davidson et al.[28] mention that views taken in 35° of obliquity and full plantar flexion are useful to evaluate lateral dome lesions. Also, Davis,[30] and Alexander and Lichtman[1] suggest that inversion stress radiographs help demonstrate these lesions, particularly of the superolateral aspect of the dome of the talus.

Finally, although part of the talar dome is obscured by the overlying medial and lateral malleoli on the lateral view, this view is important because it indicates whether the lesion is anterior or posterior on the talar dome, a finding necessary for preoperative planning.[4,95]

Mensor and Melody[83] in 1941 first described the use of tomograms in evaluating lesions in the dome of the talus. Most authors believe that tomograms provide more accurate information as to size and location of these lesions[1,4,17,24] Newberg[95] suggests the value of *poly*tomography in both the lateral and oblique planes when localizing the fracture fragment and notes that anteroposterior tomograms may obscure a small fragment because of overlapping shadows.

It is important to remember that radiographically the fragment appears much smaller than when it is seen at operation, because the chondral component is radiolucent.[95] Air contrast arthography may be useful in better defining the size of a fragment and in determining whether it is completely detached.[129,134] Additionally, air contrast arthrography may demonstrate lesions that are purely chondral.[134] Recently, Reis et al.[118] clearly demonstrated the value of high-resolution computed tomography (CT) scan for lesions of the dome of the talus. I too have found the CT scan studies valuable in selecting the best surgical approach for these lesions.

The incidence of talar dome lesions is nearly equally distributed between the medial and lateral talar dome.[44,116,125] According to Canale and Belding[16] medial lesions are usually deeper and cup shaped while lateral fragments are shallow and wafer shaped (see Fig. 24-57). The radiographic appearance of the osteochondral lesion also depends on its duration.[16,49,122,151] In acute injuries, the osteochondral fragment has sharp edges demonstrable radiographically and there is no resorption at the fracture site. When seen later in the course of the disease, the signs of nonunion may be present. These include a sclerotic margin lining the concave talar bed and fragmentation of the subchondral bone plate.[151] It is this chronic picture that suggests the term *osteochondritis dissecans*.[78,151] Finally, secondary degenerative arthritis can be found either in the medial or lateral aspect of the ankle in cases with a long history.

Davidson et al.[28] emphasize the importance of follow-up radiographs to determine the progress of healing of these lesions. They stress that early healing is by fibrocartilage which is radiolucent. Therefore the defect and the fragment may appear larger in the early follow-up films than initially.

Treatment

Acute fractures. Berndt and Harty[4] report that, following an acute injury, treatment by reduction and adequate immobilization ordinarily results in healing, while Canale and Belding[16] found that with long-term follow-up few lesions united when treated nonoperatively.

Shelton and Pedowitz[129] stress the importance of correct staging and prompt and adequate treatment to produce the best results. For healing to take place, capillaries from the remaining talar body must cross the fracture site. If immobilization is inadequate, repetitive motion at the fracture site may transect these ingrowing capillaries and result in delayed or nonunion.[4,129] They recommend treating stage I, II, and II lesions without radiographic signs of an established nonunion (i.e., sclerosis, uneven joint surfaces or arthritic changes) in a short leg non-weight-bearing cast until union is demonstrated radiographically. They believe that stage IV displaced fractures are best treated by surgical removal of the fragment to prevent deterioration of the joint.[129] Newberg[95] recommends repair of associated ligamentous damage to improve results. In stage IV fractures with associated severe osteoarthritic changes in the ankle, simple removal of the loose body may be inadequate, and ankle fusion may be necessary.[129]

Canale and Belding[16] base treatment not only on displacement but on location of the lesion. They recommended that stage I and II lesions, whether medial or lateral in location, be treated nonoperatively in a cast or patellar tendon–bearing brace. They believe that stage III lesions on the medial talar dome should be treated by the same method. If symptoms persist after this conservative treatment, surgical excision and curettement of the lesion is recommended. In stage III lesions involving the lateral dome of the talus and both medial and lateral dome stage IV lesions, treatment by immediate excision of the fragment and curettement of the defect is recommended. Rosenberg,[122] on the other hand, reports that although prolonged immobilization has frequently been used, none of the lateral fractures he treated in this manner healed. He believes therefore that lateral lesions almost always require surgical treatment and that the decision of excision of the frag-

ment, curettement, or replacement is dependent on the size of the lesion.[122]

The management of the talar dome defect left after fragment excision is controversial. Ray and Coughlin[116] believe that the defect in the talus should be saucerized and all loose fragments excised from the joint. On the other hand, O'Donoghue[100] stresses that the articular cartilage at the edge of the defect should not be saucerized, but trephined by cutting the articular cartilage vertical to the articular surface. This minimizes the size of the articular cartilage defect which has to be filled. Also, to encourage revascularization of this denuded area, he recommends the use of fine drills or Kirschner wire holes as advocated by Smillie.[133]

Long-standing lesions. In dealing with long-standing lesions, Vaughan and Stapleton[145] and Nisbet[97] recommend operative removal of the fragment and curettement of the necrotic bone, while Lindholm et al.[75] recommend conservative treatment initially. However, if symptoms persist following conservative treatment, they recommend removal of the loose bodies. In those situations in which a large fragment from the weight-bearing dome is present, they suggest replacement of the fragment using bone pegs for internal fixation. Ray and Coughlin[116] recommend that in patients in whom the lesion is discovered accidently and who have no definite symptoms referable to the lesion, operative intervention be delayed until symptoms develop or until radiographs demonstrate progression of the lesion. They note that once the diagnosis is established and the patient has symptoms referable to the site of the lesion, surgical intervention is the only satisfactory method of treatment. O'Farrell and Costello[101] report that results are better in patients in whom surgery is performed within 12 months of the onset of symptoms. They suggest drilling the base of the defect after excision of the osteochondritic fragment in an effort to promote fibrocartilage formation in the defect. Davidson et al.[28] also note that a delay in surgical removal of a loose fragment may result in or contribute to posttraumatic arthritis.

Recently, in patients in whom the roentgenographs suggest an osteochondral defect, a small-caliber arthroscope has been used to evalute the joint surface of the ankle[39,75] and hence to stage the lesion. Additionally, small loose bodies can be removed arthroscopically, which limits the degree of postoperative rehabilitation necessary.[39] Arthroscopic currettement, debridement, and drilling of the defect after loose body removal is possible and greatly reduces postoperative morbidity.[39]

Operative approach. Ray and Coughlin[116] recommend an anteromedial incision for lesions in the superomedial aspect of the talus. However, in some cases the lesion may be completely hidden beneath the medial malleolus. Exposure of these lesions can be ob-

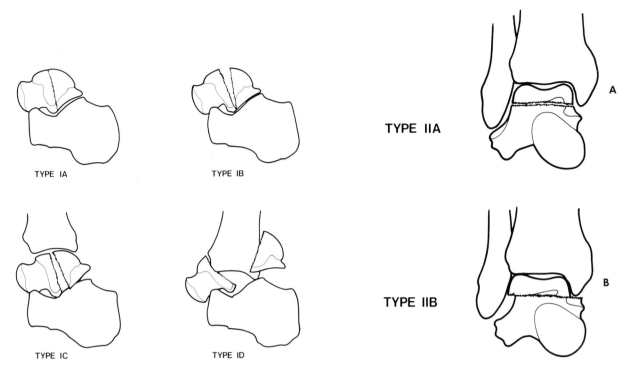

Fig. 24-63. Shearing fractures of talar body. Type IA fractures are nondisplaced. Type IB are displaced at talocrural (ankle) articulation. Type IC are displaced at *both* talocrural (ankle) and subtalar articulations. In type ID fractures, talar body fragment is completely dislocated.

Fig. 24-64. A, Nondisplaced, and **B,** displaced horizontal shearing fractures of the body of the talus.

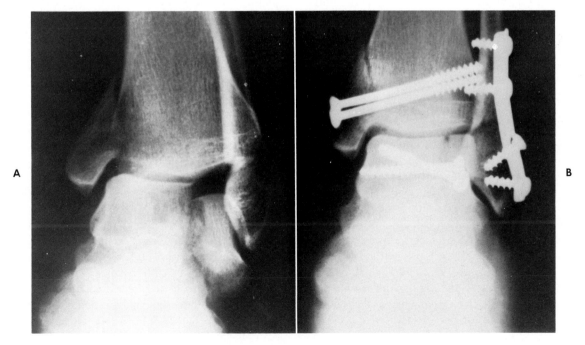

Fig. 24-65. A, Sagittal shearing fracture of talar body associated with bimalleolar ankle fracture. **B,** Treatment by open reduction and internal fixation of talus using small A-O cancellous screws.

On physical examination there is marked swelling and tenderness, particularly over the anterior aspect of the ankle.[13,43,86] Since these fractures involve both the ankle and the subtalar joints, inversion and eversion of the subtalar joint, in addition to dorsiflexion and plantar flexion of the ankle, are extremely painful. As with other injuries to the talus, the force dissipated at the time of injury is substantial, and it is not uncommon to for these fracture-dislocations to be associated with open wounds.[43] If the injury is closed, however, circulation to the overlying skin is often compromised.[86]

Radiographic examination. Routine anteroposterior, lateral, and oblique radiographs of the ankle are necessary to evaluate these injuries.[43,46,64] In all fractures of the talar body, particularly those which appear to be simple and nondisplaced, careful radiographic evaluation of the subtalar joint is essential to make certain that a subluxation of the subtalar joint is not missed.[64] Displacement at the site of a talar body fracture rarely occurs without an associated subtalar dislocation or subluxation.

Giannestras and Sammarco[46] note that the pain associated with these injuries may make it impossible to position the patient properly to obtain the necessary radiographs. Therefore they suggest that final radiographs used for the evaluation of the fracture and for treatment planning be taken in the operating room with the patient under anesthesia so that the correct views may be taken.

Minimally displaced fractures of the body of the talus may be difficult to detect on routine films; therefore polytomography (see Fig. 24-61, *B*) or CT scanning can be used to confirm the diagnosis and determine displacement.

Treatment

Group II fractures: type I (coronal or sagittal fractures)

IA and IB: nondisplaced and minimally displaced fractures. Nondisplaced (type IA) or minimally displaced (type IB) (i.e., those with less than 2 or 3 mm of displacement at the trochlear articular surface) coronal or sagittal shear fractures of the body of the talus, are best treated conservatively with a short leg non-weight-bearing cast for 6 to 8 weeks or until fracture union occurs.[13,40,43,46,106] Mindel et al.[86] reports that union occurs in 2 to 3 months with this method of treatment.

IC: displaced fractures with subtalar dislocation. In displaced shear fractures, associated subtalar dislocation is *usually* present and must be detected (type IC) (see Fig. 24-63). In displaced fractures the goal of treatment is anatomic reduction of both the displaced fracture *and* the subtalar joint.[40] Results of displaced intraarticular fractures of the body of the talus are dependent on an exact

reduction and stable internal fixation.[138] Kleiger[64] reports that in 5 of his 8 patients with displaced fractures of the talar body, the posterior subtalar joint was also dislocated. Reduction by *closed* manipulation is attempted with the patient under general or spinal anesthesia with the knee flexed to 90° and the foot held in equinus. Traction is exerted on the foot by grasping both the heel and the forepart of the foot, while countertraction is maintained at the thigh. While this traction is maintained, pressure is exerted with the thumb on the sole of the foot at the level of the displacement in an attempt to manipulate the fragments into position. Dunn et al.[40] caution against repeated forcible attempts at a closed reduction, instead preferring open reduction as recommended by Boyd and Knight.[13]

Kleiger[64] cautions that the reduction of these fractures must be accurate, because any remaining displacement in the superior articular surface may cause the distal fragment to abut against the anterior margin of the articular surface of the distal tibia and thereby block dorsiflexion. For this reason he emphasizes the importance of an absolutely true lateral radiograph after reduction to evaluate the talar body reduction.

Watson-Jones[146] advocated that the foot be kept in equinus following reduction to prevent recurrence of the subtalar displacement. Kleiger,[64] however, believes that once properly reduced, the fragments are stable in the neutral position. Following reduction, immobilization in a non-weight-bearing short leg cast is recommended until union occurs.[64,146]

ID: fractures with complete dislocation of talar body. In fractures of the talar body in which there is complete dislocation of the body from both the subtalar and ankle mortise (Type ID) (see Fig. 24-63), Watson-Jones[146] recommended closed reduction. The calcaneus is distracted from the tibia by traction on the calcaneus with the foot in equinus. The displaced fragment is then replaced by pressure of the fingers on the fragment. Watson-Jones suggested a metal pin be inserted into the talar fragment and used to manipulate it into position, while Kleiger[64] believes that using such a pin is not indicated, as it might further damage the articular cartilage.

Giannestras and Sammarco[46] recommend open reduction of these fractures after one attempt at closed reduction. Garcia and Parkes[41] prefer a medial incision with an accompanying transverse osteotomy of the medial malleolus as it provides excellent exposure of the talus and facilitates internal fixation. Additionally, this approach does not violate the deltoid ligament with its accompanying vascular supply to the talar body.[41] Once the fracture is reduced, two Kirschner wires are driven from the talar neck into the body and the medial malleolus is reattached with a screw.[43,46] Following open reduction, a cast extending from the toes to the mid-thigh with the knee in 25° of flexion and the foot in 25° of equinus is applied. The Kirschner wires are removed at 4 weeks. Weight bearing is not permitted until there is radiographic evidence of fracture union, usually in 12 to 16 weeks.

Dunn et al.[40] and Kleiger[64] suggest a lateral approach to avoid further damage to the medial artery to the talar body and to avoid the traumatized skin medially that overlies the displaced fragment.[40,64] A Kirschner wire in the calcaneus during the open reduction to supply the distraction needed for the reduction is helpful.[64] Once the reduction is obtained, Kleiger recommends the use of screw fixation from the outer surface of the distal portion of the neck into the body of the talus., while Dunn et al.[40] use Kirschner wire fixation. Kleiger[64] suggests subtalar arthrodesis in these cases in addition to open reduction to eliminate later disability and to supply an additional source of circulation to the talus, which he feels most likely will undergo aseptic necrosis. However, subtalar arthrodesis to improve circulation has not been found successful by other authors.[16]

Group II fractures: type II (horizontal fractures) (Fig. 24-64). Little has been written regarding treatment of the horizontal shear fracture (type II).[11,31] According to Bonnin,[11] these fractures can be best reduced by lateral pressure combined with skeletal traction. Immobilization in a short leg cast is used until union is present. He reports that aseptic necrosis is more likely to occur in these fractures than in fractures of the talar neck.

Group V: comminuted fractures of body of talus

Nondisplaced fractures. Pennal[106] recommends immobilization in a short leg cast for 4 to 6 weeks for nondisplaced comminuted fractures. Boyd and Knight[13] also recommend cast immobilization for comminuted fractures of the body of the talus without displacement. They caution, however, that even without displacement, later subtalar or ankle arthritis may necessitate arthrodesis.

Displaced fractures. Because of the mechanism of injury, most comminuted talar body fractures are severely displaced and rarely result in a functional ankle.[46,106] Treatment recommendations in this group depend on the degree of comminution and displacement. Boyd and Knight[13] emphasize that it is impractical to attempt open reduction in the severely comminuted fracture, and suggest talectomy as the only logical treatment. However, they emphasize that a talectomy alone usually results in poor function because of pain on weight bearing, instability, and lack of endurance, and for this reason, they prefer a tibiocalcaneal fusion after talectomy. Dunn et al.[40] also recommend primary tibiocalcaneal fusion rather than

talectomy because of the poor results following simple talectomy noted by other authors.[18,80,84,106,126]

Pennal[106] also prefers tibiocalcaneal fusion, but waits until the third or fourth week after injury in the grossly comminuted and displaced fracture.[106] Giannestras and Sammarco[46] treat such patients initially with splint immobilization and elevation in bed. Once the acute reaction to injury has subsided and the soft tissues are able to safely tolerate an operative procedure, they recommend pantalar arthrodesis, if the comminution is not too severe. Alternatively, they recommend tibiocalcaneal fusion in 5° of plantar flexion for those patients in whom the fracture is extremely comminuted.

Blair,[8] Dennis and Tullos,[34] and Lionberger et al.[76] recommend the Blair fusion for patients with a comminuted fracture of the body of the talus. Because the head and neck of the talus, which contain the anterior and middle facets of the subtalar joint, are usually not involved in these fractures, Blair recommends leaving the head and neck of the talus in situ. A sliding bone graft is taken from the anterior aspect of the tibia into the neck of the talus to effect a tibiotalar fusion. The principal advantages of this procedure are that the foot has a more normal appearance and some motion remains in the talonavicular, calcaneocuboid, and anterior talocalcaneal joints. The patient therefore is not left with a completely rigid foot and a short limb as in a tibiocalcaneal fusion.[8,34] Further discussion of the technique of the Blair fusion is in the section on Talar Neck Fractures.

Results. The only chance for good long-term results following these fractures hinges on early anatomic reduction and stable internal fixation.[138] Sneppen et al.[138] concluded that results in talar body fractures are directly related to the severity of the initial injury. They emphasize that if, at the time of initial injury, there was subluxation and articular damage to the subtalar and talotibial joints, a grave long-term prognosis is likely. Kleiger[64] emphasizes that good results following talar body fractures decrease as one progresses from a nondisplaced fracture to a fracture with complete talar body dislocation.

The most important complications following fractures of the talar body are aseptic necrosis, nonunion, malunion, stiffness, and osteoarthritis involving the ankle and/or subtalar joint.

ASEPTIC NECROSIS. The incidence of aseptic necrosis following coronal fracture of the talar body has been reported to be higher than that following talar neck fractures.[138] This might be explained by the fact that the fracture line occurs more posteriorly and may exit medially through the insertion of the deltoid ligament into the talus, thereby disrupting a source of blood supply to the body of the talus, which may remain intact in most talar neck fractures.[87,96,127] Also, the more posteriorly in the body the fracture occurs, the greater the chance for disruption of intraosseous vascular anastomoses.[32]

The incidence of aseptic necrosis in the individual groups of coronal shearing fractures (i.e., nondisplaced [IA and IB], the displaced with subtalar dislocation [IC], and the displaced with a completely dislocated talar body [ID]) has not been documented in the literature. Mindel et al.[86] report that 25% of patients with nondisplaced shearing type fractures developed aseptic necrosis.[86] They also report that aspectic necrosis developed in 50% of patients with fractures of the talar body with dislocation. They did not, however, distinguish between dislocation of the subtalar joint and complete dislocation of the talar body. Sneppen et al.[138] report that aseptic necrosis occurred in 5 of 13 displaced shearing fractures.

Garcia and Parkes,[43] quoting Hawkins, report an incidence of aseptic necrosis of 40% to 50% in patients with talar body fractures in which there is an associated subtalar dislocation. If the talar body fragment was completely dislocated, the necrosis incidence rose to 90%. It must be remembered, however, that Hawkins' work is based on fractures of the neck of the talus, which are more distal than those discussed here.

Finally, Bonnin[12] reports that, particularly in horizontal shearing fractures of the body, the incidence of aseptic necrosis is much higher than in talar neck fractures.

The incidence of aseptic necrosis following crush-type fractures is not well documented, partly because so many of these fractures are treated primarily by excision. However, Sneppen et al. (1977) report that 3 of 4 of their patients with comminuted fracture developed aseptic necrosis.

It is important to remember that, even with aseptic necrosis, up to 50% of patients may have little disability.[40,43] The principles of diagnosis, treatment, and prognosis of aseptic necrosis of the talus are more thoroughly discussed in the section on Talar Neck Fractures.

DELAYED NONUNION. Mindel et al.[86] report that all of the fractures of the body of the talus healed in an average of 3.4 months. However, union time was delayed in fractures with complete displacement and those which developed aseptic necrosis. Garcia and Parkes[43] also note a delay in union in displaced fractures, occurring in an average of 5 months, compared to 8 to 10 weeks when the talar body is not displaced.[43]

MALUNION AND OSTEOARTHRITIS. In a retrospective analysis, Sneppen et al.[138] reported that one third of displaced talar body fractures were inadequately reduced. This suggests the need to more critically analyze postreduction radiographs. Indeed, Kleiger[64] stresses the importance of evaluating the reduction on a *true lateral* radiograph to determine whether or not the superior articular surface of the talus is satisfactorily aligned. If it is not, a malunion will result in limited dorsiflexion of the ankle. The malunion also results in a step off on the trochlear articular surface, which can lead to arthritic changes in the ankle. Additionally, any residual displacement at this fracture site suggests residual subtabular subluxation and hence long-term disability (see Fig. 24-46, A).

Boyd and Knight[13] caution that traumatic arthritis involving the subtalar joint may develop even following acceptable reduction and union. They compare this to the subtalar arthritis seen following a well-reduced os calcis fracture in which minor disturbances remain at the articular surface in spite of a good reduction. They emphasize that these minor disturbances in the subtalar joint may not be seen radiographically, but may produce significant discomfort in the subtalar area. Coltart[25] also mentions late subtalar osteoarthritis following nondisplaced fractures of the talar body.

Sneppen et al.[138] documented that fractures that united with displacement resulted in osteoarthritis of the talocrural and/or subtalar joints. Additionally, 75% of fractures that united *without* displacement resulted in osteoarthritic changes. The importance of the direct relationship between osteoarthritis, malunion, and subluxation documented by these authors must be emphasized.

Other complications that may occur following talar body fracture include persistent infection, skin loss, and scar sensitivity following open fractures. Detailed discussion of these complications are included in the section on Fractures of Talar Neck.

AUTHOR'S PREFERRED METHOD OF TREATMENT

For open fractures of the talar body, management of the open wound is performed as outlined under the section on Open Fractures of the Talus. The fractures are then managed individually as described here.

GROUP II: SHEAR FRACTURES. Shearing fractures of the talar body in the coronal or sagittal plane are evaluated radiographically to determine the degree of displacement at the ankle articular surface. I have found polytomography particularly useful in evaluating the degree of displacement at the articular surface (see Fig. 24-61, B). In fractures that are truly nondisplaced or in which displacement is only 1 to 2 mm, I immobilize the ankle in the neutral position and keep the patient non-weight bearing until fracture union is noted.

In fractures with minimal displacement at the ankle articular surface and *no* subtalar dislocation, (i.e., in the range of 2 to 3 mm) I prefer closed reduction by the technique described below. I consider percutaneous Kirschner wire fixation essential following reduction to maintain stability. Patients are then kept non-weight bearing in a short leg splint. If stable fixation is obtained by percutaneous fixation, the posterior splint is removed and early range of motion exercises instituted. After motion has been restored, a short leg non-weight-bearing cast is applied. Weight bearing is allowed only when union is present. The Kirschner wires are removed at 4 to 6 weeks.

Fractures of the body of the talus with more than 3 mm displacement but *without* associated subtalar dislocation are extremely rare, and displacement at the talar articular surface of this magnitude usually requires subluxation of the subtalar joint. These patients should be treated by closed reduction (see below) with critical evaluation of both the subtalar joint and the articular surface of the ankle joint in the postreduction radiographs. Percutaneous Kirschner wire fixation or compression screw fixation of these fractures is performed. If good stability is obtained with either type of fixation, early inversion and eversion exercises are encouraged with the extremity in a posterior splint, which is removed for these exercises. Once motion has been restored, immobilization in a short leg non-weight-bearing cast at 90° is used until union occurs.

Shearing fractures of the body of the talus *with* associated subtalar dislocation are reduced by closed reduction. General or spinal anesthesia is preferred. The knee is flexed 90° over the patient's bed. Longitudinal traction on the heel and forefoot, plantar flexion, and an anterior force applied to the heel will usually reduce the fracture. The reduction is monitored under image intensification. It is important that the postreduction films be evaluated for residual subtalar and ankle joint displacement. Anatomic reduction is essential. Once the reduction has been obtained, percutaneous Kirschner wire fixation or fixation using an A-O compression screw across the fracture site is used (Figs. 24-62 and 24-65). Postoperative management is the same as mentioned above.

Patients with talar body fracture and complete dislocation of the body are considered surgical emergencies. Because the talar body is displaced and may be rotated on its deltoid pedicle, I treat these injuries *immediately* in an effort to reduce the fracture before the vessels remaining in the deltoid ligament thrombose (see Fig. 24-48). I do not attempt a closed reduction in these patients, because this has been unsuccessful in my hands. In the operating room, after the limb has been prepped and draped, a sterile Steinmann pin is placed through the calcaneus to be used for traction during the open reduction. I prefer a medial surgical approach, osteotomizing the medial malleolus to improve exposure. After malleolar osteotomy, the talus is manipulated back into position. Once an anatomic reduction has been obtained, the fracture is stabilized using A-O screws or Kirschner wires. The choice of internal fixation depends on the associated soft tissue injury. Crossed Kirschner wires are easier to insert and require less dissection; however, they do not provide the stability of an AO cancellous screw.

Following open reduction in these injuries, the limb is placed in a short leg non-weight-bearing cast. If the fracture is stable, the cast is bivalved and the patient is allowed to remove it and institute early range of motion of the ankle, subtalar, and midtarsal joints. Weight bearing is not allowed until there is radiographic evidence of fracture union. Once fracture union is obtained, weight bearing is begun.

After fractures of the talar body, patients undergo serial radiographs to detect aseptic necrosis as soon as possible. The diagnosis and treatment of aseptic necrosis after fracture of the talus is discussed completely in the section on Talar Neck Fractures.

GROUP V: COMMINUTED FRACTURES. For comminuted fractures of the body of the talus in which displacement is minimal, I prefer closed treatment. A short leg non-weight-bearing cast is used until there is evidence of fracture healing. If the fracture fragments are stable, however, early range of motion is instituted using a removable posterior splint. These patients are kept non-weight bearing until there is evidence of fracture healing.

In severely comminuted and displaced fractures of the body of the talus, I prefer the Blair fusion to a tibiocalcaneal arthrodesis. In my opinion, there is no place for a talectomy as a definitive form of treatment in these injuries. If the injury is open and severely contaminated or if the overlying skin is compromised, a talectomy is performed as an *initial* procedure. When the soft tissue has healed, a Blair fusion is performed using the technique described in the section on Fractures of Neck of Talus.

Group III: fractures of posterior process of talus

Fractures of lateral tubercle of posterior process. Cloquet in 1844 was the first to describe a fracture of the lateral tubercle of the posterior process.[22] Shepard in 1882 described an additional three cases in the English literature, and the fracture has subsequently come to be known as "Shepard's fracture."[130] Although Giannestras and Sammarco[46] report that this fracture is uncommon, Sneppen et al.[138] found fractures of the *posterior* tubercle to represent 20% of all fractures of the talar body.

Anatomy. The posterior process of the talus is com-

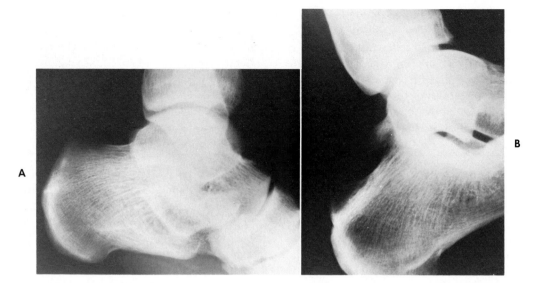

Fig. 24-66. Size of the posterolateral tubercle varies from being nearly absent (**A**), to large prominent process (**B**).

posed of the posterolateral and posteromedial tubercles, which are separated by the sulcus for the flexor hallucis longus tendon[124] (Fig. 24-43, *E*). The posterolateral tubercle is larger and more prominent than the posteromedial tubercle. The size of the posterolateral tubercle varies from a barely perceptible structure to a well-developed tubercle projecting posterolaterally from the talus[124] (Fig. 24-66).

The superior surface of the posterolateral tubercle is nonarticular and provides insertion for the posterior talofibular ligament and the talar component of the fibuloastragulocalcaneal ligament.[124] The inferior surface is in continuity with the posterior calcaneal articular surface of the talus.

Os trigonum. An accessory bone, the os trigonum, can be found in association with the posterolateral tubercle. Howse[56] stresses that the os trigonum varies in size, and one that appears to be small radiographically may in fact be much larger because of the cartilage around the bony nucleus (Fig. 24-67).

Rosenmuller in 1804 was the first to describe the os trigonum.[123] According to Sarrafian,[124] the incidence varies from 2.7% to 7.7% of specimens. The os trigonum can be present unilaterally or bilaterally and can be fused to the talus or calcaneus.[60] Geist[45] found 7 cases of unilateral os trigonum separated from the talus, with 3 of the 7 having a large posterior process of the talus in the *opposite* foot. He also noted 12 cases of large posterior processes, of which 4 were bilateral. Burman and Lapidus[14] report that an os trigonum, either fused or separated, occurs in 50% of all feet. They found the os trigonum to be unilateral in 10% of cases.

Less than 1% had a free os trigonum on one side and a fused os trigonum on the other, while 17% of patients had bilaterally fused os trigonum (i.e., the trigonal process). According to Sarrafian,[124] 10.9% of tali present a separated ossicle in the region of the os trigonum.

This ossicle has three surfaces: anterior, inferior, and posterior. The anterior surface connects with the posterolateral tubercle by fibrous, fibrocartilaginous, or cartilaginous tissue (Fig. 24-68). The inferior surface of the os trigonum articulates with the os calcis.[124] The posterior surface is nonarticular and serves as the point of attachment for structures that insert on the posterior tubercle.

The relationship of the os trigonum to the posterior tubercle varies from complete separation to complete fusion. The separation can include a notch in the margin of the posterior lateral tubercle, a groove on the articular surface, or a complete separation. A fused os trigonum is called the trigonal process and appears as a very large posterolateral tubercle[124] (Fig. 9-21, p. 220, and Fig. 24-66, *B*).

The os trigonum has created a problem in differential diagnosis since its original description.[130] Indeed, Shepard[130] reported a talus fracture in which he described a fragment located posterior to the talus, lateral to the groove for the flexor hallucis longus. He believed that this fragment of bone was torn off by the posterior fasciculus of the talofibular ligament. He did not believe that this could represent an ununited apophysis, as he believed there was only one ossific center for the talus. However, he was unable to reproduce this fracture in cadaver specimens. Turner,[144] in the same year,

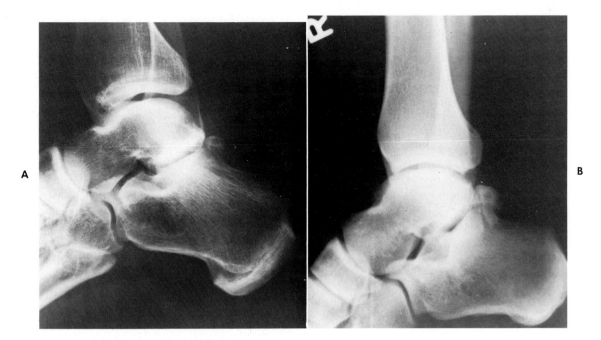

Fig. 24-67. Os trigonum varies greatly in size from a small oval structure with smooth surfaces (**A**) to a large structure involving more of subtalar joint (**B**).

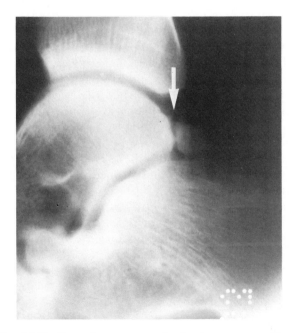

Fig. 24-68. Lateral tomogram clearly demonstrates fibrous connection (arrow) between posterolateral tubercle and os trigonum. Note sclerotic margin of adjacent os trigonum and posterolateral tubercle of talus. Width of fibrous connection does not suggest disruption.

presented the theory that the os trigonum was a secondary center of development and cited other references which agreed with his theory. Kohler and Zimmer,[68] noting the confusion among clinicians as to whether the free ossicle represents a fracture of a fused os trigonum or developmental failure of fusion of a secondary ossification center in the talus, report that the os trigonum is actually embraced on both sides by the posterior process of the talus. They believe that the posterior process is actually made up of the lateral tubercle *and* the os trigonum, both of which may unite to form the trigonal process.

McDougall[79] in an excellent anatomic study of the talus, reports that the lateral tubercle is usually the larger and is commonly referred to as the posterior process, although not infrequently the medial tubercle may be as large. He stresses that the tubercles vary considerably in size from small processes, hardly discernible on a lateral radiograph, to a prominent posterior projection. He found that in early childhood the posterior border of the talus is rounded without the projection seen in the adult talus. Secondary centers of ossification for the medial and lateral tubercles appear at the posterior margin of the talus between the ages of 8 and 11 years. These quickly unite with the main bone, usually within 1 year of their appearance. McDougall[79] notes that the lateral secondary center of ossification may be prevented from uniting with the main body of the talus and thereby produce an os trigonum, but that this occurs infrequently. Instead, he notes an *increased* incidence of the so-called os trigonum associated with age. He believes the os trigonum is secondary to repeated trauma, which results in fracture of the fused os trigonum or posterior process from the talus. Indeed, Paulos et al.[105] suggest that athletic patients have an increased incidence of posterior process fracture, with a number of these progressing to asymptomatic nonunion, which suggests an os trigonum.

Shelton and Pedowitz[129] attempt to distinguish a fracture of the posterior tubercle from the os trigonum. They too believe the os trigonum arises from failure of fusion of a secondary center of ossification on the posterior aspect of the talus with the body of the talus. They believe that the os trigonum does not involve the subtalar or ankle joint and that its separation rarely caused symptoms. However, Sarrafian[124] points out that the inferior aspect of the os trigonum contains an articular surface for the posterior talocalcaneal joint.

Therefore in the adult the os trigonum may represent either a failure of fusion of the secondary center of ossification or a fracture of the lateral tubercle of the posterior process, which develops a non-union.[79,96,105] To add to the confusion, a true os trigonum may become symptomatic because of disruption of its fibrous or fibrocartilaginous attachment to the posterior process of the talus.[59] Indeed, Moeller[88] has documented pain in the area of an established os trigonum secondary to increased activity.

The medial tubercle of the posterior process is also variable in size.[79] It provides attachment to the deep and superficial layers of the talotibial component of the deltoid ligament and forms a medial wall of the tunnel for the flexor hallucis longus.[19] According to Sarrafian,[124] this tubercle may rarely be very large and extend down over the os calcis, contributing to a talocalcaneal coalition.

Mechanism of injury. Two mechanisms of injury to the lateral tubercle of the posterior process of the talus have been presented in the literature. First, forced plantar flexion of the foot causes direct impingement of the posterior tibial plafond on the posterolateral process. This forced plantar flexion may result in a fracture of the posterolateral process, separation through the fibrous attachment of an os trigonum, or, if the os trigonum is attached to the talus by bone, a fracture of the resulting trigonal process.[51,59,64]

The second theory is that excessive dorsiflexion of the ankle, resulting in increased tension in the posterior talofibular ligament, may avulse the lateral tubercle of the posterior facet.[82] The occurrence of this fracture in the athlete who suffers a twisting injury of the ankle helps to support this mechanism.[82,105]

Clinical diagnosis. A careful history and physical examination are important to distinguish fracture of a lateral process or fused os trigonum, a disruption of the fibrous attachment of an os trigonum to the body of the talus, and an asymptomatic os trigonum. Only if the physical examination correlates with the radiographic findings is damage or injury to the lateral tubercle or os trigonum confirmed.

The patient usually gives a history of sudden uncontrolled injury to the foot, such as catching the heel on a step when going downstairs.[79] McDougall[79] notes that forced equinus from kicking a football may be responsible for the injury. Moeller[88] emphasizes that a history of repetitive microtrauma secondary to a rapid increase in weight or activity or change to a more strenuous routine may be present in the patient with a painful os trigonum. This microtrauma can lead to disruption of the fibrous attachment of the os trigonum to the body of the talus.

The patients usually complain of pain with mild swelling in the posterior aspect of the ankle.[27] The pain may be accentuated by running, jumping, or descending stairs, and symptoms of giving way may be present.[105] Schrock[126] emphasizes that pain aggravated by walking downhill or squatting on a plantar-flexed foot is suggestive of a posterior process fracture.

The clinical picture may be as helpful as the serrated edge of a fragment noted radiographically in diagnosing a fracture of the os trigonum or posterior process.[58] Clinically, tenderness is present anterior to the Achilles tendon and posterior to the talus.[59] A circumscribed area of ecchymosis just anterior to the Achilles tendon may be noted 24 to 48 hours following an acute injury.[82] Crepitation may be heard or felt with plantar flexion of the foot.[58] Pain is increased when plantar flexion stress is applied to the foot.[105] Pain can also be accentuated by resisted plantar flexion or dorsiflexion of the great toe; this is caused by the presence of the flexor hallucis longus tendon in the groove between the fractured lateral tubercle and the medial tubercle of the posterior process.[27,59,105,126]

Associated ligamentous instability is usually not clinically detectable.[105] Hamilton injects 1 ml of lidocaine into the affected area, which produces temporary relief of symptoms, in an effort to confirm the diagnosis. This is particularly useful in the patient with the clinical findings of a posterior process fracture and a radiograph suggesting an os trigonum.

Radiographic examination. A lateral radiographic view of the ankle best demonstrates the lateral tubercle of the posterior process of the talus and the os trigonum. It is well-known that the os trigonum, following a plantar flexion injury, can become symptomatic

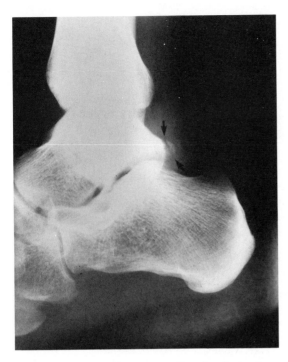

Fig. 24-69. Fracture of posterior tubercle of talus (arrow).

because of disruption of its fibrous attachment to the main body of the talus.[96] Although many authors have emphasized the importance of differentiating the os trigonum (which can be a normal variant noted radiographically) from a fracture of the posterior process, this radiographic differentiation may not be so important if the patient has a history of injury and the clinical findings suggestive of injury to the posterior process. Indeed, Jensenius[59] stresses that differentiating between an os trigonum and a fracture in the symptomatic patient is of minor *practical* importance, as the indications for excision in both instances are similar.

However, if roentgenographic differentiation is important because of a *lack* of clinical correlation, Kohler[67] describes the os trigonum as a round, oval, and three-cornered bone located behind the talus (see Fig. 24-67, A). On the other hand, in acute fracture of the posterior process of the talus the fracture surfaces should be rough and irregular (Fig. 24-69). Because the os trigonum is reported to be unilateral in over two thirds of cases,[45,79] comparison radiographs may not be of value.

Paulos et al.[105] suggest the use of a special 30° subtalar oblique view to help distinguish between an acute fracture and an os trigonum. They find that a posterior process fracture is generally larger and extends further into the body of the talus. In the acute fracture they

report that the fracture line is very different from the smooth, rounded, well-corticated os trigonum (see Fig. 24-67, A).

I have found lateral polytomes useful to delineate the connection between the posterior lateral process of the talus and the os trigonum (see Fig. 24-68). However, they rarely confirm disruption of the fibrous attachment of the os trigonum to the posterolateral process of the talus. Paulos et al.[105] were the first to show that the definitive distinction between a normal os trigonum, a traumatic separation of a normal os trigonum through its fibrous attachment to the talus, and a fractured posterior process of the talus can be made with a technetium bone scan. A positive technetium bone scan was present in all patients with a fracture of the posterior process and in those with disruption of the fibrous attachment of the os trigonum to the talus. However, it was negative in patients with a normal, asymptomatic os trigonum (Fig. 24-70). This can be quite helpful in determining if the os trigonum is responsible for a patient's posterior ankle pain.

Treatment. The recommended treatment of acute fracture of the posterior process of the talus is conservative.[27] Giannestras and Sammarco[46] suggest immobilization in a short leg walking cast with the foot in 15° of equinus for 4 to 6 weeks. Because the fracture involves the weight-bearing surface, Sneppen et al.[138] do not permit weight bearing until the fracture has healed. Even if a nonunion results, the fragment should not be removed unless the patient complains of persistent pain in the region of the fragment.[46] Paulos et al.[105] recommend casting for 6 weeks following an acute injury. For a chronic injury, they also suggest conservative treatment in a short leg cast initially. However, if symptoms persist for longer than 4 to 6 months after the initiation of conservative treatment in either acute or chronic injuries, they recommend surgical removal of the fragment.

Shelton and Pedowitz[129] suggest that anatomic reduction and rigid internal fixation by open methods followed by early range of motion would be the *ideal* treatment for a *large* fracture of the posterior process of the talus that involves a significant portion of the articular surface of the posterior facet of the subtalar joint. They concede, however, that this technique has not been reported and would be technically difficult. They therefore recommend plaster immobilization and non-weight bearing for 6 to 8 weeks until union occurs.

If symptoms of pain and decreased ankle motion persist following conservative treatment, Ihle and Cochran[58] and Paulos et al.[105] recommend surgical excision of the fracture fragment. The preferred surgical approach to the posterior process varies. Howse[56] rec-

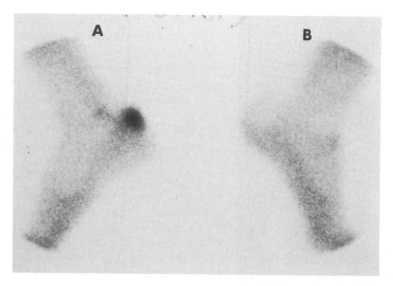

Fig. 24-70. Technitium bone scan of both feet of patient with bilateral os trigonum on radiograph. Bone scan is positive over area of right os trigonum (**A**), and negative over left (**B**). This confirms presence of disruption of fibrous attachment between talus and os trigonum in right foot. (From Paulos, L.E., Johnson, C.L., and Noyes, F.R.: Am. J. Sports Med. 11:439-443, 1983. © 1983, American Orthopaedic Society for Sports Medicine.)

ommends a medial rather than a lateral approach, because the lateral approach interferes with the peroneal tendons and may produce postoperative stiffness. However, posterolateral arthrotomy has been recommended by Ihle and Cochran,[58] McDougall,[79] and Weinstein and Bonfiglio.[147] Paulos et al.[105] state that either a posteromedial or posterolateral approach can be used for fragment excision. They stress that following surgical removal, the patient's ankle should be splinted only briefly and then a vigorous stretching and strengthening program instituted.

Results. Most authors report that conservative treatment produces relief of symptoms. However, should conservative treatment fail, they believe simple excision of the fragment will restore normal joint function.* Paulos et al.[105] report one third of their patients responded to conservative treatment and were only occasionally symptomatic. Two thirds of their patients failed initial conservative treatment consisting of 6 weeks of cast immobilization. These patients then underwent steroid injection into the os trigonum and 4 weeks of additional casting. This was successful in less than 10% of patients; the remainder required surgical removal of the posterior bony fragment. Surgical excision was effective in relieving these patients' symptoms.[145]

On the other hand, some authors report these frac-

tures may not produce the excellent results associated with other avulsion fractures. Sneppen and Buhl[137] found that of 11 patients with fractures of the posterior process, 8 developed talocrural or subtalar arthritis and that *all* 8 of these persisted with complaints of pain in the foot and prolonged disability. Jensenius[59] also reports persistent disability and discomfort in over one half of patients following this fracture.

AUTHOR'S PREFERRED METHOD OF TREATMENT

I routinely obtain anteroposterior, mortise, lateral, and 35° oblique radiographs in the patient complaining of pain in the posterolateral aspect of the ankle following injury. If the radiographs confirm a definite fracture of the lateral tubercle of the posterior process, the patient is treated in a short leg non-weight-bearing cast for 4 weeks. The toes are left free in this cast, and early range of motion to the metatarsophalangeal joints of the great toe is initiated to prevent trapping of the flexor hallucis longus tendon in the groove of the posterior process. After 4 weeks, a short leg walking cast is worn for an additional 2 weeks. At this point, immobilization is discontinued. If radiographic nonunion results, no further treatment is recommended unless the patient is symptomatic. If symptoms persist, another 4 to 6 weeks of immobilization is recommended. If symptoms persist for 6 to 8 months in patients with a nonunion, excision of the fragment is recommended. If the posterior pro-

---

*References 46, 58, 70, 79, 82, and 105.

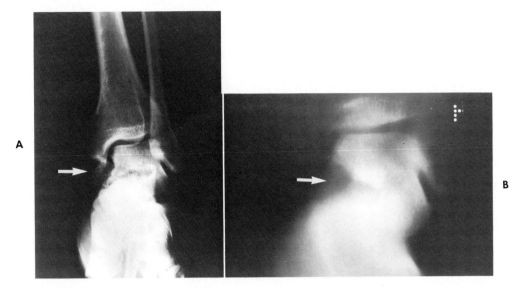

Fig. 24-71. A, Fracture of medial tubercle of posterior process. Large medial tubercle fragment is located beneath medial malleolus. **B,** Anteroposterior tomogram demonstrates fracture communicates with posterior subtalar facet.

cess fracture is very large and occupies a *substantial* portion of the posterior calcaneal facet of the talus, consideration can be given to open reduction and stable internal fixation. However, I have not seen this type of fracture in my practice.

In patients who have a history and clinical examination suggestive of injury to the posterior process and who have radiographic evidence suggesting an os trigonum or nonunion of a posterior process fracture, I obtain a technetium bone scan to determine if the nonunion or os trigonum is "hot," indicating a recent injury. These patients are treated exactly as outlined for acute fractures, with fragment excision being recommended only if conservative treatment fails.

In patients in whom conservative therapy fails and in whom significant pain on the posterolateral aspect of the ankle persists, consideration is given to surgical excision of the free fragment. Before surgical excision, the area is injected with lidocaine under radiographic control to confirm that the fragment is the actual cause of the persistent posterolateral pain. In these patients, a positive technetium bone scan is considered as contributory evidence the fragment is responsible for the pain.

I prefer the posterolateral approach for fragment excision, being careful to avoid the sural nerve. The fragment is excised and the foot immobilized in a short leg cast *only* for soft tissue healing, usually 7 to 10 days. Immediately postoperatively, flexor hallucis longus function and range of motion of the metatarsophalangeal joints of all toes is instituted. After initial immobilization for 7 to 10 days, stretching and range of motion

exercises are encouraged and weight bearing is allowed.

Fracture of medial tubercle of posterior process. Fracture of the medial tubercle of the posterior process of the talus is much more uncommon than fracture of the lateral tubercle of the posterior process. Cedell[19] in 1974 reported four cases of fracture of the medial tubercle, which he believed were secondary to avulsion of the bone fragment by the posterior talotibial ligament when the ankle is dorsiflexed and pronated.

Clinically, there is obvious swelling behind the medial malleolus with loss of the normal contour of the posteromedial ankle. Radiographic examination demonstrates a fragment of varying size situated medial and dorsal to the talus (Fig. 24-71). All patients in Cedell's this series were treated by immobilization and a soft bandage.[19] Although the injuries seemed to heal, medial pain and swelling recurred when the patients resumed sporting activities. As a result of this, 3 of the 4 patients subsequently underwent excision of the fragment with restoration of normal function.[19]

AUTHOR'S PREFERRED METHOD OF TREATMENT

Posteromedial pain in the ankle following a pronation injury to the foot should suggest avulsion of the medial tubercle of the posterior process. In these patients, careful radiographic evaluation, including polytomography (Fig. 24-71, *B*), may be necessary to document the fracture. If the fracture fragment is small and does not interfere with ankle or subtalar motion, I prefer immobi-

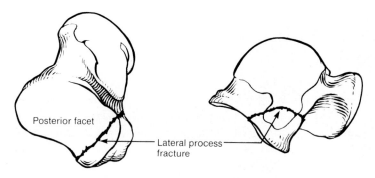

Fig. 24-72. Fracture of lateral process of talus involves talofibular component of ankle joint and also posterior facet of talocalcaneal joint.

Fig. 24-73. Lateral process serves as point of attachment for anterior talofibular, cervical, bifurcate, and talocalcaneal ligaments.

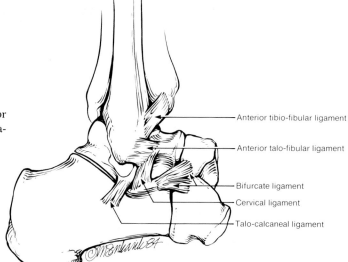

lization in a short leg non-weight-bearing cast for 4 to 6 weeks. If pain and swelling persist for 4 to 6 months following this conservative treatment, I recommend surgical excision through a posteromedial arthrotomy.

If the fragment is larger or it interferes with ankle or subtalar motion, consideration is given to open reduction and internal fixation or excision. Management after excision through a posteromedial arthrotomy is as outlined previously for lateral tubercle excision.

Group IV: fractures of lateral process of talus

Fractures of the lateral process of the talus, first described in detail by Dimon[38] in 1961, account for 24% of fractures of the body of the talus.[129] Indeed, Hawkins[52] regards this as the second most common fracture of the body of the talus. Mukherjee et al.[93] found 13 cases of fracture of the lateral process of the talus in 1,500 cases of fractures and sprains about the ankle. Several small series have been reported in the

literature, with most authors stressing that this fracture occurs more commonly than is suspected and is often overlooked.*

This fracture has been variously termed *fracture of the lateral process,*[6,21,42,52,113] *fracture of the posterior facet of the talus,*[38] and *fracture of the lateral tubercle.*[129] The diagnosis of this fracture is frequently overlooked,[21,52] and substantial disability can result.[129]

Anatomy. The lateral process of the talus is a wedge-shaped prominence that is the most lateral aspect of body of the talus and extends from the lower margin of the talar articular surface for the fibula to the posteroinferior surface of the talus[93] (Fig. 24-72). A fracture of the lateral process of the talus therefore involves both the talofibular articulation of the ankle joint and the posterior talocalcaneal articulation of the subtalar joint.[21,38,52] The degree of involvement of the talofibu-

---

*References 6, 21, 38, 42, 52, 65, 93, 106, 114, 129, and 138.

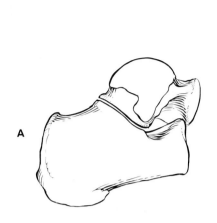
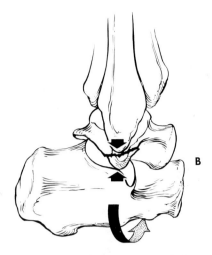

Fig. 24-74. A, Normal talocalcaneal articulation. **B,** When heel of foot is inverted, lateral shift of talar head results in upward shift of lateral process of talus on calcaneus. This produces an incongruity in posterior talocalcaneal joint. Dorsiflexion of foot then concentrates force on lateral process of talus and results in its fracture.

lar and posterior talocalcaneal joints is dependent on fracture size. Shelton and Pedowitz[129] point out that the presence of heavy cancellous trabecular bone and its horizontal orientation within the lateral process emphasize its importance in weight bearing.[129]

Additionally, the lateral process serves as a point of attachment for the lateral talocalcaneal, cervical, bifurcate, and anterior talofibular ligaments (Fig. 24-73). The lateral process of the talus is therefore an important structure that provides stability to the ankle mortise and also participates with the weight-bearing role of the distal fibula.[129]

Mechanism of injury. Several mechanisms have been postulated for this injury.[21,38]

1. The lateral process can be sheared off the posterior facet of the talus by the lateral malleolus as the foot is forced into eversion.[38] Dimon states that, because he has not seen evidence of a deltoid ligament sprain or fracture of the medial malleolus associated with this injury, this mechanism is unlikely.[38]

2. The lateral process fragment could be avulsed by the anterior talofibular or talocalcaneal ligaments[21,38] (Fig. 24-73). However, Dimon again postulates that because inversion injuries of the ankle are so common, lateral process fracture should be seen more frequently if this mechanism were a frequent cause of the injury.[38] Also, Hawkins[40] believes that since he has not noted this fracture in association with subtalar dislocations, which usually rupture the strong talocalcaneal ligament, this mechanism is unlikely.

3. Cimmino[21] reports that a direct blow can produce this fracture.

4. Most authors agree that fractures of the lateral process are the result of acute dorsiflexion and inversion of the foot.[19,42,52,93,109] Huson[57] noted that the articular surfaces of the posterior talocalcaneal joints are congruous in the standing position. However, when the heel is inverted, a lateral shift of the head of the talus results in an upward shift of the lateral process of the talus on the posterior articular surface of the calcaneus.[93] This results in the posterior talocalcaneal joint being incongruous. If the foot is then acutely dorsiflexed, force is concentrated on the lateral process of the talus (Fig. 24-74). Compression of the lateral process of the foot in inversion and dorsiflexion therefore results in the fracture.[42,93]

Mukherjee et al.[93] report that in all of their patients the injury resulted from inversion and dorsiflexion of the ankle. According to Shelton and Pedowitz,[129] the mechanism of inversion and dorsiflexion of the foot is supported by the association of this fracture with (1) anterior subtalar dislocations, (2) fractures of the talar neck, (3) adduction-type fractures of the medial malleolus, and (4) complete rupture of the lateral collateral ligament and avulsion fractures of the fibula.

Clinical diagnosis. Because the mechanism of injury and the clinical findings following lateral process fracture are identical to those of an inversion sprain of the ankle, careful evaluation of patients whose history suggests an ankle sprain is indicated if the diagnosis is to be made. Indeed, in every patient diagnosed as having an ankle sprain who is resistant to the usual conservative treatment, the radiographs must be reviewed and

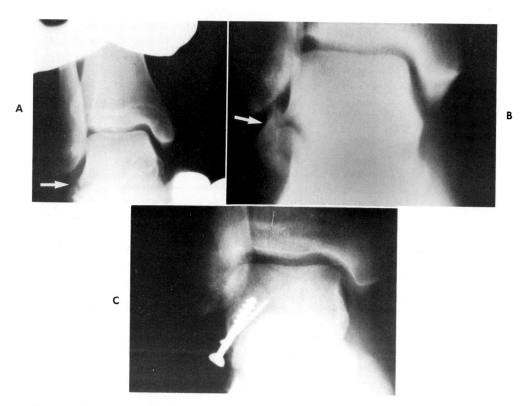

Fig. 24-75. **A,** Anteroposterior view of ankle with leg internally rotated 20° suggests large fracture of lateral process (see arrow). **B,** Polytome more clearly denotes fragment size and displacement. **C,** Open reduction and stable internal fixation of talar process fracture.

even repeated with fracture of the lateral talar process in mind.[38]

These patients are usually young males who have fallen from a height, been involved in a motor vehicle accident, or stepped in a hole.[52] The physical findings are indistinguishable from those which occur with a sprain of the anterior talofibular ligament.[38] Immediate disability with swelling and tenderness over the anterolateral aspect of the foot just anterior to the lateral malleolus is noted.[21,38,52,54] Ecchymosis in the same location may occur within 24 hours.[21] Although specific clinical signs may be masked by the associated soft tissue injury, acute local tenderness over the lateral process of the talus, located just below the tip of the lateral malleolus, is diagnostic.[93] Pain occurs with ankle dorsiflexion and plantar flexion and inversion or eversion of the subtalar joint.[21,52] Crepitus is usually not present.[52]

Radiographic examination. Generally, fractures of the lateral process of the talus can be easily demonstrated on the standard ankle series, which includes an anteroposterior, a lateral, and a mortise view.[21,93] The key to radiographic diagnosis is awareness of the injury rather than a specific radiographic view.[93]

Hawkins[52] emphasized the need for both anteropos-terior and lateral radiographs to make the diagnosis. He pointed out that in some situations the fracture may only be demonstrable on the lateral radiograph. Mukherjee et al.[93] recommend the use of an anteroposterior view taken with the ankle in neutral and the leg rotated inward 20° to demonstrate a fracture of the lateral process of the talus. This view, a variation of the mortise view, best demonstrates this fracture because the process lies almost in the frontal plane in this projection[93] (Fig. 24-75, *A*). Dimon[38] recommended routine radiographs of the ankle, but noted that, in cases of doubt, oblique radiographs consisting of an anteroposterior view with the foot in 45° of internal rotation and 30° of equinus are helpful.[38] I too have found this view useful in cases in which the fracture is not clearly visualized.

Cimmino[21] noted that the downward-directed apex of the lateral process of the talus and the upward-directed apex of sustentaculum tali are superimposed on a lateral radiograph of the ankle. He stresses that one must differentiate the two processes on the lateral view to make the diagnosis of lateral process fracture. He also emphasized that a posterior subtalar joint effusion noted on the lateral view suggests this injury.[21] He mentions

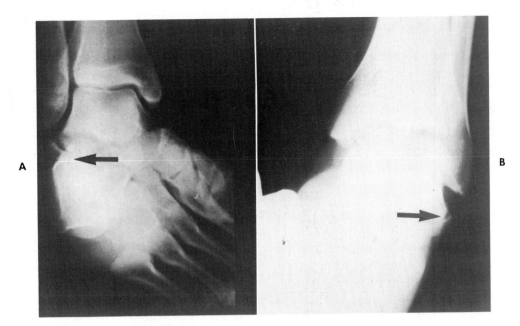

Fig. 24-76. Mortise views of the right (**A**) and left (**B**) ankles. Note radiolucency in both lateral processes, which suggests fracture. Right ankle was explored, because lesion was detected radiographically after acute inversion sprain. No defect was noted in lateral process, suggesting unfused accessory ossification center. Comparison views taken later demonstrated similar lesion in left ankle (**B**).

a congenital "ununited process" may occur and should not be mistaken for a fracture. Shelton and Pedowitz[129] also stress that normal accessory ossicles occur in the area of the lateral process and must be differentiated from fractures. I have noted an apparent accessory ossification center in one case, which caused confusion with a fracture. The presence of this lesion bilaterally helped to exclude an acute fracture (Fig. 24-76, *A* and *B*).

Evaluation of the size, amount of articular involvement, and degree of displacement of lateral process fractures can be greatly improved by the use of anteroposterior polytomograms of the talus (See Fig. 24-75, *B*). High-resolution CT scanning can also be helpful in determining fracture location, size, and displacement.[118]

Hawkins[52] reports three types of lateral process fracture: (1) type I, a simple fracture of the lateral process of the talus that extends from the talofibular articular surface to the posterior talocalcaneal articular surface of the subtalar joint; (2) type II, a comminuted fracture involving both the fibular and posterior talocalcaneal articular surface of the talus and the entire lateral process; and (3) type III, a chip fracture of the anterior and inferior portion of the posterior articular process of the talus. Type III fractures could be seen only on the lateral radiograph and are noted in the region of the sinus

tarsi. This type III fracture does not extend into the talofibular articulation.

Treatment. The size of the lateral process fracture and the degree of comminution and displacement are the critical factors in determining treatment.[54] Heckman et al.[54] and Cimino[21] report that acute nondisplaced fractures will heal with immobilization, but displaced fragments require open reduction and internal fixation or excision.

Hawkins[52] and Shelton and Pedowitz[129] recommend that closed reduction be attempted in all fractures of the lateral process of the talus. The lateral process is palpated and manipulated into an acceptable position with the foot in the neutral or everted position. Following reduction, a cast is applied from the toes to just below the knee with the foot in the neutral position. If the reduction is satisfactory, the cast is maintained for 4 weeks without weight bearing. An additional 2 weeks of cast immobilization with weight bearing is then recommended. Hawkins[52] and Shelton and Pedowitz[129] believe that this approach is also indicated for comminuted (type II) and chip (type III) fractures. Simple fractures (type I) that remain severely displaced, even after an attempted closed reduction, should be considered for open reduction and internal fixation using Kirschner wires or small compression screws.[21,52,129] Mukherjee et al.[93,114] believe a large single fragment should be reduced accurately by open reduction to restore the congruity of the subtalar joint, while small and comminuted fractures are best treated by removal.

In fractures detected late, Cimino[21] prefers a trial of immobilization, but stresses that eventually excision of the fragment will be necessary. McQueen emphasizes that simple plaster immobilization in fractures diagnosed late often produces a poor result.[114] Although Dimon[38] was unable to draw any definite conclusions regarding the best treatment, he did emphasize that, if the fracture is not recognized initially, prolonged disability will usually occur, and this disability is often *not* relieved by excision of the fragment. Mukherjee et al.[93] and Pringle and Mukherjee[114] also stressed the need for treatment soon after the injury to prevent long-term disability.

Sneppen et al.[138] stress that, whatever treatment modality is used, it is *essential* to aim at rapid normalization of function of the talocrural and subtalar joints. This can best be accomplished by a brief period of immobilization, which allows healing of the joint capsule and ligamentous structures. Thereafter active foot movement is instituted. Because these fractures invariably involve a weight-bearing joint, Sneppen et al. recommend that patients not be allowed to bear weight on the foot until there is solid union of the fracture.

Results. All series reported in the literature emphasize the importance of *early* diagnosis followed by reduction or excision to prevent long-term sequelae.[21,52,54,129,138] Pringle and Mukherjee[114] found that in their patients with poor results the injury had not been recognized for 6 to 9 months postoperatively. Hawkins[52] also found that all patients who required subtalar fusion following this injury had inadequate initial treatment. Additionally, Dimon[38] and Shelton and Pedowitz[129] stress that not only does delayed diagnosis produce disability, delayed excision of the fragment may not relieve the symptoms.

Sneppen et al.,[138] Mukherjee et al.,[93] and Pringle and Mukherjee[114] emphasize that even nondisplaced fractures of the lateral process can result in long-term disability caused by subtalar osteoarthrosis and moderate to severe discomfort on the lateral aspect of the ankle with weight bearing. Hawkins[52] reports that pain with walking or standing sufficient to warrant exploration was present in one half of his patients. He also stresses the frequency of symptomatic nonunions in the untreated patient, a finding also noted by Heckman et al.[54]

Overgrowth of bone in the region of the sinus tarsi that impinges on the calcaneus or the fibula has also been reported after this fracture.[52,54,129] Hawkins,[52] and Shelton and Pedowitz[129] conclude if there is evidence of nonunion, malunion, or overgrowth of the lateral process, excision of the fracture or subtalar fusion should be considered.

Author's preferred method of treatment. Because of the disability resulting from missed or delayed diagnosis, a high index or suspicion is *essential* in evaluating patients who present with a clinical history suggestive of lateral ankle sprain, as they may indeed have a lateral process fracture. I routinely use anteroposterior, lateral, and mortise radiographs to evaluate the lateral process. If these do not demonstrate a fracture but the clinical findings suggest one, 30° internal oblique films are taken. One must clearly see the lateral process in these patients before a fracture is excluded. If a fracture is noted on routine radiographs, polytomes or a CT scan may be necessary to determine fragment size, displacement, and comminution. I must again emphasize the importance of recognizing accessory ossicles in the region of the lateral process[55,128] (see Fig. 24-76) so they are not interpreted as fractures.

In fractures that are truly nondisplaced, I use a short leg non-weight-bearing cast for 4 weeks. This is followed by 2 weeks in a walking cast.

In my experience, displaced fractures cannot be reduced anatomically by closed means. Also, displaced fractures are associated with more severe damage to the subtalar joint. If closed reduction and prolonged casting are used in these patients, subtalar stiffness and pain often result. Therefore I choose either excision or open reduction and stable internal fixation so that early subtalar motion can be used. Open reduction and internal fixation is recommended if the fracture fragment is large enough to allow stable internal fixation (See Fig. 24-75, *C*). I have found a modified anterolateral ankle arthrotomy very acceptable. The incision begins just anterior to the fibula, 5 cm above the ankle, and progresses to the tip of the fibula, curving slightly posterior beneath the fibula. This gives excellent exposure to the lateral process. If comminution or fracture size prevent stable internal fixation, immediate excision is performed.

Following open reduction and stable internal fixation, a short leg cast is applied to allow the surgical wound to heal. Active range of motion of the metatarsophalangeal joints is encouraged in the cast to decrease swelling in the foot. The cast is removed at 2 to 3 weeks and replaced with a removable splint. Removal of the splint allows a physical therapy program that stresses subtalar and midtarsal motion. Weight bearing is allowed when there is radiographic evidence of union, usually at 6 weeks.

If the lateral process fragments are small and excision is necessary, the extremity is kept in a short leg cast for 3 weeks. Following this, active subtalar and midtarsal motion is encouraged, and progressive weight bearing is allowed within the limits of pain.

For patients who present late, i.e., 12 weeks or longer after injury, I have found that cast immobilization does not produce predictable results. Therefore in these patients I proceed directly to excision of the fragment, unless it is large and an anatomic reduction can be obtained. The likelihood of obtaining an anatomic reduction following any delay in treatment, however, is not good. The postoperative management following excision of these fractures in which the diagnosis is delayed is the same as that used for excision of an acute fracture.

REFERENCES

1. Alexander, A.H., and Lichtman, D.M.: Surgical treatment of transchondral talar-dome fractures (osteochondritis dissecans), J. Bone Joint Surg. **62A:**646-652, 1980.
2. Anderson, H.G.: The medical and surgical aspects of aviation, London, 1919, Hodder & Co.
3. Arcomano, J.P., Kamhi, E., Karas, S., and Moriarty, V.J.: Transchondral fracture and osteochondritis dissecans of talus, N.Y. State J. Med. **78:**2183-2189, 1978.
4. Berndt, A.L., and Harty, M.: Transchondral fractures (osteochondritis dissecans) of the talus, J. Bone Joint Surg. **41A:**988-1020, 1959.
5. Besson, J., and Wellinger, C.: L'osteochondrite dissequante de l'astragale a propos de 12 observations, Rev. Rhum., **34:**552-566, 1967.
6. Bigelow, D.R.: Fractures of the processus lateralis tali, J. Bone Joint Surg. **56B:**587, 1974.
7. Birt, D., and Townsend, R.: Major talar fractures, J. Bone Joint Surg. **58A:**733, 1976.
8. Blair, H.C.: Comminuted fractures and fracture dislocations of the body of the astragalus, Am. J. Surg. **59:**37-43, 1943.
9. Bobechko, W.P., and Harris, W.R.: The radiographic density of avascular bone, J. Bone Joint Surg. **42B:**626-632, 1960.
10. Bohler, L.: Treatment of fractures, ed. 5, New York, 1956, Grune & Stratton, Inc.
11. Bonnin, J.G.: Dislocations and fracture-dislocations of the talus. Br.J. Surg. **28:**88-100, 1940.
12. Bonnin, J.G.: Injuries to the ankle, Darien, Conn., 1970, Hafner Publishing Co., pp. 324-380.
13. Boyd, H.B., and Knight, R.A.: Fractures of the astragalus, South. Med. J. **35:**160-167, 1942.
14. Burman, M.S., and Lapidus, P.W.: The functional disturbances caused by the inconstant bones and sesamoids of the foot, Arch. Surg. **22:**936-975, 1931.
15. Cameron, B.M.: Osteochondritis dissecans of the ankle joint, J. Bone Joint Surg. **38A:**857-861, 1956.
16. Canale, S.T., and Belding, R.H.: Osteochondral lesions of the talus, J. Bone Joint Surg. **62A:**97-102, 1980.
17. Canale, S.T., and Kelly, F.B., Jr.: Fractures of the neck of the talus, J. Bone Joint Surg. **60A:**143-156, 1978.
18. Carmack, J.C., and Hallock, H.: Tibiotarsal arthrodesis after astragalectomy: a report of 8 cases, J. Bone Joint Surg. **29:**476-482, 1947.
19. Cadell, C.A.: Rupture of the posterior talotibial ligament with the avulsion of a bone fragment from the talus, Acta Orthop. Scand. **45:**454-461, 1974.
20. Chapman, M.W.: Fractures and fracture-dislocations of the ankle. In Mann, R.A., ed.: DuVries' surgery of the foot, ed. 4, St. Louis, 1978, The C.V. Mosby Co.
21. Cimmino, C.V.: Fracture of the lateral process of the talus, Am. J. Roentgenol. Rad. Ther. Nucl. Med. **90:**1277-1280, 1963.
22. Cloquet: Bull. Soc. Anat. Paris **19:**131, 1844.
23. Cobey, M.C.: Traumatic avascular necrosis of the talus, Clin. Orthop. **81:**180-181, 1971.
24. Coker, T.P., Jr., and Arnold, J.A.: Sports injuries to the foot and ankle. In Jahss, M.H., ed.: Disorders of the foot, vol. II, Philadelphia, 1982, W.B. Saunders Co.
25. Coltart, W.D.: "Aviator's astragalus," J. Bone Joint Surg. **34B:**545-566, 1952.
26. Cooper, A.: A treatise on dislocations, and on fractures of the joints, ed. 2, Boston, 1832, Lilly, Wait, Carter & Hendee, pp. 341-342.
27. Craig, F.S., and McLaughlin H.L.: Injuries of the foot. In McLaughlin, H.L., ed.: Trauma, Philadelphia, 1959, W.B. Saunders Co., pp. 307-317.
28. Davidson, A.M., Steele, H.D., MacKenzie, D.A., and Penny, J.A.: A review of twenty-one cases of transchondral fracture of the talus, J. Trauma, **7:**378-415, 1967.
29. Davis, F.J., Fry, L.R., Lippert, F.G., Simons, B.C., and Remington, J.: The patellar tendon-bearing brace: report of 16 patients, J. Trauma, **14:**216–221, 1974.
30. Davis, M.W.: Bilateral talar osteochondritis dissecans with lax ankle ligaments, J. Bone Joint Surg. **52A:**168-170, 1970.
31. Deetz, E.: Ueber Luxatio Pedis subtalo nach vorn mit Talusfraktur, Deutsche Ztschr. Chir. **76:**581-593, 1904.
32. DeLee, J.C.: Talar neck fracture with total dislocation of the body. Report of the Committee on Trauma of the American Orthopaedic Foot Society, Presented in Anaheim, Calif., Feb. 1983.
33. DeLee, J.C., and Curtis, R.: Subtalar dislocation of the foot, J. Bone Joint Surg. **64A:**433-437, 1982.
34. Dennis, M.D., and Tullos, H.S.: Blair tibiotalar arthrodesis for injuries of the talus, J. Bone Joint Surg. **62A:**103-107, 1980.
35. DePalma, A.F., Ahmed, I., Flannery, G., and Gandhi, O.P.: Aseptic necrosis of the talus: revascularization after bone grafting, Clin. Orthop. **101:**232-235, 1974.
36. Detenbeck, L.C., and Kelly, P.J.: Total dislocation of the talus, J. Bone Joint Surg. **51A:**283-288, 1969.
37. Deyerle, W.M., and Burkhardt, B.W.: Displaced fractures of the talus: an aggressive approach, Orthop. Trans. **5:**465, 1981.
38. Dimon, J.H.: Isolated displaced fracture of the posterior facet of the talus, J. Bone Joint Surg. **43A:**275-281, 1961.
39. Drez, D.J., Guhl, J.F., and Gollehan, D.L.: Ankle arthroscopy: technique and indications, Foot Ankle **2:**138-143, 1981.
40. Dunn, A.R., Jacobs, B., and Campbell, R.D., Jr.: Fractures of the talus, J. Trauma, **6:**443-468, 1966.
41. Fahey, J.J., and Murphy, J.L.: Dislocations and fractures of the talus, Surg. Clin. North Am. **45:**79-102, 1965.
42. Fjeldborg, O.: Fracture of the lateral process of the talus: supination-dorsal flexion fracture, Acta Orthop. Scand. **39:**407-412, 1968.
43. Garcia, A., and Parkes, J.C., II: Fractures of the foot. In Giannestras, N.J., ed.: Foot disorders: medical and surgical management, ed. 2, Philadelphia, 1973, Lea & Febiger.
44. Gatellier, J.: Juxtoretroperoneal route in operative treatment of fracture of malleolus with posterior marginal fragment, Surg. Gynecol. Obstet. **52:**67-70, 1931.

45. Geist, E.S.: Supernumerary bones of the foot: a roentgen study of the feet of one hundred normal individuals, Am. J. Orthop. Surg. **12**:403-414, 1914-1915.

46. Giannestras, N.J., and Sammarco, G.J.: Fractures and dislocations in the foot. In Rockwood, C.A., Jr., and Green, D.P., eds.: Fractures, vol. II, Philadelphia, 1975, J. B. Lippincott Co.

47. Gibson, A., and Inkster, R.G.: Fractures of the talus, Can. Med. Assoc. J. **31**:357-362, 1934.

48. Gillquist, J., Oretorp, N., Stenstrom, A., Rieger, A., and Wennberg, E.: Late results after vertical fracture of the talus, Injury **6**:173-179, 1974.

49. Gustilo, R.B., and Gordon, S.S.: Osteochondral fractures of the talus, Minn. Med. **51**:237-241, 1968.

50. Haliburton, R.A., Sullivan, C.R., Kelly, P.J., and Peterson, L.F.A.: The extra-osseous and intra-osseous blood supply of the Talus, J. Bone Joint Surg. **40A**:1115-1120, 1958.

51. Hamilton, W.G.: Stenosing tenosynovitis of the flexor hallucis longus tendon and posterior impingement upon the os trigonum in ballet dancers, Foot Ankle **3**:74-80, 1982.

52. Hawkins, L.G.: Fracture of the lateral process of the talus, J. Bone Joint Surg. **47A**:1170-1175, 1965.

53. Hawkins, L.G.: Fractures of the neck of the talus, J. Bone Joint Surg. **52A**:991-1002, 1970.

54. Heckman, J.D., McLean, M.R., and DeLee, J.C.: Fracture of the lateral process of the talus, Orthop. Trans., **5**:465, 1981.

55. Holland, C.T.: The accessory bones of the foot, with notes on a few other conditions: the Robert Jones Birth volume, New York, 1928, Oxford University Press, pp. 157-182.

56. Howse, A.J.G.: Posterior block of the ankle joint in ballet dancers, Foot Ankle **3**:81-84, 1982.

57. Huson, A.: An anatomical and functional study of the tarsal joints, Leiden, 1961, Drukkerij Luctor et Emergo.

58. Ihle, C.L., and Cochran, R.M.: Fracture of the fused os trigonum, Am. J. Sports Med. **10**:47-50, 1982.

59. Jensenius, H.: Fracture of the astragalus, Acta Orthop. Scand. **19**:195-209, 1950.

60. Kappis, M.: Weitere Beitrage zur traumatisch: Mechanischen Entstehung der "Spontanen" Knorpelablosungen (Sogen. Osteochondritis Dissecans), Deutsche Ztschr. Chir., **171**:13-29, 1922.

61. Kelly, P.J., and Sullivan, C.R.: Blood supply of the talus, Clin. Orthop. **30**:37-44, 1963.

62. Kenwright, J., and Taylor, R.G.: Major injuries of the talus, J. Bone Joint Surg. **52B**:36-48, 1970.

63. Key, J.A., and Conwell, H.E.: The management of fractures, dislocations and sprains, ed. 4, St. Louis, 1946, The C.V. Mosby Co.

64. Kleiger, B.: Fractures of the talus, J. Bone Joint Surg., **30A**:735-744, 1948.

65. Kleiger, B., and Ahmed, M.: Injuries of the talus and its joints, Clin. Orthop. **121**:243-262, 1976.

66. Kleinberg, S.: Supernumerary bones of the foot, Ann. Surg. **65**:499-509, 1917.

67. Kohler, A.: Roentgenology, ed. 2, London, 1935, Bailliere, Tindall & Cox.

68. Kohler, A., and Zimmer, E.A.: Borderlands of the normal and early pathologic in skeletal roentgenology, ed. 11, New York, 1968, Grune & Stratton, Inc.

69. Lahaut, M.: Fracture du col de l'astragale traitee par autogreffe immediate, Mem. Acad. Chir. **81**:261-264, 1955.

70. Lapidus, P.W.: A note on the fracture of os trigonum: report of a case, Bull. Hosp. Jt. Dis. **33**:150-154, 1972.

71. Larson, R.L., Sullivan, C.R., and Janes, J.M.: Trauma, surgery, and circulation of the talus: what are the risks of avascular necrosis? J. Trauma **1**:13-21, 1961.

72. Laughlin, J.E.: Injuries of the talus: a review of the literature and case presentation, J. Am. Osteopath. Assoc. **71**:334-341, 1971.

73. Lemaire, R.G., and Bustin, W.: Screw fixation of fractures of the neck of the talus using a posterior approach, J. Trauma, **20**:669-673, 1980.

74. Lieberg, O.U., Henke, J.A., and Bailey, R.W.: Avascular necrosis of the head of the talus without death of the body: report of an unusual case, J. Trauma **15**:926-928, 1975.

75. Lindholm, T.S., Osterman, K., and Vankka, E.: Osteochondritis of the elbow, ankle, and hip, Clin. Orthop. **148**:245-253, 1980.

76. Lionberger, D.R., Bishop, J.O., and Tullos, H.S.: The modified blair fusion, Foot Ankle **3**:60-62, 1982.

77. Lorentzen, J.E., Christensen, S.B., Krogsoe, O., and Sneppen, O.: Fractures of the neck of the talus, acta Orthop. Scand. **48**:115-120, 1977.

78. Marks, K.L.: Flake fracture of the talus progressing to osteochondritis dissecans, J. Bone Joint Surg. **34B**:90-92, 1952.

79. McDougall, A.: The os trigonum, J. Bone Joint Surg. **37B**:257-265, 1955.

80. McKeever, F.M.: Fracture of the neck of the astragalus, Arch. Surg. **46**:720-735, 1943.

81. McKeever, F.M.: Treatment of complications of fractures and dislocations of the talus, Clin. Orthop. **30**:45-52, 1963.

82. Meisenbach, R.: Fracture of the os trigonum: report of two cases, JAMA **89**:199-200, 1927.

83. Mensor, M.C., and Melody, G.F.: Osteochondritis dissecans of ankle joint: the use of tomography as a diagnostic aid, J. Bone Joint Surg. **23**:903-909, 1941.

84. Miller, O.L., and Baker, L.D.: Fracture and fracture-dislocation of the astragalus, South. Med. J. **32**:125-136, 1939.

85. Miller, W.E.: Operative intervention for fracture of the talus. In Bateman, J.E., and Trott, A.W., eds.: Foot and ankle, New York, 1980, Brian C. Dekker, Publishers.

86. Mindel, E.R., Cisek, E.E., Kartalian, G., and Dziob, J.M.: Late results of injuries to the talus, J. Bone Joint Surg. **45A**:221-245, 1963.

87. Mitchell, J.I.: Total dislocation of the astragalus, J. Bone Joint Surg. **18**:212-214, 1936.

88. Moeller, F.A.: The os trigonum syndrome, J. Am. Podiatry Assoc. **63**:491-501, 1973.

89. Monkman, G.R., Johnson, K.R., and Duncan, D.M.: Fractures of the neck of the talus, Minn. Med. **58**:335-340, 1975.

90. Morris, H.D.: Aseptic necrosis of the talus following injury, Orthop. Clin. North Am. **5**:177-189, 1974.

91. Morris, H.D., Hand, W.L., and Dunn, A.W.: The modified blair fusion for fractures of the talus, J. Bone Joint Surg. **53A**:1289-1297, 1971.

92. Mukherjee, S.K., and Young, A.B.: Dome fracture of the talus: a report of ten cases, J. Bone Joint Surg. **55B**:319-326, 1973.

93. Mukherjee, S.K., Pringle, R.M., and Baxter, A.D.: Fracture of the lateral process of the talus: a report of thirteen cases, J. Bone Joint Surg. **56B**:263-273, 1974.

94. Mulfinger, G.L., and Trueta, J.: The blood supply of the talus, J. Bone Joint Surg. **52B**:160-167, 1970.

95. Newberg, A.H.: Osteochondral fractures of the dome of the talus, Br. J. Radiol. **52**:105-109, 1979.

96. Newcomb, W.J., and Brav, E.A.: Complete dislocation of the talus, J. Bone Joint Surg. **30A**:872-874, 1948.

97. Nisbet, N.W.: Dome fracture of the talus, J. Bone Joint Surg. **36B**:244-246, 1954.

98. O'Brien, E.T.: Injuries of the talus, Am. Fam. Physician **12**:95-105, 1975.

99. O'Brien, E.T., Howard, J.B., and Shepard, M.J.: Injuries of the talus (Abstract), J. Bone Joint Surg. **54A**:1575-1576, 1972.

100. O'Donoghue, D.H.: Chondral and osteochondral fractures, J. Trauma **6**:469-481, 1966.

101. O'Farrell, T.A., and Costello, B.G.: Osteochondritis dissecans of the talus, J. Bone Joint Surg. **64B**:494-497, 1982.

102. Pantazopoulos, T., Galanos, P., Vayanos, E., Mitsou, A., and Hartofilakidis-Garofalidis, G.: Fractures of the neck of the talus, Acta Orthop. Scand. **45**:296-306, 1974.

103. Pantazopoulos, T., Kapetsis, P., Soucacos, P., and Gianakis, E.: Unusual fracture-dislocation of the talus: report of a case, Clin. Orthop. **83**:232-234, 1972.

104. Patzakis, M.J., Harvey, J.P., and Ivler, D.: The role of antibiotics in the management of open fractures, J. Bone Joint Surg. **56A**:532-541, 1974.

105. Paulos, L.E., Johnson, C.L., and Noyes, F.R.: Posterior compartment fractures of the ankle: a commonly missed athletic injury, Am. J. Sports. Med. **11**:439-443, 1983.

106. Pennal, G.F.: Fractures of the talus, Clin. Orthop. **30**:53-63, 1963.

107. Penny, J.N., and Davis, L.A.: Fractures and fracture-dislocations of the neck of the talus, J. Trauma **20**:1029-1037, 1980.

108. Percy, E.C.: Open fracture of the talus, Can. Med. Assoc. J. **101**:91-92, 1969.

109. Peterson, L., and Goldie, I.F.: The arterial supply of the talus: a study on the relationship to experimental talar fractures, Acta Orthop. Scand. **46**:1026-1034, 1975.

110. Peterson, L., Goldie, I.F., and Irstam, L.: Fracture of the neck of the talus: a clinical study, Acta Orthop. Scand. **48**:696-706, 1977.

111. Peterson, L., Goldie, I., and Lindell, D.: The arterial supply of the talus, Acta Orthop. Scand. **45**:260-270, 1974.

112. Pinzur, M.S., and Meyer, P.R., Jr.: Complete posterior dislocation of the talus: case report and discussion, Clin. Orthop. **131**:205-209, 1978.

113. Pirie, A.H.: Extra bones in the wrist and ankle found by roentgen rays, Am. J. Roentgenol. **8**:569-573, 1921.

114. Pringle, R.M., and Mukherjee, S.K.: Fracture of the lateral process of the talus, J. Bone Joint Surg. **56B**:201-202, 1974.

115. Ray, A.: Fractures de l'astragale (a propos de 34 observations), Rev. Chir. Orthop. **53**:279-294, 1967.

116. Ray, R.B., and Coughlin, E.J.: Osteochondritis dissecans of the talus, J. Bone Joint Surg. **29**:697-706, 1947.

117. Reckling, F.W.: Early tibiocalcaneal fusion in the treatment of severe injuries of the talus, J. Trauma **12**:390-396, 1972.

118. Reis, N.D., Zinman, C., Besser, M.I.B., et al.: High-resolution computerized tomography in clinical orthopaedics, J. Bone Joint Surg. **64B**:20-24, 1982.

119. Rendu, A.: Fracture intra-articulaire parcellaire de la poulie astragalienne, Lyon Med. **150**:220-222, 1932.

120. Roden, S., Tillegard, P., and Unander-Scharin, L.: Osteochondritis dissecans and similar lesions of the talus: a report of fifty-five cases with special reference to etiology and treatment, Acta Orthop. Scand. **23**:51-66, 1954.

121. Rogers, L.F., and Campbell, R.E.: Fractures and dislocations of the foot, Semin. Roentgenol. **13**:157-166, 1978.

122. Rosenberg, N.J.: Fractures of the talar dome, J. Bone Joint Surg. **47A**:1279, 1965.

123. Rosenmuller: Quoted in Holland, C.T.: On rarer ossifications seen during x-ray examinations, J. Anat. **55**:235-248, 1921.

124. Sarrafian, S.: Anatomy of the foot and ankle, Philadelphia, 1983, J.B. Lippincott Co., pp. 47-54, 295-297.

125. Scharling, M.: Osteochondritis dissecans of the talus, Acta Orthop. Scand. **49**:89-94, 1978.

126. Schrock, R.D.: Fractures of the foot: fractures and dislocations of the astragalus. In Pease, C.N., ed.: American Academy of Orthopaedic Surgeons Instructional course lectures, vol. 9, Ann Arbor, Mich., 1952, J.W. Edwards Co., pp. 361-365.

127. Shahriaree, H., Sajadiik, A.K , Silver, C., and Modsavi, A.: Total dislocation of the talus: a case report of a four-year follow-up, Orthop. Rev. **9**:65-68, 1980.

128. Shands, A.R., Jr., and Wentz, IJ.: Congenital anomalies, accessory bones and osteochondritis in the feet of 850 Children, Surg. Clin. North. Am. **33**:1643-1666, 1953.

129. Shelton, M.L., and Pedowitz, W.J.: Injuries to the talus and midfoot. In Jahss, M.H., ed.: Disorders of the foot, vol. II, Philadelphia, 1982, W.B. Saunders Co.

130. Shepard, F.J.: A hitherto undescribed fracture of the astragalus, J. Anat. Physiol. **18**:79-81, 1882.

131. Sisk, T.D.: Fractures. In Edmonson, A.S., and Crenshaw, A.H., eds.: Campbell's operative orthopaedics, ed. 6, vol. 1, St.Louis, 1980, The C.V. Mosby Co.

132. Skinner, H.A.: The origin of medical terms, ed. 2, New York, 1970, Hafner Publishing Co.

133. Smillie, I.S.: Osteochondritis dissecans. Loose bodies in joints. Etiology, pathology, treatment, Edinburgh, 1960, E & S Livingstone Ltd.

134. Smith, G.R., Winquist, R.A., Allan, T.N.K., and Northrop, C.H.: Subtle transchondral fractures of the talar dome: radiological perspective, Radiology **124**:667-673, 1977.

135. Sneed, W.L.: The astragalus. A case of dislocation, excision and replacement. An attempt to demonstrate the circulation in this bone, J. Bone Joint Surg. **7**:384-399, 1925.

136. Sneppen, O.: Fracture of the talus, a study of its genesis and morphology. Proceedings of the Danish Orthopaedic Society, Acta Orthop. Scand. **48**:334, 1977.

137. Sneppen, O., and Buhl, O.: Fracture of the talus. A study of its genesis and morphology based upon cases with associated ankle fracture, Acta Orthop.Scand. **45**:307-320, 1974.

138. Sneppen, O., Christensen, S.B., Krogsoe, O., and Lorentzen, J.: Fracture of the body of the talus, Acta Orthop. Scand. **48**:317-324, 1977.

139. Stealy, J.H.: Fracture of the astragalus, Surg. Gynecol. Obstet. **8**:36-48, 1909.

140. Sullivan, C.R., and Jackson, S.C.: Fracture dislocations of the astragalus in children, Acta Orthop. Scand. **27**:302-309, 1958.

141. Syme, J.: Contributions to the pathology and practice of surgery, Edinburgh, 1848, Sutherland & Knox, p. 126.

142. Taylor, R.G.: Immobilization of unstable fracture dislocations by the use of kirschner wires, Proc. R. Soc. Med., **55**:499-501, 1962.

143. Trillat, A., Bousquet, C., and Lapeyre, B.: Les fractures-separations totales du col ou du corps de l'astragale: interet du vissage par voie posterieure, Rev. Chir. Orthop. **56**:529-536, 1970.

144. Turner, W.: A secondary astragalus in the human foot, J. Anat. Physiol. **17**:82, 1882.

145. Vaughan, C.E., and Stapleton, J.G.: Osteochondritis dissecans of the ankle, Radiology **49**:72-79, 1947.

146. Watson-Jones, R.: Fractures and joint injuries, ed. 4, vol. II, Baltimore, 1955, The Williams & Wilkins Co.

147. Weinstein, S.L., and Bonfiglio, M.: Unusual accessory (bipartite) talus simulating fracture: a case report, J. Bone Joint Surg. **57A**:1161-1163, 1975.

148. Wildenauer, E.: Die Blutversorgung der Talus, Ztschr. Anat. **115**:32, 1950.

149. Winkler, H.: The treatment of trauma to the foot and ankle. In Thomson, E.M., ed.: Lectures on regional orthopaedic surgery and fundamental orthopaedic problems, Ann Arbor, Mich., 1947, J.W. Edwards Co., p. 30.

150. Yuan, H.A., Cady, R.B., and DeRosa, C.: Osteochondritis dissecans of the talus associated with subchondral cysts, J. Bone Joint Surg. **61A:**1249, 1979.
151. Yvars, M.F.: Osteochondral fractures of the dome of the talus, Clin. Orthop. **114:**185-191, 1976.
152. Zatzkin, H.R.: Trauma to the foot, Semin. Roentgenol. **5:**419-435, 1970.

Fractures of the midpart of the foot

Isolated fractures of the individual bones of the midfoot, the navicular, cuboid, and cuneiforms, are unusual.[16,17,27,31] Because of the rigidity of the midpart of the foot, injuries to it are usually a combination of fracture and/or subluxation of the adjacent joints.[16,17,34,40] This section will deal with apparent *isolated* injuries to the midtarsal bones. Discussion of associated midtarsal dislocations can be found under Injuries of the Midtarsal Joint. However, one must keep in mind during this discussion that fractures of the midtarsal bones may be associated with sprains or complete disruption of the adjacent ligaments.

FRACTURES OF TARSAL NAVICULAR

Fractures of the tarsal navicular are rare injuries.* However, navicular fractures were noted more frequently by Willson[44] than either cuboid or cuneiform fractures. Bonvallet reports that these fractures represent only about 2.6% of all fractures.[3,4]

Both Watson-Jones[41,45] and Joplin[24] divided fractures of the tarsal navicular into three types: (1) fractures of the tuberosity, (2) chip fractures of the dorsal lip, and (3) fractures of the body with or without displacement.[4,5,31] Recently, attention has been directed to a fourth group of tarsal navicular injuries, stress fractures. I prefer to include these in the classification system, which results in four types of navicular fracture (see box at right).

Anatomy

The tarsal navicular has a concave proximal articular surface for articulation with the head of the talus and a convex distal articular surface that is divided into three facets for articulation with each of the three cuneiforms.[14] There may be a fourth facet for articulation with the cuboid. Eichenholtz and Levine[14] stress that, because of the strategic location of the navicular in the medial longitudinal arch of the foot, this bone plays a major role in weight bearing during locomotion.[14] It is their opinion that the navicular, rather than the talus, acts as a keystone for vertical stress on the arch.

---

*References 7, 10, 17, 22, 27, and 31.

CLASSIFICATION OF NAVICULAR FRACTURES

1. Fractures of the tuberosity (Fig. 24-80)
2. Chip fractures of the dorsal lip (Fig. 24-78)
3. Fractures of the body
   a. Without displacement (Fig. 24-81)
   b. With displacement (Fig. 24-82)
4. Stress fractures of the navicular (Fig. 24-84)

Lehman and Eskeles[27] emphasized that the ligaments connecting the navicular to the cuneiforms are weaker than those connecting the talus to the navicular. This difference in strength between the two sets of ligaments results in disruption of the naviculocuneiform ligaments with forced plantar flexion of the foot. Disruption of naviculocuneiform ligaments permits naviculocuneiform subluxation, which results in compression fracture of the body of the navicular by the cuneiforms.

The blood supply of the navicular plays a major role in the prognosis of injury to this bone.[25] The navicular receives its blood supply from the dorsal and plantar aspects and from the tuberosity.[25,36,42] Sarrafian[36] emphasizes that direct branches enter the dorsum of the bone from the dorsalis pedis artery, while the plantar surface receives vessels from the medial plantar artery. The tuberosity, on the other hand, receives vessels from an arterial network formed by the union of the two source arteries, the dorsalis pedis and the medial plantar arteries.

Torg et al.[38] stressed that because much of the surface area of the navicular is covered by articular cartilage, only a small area of cortical bone is available for vessels to enter and leave the bone. Their microangiographic studies showed that the medial and lateral thirds of the navicular body had good blood supply, but the central one third is relatively avascular[32] (Fig. 24-77).

Sarrafian[36] emphasizes that between the ages of 20 and 65 years the number of arteries supplying the navicular decreases. Because of this decreased vascularity with increasing age, pseudarthrosis and aseptic necrosis following injury to this bone, particularly when there is extensive displacement of the fracture, increase with the age of the patient.

Radiographic evaluation

Anteroposterior, lateral, and oblique radiographs are needed to evaluate the navicular for fracture. However, Eichenholtz and Levine[14] report that fractures of the navicular may be missed even when the correct views

16. Garcia, A., and Parkes, J.C.: Fractures of the foot. In Giannestras, N.J., ed.: Foot disorders: medical and surgical management, ed. 2, Philadephia, 1975, Lea & Febiger.
17. Giannestras, N.J., and Sammarco, G.J.: Fractures and dislocations in the foot. In Rockwood, C.A., Jr., and Green, D.P., eds.: Fractures, vol. II, Philadelphia, 1975, J.B. Lippincott Co.
18. Goergen, T.G., Venn-Watson, E.A., Rossman, D.J., Resnick, D., and Gerber, K.H.: Tarsal navicular stress fractures in runners, Am. J. Roentgenol. **136**:201-203, 1981.
19. Heck, C.V.: Fractures of the bones of the foot (except the talus), Surg. Clin. North Am. **45**:103-117, 1965.
20. Henderson, M.S.: Fractures of the bones of the foot, except the os calcis, Surg. Gynecol. Obstet. **64**:454, 1937.
21. Hillegass, R.C.: Injuries to the midfoot: a major cause of industrial morbidity. In Bateman, J.E., ed., Foot science, Philadelphia, 1976, W.B. Saunders Co.
22. Hoffman, A.: Ueber die isolierte fraktur des os naviculare tarsi, Beitr. Klin. Chir. **59**:217, 1908.
23. Hunter, L.Y.: Stress fractures of the tarsal navicular, Am. J. Sports Med. **9**:217-219, 1981.
24. Joplin, R.J.: Injuries of the foot. In Cave, E.F., ed.: Fractures and other injuries, Chicago, 1958, Year Book Medical Publishers, Inc.
25. Kelly, P.J.: Anatomy, physiology and pathology of the blood supply of bones, J. Bone Joint Surg. **50A**:766-783, 1968.
26. Kohler, A., Zimmer, E.A., and Case, J.J.: Borderlands of the normal and early pathologic in skeletal roentgenology, New York, 1956, Grune & Straton, Inc., p. 723.
27. Lehman, E.P., and Eskeles, I.H.: Fractures of tarsal scaphoid: with notes on the mechanism, J. Bone Joint Surg. **10**:108, 1928.
28. McKeever, F.M.: Fractures of the tarsal and metatarsal bones, Surg. Gynecol. Obstet. **90**:735-745, 1950.
29. Morrison, G.M.: Fractures of the bones of the foot, Am. J. Surg. **38**:721, 1937.
30. Mygind, H.B.: The accessory tarsal scaphoid, Acta. Orthop. Scand. **23**:142-151, 1954.
31. Nadeau, P., and Templeton, J.: Vertical fracture-dislocation of the tarsal navicular, J. Trauma **16**:669-671, 1976.
32. Orva, S., Puranen, J., and Ala-Ketola, L.: Stress fractures caused by physical exercise, Acta Orthop. Scand. **49**:19-27, 1978.
33. Penhallow, D.P.: An unusual fracture-dislocation of the tarsal scaphoid with dislocation of the cuboid, J. Bone Joint Surg. **19**:517, 1937.
34. Perriard, M., Dieterli, J., and Jeannet, E.: Les lesions traumatiques recentes comprises entre les articulations de Chopart et de Lisfranc, incluses, Z. Unfallmed. Berufskr. **63**:318, 1970.
35. Prather, J.L., Nusynowitz, M.L., Snowdy, H.A., Hughes, A.D., McCartney, W.H., and Bagg, R.J.: Scintigraphic findings in stress fractures, J. Bone Joint Surg., **59A**:869-874, 1977.
36. Sarrafian, S.K.: Anatomy of the foot and ankle, 1983, Philadelphia, J.B. Lippincott, Co.
37. Speed, K.: A textbook of fractures and dislocations covering their pathology, diagnosis and treatment, ed. 4, Philadelphia, 1942, Lea & Febiger.
38. Torg, J.S., Pavlou, H., Cooley, L.H., Bryant, M.H., Arowoczky, S., Bergfeld, J., and Hunter, L.Y.: Stress fractures of the tarsal navicular, J. Bone Joint Surg. **64A**:700-712, 1982.
39. Towne, L.C., Blazina, M.E., and Cozen, L.N.: Fatigue fracture of the tarsal navicular, J. Bone Joint Surg. **52A**:376-378, 1970.
40. Waters, C.H., Jr.: Midtarsal fractures and dislocations. In American Academy of Orthopaedic Surgeons: Instructional course lectures, vol. 9, Ann Arbor, Mich., 1952, J.W. Edwards.
41. Watson-Jones, R.: Fractures and joint injuries, vol. 2, ed. 4, Baltimore, 1955, The Williams & Wilkins Co.
42. Waugh, W.: The ossification and vascularization of the tarsal navicular and their relationship to Kohler's disease, J. Bone Joint Surg. **40B**:765-777, 1958.
43. Wiley, J.J. and Brown, D.: Listhesis of the tarsal scaphoid, J. Bone Joint Surg. **56B**:586, 1974.
44. Wilson, P.D.: Fractures and dislocations of the tarsal bones, South. Med. J. **26**:833, 1933.
45. Wilson, J.N.: Watson-Jones fractures and joint injuries, ed. 6, Edinburgh, 1982, Churchill-Livingstone.

Fractures of the cuboid and cuneiform bones

Isolated fractures of the cuboid and cuneiform bones are quite rare.[12,13] McKeever[12] believed this was because both the cuboid and cuneiform bones occupy a protected and buttressed location in the metatarsus. When these fractures do occur, they are most frequently caused by a direct crushing force[12] or by a fall on the foot in plantar flexion with accompanying inversion or eversion.[13] Wilson[13] reported that fractures of the cuboid or cuneiform, either singly or in combination with other injuries, were of no serious significance. McKeever also reported that, because of the protected and buttressed location of these bones, displacement was seldom present and therefore reduction was usually not required.

FRACTURES OF CUBOID

Chapman[4] reports isolated fractures of the cuboid are quite rare and that they more commonly occur in conjunction with fractures of the cuneiforms or the bases of the lateral metatarsals. Garcia and Parkes[6] emphasize that fractures of the cuboid, although usually comminuted, are seldom displaced because of maintenance of position of the fracture fragments by the strong intertarsal ligaments. They stress that fractures of the cuboid are often associated with tarsometatarsal or midtarsal dislocations or subluxations and that the cuboid may also be involved in calcaneal fractures.

Hillegass[10] reports two types of cuboid injuries. The first and most frequent is avulsion fracture of the cuboid (Fig. 24-85). The second type is fractures that involve the entire body of the cuboid. Blazina and Webster[1] report an avulsion injury of the cuboid and emphasize that the location of such cortical avulsions on the lateral aspect of the foot causes them to be confused with a routine ankle sprain. Hermel and Gershon-Cohen[9] reported five cases of "nutcracker fracture of the cuboid" as examples of the second type of fracture. In these 5 cases the cuboid was caught "like a nut in a cracker" between the bases of the fourth and fifth metatarsals and the calcaneus. In each instance the toes were fixed, and the weight of the body was transmitted by the calcaneus through the cuboid and the two lateral

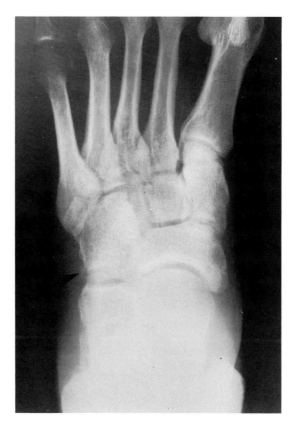

Fig. 24-85. Chip fracture of cuboid (arrow).

metatarsals.[9,11] The cuboid was thus crushed, giving rise to an impacted and comminuted fracture (Fig. 24-86). It is important to recognize that in 2 of the 5 patients reported by these authors there was an associated subluxation of Chopart's joint.

Signs and symptoms

The patient will give a history of either a direct blow to the lateral aspect of the foot or of trauma to the foot following jumping or twisting the foot beneath the body.[7,9] There is pain on the lateral border of the foot with point tenderness over the cuboid. Associated tenderness over the medial aspect of Chopart's joint suggests associated subluxation or actual dislocation of the entire midtarsal joint. Passive abduction and adduction or inversion and eversion of the foot will accentuate the pain in the midpart of the foot.

Radiographic examination

Anteroposterior, lateral, and oblique radiographs are useful in evaluating fractures of the cuboid.[7] In my experience, the oblique view is most helpful in determining not only the direction of the fracture line but also the presence or absence of displacement of the calca-neocuboid or cuboid-metatarsal joint surfaces. Evaluation of this oblique radiograph is also essential to determine the presence or absence of associated fractures of the calcaneus or metatarsals. As emphasized by Hermel and Gershon-Cohen,[9] in patients with the "nutcracker fracture" *and* an associated avulsion fracture of the navicular tubercle, midtarsal subluxation must be considered.

Treatment

Bohler[2] and Conwell and Reynolds[5] both emphasize that fractures of the cuboid rarely demonstrate displacement and therefore treatment need only be immobilization. Heck[8] also reports that displacement of such fractures is rare and healing occurs with few complications. He recommends early treatment with a short leg cast for 3 to 4 weeks followed by an adequate shoe. He warns of the late complication of a bony prominence over the dorsum of the foot in the area of the fracture that may interfere with the wearing of shoes.

Giannestras and Sammarco[7] also prefer a well-padded and molded short leg weight-bearing cast for 5 to 6 weeks following the injury. This is followed by a well-fitting longitudinal arch support for an additional 4

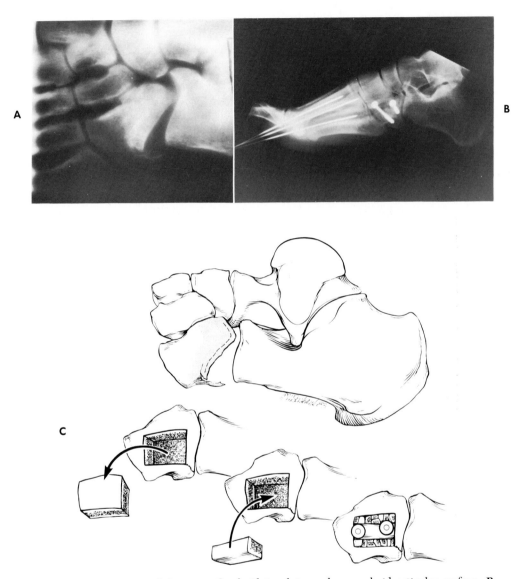

Fig. 24-86. A, Impacted fracture of cuboid involving calcaneocuboid articular surface. **B,** Open reduction and internal fixation of cuboid. Joint surface has been restored. Kirschner wires are stabilizing associated metatarsal shaft fractures. **C,** Corticocancellous strut graft was used to stabilize reduction of the articular surface. Cancellous bone was used to fill in defect.

to 6 months. They report that, although there may be some discomfort on weight bearing for several weeks after cast removal, long-term complications are unusual. Garcia and Parkes[6] recommend a below the knee walking cast for 6 to 8 weeks with progressive ambulation. These authors report that, because there is little motion in these joints normally, little or no impairment of function of this part of the foot is noted following this injury. They do stress, however, that the mechanism of these injuries, a crushing type trauma from heavy objects falling on the foot, can result in severe soft tissue damage. Therefore they stress the importance of close observation of the soft tissues in the area of the fracture in the hospital until the period of danger to the soft tissues has passed.

Hermel and Gershon-Cohen[9] recommend early midtarsal fusion for severe fractures associated with subluxation or dislocation of the cuboid. Hillegass,[10] however, believes that these injuries might respond well to an accurate open reduction and internal fixation if the cuboid articular surface is significantly displaced (Fig. 24-86).

AUTHOR'S PREFERRED METHOD OF TREATMENT

In patients with chip fractures of the cuboid, clinical and radiographic evaluation of the *medial* aspect of the midtarsal joint is essential. If there is no injury to the ligaments on the medial aspect of the midtarsal joint, treatment is based on the patient's requirements for weight bearing. If the patient needs to be ambulatory, I prefer a short leg walking cast until pain is relieved. If pain is minimal, an Ace bandage or Unna boot is used until pain has subsided. If an avulsion fracture of the navicular tubercle or medial midtarsal tenderness suggest an associated midtarsal sprain, short leg cast immobilization for 4 to 6 weeks followed by the use of a good shoe with a longitudinal arch support is recommended.

In fractures involving the body of the cuboid, particularly those of the "nutcracker" variety described by Hermel and Geshon-Cohen,[9] careful evaluation of the oblique radiographs is imperative. In these injuries residual displacement of the articular surface of the cuboid can result in persistent subluxation of the midtarsal joint and long-term arthritic changes. If a large portion of the calcaneocuboid or cuboid-metatarsal joint is displaced, consideration is given to open reduction. A longitudinal incision parallel to the sole of the foot and located over the cuboid is used, followed by open reduction and bone grafting. A corticocancellous bone graft used as a strut may be necessary because of compression of the cancellous bone of the cuboid, which results from the "nutcracker" mechanism (Fig. 24-86, *C*). Following

open reduction and reconstruction of the articular surface, range of motion to the foot is encouraged if fracture fixation is stable. Once range of motion to the foot has been restored, the foot is placed in a short leg non-weight-bearing cast for 6 weeks. The patient then wears a good shoe with a longitudinal arch support.

If the comminution is too severe or if the fracture is not significantly displaced a short leg walking cast is applied for 4 to 6 weeks, followed by the use of a shoe with an arch support. In my experience, such fractures have not resulted in long-term disability.

CUNEIFORM FRACTURES

Fractures of the cuneiform bones are quite rare.[7,10] According to Heck[8] displacement of these fractures is unusual and healing with few complications is likely.

The mechanism of injury of cuneiform fractures is usually direct trauma.[7] Therefore the treating surgeon must be cognizant of associated soft tissue trauma that may not be appreciated initially.

Signs and symptoms

The patient usually complains of pain in the area of the specific cuneiform injury. The location of tenderness helps delineate the particular cuneiform involved. As with fractures of the cuboid, inversion and eversion of the forefoot are distinctly painful.[6]

Radiographic examination

Anteroposterior, lateral, and oblique radiographs are useful in evaluating fractures of the cuneiform (Fig. 24-87). Chip fractures are usually nondisplaced, because associated intertarsal ligaments are strong and prevent their displacement.[12,13]

Treatment

Avulsion fractures are usually treated symptomatically by immobilization in a short leg weight bearing cast until pain subsides.[10] Hillegass[10] stresses that significant fracture displacement must be reduced accurately and that internal fixation may be necessary to maintain the reduction. Because of the limited motion in the normal midtarsal joint, long-term complications are not common. Buchman[3] reported osteochondritis dissecans and bipartite cuneiforms that must be distinguished radiographically from fractures. The bipartite cuneiform is most easily distinguished because of its smooth articular surfaces, whereas the irregular surfaces of a fracture should be diagnostic.

AUTHOR'S PREFERRED METHOD OF TREATMENT

In my experience, isolated fracture of the cuneiforms are rarely displaced. If a displaced fracture is present,

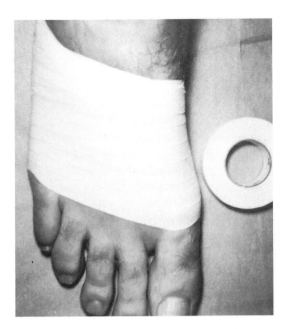

Fig. 24-89. Taping foot with ½-inch adhesive tape for nondisplaced metatarsal fracture. After taping, ambulation is begun in a postbunionectomy shoe.

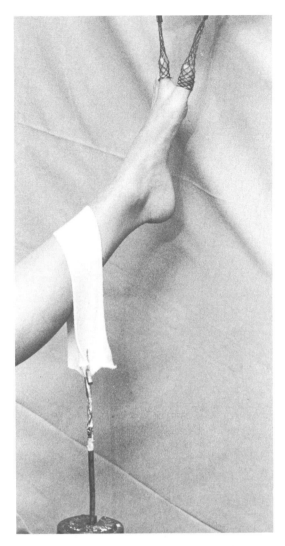

Fig. 24-90. Chinese finger traps with ankle countertraction used to reduce fracture of forefoot.

by cast immobilization. Likewise, Garcia and Parkes[20] recommend attempted closed reduction of displaced metatarsal fractures. They use Chinese finger traps applied to each toe as soon as possible after the fracture is diagnosed. After the Chinese finger traps are applied, counter-traction at the ankle usually results in satisfactory alignment of the fracture (Fig. 24-90). Following reduction of the fractured metatarsal shaft, a well-molded plaster cast is applied. The cast is first applied from the tips of the toes to the midtarsal area. Once this is allowed to set, the countertraction on the ankle is released and the cast is extended to the level of the tibial tubercle. The foot remains in this cast nonweight bearing for 4 weeks, at which time the cast is removed and radiographs are obtained. Weight bearing in a short leg walking cast is then permitted.

Giannestras and Sammarco[21] also recommend the use of Chinese finger traps in displaced metatarsal fractures. Following reduction, the foot is kept in a nonweight-bearing cast for 4 weeks. At this time the cast is changed, radiographs are taken, and the patient is allowed to begin weight bearing. If reduction by manipulation and traction is unsuccessful, open reduction and internal fixation with crossed Kirschner wires may be indicated in certain instances.[14,21] Giannestras and Sammarco[21] believe that lateral displacement of a metatarsal shaft fracture, with the exclusion of the first metatarsal, is of no great significance and does not re-

quire open reduction. Severe dorsal or plantar angulation, however, cannot be accepted.[1,21,43] Malalignment in this plane may result in abnormal pressure on the plantar aspect of the foot or in deformity of the toes resulting in painful plantar callosities.[1,21,26]

Garcia and Parkes[20] believe open anatomic reduction and fixation using Kirschner wires are necessary if closed reduction fails. Open reduction of fractures of the metatarsals is carried out through one or more longitudinal dorsal incisions.[1,38,50] Usually two adjacent metatarsal necks or shafts can be exposed adequately through one incision placed midway between and parallel to the metatarsal shafts.[1]

Johnson[28] emphasizes that if, after closed reduction, the fragments are in any degree of apposition and not displaced towards the sole, conservative treatment can be continued. Shortening, particularly in single or multiple fractures of the middle three metatarsals, is not significant according to Johnson.[28] If an unacceptable reduction is obtained, he believes that open reduction with the patient under anesthesia with intramedullary Kirschner wire fixation and early ambulatory treatment postoperatively is indicated.[28] He stresses, however, that as long as the alignment is maintained by open or closed methods, axial shortening can be accepted rather than subjecting the foot to any form of fixed traction. He believes that such fixed traction devices lead to stiffness of the forefoot, which results in more disability than the metatarsal fracture itself.

Sisk[50] recommends that isolated fractures in the metatarsal diaphysis, particularly if adjacent metatarsals are intact, be treated conservatively. He emphasizes, however, that the more distal the fracture of a metatarsal, the more definite the indication for open reduction. Open reduction and internal fixation of such fractures in the distal end of the metatarsal is most often indicated when there is significant dorsal angulation of the fracture, causing the metatarsal head to be prominent on the plantar aspect of the sole of the foot.[50] He recommends open reduction and intramedullary Kirschner wire fixation, with the wire left protruding through the skin in the area of the metatarsophalangeal joint for 3 weeks. The wire thus crosses the articular surface of the head of the metatarsal. He reports no complications from infection and minimal problems caused by stiffness of the metatarsophalangeal joint. In selected midshaft fractures undergoing open reduction, he recommends the use of a 4-5 hole plate contoured to the dorsolateral surface of the metatarsal and fixed to the bone with multiple screws.

Metatarsal neck fractures

Fractures of the *necks* of the metatarsals are usually multiple and are often displaced.[1] Persistent displacement of the metatarsal head and neck into the plantar aspect of the sole of the foot may result in plantar callosities and/or dorsal corns.[1,21,22,43] Anderson stresses the importance of an accurate reduction of these fractures to prevent such sequalae.[1] Such fractures can usually be reduced with the patient under anesthesia with use of the Chinese finger trap technique,[5] or by digital pressure under the metatarsal head with traction of the toe.[41] If a good reduction is obtained, closed treatment in a short leg walking cast may be satisfactory.[5] However, Lindholm[38] warns that maintenance of a closed reduction of a completely dislocated metatarsal neck fracture without internal fixation is uncertain.

If complete displacement with lack of apposition of the fracture surfaces and plantar displacement of the

head and neck fragment persists following attempted closed reduction, open reduction is indicated.[28,38] Sisk,[50] and Goldstein and Dickenson[23] use a longitudinal dorsal incision, because it will usually allow access to adjacent metatarsal necks.[50] In these more distal fractures, Sisk prefers the use of intramedullary Kirschner wire fixation. Using this technique, the proximal end of the distal fragment is lifted out of the wound and the toes are held in dorsiflexion. The Kirschner wire is inserted into the medullary canal of the distal fragment and advanced distally until the point emerges through the skin in the area of the metatarsophalangeal joint. The wire is then withdrawn through the skin until its end is even with the fracture site. The fracture is then reduced and the wire drilled proximally until it meets resistance at the base of the metatarsal. The wire is left protruding through the skin, and a small dressing is applied over the ends of the wire. The foot is immobilized in a cast from the tibial tuberosity to the toes with protection of the wire to prevent it from coming in contact with the plaster. The wires are removed at 3 weeks, and a walking cast is applied.[23,50]

Lindholm has modified intramedullary Kirschner wire fixation to prevent leaving the wire out of the skin and thence going through the metatarsophalangeal joint.[38] The major drawback to leaving the Kirschner wires exiting the skin is that it exposes the metatarsophalangeal joint to infection and may result in impairment of motion of the metatarsophalangeal joint. In Lindholm's technique, the fracture is exposed through a dorsal incision and a Kirschner wire is drilled into the *proximal* fracture fragment. Enough of the wire is left exposed from the distal end of the proximal fracture fragment to engage the distal fragment. The distal fragment, like a cup, is then pressed against the proximal fragment and Kirschner wire. The wound is closed, and the foot is placed in a well-fitting plaster cast. Weight bearing is permitted after 2 weeks. The cast is kept in place until bony union is assured. The Kirschner wires in these instances are left permanently within the metatarsal. Lindholm has noted no problems with corrosion of the implants or other difficulty by leaving them in the metatarsals.[38]

Fractures of the metatarsal heads are uncommon. Blodgett[5] recommends skeletal traction by use of a transverse Kirschner wire through the proximal or middle phalanx, or by pulp wire traction for shatter-type fractures. The traction is maintained by a rubber band attached to an outrigger mounted on a below-the-knee cast. Such traction is maintained for 7 weeks with limited weight bearing on the forefoot for 10 to 12 weeks. Following this treatment, Blodgett states that only limited metatarsophalangeal flexion can be expected.[5]

AUTHOR'S PREFERRED METHOD
OF TREATMENT

Metatarsal shaft fractures

Nondisplaced fractures. I agree with Johnson[28] and Irwin[27] concerning the importance of early weight bearing in the treatment of metatarsal fractures to help minimize long-term disability. In nondisplaced fractures of the *first* metatarsal, I prefer a short leg walking cast well molded beneath the first metatarsal. Weight bearing is begun in 7 to 10 days. This cast is removed when there is evidence of healing. The foot is then placed in a stiff-soled shoe with good arch support.

In nondisplaced fractures of the lateral four metatarsals, I prefer either using a short leg walking cast or taping the foot with ½-inch adhesive tape and using a bunion-type shoe (see Fig. 24-89). The choice is dependent on the patient's employment requirements. A stiff-soled walking shoe or boot with a good arch support is used when comfort allows.

Displaced fractures. In patients with displaced metatarsal fractures, I strongly recommend extensive evaluation of the soft tissues to determine the degree of associated damage. If soft tissue damage is significant, consideration is given to placing the foot in a bulky dressing. The foot is elevated and ice is applied until subsidence of the swelling permits more aggressive fracture treatment.

In displaced fractures of the first metatarsal shaft I recommend reduction of all angulation in the dorsal plantar plane. Additionally, comminution of fractures of the first metatarsal may result in shortening and can accentuate callosities beneath the second metatarsal. In displaced fractures of the first metatarsal, I attempt a closed reduction using the Chinese finger traps. If comminution has resulted in shortening of the metatarsal and the length can be restored, I use transfixing pins from the first to the second metatarsal to maintain the length of the metatarsal. In displaced fractures that cannot be reduced by these closed methods, open reduction through a dorsal incision and fixation using crossed Kirschner wires are used. Following reduction and internal fixation, the foot is kept in a non-weight-bearing short leg cast for 4 weeks, followed by a walking cast for 2 additional weeks. The Kirschner wires are removed between the fourth and sixth weeks.

In displaced fracture of the shaft of one of the lateral four metatarsals, closed reduction is attempted using Chinese finger traps applied to the involved digit (see Fig. 24-90). If a reduction is obtained, consideration is given to percutaneous Kirschner wire fixation to an adjacent intact metatarsal, particularly when the fractured metatarsal is the fifth. Following reduction, the foot is placed in a short leg cast. Weight bearing is allowed after the second week of immobilization. In my opinion, an accurate reduction is more critical in the dorsal-plantar plane than the mediolateral plane. If dorsal-plantar angulation causing plantar prominence of the metatarsal head persists following closed reduction, I prefer open reduction and internal fixation using either longitudinal intramedullary or crossed Kirschner wires for stability. In patients in whom there is more than one displaced metatarsal fracture, internal fixation either by percutaneous methods or by open reduction may be necessary because of the loss of the splinting affect of adjacent metatarsals.

Following open reduction and internal fixation of these metatarsal shaft fractures, patients are kept non-weight bearing in a short leg cast for 2 weeks. Weight bearing is then initiated for an additional 6 weeks. The Kirschner wires are removed between 4 to 6 weeks.

Metatarsal neck fractures

In evaluating fractures of the necks of the metatarsals, the oblique and sesamoid views help to demonstrate the degree of plantar displacement of the metatarsal head. If the metatarsal head and neck fragment is displaced, I attempt closed reduction using the Chinese finger traps for traction and direct digital pressure beneath the metatarsal head to reduce the displacement. A short leg cast with a toe plate and molded beneath the metatarsal heads is applied while the traction is in place. If the reduction is maintained in the cast, the patient is treated weight bearing in the cast for 4 to 6 weeks, followed by the use of a stiff-soled shoe. If the reduction is not acceptable by these methods or is unstable and redisplaces in the cast, percutaneous Kirschner wire fixation of the fracture, while it is in the Chinese finger traps, is attempted (Fig. 24-91). If this fails, open reduction through a dorsal incision and intramedullary Kirschner wire fixation, after the method of Sisk are used.[50] It is important to emphasize that these Kirschner wires are left in place only 3 weeks and then removed. The patient is allowed to begin weight bearing in a short leg cast when swelling subsides. Following removal of the wires, the foot is managed for an additional 2 weeks in a cast and then transferred to a stiff-soled shoe.

Metatarsal base fractures

Fractures at the base of the metatarsals are not common. If the fracture fragments of the metatarsal base are displaced and large enough to permit internal fixation, I recommend an attempted closed reduction. Care must be taken in evaluating the radiographs to make sure that an associated dislocation of the involved joint is not missed (see Fig. 24-88). Traction using the Chinese finger traps is applied. If the articular surface reduces, percutaneous Kirschner wire fixation, either

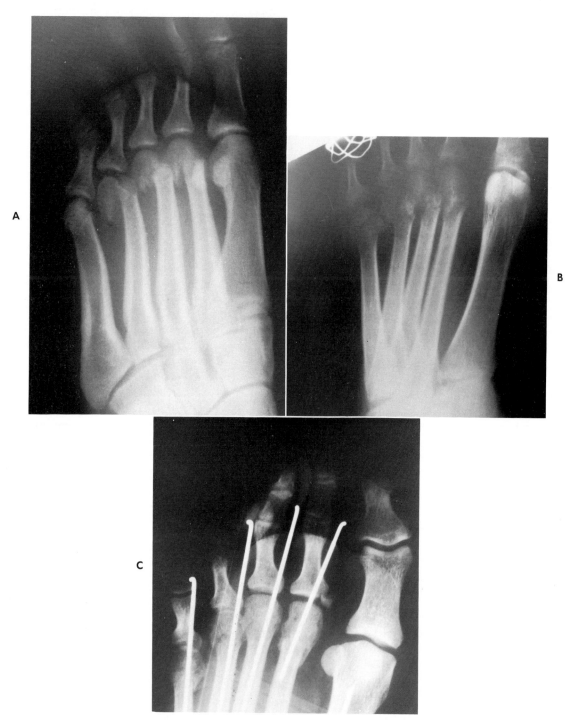

Fig. 24-91. A, Displaced fractures of second through fifth metatarsal necks. **B,** Closed reduction with Chinese finger traps. **C,** Percutaneous Kirschner wire fixation.

transarticularly or into an adjacent intact metatarsal, is performed. If persistently displaced fracture fragments are large enough to permit internal fixation or if there is an associated dislocation of the involved joint (not the entire tarsometatarsal joint, only a single tarsometatarsal joint) that cannot be reduced closed, an open reduction is performed. The goals of open reduction are (1) to restore dorsal-plantar displacement of the metatarsal to prevent later callosities beneath the forefoot and (2) to restore the articular surface of the involved tarsometatarsal joint. This is particularly important in the first and fifth metatarsals. After open reduction, the foot is treated in a weight-bearing short leg cast for 4 weeks then transferred to a shoe with a molded arch. Because of the limited motion in normal tarsometatarsal joints, open reduction does not usually result in significant loss of motion. However, connecting the subluxation of the joint, in my experience, has helped decrease the problem with painful degenerative arthritis in these joints.

If the comminution is too severe to permit open reduction and internal fixation, a closed reduction and application of a short leg cast, *well molded* in the arch to support the injured metatarsal base, is applied. The foot is kept non-weight bearing for 2 to 4 weeks. Weight bearing in a similar cast is then instituted. The patient is then changed to a stiff-soled shoe with a good arch support. Later, arthrodesis of the injured joint may be required if pain persists.

FRACTURES OF BASE OF FIFTH METATARSAL

Fractures of the base of the fifth metatarsal are treated here as a separate group for two reasons: (1) they are the most common type of metatarsal fractures,[21] and (2) there is confusion in the literature as to their treatment. Fractures of the base of the fifth metatarsal have been classically termed *Jones fractures* after Sir Robert Jones described the injury in his own foot in 1902.[30] However, as stressed by Kavanaugh et al.[31] there is confusion as to exactly which fracture Jones described. Jones actually described a transverse *diaphyseal* fracture of the fifth metatarsal, ¾ of an inch from the base. This fracture is a less common injury than avulsion of the fifth metatarsal tuberosity, with which the Jones fracture has been confused.[30,48] The transverse proximal diaphyseal fracture described by Jones often goes on to delayed or nonunion.[2,11,31] In addition to confusion as to the anatomical location of the fracture, recently Zelko et al.,[58] Kavanaugh et al.,[31] and DeLee et al.[13] have reported difficulty in treating fractures of the proximal fifth metatarsal diaphysis in which the diagnosis was initially overlooked. Stress fractures in this area are also difficult to treat.[13,31,58]

Table 8. Stewart's classification of fractures of the base of the fifth metatarsal[52]

Type		Description
1	A	Fracture of the junction of the shaft and base (See Fig. 24-92, *A*)
	B	Comminuted
2	A	Fracture of the styloid process without articular involvement (Fig. 24-93)
	B	With joint involvement (Fig. 24-94)

In an effort to clarify fractures of the base of the fifth metatarsal, Stewart[52] introduced a classification of these fractures (See Table 8). Type 1 fractures are at the junction of the metatarsal shaft and the base. This type is subdivided into two groups: noncomminuted fractures (1A) and fractures with comminution (1B). Type 2 fractures are those which involve the only styloid process. This type is also subdivided into two groups: those with joint involvement (2B) and those without (2A). Stewart formulated treatment recommendations based on this classification system.

Zelko et al.[54] and Torg et al.[58] divided fractures of the fifth metatarsal occurring at the metaphyseal-diaphyseal junction into four subgroups based upon their clinical history *and* initial radiographic findings.[58] Group 1 includes patients with an acute traumatic injury and no prior symptoms (Fig. 24-92, *A*). Radiographs demonstrate an acute fracture line with no chronic changes. Group 2 includes patients who sustain an acute injury but who previously have had mild symptoms on the lateral border of the foot (Fig. 24-92, *B*). Radiographs demonstrate a lucent fracture line with some periosteal reaction. Group 3 includes patients who sustain traumatic reinjury after one or more previous injuries. Radiographs in these patients demonstrate a lucent fracture line with periosteal reaction and often intramedullary sclerosis (Fig. 24-92, *C*). Finally, Group 4 includes patients who have a history of chronic pain or multiple injury episodes. Radiographs demonstrate a lucent fracture line with sclerotic margins (Fig. 24-92, *D*).

In an effort to simplify the discussion of these injuries, I prefer to use a classification system that incorporates both that of Stewart[42] and Zelko et al.[58] (Table 9)

I view these fractures as being of three distinct types, I, II, and III. Type IA includes nondisplaced *acute* fractures at the junction of the shaft and base. Type IB includes *acute* comminuted fractures at the junction of the metatarsal shaft and base. Type II includes fractures at the junction of the metatarsal shaft and base with clinical and radiographic evidence of pre-

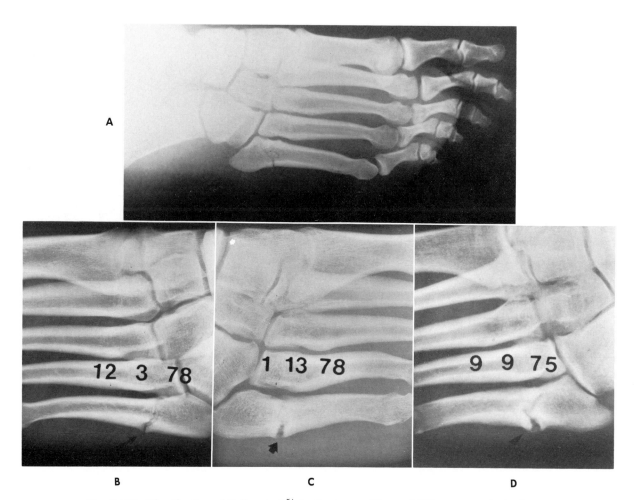

Fig. 24-92. Classification of Zelko et al.[54] for fractures of base of fifth metatarsal. **A,** Group 1: acute fracture of proximal diaphysis of fifth metatarsal. **B,** Group 2: acute fracture of proximal diaphysis of fifth metatarsal. Note preexisting periosteal reaction. **C,** Group 3: fracture of proximal diaphysis of fifth metatarsal. Note lucent fracture line and periosteal reaction. **D,** Group 4: fracture of proximal diaphysis of fifth metatarsal. Note lucent fracture line, periosteal reaction, and intermedullary sclerosis. See text for more complete description of each group. (From Zelko, R.R., Torg, J., and Rachun, A.: Am. J. Sports Med. 7:95-101, 1979. © 1979, American Orthopaedic Society for Sports Medicine.)

Table 9. Author's classification of fractures of the base of the fifth metatarsal

Type		Description
I		Acute fractures at the metaphyseal-diaphyseal junction
	A	Nondisplaced (Fig. 24-92, A)
	B	Displaced and/or comminuted
II		Fractures at the metaphyseal-diaphyseal junction with clinical and/or radiographic evidence of previous injury (i.e., pain, sclerosis, etc.) (Fig. 24-92, B to D)
III		Fractures of the styloid process of the fifth metatarsal
	A	*Without* involvement of the fifth metatarsocuboid joint (Fig. 24-93)
	B	With involvement of the fifth metatarsocuboid joint (Fig. 24-94)

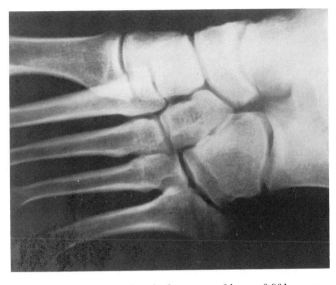

Fig. 24-93. Fracture of styloid process of base of fifth metatarsal without articular involvement.

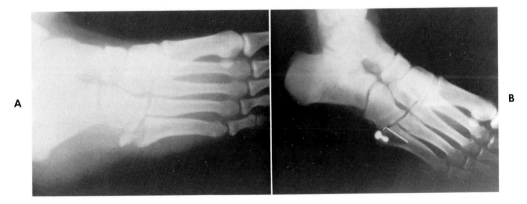

Fig. 24-94. A, Fracture of styloid process of base of fifth metatarsal with joint involvement. **B,** Open reduction and internal fixation to restore articular conguity.

vious injury. To be classified a type II fracture, the patient must have a history of prodromal symptoms along the lateral aspect of the foot before the acute fracture and/or a radiograph suggesting chronic reaction to stress, i.e., a radiolucent fracture line, periosteal reaction, heaped-up callus on the lateral cortical margin, and intramedullary sclerosis that obviously preceded the acute episode of pain[13] (Fig. 24-92, *D*). Type IIIA includes fractures of the styloid process without joint involvement, and type IIIB includes fractures of the styloid process with involvement of the fifth metatarsocuboid joint.

Stress fractures involving the proximal shaft of the fifth metatarsal distal to the tuberosity (type II) are different in their behavior from other metatarsal stress fractures. Zelko et al.[58] found them to be slow to heal, predipoded to reinjury, and often causing prolonged disability, particularly in young athletes.[58] Kavanaugh et al.[31] also stressed that this injury frequently occurs in young athletes and may be the source of prolonged disability. Its occurrence in basketball players has been emphasized by several authors.[13,31] Kavanaugh et al.[31] found that 41% of patients with fractures of the fifth metatarsal related a history of discomfort over the lateral aspect of the foot at least 2 weeks *before* the radiographic evidence of the fracture (type II). Zelko et al.[58] found radiographic evidence of a lucent fracture line with periosteal reaction in 14 of 21 patients at the time of initial fracture.

Anatomy

Because of the articulations between the base of the fifth metatarsal and the cuboid and between the bases of the fifth and fourth metatarsals, fractures of the base of the fifth metatarsal can be intraarticular in either of these two joints.[52]

Jones[30] stressed that the base of the fifth metatarsal is closely bound to the cuboid and to the fourth metatarsal by strong ligaments on every side. He believed these ligaments were so strong that dislocation of the metatarsal base at the time of fracture was "the rarest of accidents." He did not mention the function of the insertion of the peroneus brevis tendon in this fracture. Kavanaugh et al.,[31] based on the anatomic dissection of five fresh specimens, confirmed Jones' observations on the thickness and strength of these ligaments. They stressed that the diaphyseal fracture reported by Jones occurs 0.5 centimeters distal to the splayed insertion of the peroneus brevis and almost invariably just distal to the joint between the fourth and fifth metatarsals. It was their opinion that the firm capsular attachments of the metatarsocuboid joint helped to stabilize the joint, thereby concentrating fracture forces at the metaphyseal-diaphyseal junction. The strong tendon of the per-

oneus brevis inserts on the dorsolateral aspect of the base of the fifth metatarsal over a relatively large area. This insertion has given rise to the theory that avulsion fractures occur because of contracture of this muscle.[21,47]

The base or proximal end of the fifth metatarsal presents a flair, the tuberosity, which protrudes down and laterally beyond the surfaces of the shaft of the metatarsal and the adjacent cuboid.[12] Dameron[12] emphasized the individual variations in the size and shape of this tubercle. Stewart noted that the amount the styloid process overhangs the metatarsocuboid joint appears to vary and to invite isolated fractures when it is relatively long.[52]

Carp[6] in discussing delayed union of fractures of the fifth metatarsal, presented the thesis that poor blood supply to the shaft of the fifth metatarsal was responsible for the tendency to delayed union.

Mechanism of injury

Jones' original description[29,30] clearly delineated the mechanism of his own injury:

> While dancing, I trod on the outer side of my foot, my heel at the moment being off the ground. Something gave midway down my foot, and I at once suspected a rupture of the peroneus longus tendon.

Since that description, both direct and indirect mechanisms of injury have been given responsibility for this fracture.[21] The marked prominence of the tuberosity of the fifth metatarsal beyond the lateral line of the shaft of the metatarsal on the lateral border of the anterior two thirds of the foot make it particularly at risk to direct trauma.[21,42]

Fractures of the tuberosity of the fifth metatarsal by indirect violence are more common, possibly secondary to the number of structures that attach to this prominence.[8] These include the peroneus brevis tendon, a portion of the adductor digiti quinti muscle, the outer portion of plantar fascia, occasionally the abductor ossei metatarsi quinti muscle, and finally the flexor brevis minimi digiti muscle.[8] Lichtblau[37] has stressed the importance of the active role played by the peroneus brevis tendon in pulling the base of the metatarsal away from the shaft. According to him, because the peroneus brevis muscle contracts during stance phase, it is already contracted when an inversion stress is applied to the weight-loaded and plantar-flexed foot. Because of its insertion into the base of the fifth metatarsal, the tendon of the peroneus brevis holds firmly as the shaft is pulled away from it. Avulsion of the base from the rest of the fifth metatarsal is the result. Giannestras and Sammarco[21] also note that a plantar-flexion inversion

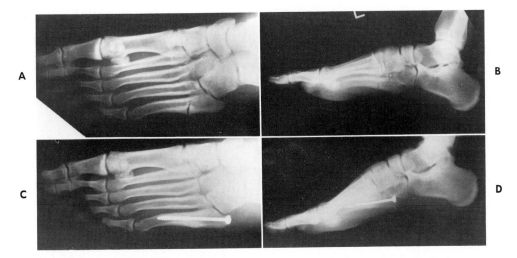

Fig. 24-97. **A,** Oblique and **B,** lateral radiographs of stress fracture of base of fifth metatarsal. **C,** Lateral and **D,** oblique radiographs demonstrating intramedullary axial screw and healed fracture.

metaphyseal-diaphyseal junction with evidence of preexisting stress reaction of bone), is based on the patient's level of activity. In the high-performance athlete, I use axial intramedullary screw fixation as demonstrated in Fig. 24-97. Following axial screw fixation, the patient is treated in a short leg non-walking cast for 2 weeks. The cast is then removed, and the foot is placed in a hard-soled shoe. Either a wooden shoe of the postbunionectomy type or a standard tennis shoe with a semiflexible steel sole insert is used to protect the foot. Progressive weight bearing is then begun. Patients are usually allowed to return to competitive sports when pain over the fifth metatarsal and the incision is gone. A soft-sole insert with protective padding over the lateral border of the foot at the base of the fifth metatarsal will prevent pressure over the screw head or under the fifth metatarsal head when the patient returns to activity.

In patients whose activity level is minimal, I use a period of immobilization in a short leg walking cast. Following casting the decision for intramedullary screw fixation is based on progression towards union. I have not used bone grafting of the fracture site in treatment of type II fractures.

In type IIIA fractures (in which the fracture is extraarticular and involves the tuberosity of the base of the fifth metatarsal), I prefer symptomatic treatment. The foot is strapped with or without a sturdy arch support until the patient becomes asymptomatic. In patients with marked displacement of the fracture, a short leg walking cast is used until pain allows treatment by strapping. In all cases, plaster immobilization is used *only* in patients in whom strapping or arch supports do

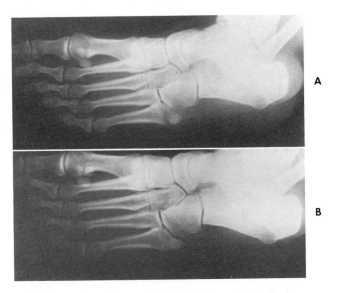

Fig. 24-98. **A,** Displaced intraarticular fracture of styloid process of base of fifth metatarsal. **B,** Fracture healed in displaced position. Patient is asymptomatic.

not alleviate pain. Weight bearing is begun as soon as the patient's pain allows it.

In patients with type IIIB fractures (fractures of the tuberosity involving the fifth metatarsocuboid joint), treatment is based on the patient's level of activity. In the highly competitive athlete, open reduction to restore articular congruity is recommended (see Fig. 24-94). However, in the majority of patients I have found that very little disability results from allowing the fracture to heal in the displaced position (Fig. 24-98). Should such a malunion produce symptoms, excision of the displaced fragment and advancement of the peroneus brevis tendon is undertaken.

STRESS FRACTURES OF METATARSAL DIAPHYSIS

Stress fractures are defined as spontaneous fractures of normal bone that result from a summation of stresses, any one of which by itself is harmless.[17,35] These fractures occur in the normal bones of healthy people involved in everyday activities.[15,17] Devas notes that these patients do not report a history of a specific injury.[15] Although stress fractures have been reported at many different sites, the metatarsals are among the best known sites of the stress fractures.[15] These fractures have been termed *march fractures* because of their frequent occurrence in military personnel.[4,20]

The distribution of stress fractures of the metatarsal diaphysis is variable, but they are noted most commonly in the second and third metatarsals.[19,42] Bernstein and Stone[4] found the second metatarsal most frequently involved, followed closely by the third metatarsal. The first, fourth, and fifth metatarsals were less frequently involved. Levy, however, found the order of frequency of stress fractures to be the second, third, first, fourth, and finally the fifth metatarsal.[35] Levy notes that the reason first metatarsal stress fractures are so rarely reported is their differing appearance radiographically.[35]

The etiology of these fractures is not completely understood, but it is felt to be recurrent microfractures of the involved bone.[21] As with stress fractures in other locations, force is applied to the bone in a normal physiologic manner, but the frequency and magnitude of the force is increased.[21] The physiologic response of the bone to this stress on a microscopic level is increased osteoclastic and osteoblastic activity. If such altered stress is given time to heal, the bone will remodel to accommodate the forces according to Wolff's law.[21] However, repetitive microfractures that are not given an opportunity to heal will produce a stress fracture across the shaft of the bone.

Predisposing conditions and activities

Congenital shortening of the first metatarsal has been suggested as a predisposing condition in the development of stress fractures of the second and third metatarsals.[3,56] However, Drez et al. were unable to show that the length of the first metatarsal in patients with stress fractures differed significantly from that in a randomly selected control group.[16] The occurrence of metatarsal stress fractures of the lateral metatarsals following Keller or Mayo bunion operations has been reported by Ford and Gilula.[18] Battey[3] theorized that the shortened first metatarsal, the posterior displacement

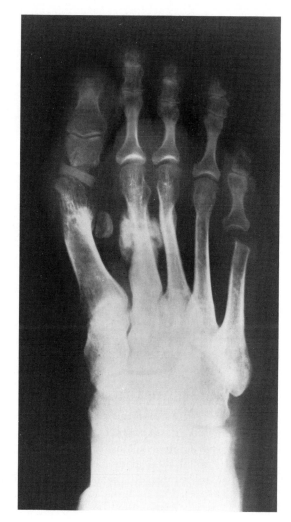

Fig. 24-99. Stress fractures of second and third metatarsal shafts after Keller bunionectomy with Silastic implant.

of the sesamoids caused by the loss of insertion of the flexor hallucis brevis, and hypermobility of the first ray following the Keller procedure all predisposed the foot to stress fractures of the lesser metatarsals[22,32] (Fig. 24-99).

Stress fractures are also commonly noted in new military recruits who undergo intensive training to which the bones of the foot are not adapted.[4,15] With the current enthusiasm for sports, particularly jogging, metatarsal stress fractures are being seen with increasing frequency in normal healthy young patients.[9,10]

Diagnosis

The most common presenting complaint is pain on a long march or with increased running on hard pavement.[20] The pain is usually described as an aching or soreness in the foot.[35,42,56] Although the pain is de-

direct trauma. In these situations the neurovascular status of the toe distal to the open fracture may be in jeopardy because of the fracture and the accompanying crushing of the soft tissues.

RADIOGRAPHIC FINDINGS

Anteroposterior, oblique, and lateral radiographs of the *toe* (not the foot) are necessary to delineate fracture location and displacement of the fracture. Although comminution is frequently present, most of these fractures are not significantly displaced, unlike fractures of the fingers.[6,7,9] Fractures of the hallux phalanges, however, are more commonly displaced. Jahss[10] emphasizes that fractures of the great toe vary from a mildly displaced fracture of the medial or lateral margin of the distal portion of the proximal phalanx to a frank fracture-dislocation. He stresses the importance of critically evaluating radiographs of the great toe to distinguish between simple fractures and fracture-dislocations involving the proximal phalanx. In these fractures, it is essential to have a *true* lateral radiograph of the hallux. Jahss also points out the value of magnification of radiographs to demonstrate fractures of the toes.[10] Radiographs taken with traction applied to hallux are often helpful in further evaluating the fracture (see Fig. 24-103, *B*).

TREATMENT

If an open fracture of the lesser toes is present, the wound should be irrigated and debrided just as any other open fracture.[5,6] Consideration is given to the use of intramedullary Kirschner wire fixation in cases in which severe soft tissue damage is present. Antibiotics

are given for 48 hours after initial irrigation and debridement. If the hallux is involved, the indications for internal fixation of the articular surface are the same as listed in this section.

In closed fractures, treatment recommendations depend on the digit involved.

Hallux phalangeal fractures

Fractures of the distal phalanx of the great toe are most often caused by dropping heavy objects on the toe.[12,14] This often results in comminution.[5] Subungual hematomas are usually present and can be relieved by drilling the nail bed.[7,11] Avulsion of the nail to decompress subungual hematoma is not warranted.[2]

In simple fractures of the phalanges of the great toe without displacement (Fig. 24-102), Cobey recommends treatment with a metatarsal bar. Alternatively, the great toe can be bound to the adjacent two toes for stability and ambulation initiated in a stiff soled shoe.[3] Johnson stresses the necessity for simple treatment of nondisplaced phalangeal fractures by protective splinting (usually to an adjacent toe), symptomatic medication, and immediate ambulation.[11]

Jahss[10] reports that displaced fractures of the hallux phalanges (when treated *early*) can usually be reduced closed with traction and local anesthetics and that the reduction can usually be maintained in a plaster boot. He recommends treatment by adhesive strapping of minor angulation or minor displacement of fractures through the condylar neck.

When hallux phalangeal fractures are displaced and reduction cannot be obtained by manipulation, Chapman suggests open reduction.[3] Taylor[14] stresses the im-

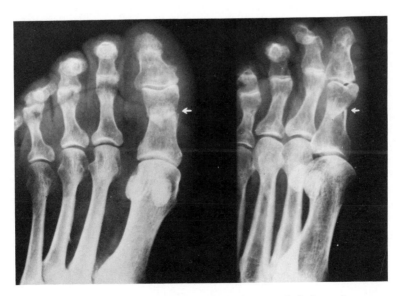

Fig. 24-102. Nondisplaced fracture (arrows) of proximal phalanx of great toe.

portance of maintaining the nail in treating fractures of the distal phalanx of the hallux. He believes it serves as an important splint to the broken phalanx and also that its removal exposes a tender area that will prevent the patient from returning to work for some weeks.[14] He recommends the use of a plaster of paris "thimble" enclosing the whole toe to provide immobilization of these fractures. Blodgett[2] recommends treating crush fractures of the terminal phalanx of the great toe with elevation and ice, followed by a cut-out shoe with a stiff sole. Heck[8] stresses that reduction is not always possible in such comminuted fractures, but care should be taken to place the toe in a functional position. If a crushing-type fracture of the great toe is open and severely comminuted and involves the majority of the distal phalanx with extensive soft tissue loss, debridement of the wound, nail excision, and a terminal Symes amputation may be indicated.[7]

If there is displacement of single fractures of the proximal or distal phalanx of the great toe, every attempt should made to correct the displacement.[6,10] Isolated medial or lateral condylar fractures or fracture-dislocations, typically seen in stubbing injuries, are unstable. Zrubecky[16] recommended open reduction and Kirschner wire stabilization of these unstable fractures (Fig. 24-103). Jahss[10] stresses that displaced fractures of the great toe phalanges, particularly those associated with dislocations of the adjacent joint, require *anatomic* reduction. Although outrigger pulp or skeletal traction has been advised in the presence of instability of these fractures,[5,8,9] Zorzi and Grisostomi consider this unnecessary and potentially dangerous, possibly leading to infection or vascular impairment of the digit.[15] Johnson[11] also cautions against such overtreatment of these injuries.

Lesser toe phalangeal fractures

In fractures involving the second, third, fourth, and fifth toe phalanges, Giannestras and Sammarco[7] believe moderate displacement is of no great significance. Although they recommend an attempt at reduction, they believe one need not be concerned if an anatomic reduction is not obtained, as long as the general alignment of the toe is satisfactory.[6,7] They treat these injuries by placing a single layer of sheet wadding between the involved toe and two adjacent toes. The toes are then strapped together with adhesive tape, with care taken not to compromise the circulation.[7] Ambulation is permitted in a stiff-soled shoe with the toe cut out. They emphasize that if the displacement is gross or if dislocation of the adjacent joint is present closed reduction with or without Kirschner wire fixation may be indicated.[7] Chapman[3] emphasizes that displacement of a fracture of the phalanges, particularly of the middle three toes, is rare, but when it does occur it can usually be reduced even without an anesthetic (Fig. 23-104). He too recommends adhesive strapping to the adjacent two toes for approximately 4 weeks and stresses *immediate* ambulation in a shoe with a semirigid sole.

Cobey[4] felt that most of the pain associated with a fractured toe results from dorsiflexing the toes with walking. In his opinion, neither taping adjacent toes together nor a hard leather sole will prevent this dorsiflexion. He therefore recommends the use of a metatarsal bar made from tongue blades and taped to the bottom of the shoe. The patient then begins early ambulation. He found that this method functionally immobilized the toes and the metatarsophalangeal joint without permanently altering the shoe. The use of tongue blades also eliminates the need for an expensive metatarsal bar.

On the other hand, Blodgett stresses that fractures of the proximal phalanx of the second through the fourth toes are prone to plantar angulation.[2] If this angulation persists, painful plantar pressure areas may develop under the toe and require operative correction.[2] He emphasizes that aggressive treatment of fractures of the proximal phalanx of the lesser toes is essential to prevent such deformity.[2] He suggests immobilization in flexion with Kirschner wire fixation or traction obtained by skin traction, pulp traction, or skeletal traction through the middle or distal phalanx. When severe comminution occurs, however, he recommends the use of adhesive taping to adjacent toes.[2] He stresses that such fractures need only be held in alignment by the tubular soft tissue of the toe and that full recovery of joint motion in the toe is not required for full walking function and shoe wearing. Johnson[11] strongly emphasizes the danger in overtreating and overprotecting patients with fractures of the phalanges, a practice which may result in long-term complications.

Long-term sequalae from phalangeal fractures of the

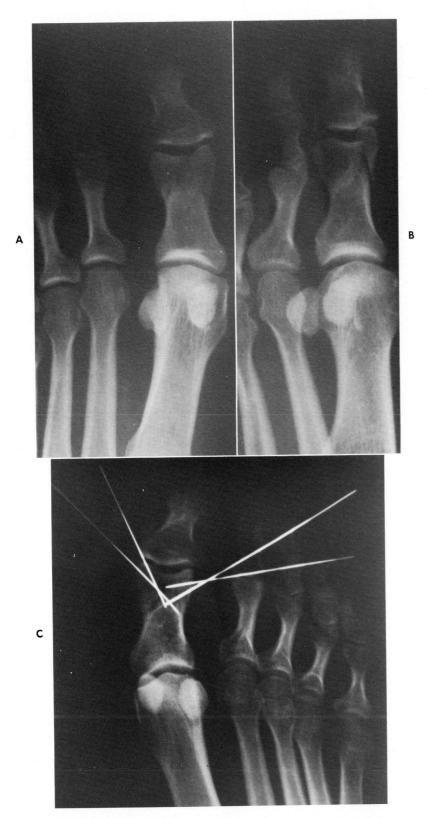

Fig. 24-103. A, Displaced fracture of both condyles of proximal phalanx of hallux. **B,** Radiograph taken with traction applied to better demonstrate fracture anatomy. **C,** Open reduction and internal fixation of fracture with Kirschner wires. Wires are cut off beneath skin and removed between 4 and 6 weeks. Note restoration of articular surface.

A   B   C

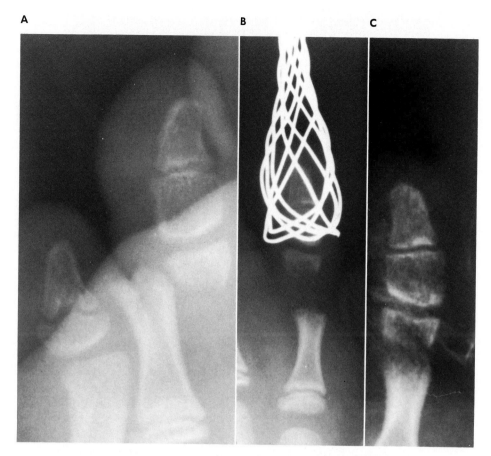

Fig. 24-104. A, Displaced fracture of proximal phalanx of third toe. **B,** Closed reduction using Chinese finger traps. Note distraction at fracture site. **C,** Stabilization by taping to adjacent toe. Alignment of fracture is excellent.

lesser toes are rarely reported. Angulation at the fracture site with malunion may result in a painful plantar pressure area under a toe, particularly when a fracture involves the proximal phalanx of the second through the fourth toe.[2] Such plantar pressure areas may require later operative correction.[2,12] However, according to Johnson, disability from stiffness, swelling, and occasional Sudek's atrophy resulting from the more aggressive types of therapy are more significant in regard to long-term disability.[11]

AUTHOR'S PREFERRED METHOD OF TREATMENT

In patients with open fractures involving the toes, thorough irrigation and debridement like that indicated in open fractures of the major bones is performed. With extensive soft tissue damage, I prefer axial Kirschner wire fixation as a splint to provide stability for soft tissue healing. If such open fractures involve the metatarsophalangeal or interphalangeal joint of the great toe, an anatomic reduction and Kirschner wire fixation is performed at the time of initial debridement. The patient is treated initially in a short leg cast and transferred to a stiff-soled shoe when swelling and pain permit.

Hallux phalangeal fractures

In nondisplaced simple fractures of the great toe, the foot is placed in a short leg walking cast with a toe plate until swelling and pain allow the use of a stiff-soled shoe with a high toe box.

In crushing injuries of the hallux phalanges in which there is comminution and no involvement of the interphalangeal joint, most attention is directed to care of the soft tissues. The subungual hematoma is drained after sterile preparation, and the foot is placed in a short leg cast with *immediate* ambulation.

In displaced fractures of the hallux, a closed reduction is attempted. If this is unsuccessful, open reduction and internal fixation are recommended. This is

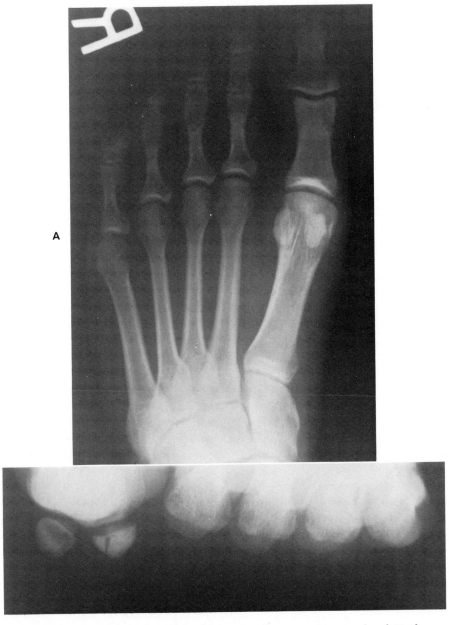

Fig. 24-108. Anteroposterior (**A**) and axial (**B**) views of patient with osteochondritis dissecans of fibular sesamoid. Note increased density. Patient is nonathletic and had spontaneous onset of pain.

Finally, a fractured sesamoid must be distinguished from osteochondritis dissecans of the first metatarsal sesamoid.[16,27] The radiographic findings in this condition are fragmentation, irregularity, and modeling of the sesamoid.[16] The axial view of the metatarsal head shows these changes, which may not be visible on standard anteroposterior projections[12,16] (see Fig. 24-108). The medial sesamoid is most commonly involved in osteochondritis and in fracture, and therefore the differentiation between the two is critical.[12]

TREATMENT
Nonoperative treatment

Initially, it is important to inform the patient that fractures of the sesamoids may be resistant to treatment and that symptoms are apt to persist for a long time.[8,21]

The treatment most frequently recommended following this injury is rest and protection of the first metatarsal head from weight bearing.[1,10,20]

Chapman immobilizes the fracture for 3 weeks with the metatarsophalangeal joint in a flexed position.[5] If this fails to relieve the symptoms, excision is recommended.[5] Coker and Arnold[6] also use cast immobilization for 3 weeks. If symptoms persist after 8 weeks of treatment, the fractured sesamoid may be excised.[6] Hobart[13] recommends the patient be kept off the injured foot and that it be immobilized until the fracture is healed, a period that he believes to be between 3 and 6 weeks. He recommends immobilization in a plaster of paris cast that includes the great toe during this period. However, Giannestras and Sammarco[11] believe that only in cases with severe pain is a short leg weight-bearing cast necessary.

Other authors have not recommended cast immobilization. Bizarro recommended the use of a metatarsal bar on the sole of the shoe, a trick he learned from Sir Robert Jones.[1] Morrison recommends an anterior arch support to remove the weight from the tender area for 1 to 2 months.[19] If symptoms persist, he recommends excision. Garcia and Parkes[10] also recommend the use of a comma-shaped metatarsal pad in the shoe to relieve pressure on the plantar aspect of the first metatarsal head or the use of a transverse metatarsal bar for a period of 6 to 8 weeks after the injury.

Orr[20] cautions that unless rest is prolonged, the patient may remain symptomatic. He therefore recommends a shoe with a depression on the inner sole designed to relieve pressure under the first metatarsal head for prolonged periods. He states that if the area is still tender after a reasonable period of conservative treatment, the sesamoid fragments should be excised. Giannestras and Sammarco[11] recommend a stiff-soled shoe and metatarsal pad with an elevation behind the head of the metatarsal to relieve pressure on the plantar aspect of the first metatarsal head. Although this fracture may unite with bony union if treated for an extended period, Brugman believes that the resulting callus may be a source of pain for some time after the use of the foot has been resumed, unless protective pads are used.[3]

Operative treatment

Although Brugman mentions immediate removal of the fractured sesamoid in an effort to decrease the morbidity from this fracture, no other authors recommend such aggressive initial treatment.[3] However, in cases with persistent disability after a reasonable period of conservative therapy, most authors recommend excision of the involved sesamoid.[5,6,10,11,20] The indications commonly given for sesamoid excision include: (1) painful nonunion, (2) prolonged pain in spite of conservative treatment, and (3) the development of posttraumatic degenerative changes on the sesamoid articular surface. Although Orr[20] credits Speed with suggesting that

both sesamoids be removed in these situations because of subsequent degenerative changes in the remaining sesamoid, Blodgett[2] confirms my experience that excision of only the fractured sesamoid is indicated.[2]

Several authors have emphasized the importance of placing the surgical incision so as to avoid painful scar formation.[19,25] Van Hal et al.[25] report the use of a medial longitudinal plantar incision to remove the medial sesamoid. However, care must be taken that the digital nerve be visualized and protected. Although Van Hal et al.[25] approach the fibular sesamoid through a plantar incision between the first and second metatarsal heads, a dorsal web-splitting incision between the first and second metatarsal heads will avoid a plantar scar and is safer. McBride recommends division of the strong intersesamoid ligament as early as possible in the procedure to allow easier mobilization and removal of the sesamoid.[2] Additionally, the sesamoid must be carefully shelled out of the tendon of the flexor hallucis brevis to prevent the later development of a cock-up deformity of the hallux.[11,22]

AUTHOR'S PREFERRED METHOD OF TREATMENT

A complete set of radiographs, including anteroposterior, oblique, and axial views of the sesamoid, is essential in evaluating injuries to these bones. The axial views are particularly helpful in distinguishing between osteochondritis dissecans, a bipartite sesamoid, and a fracture with displacement. Although I strive to distinguish between an acute fracture and a bipartite sesamoid, the conservative treatment I use for a painful bipartite sesamoid and for a fractured sesamoid are similar.

For patients who suffer a fracture of the sesamoid, I prefer a short leg walking cast with the walking heel placed so that all weight is transferred from beneath the first metatarsal head to a more posterior location. This cast is usually worn for 2 to 3 weeks. The foot is then placed in a stiff-soled shoe with a metatarsal pad placed behind the head of the first metatarsal to relieve pressure from the plantar aspect of the first metatarsal head. The patient is warned that total relief of symptoms may require 4 to 6 months, during which a metatarsal support is essential.

If significant symptoms persist after 6 months of conservative treatment, excision of the involved sesamoid is recommended. I prefer a medial longitudinal approach for tibial sesamoid excision and a dorsal incision between the first and second metatarsals for fibular sesamoid excision. Care is taken to protect the digital nerves with both incisions.

STRESS FRACTURES OF SESAMOIDS

Although Golding in 1960 alluded to hallux sesamoid stress fractures,[12] he did not provide histologic documentation of his cases. Scranton and Rutkowski[22] in 1980 reported the histology of a sesamoid excised from a runner, but they concluded the microscopic findings were indistinguishable from a nonunion or bipartite sesamoid. Van Hal et al.[25] reported four cases of stress fractures of the hallux sesamoid with histologic confirmation of the diagnosis. According to these authors, theirs were the first histologically documented cases of sesamoid stress fractures. Van Hal et al.[25] stressed that these patients have a history of the insidious onset of pain in the area of the first metatarsophalangel joint during and/or after athletic activity. The pain is usually relieved by rest. The pain is accentuated by palpation and hyperextension of the first metatarsophalangeal joint. Importantly, there is no history of a specific episode of foot trauma. The clinical differential diagnosis includes sesamoiditis and metatarsalgia.[22,25] Failure to recognize and treat the sesamoid stress fracture can lead to prolonged disability.[24]

If a stress fracture is suspected, Van Hal et al.[25] suggest weight-bearing anteroposterior, lateral, and axial radiographs at 3-week intervals. They emphasize that delay in diagnosis is likely if radiographs initially interpreted as being negative are not repeated. The authors also emphasize the importance of distinguishing stress fractures from the multipartite sesamoid.[12,15,25] Bone scans may demonstrate characteristic increased bony activity in the area of the first metatarsophalangel joint, while the multipartite sesamoid will be "cold" on scan.[25]

Although most stress fractures heal when the precipitating activity is limited, sesamoid stress fractures seem to behave differently.[25] None of the fractures presented by Van Hal et al.[25] healed despite 6 weeks of casting and/or 4 to 6 months of inactivity. The authors report that often persistent symptoms led to excision of the involved sesamoid before relief was obtained. However, following excision, all of their patients returned to athletic activities. They believe the anatomic location and biomechanic function of the sesamoids leads to the failure of nonoperative treatment.

Van Hal et al. recommend that all stress fractures of the sesamoids be treated immediately in a cast for 6 weeks, at which time new radiographs are taken and the foot recasted if necessary. Excision of the involved sesamoid is reserved for cases in which the fracture does not heal with casting or the athlete does not desire further casting.[25] Three patients in their series returned to prefracture activities without symptoms in an average of 10 weeks after excision. None of the patients had a loss of great toe flexion power as the result of sesamoid excision.[25]

AUTHOR'S PREFERRED METHOD OF TREATMENT

In patients at risk for a sesamoid stress fracture, early diagnosis is essential. If initial radiographs are negative, they are repeated in 3 weeks. If the second set of radiographs is negative, a bone scan is recommended.

Once the diagnosis has been confirmed, I prefer to treat these patients in a short leg cast with a toe plate to relieve the stresses on the metatarsophalangeal joint for 6 weeks. If the fracture is not healed, a second 6-week period is recommended. Following casting, a soft insert is placed behind the sesamoids in the arch of the foot to relieve the stress of weight bearing on the first metatarsophalangeal joint. If symptoms persist following this sequence of conservative therapy, excision is recommended.

REFERENCES

1. Bizarro, A.H.: On the traumatology of the sesamoid structures, Ann. Surg. 74:783-791, 1921.
2. Blodgett, W.H.: Injuries of the forefoot and toes. In Jahss, M.H., editor: Disorders of the foot, vol. 2, Philadelphia, 1982, W.B. Saunders Co.
3. Brugman, J.C.: Fractured sesamoids as a source of pain around the bunion joint, Milit. Surg. 49:310-313, 1921.
4. Burman, M.S., and Lapidus, P.W.: The functional disturbance caused by the inconstant bones and sesamoids of the foot, Arch. Surg. 22:936-975, 1931.
5. Chapman, M.W.: Fractures and dislocations of the ankle and foot. In Mann, R.A., editor: DuVries' surgery of the foot, ed. 4, St. Louis, 1978, The C.V. Mosby Co.
6. Coker, T.P., Jr., and Arnold, J.A.: Sports injuries to the foot and ankle. In Jahss, M.H., editor: Disorders of the foot, vol. 2, Philadelphia, 1982, W.B. Saunders Co.
7. Colwill, M.: Disorders of the metatarsal sesamoids, J. Bone Joint Surg. 52B:390, 1970.
8. Feldman, F., Pochaczevsky, R., and Hecht, H.: The case of the wandering sesamoid and other sesamoid afflictions, Radiology 96:275-284, 1970.
9. Freiberg, A.H.: Injuries to the sesamoid bones of the great toe, J. Bone Joint Surg. 2:453-465, 1920.
10. Garcia, A., and Parkes, J.E.: Fractures of the foot. In Giannestras, N.J., editor: Foot disorders: medical and surgical management, Philadelphia, 1973, Lea & Febiger.
11. Giannestras, N.J., and Sammarco, G.J.: Fractures and dislocations in the foot. In Rockwood, C.A., Jr., and Green, D.P., editors: Fractures, vol. 2, Philadelphia, 1975, J.B. Lippincott Co.
12. Golding, C.: Museum pages. V. The sesamoids of the hallux, J. Bone Joint Surg. 42B:840-843, 1960.
13. Hobart, M.H.: Fracture of sesamoid bones of the foot, J. Bone Joint Surg. 11:298-302, 1929.
14. Hubay, C.A.: Sesamoid bones of the hands and feet, Am. J. Roentgenol. 61:493-505, 1949.
15. Inge, G.L., and Ferguson, A.B.: Surgery of the sesamoid bones of the great toe, Arch. Surg. 21:456-489, 1933.
16. Ifeld, F.W., and Rosen, V.: Osteochondritis of the first metatarsal sesamoid, Clin. Orthop. 85:38-41, 1972.
17. Kelikian, H.: Hallux valgus, allied deformities of the forefoot and metatarsalgia, Philadelphia, 1965, W.B. Saunders Co.
18. Kewenter, Y.: Die Sesameine des Metatarso-phalangeal Gelenks des Menschein, Acta. Orthop. Scand. 2:1-108, 1936.

19. Morrison, G.M.: Fractures of the bones of the feet, Am. J. Surg. **38**:721-726, 1937.
20. Orr, T.G.: Fracture of the great toe sesamoid bones, Ann. Surg. **67**:609-612, 1918.
21. Powers, J.H.: Traumatic and developmental abnormalities of the sesamoid bones of the great toes, Am. J. Surg. **23**:315-321, 1934.
22. Scranton, P.E., and Rutkowski, R.: Anatomic variations in the first ray. Part B. Disorders of the sesamoids, Clin. Orthop. **151**:256-264, 1980.
23. Sisk, T.D.: Fractures. In Edmonson, A.S., and Crenshaw, A.H., editors: Campbell's operative orthopaedics, ed. 6, vol. 1, St. Louis, 1980, The C.V. Mosby Co.
24. Sundt, H.: On partition of the sesamoid bones of the lower extremities, Acta. Orthop. Scand. **15**:59-138, 1944.
25. Van Hal, M.E., Keene, J.S., Lange, T.A., and Clancy, W.G.: Stress fractures of the sesamoids, Am. J. Sports Med. **10**:122-128, 1982.
26. Wilson, D.W.: Fractures of the foot. In Klenerman, L., editor: The foot and its disorders, ed. 2, Oxford, England, 1982, Blackwell Scientific Publications.
27. Zimmer, E.A.: Borderlands of the normal and early pathologic in skeletal roentgenology, New York, 1968, Grune & Stratton, Inc., pp. 531-534.

Dislocations about the talus

Dislocations about the talus without fracture are classified into three types (see the box at right). The first is talocrural dislocation in which the talus is dislocated from the ankle mortise but the subtalar and midtarsal joints remain intact (Fig. 24-109) (the talocrural dislocation is not discussed in this chapter, but is included in Chapter 23.) The second is subtalar dislocation, in which the calcaneus is dislocated from the intact talus but the relationship of the talus with ankle mortise and midtarsal joints remains intact. The third is total dislocation of the talus in which the relationship of the talus

DISLOCATIONS ABOUT THE TALUS WITHOUT FRACTURE	
Type 1	Talocrural dislocation
Type 2	Subtalar dislocation
Type 3	Total dislocation of the talar body

with both the ankle and the subtalar joints is disrupted. The last two types of talar dislocations will be discussed in this section.

SUBTALAR DISLOCATIONS

Subtalar dislocation of the foot is an injury in which both the talocalcaneal and talonavicular joints are simultaneously dislocated. This injury is unassociated with a fracture of the neck of the talus.[9,12] The tibiotalar and calcaneocuboid joints remain intact.[37,44] Barber et al.[2] felt that the term *peritalar dislocation of the foot* more accurately describes this condition. These dislocations have also been designated subastraglar,[45] subastragaloid,[43] and talocalcaneal-navicular dislocations.[14]

Subtalar dislocations unassociated with regional fractures are uncommon injuries.* Leitner[29,30] and Smith[45] reported these dislocations to compromise 1% of all traumatic dislocations. Additionally, Pennal[41] reported that they comprise only 15% of all injuries to the talus.

Dufaurest and Judcy[11] were the first to report subtalar dislocations in 1811. Broca[4] in 1853 classified subtalar dislocations as medial, lateral, and posterior.

*References 1, 3, 9, 10, 44, 46, and 49.

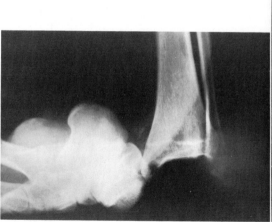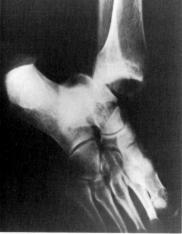

Fig. 24-109. Type I: talocrural dislocation.

Malgaigne[34] in 1855 added anterior dislocations to this classification. However, Fahey and Murphy[14] state that while posterior and anterior dislocations have been described, they usually are considered as part of the displacement present in the more common medial or lateral dislocations.

Most authors, however, have preferred to use the classification of Broca and Malgaigne.[9,17,32,44] Medial dislocations make up, by far, the majority of the subtalar dislocations.* According to Dunn,[12] Smith,[45] and Vincenti,[48] the frequency of occurrence in decreasing order is medial, lateral, posterior, and finally anterior dislocation. Larsen[28] reports that of all subtalar dislocations medial dislocations make up 59%, lateral dislocations 23%, posterior dislocations 11%, and anterior dislocations 7%. Patients suffering from this injury vary in age from 10 to 70, with men being affected from 3 to 10 times more frequently than women.[44]

Anatomy

The subtalar joint consists of three facets, anterior, medial and posterior through which the talus and calcaneus articulate.[5] The talus and calcaneus are united by the strong interosseous talocalcaneal ligament in the sinus tarsi.[5,44] A fibrous capsule also connects the adjacent articular margins of the three talocalcaneal facets.[44] Medially, the superficial portions of the deltoid ligament, and laterally, the calcaneofibular ligament, supplement talocalcaneal stability.[5,44] Finally, the talus and navicular are united by a weak talonavicular capsule. All of these structures must be disrupted for a subtalar dislocation to occur. Additionally, the closely contoured surfaces of the subtalar joint afford significant stability to the joint, particularly regarding anteroposterior displacement.[44] Because of this bony stability, fractures involving the lateral process and posterior tubercles of the talus are often associated with subtalar dislocations.[9,44]

Buckingham reports that the head of the talus appears between the extensor hallucis longus and the long toe extensors in medial subtalar dislocations, resting either on the navicular or cuboid bone.[5] In lateral dislocations the prominent head of the talus is palpable over the medial aspect of the foot, while the heel is displaced laterally.[5] He termed the medial dislocation in which the forepart of the foot is dislocated medially the *acquired clubfoot*, while the lateral dislocation is occasionally called the *acquired flatfoot*.[5]

Mechanism of injury

The mechanism of a medial subtalar dislocation is plantar flexion of the foot with forceful inversion of the

---

*References 9, 12, 14, 17, 25, and 30.

forefoot.[5] This results in the neck of the talus pivoting with the sustentaculum tali as a fulcrum. This movement produces a dislocation of the talonavicular joint followed by dislocation of the subtalar joint.[5,14-16,28,36] The less common lateral dislocation occurs with plantar flexion of the foot accompanied by forceful eversion of the forefoot. This results in the anterolateral corner of the talus pivoting over the anterior calcaneal process as a fulcrum.[14,36,38] The head of the talus is forced through the talonavicular capsule, and the calcaneus is dislocated laterally.[44]

Giannestras and Sammarco[16] emphasize that the actual forces required to produce subtalar dislocations are not necessarily great. Kleiger and Ahmed[26] emphasize that even with minor injuries the cartilage of the articular surfaces may be fractured or contused along with *or* independent of fractures involving the subchondral bone. This concept is particularly important when considering long-term sequalae. However, as the amount of force producing the dislocation increases, so does the incidence of poor results caused by increased soft tissue and bony damage.

Grantham[17] termed medial subtalar dislocation *basketball foot* because the majority of the patients he reported were injured while playing basketball. This mechanism, involving plantar flexion and inversion, is less forceful. This is evidenced by the excellent range of motion of the subtalar joint and minimal radiographic evidence of subtalar arthritis at follow-up.[17] On the other hand, injuries secondary to motor vehicle accidents or falls from heights are more often associated with more initial trauma, a higher incidence of associated intraarticular fractures, and usually a poorer clinical result.[9]

Clinical diagnosis

Although the patient may give a history of severe trauma to the foot,[15,44] Grantham[17] and DeLee and Curtis[9] emphasized that subtalar dislocations, particularly medial, can occur secondary to minor trauma such as a missed step. The patient usually complains of pain about the hindfoot.[16] The entire foot is swollen, and any motion of the ankle and subtalar joint is painful.[15,16] There is a complete loss of the normal bony contours of the foot in the region of the ankle joint.[15]

The clinical appearance of the foot is an excellent key to the type of subtalar dislocation. In medial subtalar dislocations the foot is plantar flexed, adducted, and supinated, and the head of the talus is prominent over the dorsolateral aspect of the foot[14,44,47] (Fig. 24-110, A). The overlying skin may appear blanched.[14] The heel is noted to be displaced medially in relation to the long axis of the leg.[44,47] Additionally, the toes may be dorsiflexed.[14] The lateral border of the foot appears long, while the medial border appears short.[14] In lat-

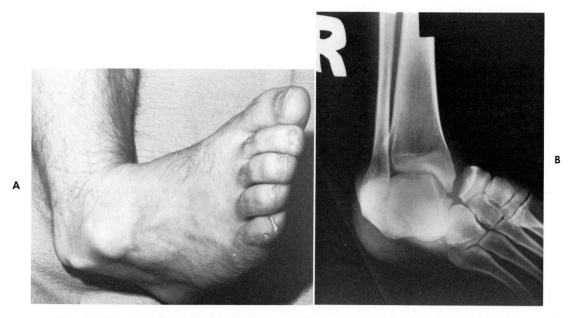

Fig. 24-110. A, Medial subtalar dislocation. **B,** Radiograph of medial subtalar dislocation. (From DeLee, J.C., and Curtis, R.: J. Bone Joint Surg. **64A:**433-437, 1982.)

eral subtalar dislocations, the foot appears pronated and abducted, and the toes may appear in the plantar-flexed position.[14] The prominent talar head is palpable medially, and the heel is lateral to the long axis of the leg[44,47] (Fig. 24-111). In posterior dislocations, the foot is shortened and the heel projects posteriorly, but the normal longitudinal axis of the foot with the lower leg is maintained.[28,44] In anterior dislocations, the heel is flattened, and the foot appears to be extended while maintaining its normal longitudinal orientation[28,44] (Fig. 24-112). Any of the four types of subtalar dislocation may present as an open injury. Additionally, the displacement of the dislocation may result in compromise of circulation to the overlying skin[14,16,44] and necessitate immediate reduction to prevent necrosis.

Radiographic diagnosis

Anteroposterior, lateral, and oblique radiographs of the foot are the *minimum* views required for complete evaluation of a subtalar dislocation.[15,16,44] Routine radiographs reveal the talus to be in a flexed position and the forefoot and os calcis to be displaced medially, laterally, anteriorly, or posteriorly depending on the particular type of dislocation.[9,15,16] Barber et al.[2] stressed the use of a superoinferior view of the foot to clearly demonstrate the absence of the head of the talus in the cup of the navicular.

The foot is displaced medially in a medial dislocation, revealing the plantar articulations of the talus without the calcaneus beneath it (see Fig. 24-110, *A*). In the

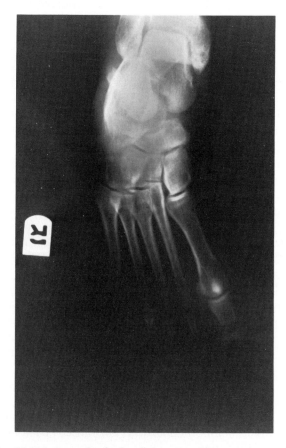

Fig. 24-111. Lateral subtalar dislocation. (From DeLee, J.C., and Curtis, R.: J. Bone Joint Surg. **64A:**433-437, 1982.)

flexed, the heel pulled plantarward, and the foot dorsiflexed as a unit. In a pure anterior dislocation the foot is plantar flexed, the heel pulled forward, and then the entire foot is pushed posteriorly as a unit. Following closed reduction, a repeat set of radiographs is obtained and careful evaluation of the subtalar joint for accurate reduction is performed. If no associated intraarticular fractures are seen on routine films, polytomography is recommended. If large intraarticular fractures are present, consideration is given to open reduction and internal fixation or to excision. In patients with small intraarticular fractures that prevent an anatomic reduction of the subtalar joint, excision is recommended.

If closed reduction with the patient under general anesthesia fails, I proceed directly to an open reduction. In an irreducible medial dislocation I use a surgical incision parallel to the long axis of the foot placed over the talar head, which is easily palpated. This allows direct access to the extensor retinaculum and extensor digitorum brevis, which are most likely to be the obstacles to reduction. In an irreducible lateral dislocation, I prefer an incision over the sinus tarsi. This allows exposure of both the subtalar and midtarsal joints and direct visualization of the neck of the talus and the commonly obstructing posterior tibial tendon. In patients with irreducible anterior or posterior dislocations, a longitudinal incision parallel to the sole of the foot and just below the distal fibula is used. This allows direct access to the subtalar joint, which can then be reduced under direct vision.

Following reduction of the dislocation and careful radiographic evaluation, the foot is placed in a short leg nonwalking cast for 3 weeks. The cast is well-molded in the arch of the foot, but extends only to the metatarsophalangeal joints. Range of motion exercises to the metatarsophalangeal joint are begun *immediately*. At 3 weeks the cast is removed and the patient begun on subtalar and ankle motion using both active and active-assisted methods. Intermittent soaking or swimming pool exercises may be added.[27] If associated fractures are present, the I prefer a short period of immobilization, 3 to 4 weeks, followed by early range of motion as mentioned previously. The only indication I have for a longer period of immobilization is a patient in whom excision or comminution of fracture fragments has rendered the joint unstable. This determination is made at the time of the initial reduction and may require immobilization from 4 to 6 weeks.

During the rehabilitation phase, if subtalar or midtarsal motion does not appear to be progressing satisfactorily, I have used manipulation with the patient under anesthesia up to 3 months after injury. I have noted a significant improvement in the range of motion following this regime.

In patients in whom an open dislocation is present, extensive irrigation and debridement are carried out *before* reduction of the dislocation. Performing an irrigation and debridement before reduction allows access to the subtalar and talonavicular joints. Once the irrigation and debridement are completed, a reduction under direct vision is performed. A second irrigation and debridement of equal thoroughness is then performed. The wound is left open and a delayed primary closure is performed at 5 to 7 days. The period of immobilization and postoperative management are identical to those for patients with closed injuries.

REFERENCES
Subtalar dislocations

1. Atsatt, R.F.: Subastragalar dislocation of the foot, J. Bone Joint Surg. **13**:574-577, 1931.
2. Barber, J.R., Bricker, J.D., and Haliburton, R.A.: Peritalar dislocation of the foot, Can. J. Surg. **4**:205-210, 1961.
3. Bohler, L.: The treatment of fractures, vol. 3, ed. 5, New York, 1958, Grune and Stratton, Inc.
4. Broca, P.: Memoire sur les luxations sous-astragaliennes, Mem. Soc. Chir. **3**:566-656, 1853.
5. Buckingham, W.W.: Subtalar dislocation of the foot, J. Trauma **13**:753-765, 1973.
6. Chapman, M.W.: Fractures and fracture-dislocations of the ankle and foot. In Mann, R.A., editor: DuVries' surgery of the foot, ed. 4, St. Louis, 1978, The C.V. Mosby Co.
7. Christensen, S.B., Lorentzen, J.E., Krogsoe, O., and Sneppen, O.: Subtalar dislocation, Acta. Orthop. Scand. **48**:707-711, 1977.
8. Coltart, W.D.: "Aviator's astragalus," J. Bone Joint Surg. **34B**:545-566, 1952.
9. DeLee, J.C., and Curtis, R.: Subtalar dislocation of the foot, J. Bone Joint Surg. **64A**:433-437, 1982.
10. Detenbeck, L.C., and Kelly, P.J.: Total dislocation of the talus, J. Bone Joint Surg. **51A**:283-288, 1969.
11. Dufaurest, P.: Luxation du pied en dehors, compliquee de l'issue de l'astragale a travers le capsule et les tequmens dechires, J. Med. Chir. Pharm. **22**:348-355, 1811.
12. Dunn, A.W.: Peritalar dislocation, Orthop. Clin. North Am. **5**:7-18, 1974.
13. Dwyer, F.C.: Causes, significance and treatment of stiffness of the subtaloid joint, Proc. R. Soc. Med. **69**:97-102, 1976.
14. Fahey, J.J., and Murphy, J.L.: Dislocations and fractures of the talus, Surg. Clin. North Am. **45**:79-102, 1965.
15. Garcia, A., and Parkes, J.C.: Fractures of the foot. In Giannestras, N.J., editor: Foot disorders: medical and surgical management, ed. 2, Philadelphia, 1973, Lea & Febiger.
16. Giannestras, N.J., and Sammarco, G.J.: Fractures and dislocations in the foot. In Rockwood, C.A., and Green, D.P., editors: Fractures, Philadelphia, 1975, J.B. Lippincott Co.
17. Grantham, S.A.: Medial subtalar dislocation: five cases with a common etiology, J. Trauma **4**:845-849, 1964.
18. Gross, R.H.: Medial peritalar dislocation: associated foot injuries and mechanism of injury, J. Trauma **15**:682-688, 1975.
19. Haliburton, R.A., Barber, J.R., and Fraser, R.L.: Further experience with peritalar dislocation, Can. J. Surg., **10**:322-324, 1967.
20. Hauser, E.D.W.: Management of lesions of the subtalar joint, Surg. Clin. N. Am. **25**:136-160, February, 1945.
21. Heppenstall, R.B., Farahvar, H., Balderston, R., and Lotke, P.: Evaluation and management of subtalar dislocations, J. Trauma **20**:494-497, 1980.

22. Inman, V.T.: The joints of the ankle, Baltimore, 1976, The Williams & Wilkins Co.

23. Inman, V.T., and Mann, R.A.: Principles of examination of the foot and ankle. In Mann, R.A., editor: DuVries' surgery of the foot, ed. 4, St. Louis, 1978, The C.V. Mosby Co.

24. Judcy, P.: Observation d'une luxation metatarsienne, Bull. Fac. Med. Paris, **11**:81-86, 1811.

25. Kenwright, J., and Taylor, R.G.: Major injuries of the talus, J. Bone Joint Surg. **52B**:36-48, 1970.

26. Kleiger, B., and Ahmed, M.: Injuries of the talus and its joints, Clin. Orthop. **121**:243-261, 1976.

27. Lapidus, P.W., and Guidotti, F.P.: Immediate mobilization and swimming pool exercises in some fractures of the foot and ankle bones, Clin. Orthop. **56**:197-206, 1968.

28. Larsen, H.W.: Subastragalar dislocation (luxatio pedis sub talo): a follow-up report of eight cases, Acta. Chir. Scand. **113**:380-392, 1957.

29. Leitner, B.: Behandlung und Behandlungsergebnisse von 42 frischen Fallen von Luxatio pedis sub talo im Unfallkrankenhaus Wien in den Jahren 1925-1950, Ergeb. Chir. Orthop. **37**:501-577, 1952.

30. Leitner, B.: Obstacles to reduction in subtalar dislocations, J. Bone Joint Surg. **36A**:299-306, 1954.

31. Loup, J.: Luxation ouverte sous-astragalienne, Ann. Chir. **27**:993-995, 1973.

32. Mac, S.S., and Kleiger, B.: The early complications of subtalar dislocation, Foot Ankle **1**:270-274, 1981.

33. McKeever, F.M.: Treatment of complications of fractures and dislocations of the talus, Clin. Orthop. **30**:45-52, 1963.

34. Malgaigne, J.F., and Burger, C.G.: Du knochenbruche and verrenkungen, Stuttgart, 1856, Reiger.

35. Mindell, E.R., Cisek, E.E., Kartalian, G., and Dziob, J.M.: Late results of injuries to the talus, J. Bone Joint Surg. **45A**:221-245, 1963.

36. Monson, S.T., and Ryan, J.R.: Subtalar dislocation, J. Bone Joint Surg. **63A**:1156-1158, 1981.

37. Mulroy, R.D.: The tibialis posterior tendon as an obstacle to reduction of a lateral anterior subtalar dislocation, J. Bone Joint Surg. **37A**:859-863, 1955.

38. O'Brien, E.T.: Injuries of the talus, Am. Fam. Physician **12**(5):95-105, 1975.

39. Parkes, J.C., II: Injuries of the hindfoot. Clin. Orthop. **122**:28-36, 1977.

40. Pavlov, H.: Ankle and subtalar arthrography. Clin. Sports Med. **1**:47-69, 1982.

41. Pennal, G.F.: Fractures of the talus, Clin. Orthop. **30**:53-63, 1963.

42. Plewes, L.W., and McKelvey, K.G.: Subtalar dislocation, J. Bone Joint Surg. **26**:585-588, 1944.

43. Shands, A.R., Jr.: The incidence of subastragaloid dislocation of the foot with a report of one case of the inward type, J. Bone Joint Surg. **10**:306-313, 1928.

44. Shelton, M.L., and Pedowitz, W.J.: Injuries to the talus and midfoot. In Jahss, M.H., editor: Disorders of the foot, vol. 2, Philadelphia, 1982, W.B. Saunders Co.

45. Smith, H.: Subastragalar dislocation, J. Bone Joint Surg. **19**:373-380, 1937.

46. Soustelle, J., Meyer, P., and Sauvage, Y.: Luxation sousastragalienne fermee, Lyon Chir. **60**:119, 1964.

47. Straus, D.C.: Subtalus dislocation of the foot: with report of two cases, Am. J. Surg. **30**:427-434, 1935.

48. Vincenti, F.R.: Subtalar dislocations, Paper presented at the Western Orthopaedic Association Meeting, Houston, 1975.

49. Von Vogt, H.: Drei seltene Verrenkungsformen im talusbereich, Schweiz. Med. Wochenschr. **89**:1005, 1959.

50. Wilhelm, B., and Komanov, I.: Subtalus luxation of the foot, Lijec. Vjes. **94**:283-286, 1972.

51. Wright, P.E.: Dislocations. In Edmonson, A.S., and Crenshaw, A.H., editors: Campbell's operative orthopaedics, vol. 1, ed. 6, St. Louis, 1980, The C.V. Mosby Co.

TOTAL DISLOCATION OF TALUS

Total dislocation of the talus, in which the talus is dislocated both from the ankle joint and from the rest of the foot, is extremely unusual, accounting for no more than 10% of all major talar injuries.[13] Indeed, Coltart[2] was able to find only 9 cases of total dislocation in 228 major talar injuries. Two thirds of these were open injuries, and all were the result of aircraft accidents. Detenbeck and Kelley[4] in 1969 reported an additional 9 cases, 7 open. Most of the literature consists of isolated case reports,* with no one author having extensive experience with these injuries.

Mechanism of injury

Leitner[9] believes that total dislocation of the talus actually represents the end-point in the spectrum of supination or pronation injury to the ankle. According to Leitner[9] a first-degree supination injury to the ankle results in a medial subtalar dislocation, while the second-degree supination injury results in medial subtalar dislocation and talocrural subluxation. Finally, the third-degree supination injury results in total *lateral* dislocation of the talus. A first-degree pronation injury, on the other hand, results in a lateral subtalar dislocation, while the second-degree pronation injury results in a lateral subtalar dislocation *and* a talocrural subluxation.[9] The third-degree pronation injury results in total *medial* dislocation of the talus. Therefore the position of the talus in a total talar dislocation gives an indication as to whether supination or pronation was the mechanism of injury.[9] Leitner reports that supination injuries are much more common than pronation injuries; therefore lateral talar dislocations are more common than those that occur medially.[9]

Pinzur and Meyer[15] in 1977 reported a case of complete posterior dislocation of the talus. The posterior location of the talar body in this case suggests that neither pronation or supination is the mechanism of injury. Instead, this injury was accompanied by diastasis of the ankle and a fracture of the anterior process of the calcaneus, suggesting that severe dorsiflexion and forward displacement of the foot onto the leg were the mechanisms of injury.

Finally, Pennal[14] reports that total dislocation of the talus is a result of a severe plantar-flexion and inversion force on the foot. He believes that extreme plantar flex-

---

*References 1, 4, 7, 9, 10, 12-14, 17, and 18.

ion causes a forward dislocation of the foot at the ankle joint with complete rupture of the collateral ligaments. As this force continues, an additional inversion stress will cause disruption of the talocalcaneal ligaments. As the displaced foot recoils, the detached talus remains rotated, lying anterior to the lateral malleolus.

Clinical diagnosis

According to Coltart[3] and Detenbeck and Kelley,[4] 75% of these injuries are open. The open wound consists of an irregular laceration, and the patient may actually come for medical attention with his talus wrapped in a handkerchief.[13]

In patients with a closed injury, physical examination will reveal marked inversion of the foot with a prominence located *anterior* to either the lateral or medial malleolus or posteriorly.[9,12,15,20] The skin over the prominence of the talus is tented and blanched.[12,14] The posterior and anterior neurovascular bundle may be compromised by the dislocation, leading to signs and symptoms of ischemia in the foot when it is first seen.[1,4]

Radiographic diagnosis

Total dislocation of the talus is easily visualized on anteroposterior, lateral, and oblique views of the foot. However, Segal and Wasilewski[17] documented a complete talar dislocation that initially presented only as a talocrural dislocation. Only after stress radiographs were taken was it apparent that the connections of the talus to the calcaneus and midtarsal joints had been disrupted. The associated dislocations had apparently spontaneously reduced. These authors therefore emphasize the need for stress radiographs to test the integrity of the of the ligaments of the talonavicular and talocalcaneal articulations when a talocrural dislocation is evident radiographically.[17]

Treatment

Following total dislocation of the talus, most authors prefer open or closed reduction in an effort to preserve function of the joint and length of the extremity.[5,11-13,20,22] On the other hand, Detenbeck and Kelley[4] advocated primary excision of the talus and tibiocalcaneal fusion in an effort to prevent the long-term sequalae of infection that may follow open reduction.

All major vascular connections to the talus are usually disrupted in total dislocation of the talus, thereby leaving it completely avascular. However, incomplete dislocations and occasionally total dislocations may spare some ligamentous attachments to the talus, particularly the deltoid ligament, which explains why aseptic necrosis does not occur in all of these patients.[11,12,19] Segal and Wasilewski[17] found despite total dislocation of the talus in their patient that the lateral malleolus remained attached by ligamentous tissue to the talus, thereby providing a blood supply to the talus and preventing the development of aseptic necrosis.

In closed injuries, immediate reduction is essential to remove pressure on the overlying skin. Pennal[14] reports a successful closed reduction of a total dislocation of the talus; however, aseptic necrosis later developed and required tibiocalcaneal fusion. Newcomb and Brav[12] also report successful closed reduction of a complete dislocation of the talus. They recommend spinal anesthesia for muscle relaxation, followed by the insertion of a Kirschner wire through the calcaneus to be used as a traction pin. Countertraction is obtained through a Steinmann pin inserted through the distal tibia. These two pins are used to achieve the distraction of the ankle joint space, which is necessary to allow reduction of the talus.[11,12,14] Once this distraction is obtained, pressure in a posteromedial direction over the laterally dislocated talus may force the displaced bone back into the ankle mortise. Newcomb and Brav[12] recommend removal of the Kirschner wires following the reduction. Following closed reduction, the talus is usually stable. The authors recommend a long leg cast for 4 weeks.[12] Shelton and Pedowitz[20] caution against attempting ligamentous repair, particularly of the deltoid ligament, following successful closed reduction for fear of further compromise to the damaged overlying skin.

If closed reduction of a total dislocation of the talus is unsuccessful, open reduction is indicated. Shelton and Pedowitz[20] recommend the use of skeletal traction provided by Kirschner wires through the calcaneus and tibia in a manner similar to that used for closed reduction. An incision is made over the displaced talus, and the reduction is performed under direct vision. They strongly recommend capsular repair in an effort to cover exposed joint surfaces, since later skin necrosis may develop.[20] They suggest leaving the skin open and delaying primary closure in an effort to minimize skin necrosis. When closure cannot be obtained within 5 days, they encourage coverage by myocutaneous or free flap, because wounds left open more than 7 days may become infected.[20]

Up to 75% of these cases present as open injuries, with the open wounds being of a crushing, bursting type.[2,4] The margins of the wound are often ischemic with early necrosis and are usually severely contaminated. O'Brien[13] cautions against discarding the talus in these open dislocations. He recommends that the wound and the talus be extensively cleansed and the talus replaced in its proper position using Kirschner wires to maintain the reduction. He recommends that the skin be left open and closed secondarily. He believes that the talus should not be discarded unless an infection intervenes or primary treatment is extremely delayed. Following extensive debridement of the skin edges, Shelton and Pedowitz[20] also recommend replacement of the talus, leaving the wound open for delayed closure. If delayed closure is not possible, either free or regional myocutaneous flaps may be necessary to cover the skin defect in an effort to prevent the development of talar osteomyelitis. After reduction, Shelton and Pedowitz[20] recommend a long leg cast for 4 weeks followed by further immobilization in a short leg cast. They recommend the patient be followed closely for the development of Hawkin's sign indicating talar aseptic necrosis.[6] A more complete discussion of the diagnosis and treatment of aseptic necrosis is found in the section on Fractures of the Neck of the Talus.

Detenbeck and Kelley[4] reported 9 cases of total dislocation of the talus in which there were *no* successful closed reductions. In spite of open reduction, infection occurred in 8 of their 9 patients, with the result that 7 required talectomy. As a result of this experience, these authors recommend a more aggressive approach to this injury that includes talectomy and tibiocalcaneal arthrodesis as their initial treatment. These authors[4] and Pennal[14] report that talectomy alone is not satisfactory because of progressive pain, varus deformity, and weakness of the foot that results after talectomy. However, Shelton and Pedowitz[20] caution that tibiocalcaneal fusion results in significant shortening of the limb and decrease in foot height, and therefore, they suggest pantalar arthrodesis as a salvage procedure for posttraumatic arthritis.

Complications

Soft tissue infection. Shelton and Pedowitz[20] stress the importance of wound debridement and leaving skin open primarily to avoid infection. If early soft tissue infection occurs, prompt debridement and closure performed when the infection is controlled will help to prevent septic arthritis and talar osteomyelitis, which usually require talectomy for salvage.

Osteomyelitis. The fact that 8 of 9 patients reported by Detenbeck and Kelley[4] became infected following total dislocation of the talus emphasizes the importance of *early* adequate debridement and reduction. If the patient presents with an infection involving the talus following this injury, excision of the body of the talus with tibiocalcaneal arthrodesis is an acceptable salvage procedure.[4] Only rarely can the talar body be salvaged if it is infected. Even though tibiocalcaneal fusion resulted in a shortened extremity, it did not cause significant disability in their patients.[4] However, when talectomy alone was used, pain and giving way were significant complications.

Aseptic necrosis. Aseptic necrosis may occur following total dislocation of the talus. Shelton and

Pedowitz[20] emphasize that revascularization following this injury may be slow because of the large area covered with articular cartilage that limits access for revascularization. However, the medial talar attachment of the deltoid ligament is an important route of talar revascularization. The fact that revascularization often begins medially supports the importance of this soft tissue attachment.[4,8,14] It is essential to emphasize that even though a patient develops aseptic necrosis, good to fair function may result, particularly if it is without collapse. (For further discussion of talar aseptic necrosis see the section on Talar Neck Fractures.)

Posttraumatic arthritis. Posttraumatic arthritis may occur in the subtalar, midtarsal, and/or ankle joint, depending on the severity of the initial injury, whether the initial injury was open or closed, and the presence or absence of aseptic necrosis.[4,8,14] Degenerative arthritis following this injury is best treated by arthrodesis of the involved joints, whether by triple or pantalar arthrodesis. The management of posttraumatic arthritis of the subtalar, midtarsal, and ankle joints is discussed under Talar Neck Fractures, Complications.

AUTHOR'S PREFERRED METHOD OF TREATMENT

A closed total dislocation of the talus is considered a surgical emergency. The patient is brought to the operating room and prepped using sterile technique for an open reduction. A Kirschner wire is placed through the calcaneus and a Steinmann pin in the distal tibia to apply traction. Traction is applied under image intensification to distract the joint. One attempt is made at a closed reduction by manipulating the displaced talus in a posteromedial or posterolateral direction (depending on whether talar body displacement is anteromedial or anterolateral). If this is unsuccessful, an immediate open reduction with incision directly over the displaced talus is done. Once the talus is exposed, distraction is again obtained by use of the pins in the tibia and calcaneus, and the talus is manipulated back into the ankle mortise.

Following closed reduction, the foot is placed in a long leg bent-knee cast for 4 weeks. This is followed by a short leg cast for an additional 2 weeks. Weight bearing in a patellar tendon–bearing brace is begun at 6 weeks if swelling allows. Although these injuries have a high incidence of aseptic necrosis, the fact that revascularization of the talus may require more than 2 years makes prolonged non-weight bearing impractical.

If an open reduction is performed, the capsule is closed over the displaced talus, but the skin and subcutaneous tissues are left open. The patient is brought back to the operating room in 3 to 5 days for a delayed primary closure. Delayed wound closure is recom-

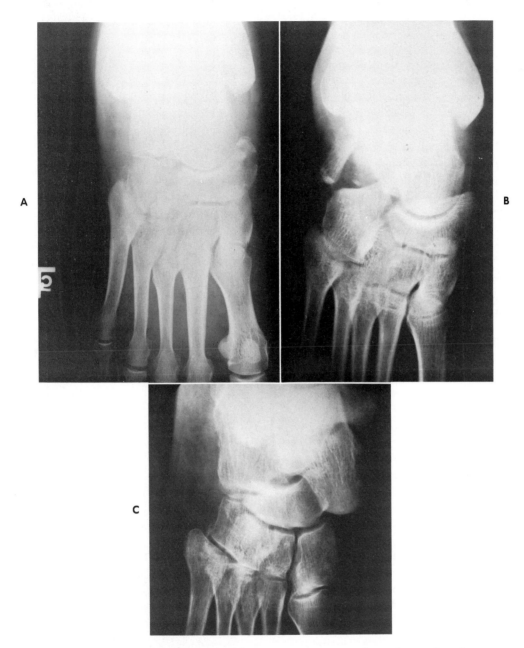

Fig. 24-118. Lateral injuries. **A,** Lateral fracture sprain. Note avulsion of navicular tuberosity and impaction fracture of cuboid. **B,** Lateral fracture-subluxation. Note comminution of anterior process of os calcis and subluxation of midtarsal joint. **C,** Lateral swivel dislocation. Lateral dislocation of talonavicular joint with calcaneocuboid joint intact. (From Main, B.J., and Jowett, R.L.: J. Bone Joint Surg. **57B:**89-97, 1975.)

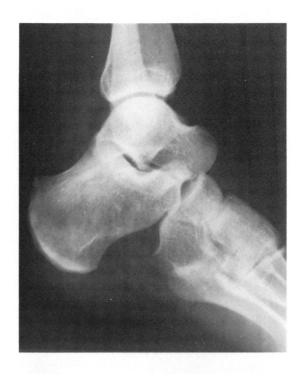

Fig. 24-119. Plantar dislocation. Subtalar joint is intact. (From Main, B.J., and Jowett, R.L.: J. Bone Joint Surg. **57B:**89-97, 1975.)

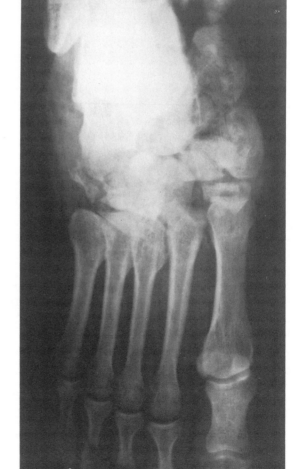

Fig. 24-120. Crush injury with severe comminution of tarsal bones. (From Main, B.J., and Jowett, R.L.: J. Bone Joint Surg. **57B:**89-97, 1975).

stopped when the inferior medial portion of the cuboid impinges on the end of the coronoid fossa of the os calcis.[22A] The motion of pronation-abduction-extension is blocked when the anterior process or beak of the os calcis impinges on the cuboid.[22A]

Motion through the talonavicular joint includes pronation with minimal abduction-extension and supination with minimal adduction-flexion.[22A] The talonavicular and calcaneocuboid joints function in unison with the subtalar joint to produce inversion and eversion.[24]

The calcaneocuboid joint is stabilized by the medial calcaneocuboid ligament, the dorsolateral calcaneocuboid ligament, and the inferior calcaneocuboid ligament.[22A] The talonavicular joint is stabilized by the talonavicular ligament, which occupies the interval between the superior medial calcaneonavicular ligament and the lateral calcaneonavicular ligament. These ligaments help to stabilize the midtarsal joint and are responsible for the avulsion fractures that occur in association with subluxation or dislocation of this joint.[22A]

Jones[17] stressed that the medial longitudinal arch of the foot consists of elements articulating with each other through curved surfaces, a fact that provides elasticity to the medial longitudinal arch because of its ability to "give and bend." However, the arch becomes less elastic toward the lateral border of the foot, resulting in a more static, rigid relationship important to foot stability. Hence, although the medial longitudinal arch permits elasticity, lateral arch rigidity is responsible for the fact that these injuries are relatively uncommon.

MECHANISM OF INJURY

Dewar and Evans[5] believe the mechanism of occult fracture-subluxation of the midtarsal joint is forced abduction, which results in an avulsion fracture of the navicular with the fragment remaining attached to the posterior tibial tendon. The forefoot, freed on the medial arch, swings further into abduction and produces a compression fracture involving the calcaneocuboid joint. Fractures of the tubercle or body of the navicular associated with midtarsal dislocations were also noted by Kenwright and Taylor,[18] a fact which supports this mechanism. This mechanism results in an unstable fracture-subluxation of the midtarsal joint.[5,18]

Main and Jowett[21] used the direction of the deforming force and resultant displacement to formulate their classification. Therefore the mechanism of injury is considered in the treatment of each type of midtarsal injury. Medial fracture-sprains, subluxations, and dislocations are produced by inversion strains or adduction stress to the forefoot. Medial swivel dislocations are produced by a medial force to the forefoot (secondary to a fall), which disrupts the talonavicular joint and leaves the calcaneocuboid joint intact. The foot rotates

medially on the calcaneocuboid joint but does not invert or evert.

Longitudinal injuries result from forces being applied to the metatarsal rays with the ankle in fixed plantar flexion. This compresses the navicular between the head of the talus and the cuneiforms. The exact fracture pattern is dependent on the magnitude of the force and the degree of ankle plantar flexion.

Lateral fracture-sprains and subluxations result from valgus forces being applied to the forefoot (usually in a fall). This mechanism is the same as that proposed by Dewar and Evans.[5] Lateral swivel dislocations are produced by a valgus and rotational force (i.e., a missed step), which causes a lateral dislocation of the talonavicular joint while the calcaneocuboid joint remains intact.

Plantar fracture-sprains and fracture-subluxations or dislocations result when plantar-directed forces are applied to the dorsum of the forefoot, such as occurs when the foot is twisted beneath the body in a fall.

Finally, crush injuries of the midtarsal joint result when direct crushing forces are applied to the plantigrade foot.

DIAGNOSIS

Although severe crushing often produces midtarsal joint injury[21] the history of a minor injury to the foot, either a missed step or an inversion sprain, should suggest a midfoot injury. Inability to bear weight on the injured foot is a frequent complaint.[13] In patients with a complete dislocation, the forefoot deformity is easily noted.[22] The clinical appearance of the foot (i.e., fixed inversion and equinus of the forefoot, plantar flexion of the forefoot) is dependent on the type of dislocation present.[21] An open laceration on the dorsum of the foot following a crushing injury should suggest the possibility of midtarsal joint involvement.[7]

In patients with pain in the midtarsal area but no overt clinical deformity, a physical examination is mandatory to evaluate occult midtarsal fracture-subluxations[5,13] There is usually slight swelling on the dorsum of the midtarsal joint.[9,13,25] Ecchymosis on the medial and lateral aspects of the foot with encroachment on the sole strongly suggests this injury.[5] Pain is elicited with any attempt at midtarsal motion.[25] Point tenderness over the calcaneocuboid and talonavicular joint is absolute evidence that midtarsal joint injury has occurred and makes further radiographic evaluation of the joint essential.[5,13] Localization of the exact point of tenderness helps differentiate this injury from the ankle sprain, an entity with which it is often confused.[5] Palpation may reveal prominence of the talar head, navicular tubercle, or cuboid.[9] Stress applied to the midtarsal joint will usually produce severe pain.

Dewar and Evans[5] report that cases seen late present

with pain on weight bearing, a fullness on the medial side of the foot, and depression of the midtarsal joint.[5]

RADIOGRAPHIC FINDINGS

Radiographic diagnosis of injuries to the midtarsal joint can be difficult because of their rarity, which results in a lack of familiarity with these injuries.[24] Quality anteroposterior, lateral, and oblique radiographs of the foot and ankle are essential in confirming the diagnosis.[6,7] As with other injuries of the foot, frank dislocation is easily recognized; however, the occult midtarsal fracture-subluxation, stressed by Dewar and Evans,[5] may be overlooked unless it is considered when reviewing the films.[7] Because midtarsal fracture-subluxation is often mistaken for an ankle sprain, Dewar and Evans[6] believe oblique radiographs of the foot should be taken in addition to routine views of the ankle.

When evaluating the radiographs to plan treatment, one must consider two points: (1) the degree of subluxation or displacement of the midtarsal joint, and (2) the degree of involvement of the articular surfaces of the talonavicular and/or calcaneocuboid joint.

London[19] describes a special view of the midtarsal joint to diagnose fracture-subluxation in this area. In this special oblique view, the roentgen beam is centered on the talonavicular joint in the plane of the metatarsals and at right angles to the long axis of the foot. He finds this view helpful in more clearly delineating the talonavicular joint.[19] Polytomography and computed tomography may be useful in delineating the degree of displacement of the articular surface of either the navicular or cuboid associated with these subluxations.[24]

When routine radiographs reveal avulsion or flake fractures of the cuboid, navicular, or talus, one should *not* assume these are isolated injuries but consider them as *definite* evidence of injury (subluxation or spontaneously reduced dislocation) to the midtarsal joint.[5,21] Stress radiographs taken with the forefoot first in abduction and then adduction may be helpful in confirming an associated fracture-subluxation or a spontaneously reduced dislocation. If pain is severe, anesthetics may be required for these stress radiographs.

Finally, careful evaluation of the post reduction roentgenographs to ensure reduction of *all* components of the midtarsal injury is critical to avoid minor degrees of persistent subluxation.

TREATMENT

Treatment of injuries to the midtarsal joint has classically been by closed methods. Kenwright and Taylor[18] recommend closed reduction and immobilization in a below-the-knee cast with the foot in a plantigrade position. Weight bearing is allowed after an average of 5 weeks, and immobilization is discontinued after 8 weeks. They recommend open reduction in cases in which closed reduction is not successful. In severe, unstable, fracture-dislocations, they recommend open reduction and fixation with a Kirschner wire.

Dewar and Evans,[5] in discussing the occult fracture-subluxation of the midtarsal joint, recommend reduction of the subluxation, reattachment of the avulsed navicular fragment, and calcaneocuboid arthrodesis in patients who are seen early. Treatment by plaster immobilization alone following closed reduction resulted in persistent disability in their series.[5]

On the other hand, Stark[25] recommended that occult fracture-subluxations of the midtarsal joint associated with fracture of the navicular tubercle be treated conservatively *if* the patient is seen early and is able to invert the foot against resistance. He used a short leg cast and allowed walking after the first week. The cast was removed at 3 weeks and the patient allowed to bear weight. He believes the fracture of the navicular tubercle can be ignored if the patient is able to invert the foot adequately, a finding that suggests the remaining slips of the tibialis posterior tendon are intact.

Hillegass[14] emphasizes that accurate reduction is the key to successful treatment. He recommends internal fixation when instability is present following the reduction. In patients with severe fractures, he gives consideration to early midtarsal arthrodesis.[14]

Friedmann[10] reported primary arthrodesis in a patient in whom tibial strut graft was used in the midtarsal area to bridge a gap between the anterior portion of the talus and the first cuneiform that resulted from comminution of the talus and navicular. Although this case was not a simple midtarsal dislocation, the use of a graft to restore the length of the medial longitudinal arch is an important principle.

Both Main and Jowett[21] and Shelton and Pedowitz[24] stress the importance of accurately reducing all midtarsal injuries to prevent long-term sequelae. By far the most complete discussion of treatment of midtarsal joint injuries is that of Main and Jowett.[21] In medial fracture-sprains and fracture-subluxations or dislocations, they recommend empirical treatment with strapping or a plaster cast *after* reduction of dislocation. Their only failures occurred when reduction was not obtained. Shelton and Pedowitz[24] believe these injuries are potentially unstable and therefore recommend plaster immobilization in a short leg cast for 6 weeks, followed by 2 weeks in a walking plaster. They recommend percutaneous Kirschner wire stabilization when swelling, circulatory problems, or skin conditions prevent adequate plaster immobilization. Medial swivel dislocations are treated by closed reduction and immobilization by Main and Jowett.[21] Shelton and Pedowitz[24] recommend treating these medial swivel dislocations by anatomic reduction, which usually requires an open reduction because of interposed soft tissue.[24] Following open reduction, a non-weight-bearing cast is used for 6 weeks with or without Kirschner wire fixation.

In longitudinal injuries, Main and Jowett[21] demonstrated a direct relationship between displacement on the standard radiographs, the severity of injury, and failure to obtain a reduction and the clinical result. In undisplaced fractures, simple plaster immobilization produced a good result. In displaced fractures, reduction by closed or open means followed by plaster immobilization was used.[21] They do not recommend early arthrodesis in these patients. Shelton and Pedowitz[24] recommend prompt anatomic reduction of displaced fractures followed by temporary Kirschner wire fixation.

In lateral injuries, Main and Jowett[21] used closed reduction and cast immobilization or strapping. They noted that the prognosis after lateral fracture-sprains, fracture-subluxations, and dislocations is worse than following medial injuries. This is because of involvement of the lateral stabilizing arch of the foot and the calcaneocuboid joint. Shelton and Pedowitz[24] believe lateral fracture-sprains are potentially unstable and recommend treatment by plaster immobilization for 6 weeks. In fracture-subluxations and dislocations, the injury usually produces subluxation of the talonavicular joint and comminution of the anterior column of the calcaneus or the cuboid which results in collapse of the lateral longitudinal arch.[24] Comminution of the calcaneocuboid joint in these instances is a major problem. They recommend open reduction but state that it does not guarantee restoration of a smooth and stable articulation. In lateral swivel dislocations they suggest closed reduction and cast immobilization.

Plantar injuries are treated by closed reduction and plaster immobilization by Main and Jowett.[21] Shelton and Pedowitz[24] recommend closed reduction followed by immobilization for 6 to 8 weeks for plantar fracture-subluxations and dislocations. If closed reduction is not successful, open reduction and temporary fixation of the talonavicular joint with Kirschner wires is recommended.[24]

In crushing injuries of the midtarsal joint, anatomic fixation of the comminuted fractures is not possible or practical. Despite persistent displacement, Main and Jowett[21] found that none of their patients required secondary surgery.

Main and Jowett[21] do not recommend early arthrodesis as has been recommended by Watson-Jones[28] and Dick[6] following midtarsal injuries. However, for persistent symptoms following medial or longitudinal injuries, they found triple arthrodesis better than talonavic-

ulocuneiform arthrodesis or midtarsal arthrodesis for this injury. A naviculocuneiform arthrodesis in addition to the triple arthrodesis, as suggested by Friedman,[10] did not seem warranted in their experience.[21,23]

COMPLICATIONS

Pennal[22] clearly documented that midtarsal dislocations unassociated with fractures had minimal disability at late review. However, dislocations associated with even marginal fractures resulted in varying degrees of disability.

Dewar and Evans[5] stressed the importance of early recognition and treatment of the occult fracture-subluxation to avoid long-term disability. In their series only one patient was seen in the first week of injury, the remaining patients were initially misdiagnosed as ankle sprains. In the cases diagnosed late, it was necessary to correct the deformity, fuse the calcaneocuboid joint, and elongate the lateral side of the foot to correct length lost because of the compression fracture involving the calcaneocuboid joint. Early diagnosis and correct treatment should prevent these problems.

Hooper and McMaster[14] reported a case of recurrent subluxation of the midtarsal joint *despite* adequate immobilization. Recurrent subluxation has previously been associated with inadequate immobilization and hypermobility of the joints,[15] but in their case, the patient was adequately immobilized and there were no signs of systemic ligamentous laxity.

Because of the direct relationship of inadequate reduction and poor results,[5,21,24] obtaining *and* maintaining an anatomic reduction are necessary to obtain a good result. Fahey and Murphy[9] reported recurrent subluxation requiring triple arthrodesis in a patient treated by open reduction *without* internal fixation. Therefore percutaneous fixation should be considered in cases where stability is in question.[24]

Shelton and Pedowitz[24] report that both medial and lateral fracture-sprains, when treated correctly, seldom produce long-term disability. However, medial and lateral fracture-subluxations or dislocations are associated with a greater degree of articular damage of both the talonavicular and calcaneocuboid joints and therefore may result in persistent long-term disability, even with adequate treatment. Similarly, their longitudinal and crush injuries, both representing increasing degrees of articular cartilage damage at the midtarsal joint, were noted to have increased disability. They reported midtarsal thickening, stiffness, swelling, and a loss of the longitudinal arches following crush injuries, which may require shoe modifications on a long-term basis.[22] They mentioned the possibility of avascular necrosis of the navicular following this type of injury. Kenwright and Taylor[18] also report that these navicular fractures can lead to talonavicular arthritis, which may require arthrodesis. They stress, however, the development of aseptic necrosis of the navicular may not preclude a good result.[18]

Main and Jowett[18] distinguish between pure longitudinal and longitudinal medial injuries. In pure longitudinal injuries unreduced severe displacement produces a poor result, while in longitudinal medial injuries severe displacement may still allow a satisfactory result. This is because in the longitudinal medial group the arch is usually preserved, although displaced medially.

Dewar and Evans[5] and Main and Jowett[18] stress that the disability following lateral fracture-subluxations or dislocation is best treated by calcaneocuboid arthrodesis rather than a triple arthrodesis. However, following medial or longitudinal injuries, they suggest triple arthrodesis rather than talonaviculocuneiform[23] arthrodesis.

AUTHOR'S PREFERRED METHOD OF TREATMENT

Grossly evident midtarsal dislocations and fracture-dislocations should be obvious to any examiner. However, a high index of suspicion is essential in diagnosing fracture-sprains and fracture-subluxations involving the midtarsal joint. A clinical examination that documents tenderness in the area of the talonavicular and/or calcaneocuboid joints following a twisting injury to the foot *demands* clear anteroposterior, lateral, and oblique radiographs of the foot.

Avulsion or marginal fractures in the area of the talonavicular or calcaneocuboid joint noted on routine radiographs suggest the diagnosis of a midtarsal fracture-sprain, fracture-subluxation, or spontaneously reduced fracture-dislocation. I have found the special oblique radiograph demonstrated by London[19] helpful in documenting the degree of associated damage to the navicular and cuboid. Additionally, polytomography and/or computed tomography are occasionally used to evaluate associated intraarticular fractures.

In cases of fracture-sprain, subluxation, or suspected spontaneously reduced dislocation, I consider evaluation of midtarsal joint stability *essential*, as the degree of stability determines my treatment decision. Stress radiographs are helpful in demonstrating the degree of associated ligamentous injury. If pain or swelling prevent this stress examination, I consider examination with the patient under anesthesia to document the presence or absence of instability. I will discuss specific treatment recommendations using the classification of Main and Jowett.[21]

Medial injuries

Medial fracture-sprains, although clinically stable, have the potential to displace. Therefore I treat these injuries in a short leg walking cast with the foot in neutral position for 4 weeks. Following this, a hard-soled shoe with a longitudinal arch support is recommended until the patient is pain free. In medial fracture-subluxation or dislocation, I take great care to ensure that an anatomic reduction is obtained. Because of the instability inherent in these injuries, I prefer percutaneous Kirschner wire stabilization and immobilization in a short leg cast. These patients are kept non-weight-bearing for 3 weeks, followed by 3 weeks in a weight bearing cast. In medial swivel dislocations, I attempt a closed reduction. If the reduction is not anatomic, I proceed directly to an open reduction. Following closed or open reduction, percutaneous Kirschner wire fixation of the talonavicular joint is performed. The foot is immobilized in a short leg non-weight-bearing cast for 6 weeks. A hard-soled shoe and good arch support are then recommended.

Longitudinal injuries

Longitudinal nondisplaced fractures are treated with immobilization in a short leg walking cast for 4 to 6 weeks. In cases with displaced fractures of the navicular, open reduction and internal fixation with A-O screws or Kirschner wires is considered, based on the degree of comminution. This is followed by immobilization in a short leg cast for 6 weeks. The patient is advised of the possibility of aseptic necrosis of the navicular and of degenerative arthritis of the talonavicular joint after this injury. A longitudinal arch support is usually needed on a long-term basis. Aseptic necrosis of the navicular without collapse may not require later treatment. I am unaware of any *documented* successful method of preventing collapse once aseptic necrosis is noted.

Lateral injuries

Lateral fracture-sprains are treated in a short leg walking cast for 4 to 6 weeks. Fracture-subluxations, on the other hand, are usually associated with comminution of the lateral column of the foot, i.e., either the anterior portion of the calcaneus or the cuboid. In my experience with these injuries, comminution of the calcaneocuboid joint has led to long-term disability. Therefore careful evaluation by polytomography is undertaken to see if reconstruction of the articular surface of the cuboid is possible. If open reduction is possible, it is followed by short leg non-weight-bearing cast immobilization for 6 weeks. This is followed by an intensive period of physical therapy and ambulation in a stiff-soled shoe. If comminution of the articular surface is too severe, closed reduction and immobilization in a short leg non-weight-bearing cast for 3 to 6 weeks is used. Long-term disability may require calcaneocuboid fusion.

Lateral swivel dislocations are treated by closed reduction followed by immobilization in a short leg cast for 6 weeks. Progressive weight bearing is then instituted.

Plantar injuries

Plantar fracture-subluxations and dislocations are treated by closed reduction and plaster immobilization for 6 weeks. In those cases in which closed reduction is not possible, I proceed to open reduction and percutaneous Kirschner wire fixation of the talonavicular and calcaneocuboid joints. A short leg non-weight-bearing cast, is used for 6 weeks, at which time the Kirschner wires are removed and weight bearing and a stiff-soled shoe or short leg cast is then instituted.

Crushing injuries

In crushing injuries of the midfoot I attempt a closed reduction. Because of instability, I prefer Kirschner wire stabilization. Any swelling is allowed to subside before a cast is applied. My decision to attempt an open reduction is based on the ability to obtain anatomic reduction of the fracture fragments. Usually this is not possible because of severe comminution. Therefore immobilization of these comminuted injuries with attention to molding of the arch in a non-weight-bearing cast for 4 to 6 weeks, followed by a stiff-soled shoe with a longitudinal arch support, is recommended.

The use of percutaneous Kirschner wires to prevent redislocation of these injuries, which may occur in a cast as swelling subsides, should be considered in all cases. In all midtarsal injuries, the short leg cast leaves the metatarsophalangeal joints free to allow early motion. After cast immobilization, range of motion exercises and swimming pool or hydrotherapy may be useful. The long-term use of a stiff-soled shoe with a longitudinal arch support may be necessary.

REFERENCES

1. Bohler, L.: The treatment of fractures, vol. 3, ed. 5, New York, 1958, Grune & Stratton, Inc.
2. Boidard, C.A.N.: Contributiona l'etude des luxations astragalo-scaphoidiennes, Master's thesis, University of Bordeaux, France, 1939.
3. Chapman, M.W.: Fractures and fracture-dislocations of the ankle and foot. In Mann, R.A., editor: DuVries' surgery of the foot, ed. 4, St. Louis, 1978, The C.V. Mosby Co.
4. Conwell, H.E., and Reynolds, F.C. Key and Conwell's management of fractures, dislocations and sprains, ed. 7, St. Louis, 1961, The C.V. Mosby Co.
5. Dewar, F.P., and Evans, D.C.: Occult fracture-subluxation of the midtarsal joint, J. Bone Joint Surg. 50B:386-388, 1968.
6. Dick, I.L.: Occult fracture-dislocation of the tarsal navicular, Proc. R. Soc. Med. 35:760, 1942.
7. Dixon, J.H.: Letter, Injury 10:251, 1979.
8. Drummond, P.S., and Hastings, D.E.: Total dislocation of the cuboid bone, J. Bone Joint Surg. 51B:716-718, 1969.
9. Fahey, J.J., and Murphy, J.L.: Dislocations and fractures of the talus, Surg. Clin. North Am. 45:79-102, 1965.
10. Friedmann, E.: Key graft fixation in mid-tarsal fracture dislocation, Am. J. Surg. 96:81-83, 1958.
11. Giannestras, N.G., and Sammarco, G.J.: Fractures and dislocations in the foot. In Rockwood, C.A., Jr., and Green, D.P., editors: Fractures, Philadelphia, 1975, J.B. Lippincott Co.
12. Gilland, F.A.E.: Les luxations isolees du scaphoid tarsien, Master's thesis, University of Nancy, France, 1936.
13. Hermel, M.B., and Gershon-Cohen, J.: The nutcracker fracture of the cuboid by indirect violence, Radiology 60:850-854, 1953.
14. Hillegass, R.C.: Injuries to the mid foot: a major cause of industrial morbidity. In Bateman, J.E., editor: Foot science, Philadelphia, 1976, W.B. Saunders Co.
15. Hooper, G., and McMaster, M.: Recurrent bilateral mid-tarsal subluxations, J. Bone Joint Surg. 61A:617-619, 1979.
16. Jaslow, I.A.: Fracture-dislocation of the mid-tarsal and cuboideonavicular joints, J. Bone Joint Surg. 28:386-388, 1946.
17. Jones, F.W.: Structure and fixation as seen in the foot, London 1944, Baiolliere, Tindall and Cox, p. 246.
18. Kenwright, J., and Taylor, R.G.: Major injuries of the talus, J. Bone Joint Surg. 52B:36-48, 1970.
19. London, P.S.: Wrinkle corner: a special view for midtarsal fracture-subluxation, Injury 5:65, 1973.
20. McLaughlin, H.L.: Trauma, Philadelphia, 1959, W.B. Saunders Co.
21. Main, B.J., and Jowett, R.L.: Injuries of the mid-tarsal joint, J. Bone Joint Surg. 57B:89-97, 1975.
22. Pennal, G.F.: Fractures of the talus, Clin. Orthop. 30:53-63, 1963.
22a. Saffafian, S.K.: Anatomy of the foot and ankle: descriptive, topographic, functional, Philadelphia, 1983, J.B. Lippincott Co.
23. Seymour, N.: The late results of naviculo-cuneiform fusion, J. Bone Joint Surg. 49B:558-559, 1967.
24. Shelton, M.L., and Pedowitz, W.J.: Injuries to the talus and midfoot. In Jahss, M.H., editor: Disorders of the foot, vol. 2, Philadelphia, 1982, W.B. Saunders Co.
25. Stark, W.A.: Occult fracture-subluxation of the midtarsal joint, Clin. Orthop. 93:291-292, 1973.
26. Van Hove, R.: Luxation partielle de l'articulation de Chopart, Acta Orthop. Belgica 23:67-72, 1957.
27. Waters, C.H.: Midtarsal fractures and dislocations. In American Academy of Orthopaedic Surgeons: Instructional course lectures, vol. IX, Ann Arbor, Mich., 1952, J.E. Edwards, pp. 368-374.
28. Watson-Jones, R.: Fractures and joint injuries, vol. 2, ed. 4, Baltimore, 1955, The Williams & Wilkins Co.
29. Weh, R.: Ueber die isolierte luxation in talonaviculargelenk, Masters thesis, University of Munich, 1939.
30. Willigens, J.E.F.: Contribution a l'etude de la luxation du scaphoid tarsien, Master's thesis, University of Nancy, France, 1936.

Tarsometatarsal dislocations

The tarsometatarsal joint, consisting of the bases of the five metatarsals and their articulations with the three cuneiforms and the cuboid is named after Jacques Lisfranc, a French surgeon in the army of Napoleon who originally described an amputation through that joint.[9,22,30,40] According to Cassebaum,[9] Lisfranc never actually wrote on the subject of fracture-dislocation of the tarsometatarsal joint, his name being attached to the dislocation simply because he described the amputation.

Dislocations and fracture-dislocations of the tarsometatarsal joint are rare injuries and are reported to occur at the rate of 1 person per 55,000 per year.[1,20,30,43] English[20] reports that only 0.2% of all fractures involve this joint. However, Del Sel[16] feels that this injury is more common than is generally supposed. Lenczner et al.[37] Bassett, and O'Regan[42] report that the injury was more common when the horse was the major means of transportation. In those days, being dragged by a horse with a foot caught in the stirrup was the common method of the injury. Today, motorcycle accidents produce a similar mechanism of injury.[17] Also, an increase in the incidence of motor vehicle accidents is believed by Lenczner et al.[37] to be responsible for an increasing incidence of injuries to the tarsometatarsal joint today. Wilson[53] reports that now 64% of all the tarsometatarsal joint injuries are the result of road traffic accidents. Additionally, Coker and Arnold[12] and O'Donoghue[44] report injuries to the tarsometatarsal joints are occurring with increasing frequency in athletic events.

Because the metatarsals may be displaced with or without an associated fracture and because they may be displaced in a dorsal, ventral, medial, or lateral direction (or any combination of these directions) in relation to the hindfoot, a working classification is essential in understanding the diagnosis and treatment of these injuries.[43] It is important to distinguish between a total dislocation, in which all the metatarsals are dislocated, and partial dislocations, in which some but not all of the metatarsals are dislocated from the tarsometatarsal joint.[40,54]

Although these dislocations exhibit a great deal of individual variation, in general they have similar patterns of displacement.[10] Various classifications of tarsometatarsal dislocations have been presented.[11,18,30,42-44] Quenu and Kuss[44] proposed a classification that is both simple and useful. They divided all these injuries into three types of dislocations: (1) homolateral dislocations, in which all five metatarsals are displaced in the coronal plane; (2) isolated dislocations, in which one or two metatarsals are displaced in the coronal plane; and (3) divergent dislocations, in which there is separation between the first and second metatarsals and the displacement occurs in the sagittal as well as the coronal plane. The simplicity of this classification system has made it attractive to many authors reporting tarsometatarsal injuries.[2,25,36]

Alternatively, O'Regan[42] uses a very simple classification system based on displacement. Uniform dislocations are those in which all the metatarsals are displaced in the same direction, while divergent dislocations are those in which the first metatarsal moves medially away from the remaining four metatarsals. He emphasizes that the deformity may involve one, all, or any combination of the metatarsals. O'Regan[42] and Granberry and Lipscomb[28] emphasized that fractures involving the tarsometatarsal joint are usually present with these dislocations.

Hardcastle et al.[30] used the classification of Quenu and Kuss[44] as a basis for classification that they developed and on which they believe treatment can be based (Fig. 24-121).

  I. Type A (Total): In these injuries there is incongruity of the entire tarsometatarsal joint. The displacement is in one plane, which may be sagittal, coronal, or combined.

 II. Type B (Partial): In these injuries there is incongruity of a part of the tarsometatarsal joint. The displaced segment is in one plane, which may be either sagittal, coronal, or combined. There are two types of partial dislocations whose treatment and prognosis differ:

    A. Medial dislocations: Displacement affects the first metatarsal either in isolation or combined with displacement of one or more of the second, third, or fourth metatarsals.

    B. Lateral dislocations: Displacement affects one or more of the lateral four metatarsals. The first metatarsal is not affected.

III. Type C (Divergent): In these injuries there may be partial or total incongruity. On the anteroposterior radiograph the first metatarsal is displaced medially, and any combination of the lateral four metatarsals is displaced laterally. Sagittal displacement also occurs in conjunction with a coronal displacement.

I prefer to use the classification of Hardcastle et al.[30] because of its relationship to the indicated treatment.

ANATOMY

The tarsometatarsal joint consists of the five metatarsal bones, three cuneiforms, and the cuboid. The medial three metatarsals articulate individually with one of the three cuneiforms. The cuboid articulates with the fourth and fifth metatarsals. The second metatarsal is the longest of all metatarsals, and the second cuneiform is the shortest of the cuneiforms. This produces an indentation in the line of the cuneiforms into which the long second metatarsal fits[36] (Fig. 24-122, A). Lenczner et al.[37] emphasize that the stability of the second metatarsal base is the key to the structure of the tarsometatarsal joint. The second metatarsal has a broader dorsal surface and a narrow ventral surface, which make this bone resemble the keystone of a Roman arch in shape, position, and function[5a,37] (Fig. 24-122, B). Because of its recessed position between the medial and lateral cuneiforms, the second metatarsal articulates with all three cuneiforms.[8] Cain and Seligson[8] also re-

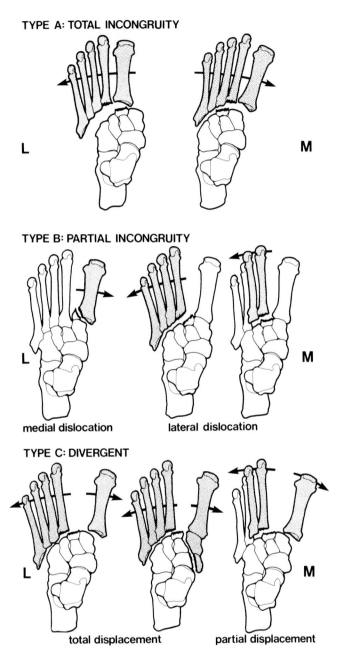

Fig. 24-121. Classification of Lisfranc fracture-dislocations. (Redrawn from Hardcastle, P.H., Reschauer, R., Kutscha-Lissberg, E., and Schoffmann, W.: J. Bone Joint Surg. **64B**:349-359, 1982.)

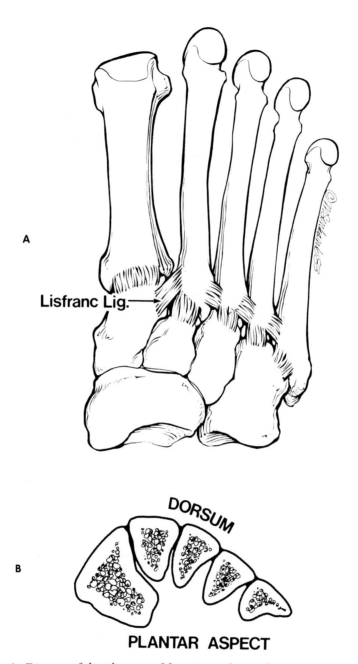

Fig. 24-122. A, Diagram of dorsal aspect of foot. Base of second metatarsal is mortised between three cuneiforms. Second, third, and fourth metatarsals are connected to each other by dorsal and plantar transverse ligaments. There is no transverse ligament between bases of first and second metatarsals. Lateral four metatarsals are attached to first cuneiform by obliquely placed Lisfranc's ligament. B, Transverse section of metatarsals. Note dorsum of second metatarsal is wider than plantar aspect.

port that the second metatarsal holds the keystone position of the tarsometatarsal joint and that no significant dislocation of the metatarsals or cuneiforms can occur unless this keystone is disrupted.

Anderson[2] reports that it is indeed rare to see a tarsometatarsal dislocation without fracture of the base of the second metatarsal, and Aitken and Poulson[1] emphasize that only if the recess is unusually shallow can a dislocation occur without a fracture of the second metatarsal. Additionally, Cain and Seligson[8] believe the second cuneiform is an important element in the integrity of the transverse arch of the foot. Along with its nonmobile articulation with the second metatarsal, it constitutes the longitudinal axis of the foot.

In addition to the stability provided by the bony anatomy, the ligamentous structures of the tarsometatarsal joint are instrumental in instability. The second, third, fourth, and fifth metatarsal bases are bound to each other by transverse ligaments located on both the dorsal and plantar aspects of the joint. The plantar ligaments support the arch and are much stronger than the dorsal ligaments.[13] There is no ligament between the bases of the great and second metatarsals; instead, the four lesser metatarsals are attached primarily to the first cuneiform by an obliquely placed plantar and dorsal ligament. This oblique ligament, termed *Lisfranc's ligament*,[34] is important because it is responsible for the avulsion fractures of the base of second metatarsal so frequently seen in these fracture-dislocations.[2] The oblique ligament of Lisfranc is so placed that when an abduction force is applied to the metatarsus it results in rupture or avulsion of the ligamentous insertion or fracture of the base of the second metatarsal, which permits lateral dislocation of the foot.[13]

The first metatarsal is secured to the medial cuneiform by ligaments that lie in an axial direction (Fig. 24-122, A). These ligaments permit marked abduction before they yield, and great force is necessary to disrupt their attachments.[13] The insertion of the anterior tibial tendon on the medial aspect of the proximal first metatarsal and of the peroneus longus tendon into the lateral aspect of the proximal first metatarsal are both factors that add to the security of the first metatarsocuneiform joint.

The structures on the sole of the foot, including the plantar fascia, the intrinsic foot muscles, and the stronger plantar tarsometatarsal ligaments, make plantar dislocation unlikely. On the other hand, the soft tissue overlying the dorsal aspect of these joints is rather scant.[1,2] These anatomic facts are responsible for displacement being most always dorsal and lateral.[6]

Finally, the location of the junction of the dorsalis pedis artery with the plantar arterial arch at the proximal end of the space between the first and second metatarsals places this artery at risk of injury with any type of tarsometatarsal dislocation.[26]

MECHANISM OF INJURY

The forces responsible for tarsometatarsal dislocation can be classified as direct and indirect.* A direct force such as a truck running over the foot or a heavy weight being dropped directly on the foot,[36] result in plantar dislocation[31,36,42] of the metatarsal bases. Secondary medial or lateral displacement may occur, depending on the exact nature of the applied force.[30] The mechanism of direct force produces extensive soft tissue damage, and multiple associated fractures may be common.

The application of indirect force can also produce tarsometatarsal dislocations.[9,34,51,53] Jumping onto the plantar-flexed foot or the application of a force up through the toes of a foot positioned in equinus can also result in the most common displacement, dorsal and lateral.[9] Jeffreys reported two patterns of indirect injury.[34] First, simple lateral dislocation of the forefoot can be produced by pronation of the hindfoot with a fixed forefoot position. Second, a medial dislocation of the first metatarsocuneiform joint can be produced by supination of the hindfoot with a fixed forefoot. This mechanism is followed by complete dislocation of the forefoot after fracture of the second metatarsal.[34]

Wiley[51] believes the pattern of the fractured metatarsals and the configuration of the tarsometatarsal joint suggest that the mechanism involved in producing tarsometatarsal dislocations is either violent abduction or plantar flexion of the forefoot. When the forefoot is violently abducted, the brunt of the force is concentrated on the fixed base of the second metatarsal. As the remaining metatarsals slide in mass, the second metatarsal cannot move until it fractures. If significant lateral displacement of the metatarsals occurs the cuboid bone may be crushed. Fractures of the cuboid and second metatarsal bones are therefore pathognomonic of this abduction-type of tarsometatarsal disruption[31,51] (Fig. 24-123). According to Wiley,[51] plantar-flexion injuries occur in two ways. The first is a force applied to the heel along the axis of the foot when the toes are fixed. This mechanism, described in the early literature, occurred when cavalrymen were thrown from their horses. As the horse tumbled to the ground, it fell on the soldier and pinned his foot to the ground. Second, plantar flexion of the foot is commonly noted in motor vehicle accidents, a situation that is far more common in today's society.[34,51] In this instance, the ankle is in a plantar-flexed position, and the foot becomes part of a long lever arm consisting of the entire lower leg. With

---

*References 25, 30, 31, 34, 36, 42, 51, and 53.

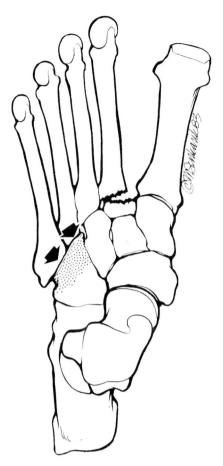

Fig. 24-123. Fractures of cuboid and second metatarsal bones are pathognomonic signs of tarsometatarsal disruption.

the lower leg and foot in the same linear axis, a force applied to the end of the foot is transmitted up this axis. If the line of this force is dorsal to the tarsometatarsal joint, the weak dorsal ligament of the joint disrupts as the force increases. The entire joint complex may dislocate with or without associated fractures. Associated rotation at the time of application of this plantar flexion force can result in various combinations of associated fractures.[26,34]

Finally, Wilson[53] demonstrated that tarsometatarsal injuries can result from eversion, inversion, and plantar flexion. Forefoot eversion (pronation) produces two stages of tarsometatarsal injury.[53] The first stage is medial dislocation of the first metatarsal bone alone (the "isolated dislocation"). The second stage, produced by more eversion, consists of medial dislocation of the first metatarsal *and* dorsilateral dislocation of the four lesser metatarsal bones (the "divergent dislocation"). Forefoot inversion (supination) also produces two stages of injury. The first consists of dorsilateral dislocation of up to four lesser metatarsal bones. The second stage con-

sists of dorsilateral dislocation of all five metatarsal bones. Finally, pure plantar-flexion force without rotation produce variable fracture patterns.

In summary, it is important to recognize that these injuries are not the result of simple inversion, eversion, or plantar flexion mechanisms. They result from a combination of these forces along with rotation along the axis of the foot. Therefore the injuries may occur with or without fracture, depending on the twisting forces simultaneously applied.[25] The importance in understanding these various mechanisms of injury is that at times the dislocation may have spontaneously reduced, and the only clue to the extent of the injury may be the fracture pattern of the tarsal and metatarsal bones.[25]

DIAGNOSIS

Injuries to the tarsometatarsal joints may be overlooked in two groups of patients. First, in the multiply injured patient with severe trauma to other organ systems, closed injuries of the forefoot frequently go undiagnosed.[2,5A,6] In cases of gross displacement of the metatarsals, the diagnosis is evident. However, the less severely displaced subluxations and dislocations that spontaneously reduce are likely to be overlooked without a careful physical examination.[5A,50] This may result in considerable disability.[9] In the less severely displaced subluxations, the clinical and radiographic findings may be subtle and go unrecognized, particularly when attention is focused to more severe injuries and to other parts of the body.[50] Finally, simple sprains of the tarsometatarsal joints with or without minimal widening between the first and second metatarsal bases do occur, and their recognition is essential for proper treatment.[12]

The signs and symptoms in tarsometatarsal dislocation vary greatly, depending on the degree of displacement.[2] As mentioned, spontaneous reduction is not unusual and can complicate the diagnosis.[2] The patient usually complains of severe pain in the midpart of the foot and at times relates of a feeling of paresthesia.[2,25] The patient complains of the inability to bear weight on the foot.[6]

Swelling and associated deformity of the foot are obvious in complete dislocation.[3,38,40,41] The deformity of the foot consists of forefoot equinus, forefoot abduction, and prominence of the medial tarsal area.[6] If the patient is not seen until 2 or more hours after the accident, gross ecchymosis and swelling of the foot are present.[5a,25] Giannestras and Sammarco[25] report that swelling of the foot may occur as soon as 2 hours following the injury. If the injury is seen early before swelling, shortening and displacement of the forefoot may be noticeable.[2,25] There is diffuse tenderness across the tarsometatarsal joint, and marked pain is experienced on passive motion.[2,5] According to Anderson,[2] almost all of these injuries are closed unless they are associated with a crushing blow by the direct mechanism of injury.

The dorsalis pedis pulse may or may not be palpable.[25] Both Gissane[26] and Groulier and Pinaud[29] reported cases of tarsometatarsal dislocation that required amputation. Although the dislocation occurs at the point of communication between the dorsalis pedis artery and the plantar arch and can result in damage to this communication, Gissane[26] believed that this arterial injury does not endanger the life of the foot unless the posterior tibial or lateral plantar artery is also damaged.[16,26] However, one must consider these injuries as orthopaedic emergencies requiring prompt reduction to prevent further swelling and vascular compromise.

RADIOGRAPHIC EVALUATION

Radiographs taken in three planes, anteroposterior, lateral, and 30° oblique, are essential to diagnose the initial displacement and to assess whether the reduction is anatomic.[25,30] It is important to include the entire foot and ankle so that associated injuries are not missed.[30] Granberry and Lipscomb[28] reported that in only 8 of 25 cases were tarsometatarsal dislocations not associated with significant fractures. They stress that associated fractures are probably present in all tarsometatarsal dislocations even though they cannot be demonstrated radiographically.

Aitken and Poulson[1] report that fractures of the base of the second metatarsal and compression fractures of the cuboid are the fractures most commonly associated with tarsometatarsal dislocations. Indeed, LaTourette et al.[36] report that fractures of the base of the second metatarsal, consisting of either a large or small fragment, are present in 90% of all tarsometatarsal dislocations.

Because of the possibility that a fracture-dislocation has spontaneously reduced and the existence of subluxation in which the dislocation is not complete, radiographic hints that suggest tarsometatarsal injury are important to note. A fractured base of the second metatarsal with any displacement should suggest an injury to Lisfranc's joint.[25] Cain and Seligson[8] report that the presence of an avulsion fracture of the medial pole of the navicular suggests a tarsometatarsal joint injury. Schiller and Ray[46] suggest that the presence of an isolated medial cuneiform dislocation should also suggest the presence of an unrecognized spontaneously reduced tarsometatarsal injury. Coker and Arnold[12] suggest that a fracture of the base of the second metatarsal, a fracture of a cuboid, and the loss of a few degrees of varus of the first metatarsal are all clues that a tarsometatarsal dislocation has occurred. If one suspects a spontaneously reduced dislocation by the presence of

such associated fractures, further evaluation by the use of comparative or stress radiographs is essential.

Anderson[2] initially emphasized the importance of evaluating the relationship of the metatarsals to the cuneiforms and fractures of the base of the second metatarsal in patients with tarsometatarsal injuries. Evaluation of the relationship of the metatarsal bases with the cuneiforms and cuboid is essential, not only in detecting subluxations of this joint but also in evaluating the quality of reduction. Giannestras and Sammarco[25] state that the lateral two or three metatarsals tend to be somewhat variable in relation to the lateral cuneiform and cuboid, and that this relationship is less reliable in diagnosising dislocations.[25]

Foster and Foster[22] reviewed the radiographs of 200 feet. They found the most consistent relationship at the tarsometatarsal joint was the alignment of the medial edge of the base of the second metatarsal with the medial edge of the second cuneiform on the frontal or oblique views. They felt that a space between the first and second metatarsal is of itself not evidence of a dislocation unless there is a step-off at the base of the second metatarsal and second cuneiform. Although the medial aspect of the base of the fourth metatarsal is usually aligned with the medial edge of the cuboid, these authors found a slight step-off (1 to 2 ml) in several cases without injury. They found that the base of the first metatarsal usually aligns with the lateral edge of the first cuneiform but that variations occur, particularly when the diameter of the metatarsal base is smaller than that of the medial cuneiform. These authors stress that the base of the third metatarsal usually aligns with the medial aspect of the third cuneiform but that this junction may be difficult to see on routine views. Foster et al.[22] also emphasize that the position of the fifth metatarsal is often difficult to assess.

Stein[47] reported that dislocation can be readily appreciated when all four lateral metatarsals move as a group. However, he stresses that it is not unusual to see intermetatarsal ligamentous disruption. In these instances, evaluation of the position of only one metatarsal can lead to a missed diagnosis. Stein[47] therefore believes it is essential for the clinician to assess the anatomic position of *all five* metatarsal shafts as they articulate with the tarsal bones. He reviewed 100 radiographic studies of the foot and observed the following constant anatomic relationships:

1. The medial border of the fourth metatarsal always forms a continuous straight line with the medial border of the cuboid on the medial oblique view (Fig. 24-124).
2. The intermetatarsal space between the third and fourth metatarsals is continuous with the intertarsal space between the lateral cuneiform and the

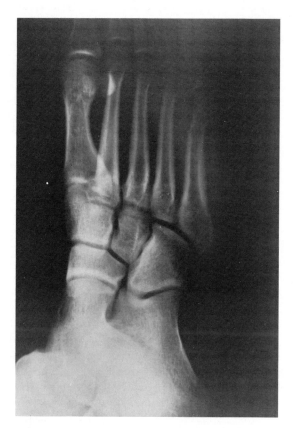

Fig. 24-124. Medial oblique view of foot. *1*, Medial border of cuboid and fourth metatarsal form continuous line. *2*, Lateral border of third metatarsal forms continuous line with lateral border of third cuneiform. *3*, Intermetatarsal space between second and third metatarsals is continuous with intertarsal space between the middle and lateral cuneiforms.

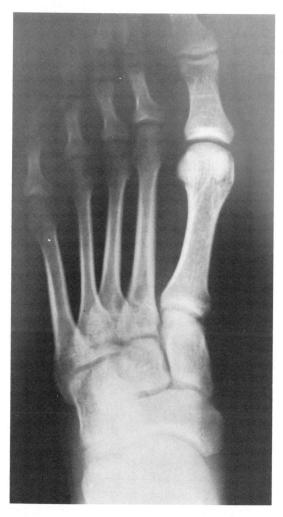

Fig. 24-125. Anteroposterior view of foot. *1*, Medial border of second metatarsal forms continuous straight line with medial border of middle cuneiform. *2*, Intermetatarsal space between first and second metatarsals is continuous with intertarsal space between medial and middle cuneiforms. *3*, First metatarsal is aligned with medial cuneiform medially and laterally.

cuboid. Therefore the lateral border of the third metatarsal shaft forms a straight line with the lateral border of the lateral cuneiform (Fig. 24-124).

3. On the medial oblique view, the intermetatarsal space between the second and third metatarsals is continuous in a straight line with the intertarsal space between the lateral and middle cuneiforms (Fig. 24-124).

4. On the anteroposterior view, the medial border of the second metatarsal forms a continuous straight line with the medial border of the middle cuneiform (Fig. 24-125).

5. Therefore the intermetatarsal space between the first and second metatarsals is continuous with the intertarsal space between the medial and middle cuneiform (Fig. 24-125).

6. The first metatarsal aligns itself with a medial cuneiform medially and laterally (Fig. 24-125).

Stein[47] stresses that these relationships are constant regardless of the rotation of the foot when the radio-

graphs are taken. He also emphasizes that it is difficult to assess the position of the fifth metatarsal in relationship to the cuboid. However, the fourth and fifth metatarsals almost always move as a unit in their relationship to the cuboid, even if there is a disruption of the intermetatarsal ligaments between the third and fourth metatarsals. Therefore an evaluation of the position of the fourth metatarsal will be satisfactory in assessing the position of the fifth.

Stein stresses that a lateral view of the foot is essential to complete the radiographic evaluation, since dorsal subluxation of the metatarsal bases (particularly the second and third metatarsals) may not be readily apparent on the anteroposterior or oblique views of the foot.

Additionally, Brown and McFarland[7] emphasized that in most tarsometatarsal dislocations the naviculocuneiform joint remains intact while the metatarsals are displaced. However, occasionally the naviculocuneiform joint is disrupted in conjunction with tarsometatarsal fracture-dislocations. This results in complete dislocation of the medial cuneiform with a Lisfranc's dislocation.[7] Cain and Seligson[8] stressed the importance of recognizing this variation of a tarsometatarsal dislocation, because it is essential to reduce the medial cuneiform *before* the tarsometatarsal dislocation can be reduced.

Finally, English[20] emphasizes the importance of evaluating the metatarsophalangeal joints on the radiographs of patients with tarsometatarsal dislocations. One is likely to overlook a dislocation of the metatarsophalangeal joint because of the more obvious dislocation of the tarsometatarsal joint. He refers to this injury combination as the "linked-toe dislocation of the metatarsal bone." He stresses the importance of recognizing the metatarsophalangeal joint dislocation, because reduction of this dislocation is dependent on accurate reduction of the fracture-dislocation of the base of the metatarsal.

TREATMENT

The goal of treatment of fracture-dislocations of the tarsometatarsal joints is the restoration of a painless and stable plantigrade foot.[27] Geckeler[24] emphasized that these injuries cause permanent pain and disability unless reduced early and completely. Although there have been reports of minimal symptoms following minimal or no treatment and persistent subluxation,[1,34,37] most recent authors emphasize that reduction of the dislocation is essential for a good result.* Key and Conwell[35] stress that an anatomic reduction is a prerequisite for a painless, functioning foot.

Closed reduction should be attempted as soon as possible.[27] If manipulation is carried out immediately, the reduction may be accomplished easily, unless a chip fracture interferes.[9,10] Cain and Seligson[8] carefully outlined the technique of manipulative reduction of these injuries. The first step is to restore the length of the foot. They accomplish this by manually pulling on the metatarsals while the heel is fixed. Once the length is restored, the second metatarsal is reduced into its mortise, thereby reestablishing the transverse arch of the midfoot.[8] Collett et al.[13] also emphasize the importance of applying uniform traction as an essential part of the reduction. They recommend the use of woven wire traps (Chinese finger traps) placed over the toes.

*References 5a, 9, 16, 25, 27, and 28.

The patient is placed in the *prone* position with the foot projecting beyond the end of the table. Anderson[2] also recommends the use of Chinese finger traps applied to the toes to obtain traction. Once the metatarsals are out to length, manipulation of the metatarsals into their proper position is performed. Fitte and Garacotche[21] also use traction, obtained with pins through the metatarsals and calcaneus.

Anderson[2] believes that, although most of these dislocations can be reduced closed, they are unstable. In patients in whom the reduction is not stable, he recommends percutaneous pin fixation to maintain the reduction. He prefers two Steinmann pins, one fixing the first metatarsal to the medial cuneiform and a second fixing the fifth metatarsal to the cuboid. He recommends that radiographs be taken before cast application to be certain that the reduction and the percutaneous pin fixation are accurate. Bassett[5a] also recommends Kirschner wire stabilization to prevent displacement after initial reduction. Foster and Foster[22] believe that if anatomic or near-anatomic alignment is achieved by closed means, cast immobilization can be used. They recommend the use of percutaneous Kirschner wire fixation only in cases of unstable reduction. Following successful reduction with or without percutaneous fixation, the foot is placed in a short leg cast. Cassebaum[9] recommends non-weight bearing for 6 to 8 weeks following reduction. Loss of reduction may develop when weight bearing is initiated too early.[6]

Hardcastle et al.[30] recommend attempted closed reduction by longitudinal traction. If the reduction is adequate, they recommend stabilization with percutaneous Kirschner wires. In their type A injuries (those with total incongruity), two Kirschner wires are necessary for stability, one from the first metatarsal to the medial cuneiform and the second laterally from the fifth metatarsal to the cuboid. In their type B injuries (partial displacements), those of the lateral segment need only a single Kirschner wire for stability. However, if the first metatarsal is displaced, the injury is inherently unstable, and two wires are required. In their type C injuries (divergent displacements), one or two Kirschner wires are necessary to stabilize the medial fragment, with another single wire used for the lateral displacement. Fixation by percutaneous Kirschner wires as well as external immobilization are both often necessary. This is because of both the initial instability of the reduction and the subsequent loss of position that may develop when the decrease in swelling invalidates the support of the cast.

After the manipulation is performed, a careful radiographic evaluation is undertaken to ascertain that an anatomic reduction has been obtained. Collett et al.[13] emphasize that the reduction must be anatomic on the

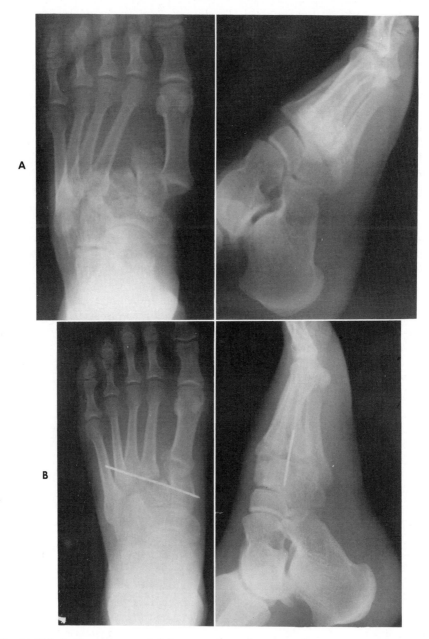

Fig. 24-126. A, Tarsometatarsal dislocation. **B,** Inadequate reduction. Note persistent lateral subluxation of second, third, fourth, and fifth metatarsal bases.

anteroposterior, lateral, *and* oblique views, because the dislocation occurs in all three planes. Evaluation of the relationship of the base of the metatarsals to the cuneiform and cuboids as outlined under Radiographic Evaluation is *essential* (Figs. 24-124 and 24-125). Wilson[53] found that of 14 patients who had undergone a closed reduction and were subsequently treated conservatively, only 1 had an *anatomic* reduction, and that in half of the patients a residual displacement of 5 mm or more was present. This stresses the importance of an accurate radiographic evaluation of the closed reduction.

Tarsometatarsal fracture-dislocations that are irreducible by closed means have been reported by several authors.[15,19,38a] Lowe and Yosipovitch[38a] reported an irreducible tarsometatarsal dislocation in which the closed reduction was blocked by a slip of the tibialis anterior tendon trapped between the medial and middle cuneiform. Holstein and Joldersma[32] also reported a case in which the tibialis anterior had become displaced between the first and second cuneiforms. DeBenedetti et al.[15] emphasized that irreducible dislocation secondary to the interposition of the tibialis anterior tendon occurs only with lateral dislocations of the first metatarsal. The presence of such a dislocation on preoperative radiographs might therefore suggest the need for an open reduction. Engber and Roberts,[19] Ballerio,[5] and Huet and Lecoeur[35] report that a superiorly dislocated peroneus longus tendon may act as an obstruction to reduction of the lateral tarsometatarsal joints in a tarsometatarsal fracture-dislocation. Open reduction to remove the trapped tibialis anterior or peroneus longus tendon is the treatment of choice.[15,19]

Lenczner et al.[37] noted that in cases of dorsolateral dislocation with an avulsion fracture of the base of the second metatarsal, the avulsed fragment may act to prevent an anatomic reduction of the metatarsal base within the cuneiform mortise, resulting in persistent subluxation of the metatarsal. In their opinion, the avulsion fracture remained attached to Lisfranc's ligament and therefore was held firmly within the mortise and could not be displaced by closed manipulation to allow the metatarsal base access to the mortise. In such cases, they recommend the fragment be excised at open reduction.

Geckeler[24] believed it was nearly impossible to reduce dislocations of the tarsometatarsal joint by manipulation and therefore recommended operative treatment. He was the first to recommend the use of Kirschner wires for stabilization of the dislocation following open reduction. After open reduction he recommended the use of a short leg cast. The Kirschner wires were removed after several weeks when soft tissue stability permitted. Wilson[53] also finds manipula-

tive reduction undependable. He therefore recommends that, unless anatomic reduction was obtained, open reduction and transfixation with Kirschner pins be the treatment of choice. He recommends leaving the wires in for 6 weeks, after which time the patient begins weight bearing. Anderson[2] also recommends open reduction and internal fixation with Kirschner pins in cases in which an anatomic closed reduction is not obtained. The patient is kept in a non-weight-bearing cast for 6 weeks followed by a short leg walking cast for an additional 3 to 4 weeks. He recommends longitudinal arch support for an additional 6 to 12 months. The percutaneous Kirschner wire fixation is to stabilize grossly unstable dislocations and also to allow maintenance of reduction during the period swelling decreases, in which a cast might not supply necessary stability to prevent redislocation.

For patients in whom there is a dislocation of the medial cuneiform bone in conjunction with a tarsometatarsal fracture-dislocation, Brown and McFarland[7] and Holstein and Joldersma[32] recommend primary open reduction through a dorsal incision centered between the first and second cuneiforms because of their lack of success with closed reduction. Following open reduction, Giannestras and Sammarco[25] recommend a short leg cast molded well about the foot. The cast and pins are removed at 6 to 8 weeks, and weight bearing with a properly fitted arch support is permitted. These authors also stress that they have not seen a single patient who had any persistent dislocation that did not subsequently require an arthrodesis of the involved joint.

Del Sel[16] recommends primary open reduction and temporary internal fixation by percutaneous wires in patients with tarsometatarsal fracture dislocations. He recommends the use of an incision in the first interosseous space with evacuation of the blood clot located there. In some cases a second incision is necessary to reduce the second and third metatarsals. He recommends debriding the tarsometatarsal joint of bits of cartilage, soft tissue, and bone and then stabilizing the reduction using percutaneous Kirschner wires. The wires are left in place for 2 to 4 weeks. After the wires are removed the patients are encouraged to walk in a below-knee cast. Tondeur[49] also advises open reduction and internal fixation of tarsometatarsal dislocations.

Wright[55] recommends longitudinal incisions on the dorsum of the foot for open reduction. He cautions, however, against the use of multiple incisions, particularly in patients in whom crushing has been extensive. After debriding the joint, he uses multiple Kirschner wires or staples to stabilize the dislocation. If Kirschner wires are used, they are left long enough to allow palpation and subsequent removal. Patients are treated in a short leg cast from the tip of the toes to the tibial tuberosity and are kept non-weight bearing for 3 weeks, and following this a short leg walking cast is applied. The Kirschner wires are removed at 4 to 6 weeks. The foot is maintained in a cast for a total of 3 weeks, after which an arch support is used for an additional 3 months. Wilppula[52] also recommends the use of a longitudinal incision between the first and second metatarsals on the dorsum of the foot. He found that when the first and second metatarsals are reduced the remainder of the metatarsals easily fall into place. He also uses Kirschner wire fixation from the metatarsals into the tarsal bones for stability.

Hardcastle et al.[30] believe that an *absolute* indication for open reduction is vascular insufficiency that does not improve after a closed reduction. In this situation, he agrees with Gissane[26] that both the dorsalis pedis and posterior tibial arteries must be explored at the time of open reduction. For open reduction, Hardcastle et al.[30] recommend the use of longitudinal incisions, the first between the first and second metatarsals, with accessory incisions located more laterally over the tarsometatarsal joint. They found that, following reduction and stable internal fixation, weight bearing as soon as the swelling subsided did not affect the final outcome, provided the foot was protected in a plaster cast and the reduction was stabilized with internal fixation. It was their opinion that such early weight bearing decreased the period of disability.

Granberry and Lipscomb[28] also recommend open reduction and internal fixation if an anatomic reduction is not obtained by closed means. Additionally, they suggest fusion of the involved joints in patients who require open reduction. This is because 11 of their 25 cases eventually required arthrodesis. Hardcastle et al.[30] suggest that primary arthrodesis may have a place in injuries where there is considerable comminution and maintenance of reduction is difficult. However, they had no experience with the technique. Primary arthrodesis is not supported by other authors.

RESULTS

Aitken and Poulson[1] report that although posttraumatic arthritis and ankylosis of the tarsometatarsal joints were common they were not a source of discomfort and disability in the majority of their patients. Indeed, they did not see the need for a tarsometatarsal fusion in their patients at follow-up. On the contrary, LaTourette et al.[36] found that all patients complained of some degree of discomfort in the foot following tarsometatarsal injury. Additionally, the majority of his patients complained of swelling.

Obtaining and maintaining an anatomic reduction is believed to be of major importance in avoiding the degenerative changes that may require surgery at a later

date.[25] LaTourette et al.[36] evaluated their results using gait analysis by foot switches attached to the sole of the patient's shoes.[14,39,45] They concluded that anatomic reduction and early ambulation produce better results. Wilson[53] too found the most critical factor in preventing late deformity, stiffness, and degenerative arthritis to be an anatomic reduction obtained by either closed or open means. Wilppula[52] demonstrated that although an anatomic result was no guarantee of a symptom-free foot, in general a good anatomic result usually produced a good functional result. Additionally, he reported that symptoms of degenerative arthritis in the tarsometatarsal joint tended to subside gradually during a period of several years follow-up. He found no need for arthrodesis as a salvage procedure in his patients, although he suggested that early arthrodesis might have accelerated their recovery. He also found that half of his patients had limitation of motion in the foot, and suggested that intensifying the mobilizing exercises during treatment could reduce this disability.

Lenczner et al[37] report that the majority of their poor results were secondary *either* to failure to *obtain* an adequate reduction or failure to *maintain* the reduction of the tarsometatarsal injury. This stresses the importance of stable fixation after reduction to prevent redislocation during the period of immobilization.[5a] Finally, Jeffreys[34] emphasizes that although accurate reduction is essential to prevent long-term disability, the late development of osteoarthritis may be determined by the damage sustained by the articular cartilage at the time of the injury. Therefore in certain cases the osteoarthritis may develop in spite of the method of treatment selected.

AUTHOR'S PREFERRED METHOD OF TREATMENT

The importance of early diagnosis and treatment of injuries to the tarsometatarsal joints cannot be overemphasized. Anteroposterior, oblique, and lateral radiographs will demonstrate frank dislocation of the tarsometatarsal joints. However, careful evaluation of radiographs is essential to detect the subtle signs of a subluxation of the tarsometatarsal joint or of a complete tarsometatarsal dislocation that has spontaneously reduced. When the clinical examination indicates tenderness at the tarsometatarsal joint, a full radiographic evaluation of the joint is essential. If such an injury is suspected, I use stress radiographs, possibly with an anesthetic, to determine the degree of instability.

Once the diagnosis of tarsometatarsal dislocation is confirmed, I prefer initially to attempt a closed reduction. In my experience, the earlier a reduction is attempted the more likely that an anatomic reduction will be obtained by closed methods. Traction is obtained with the patient in the supine position by suspending the leg with Chinese finger traps applied to the toes. A counterweight is placed over the ankle. Once the tarsometatarsal joints have been restored to length by traction, manipulation in the dorsoplantar plane is performed. Radiographic evaluation is then performed to ascertain the quality of the reduction. Anatomic reduction of the relationship of *each* of the metatarsals to their respective cuneiform or cuboid is demanded. If such a reduction is obtained, I use two percutaneous Kirschner wires, one from the first metatarsal into the medial cuneiform and the second from the fifth metatarsal into the cuboid to stabilize the dislocation (Fig. 24-127). The question of whether or not a closed reduction is stable or not is *not* considered in determining whether or not Kirschner wire fixation is needed. In my opinion, all of these injuries that are *dislocated* initially require Kirschner wire stabilization.

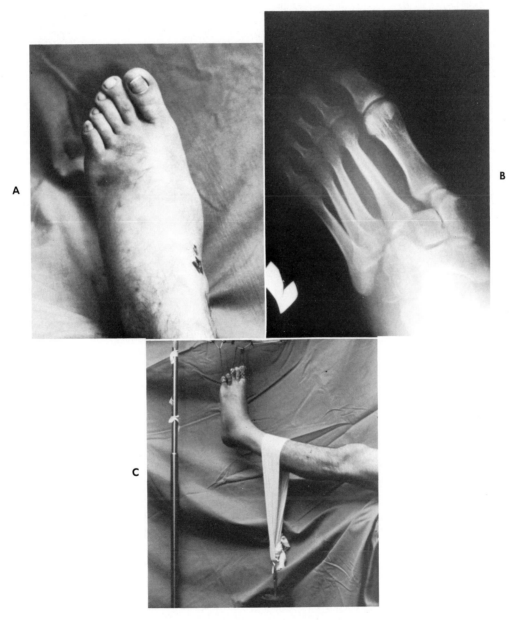

Fig. 24-127. Tarsometatarsal dislocation. **A,** Clinical appearance of injured foot. **B,** Anteroposterior radiograph demonstrating dislocation of tarsometatarsal joint. **C,** Method of closed reduction with Chinese finger traps for fixed traction.   *Continued.*

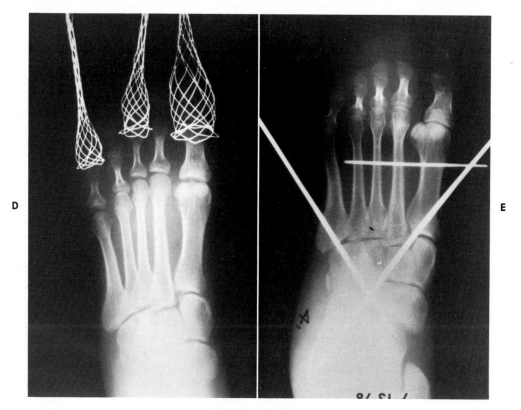

Fig. 24-127, cont'd. D, Radiograph of foot in traction after manipulative reduction. Tarso-metatarsal joint is restored. **E,** Percutaneous Kirschner wire fixation to stabilize tarsometa-tarsal reduction.

In patients with minor degrees of subluxation of the tarsometatarsal joint, Kirschner wire fixation is reserved only for those in whom cooperation with the postreduction regimen is questionable.

Following reduction and stabilization, the foot is placed in a short leg nonwalking cast for 2 weeks. The toes are left free at the end of the cast to encourage exercises of the metatarsophalangeal joints. At 2 weeks the nonweight-bearing cast is removed and a new short leg cast, well-molded in the arch, is applied and partial weight bearing allowed. This cast and the pins are removed at 6 to 8 weeks. At this point the foot is placed in a good shoe with a longitudinal arch support for an additional 9 to 12 months.

If the reduction is not anatomic radiographically, I proceed to an open reduction. I prefer an incision over the first tarsometatarsal joint. Subsequent parallel longitudinal incisions are used, usually between the third and fourth metatarsals, to expose the remainder of the tarsometatarsal joints. Anatomic reduction of these joints is obtained, and percutaneous Kirschner wire fixation as outlined previously is used. Usually debridement of small articular cartilage and osseous fragments is necessary to effect the reduction. In patients in whom there is a gross amount of swelling at the time of open reduction, interosseous decompression fasciotomies are performed between each of the metatarsals in an effort to decrease fibrosis in the foot.

The postoperative management following open reduction and internal fixation is identical to that recommended following closed reduction and percutaneous fixation.

If there is vascular compromise, I consider reduction of the dislocation an emergency. If clinical signs of insufficiency persist after anatomic reduction by open or closed means, an arteriogram is performed to evaluate the posterior tibial and lateral plantar artery. I obtain vascular surgery consultation in these instances. Consideration is given to interosseous fasciotomy if the arteriograms show patency of the vessels.

Open dislocations are treated by irrigation and debridement *before* reduction. Anatomic reduction is then obtained under direct vision, and the dislocation is stabilized with percutaneous Kirschner wires. A second debridement and irrigation are performed in 48 to 72 hours and the wounds are left open. A short leg nonweight-bearing cast is applied. At 5 to 7 days, the wounds are closed secondarily. The postoperative man-

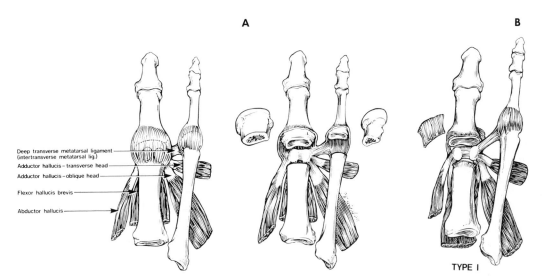

Fig. 24-128. A, Normal anatomy of first metatarsophalangeal joint. Note relationship of deep transverse metatarsal ligament and conjoined tendon of adductor hallucis and lateral head of flexor hallucis brevis. **B,** Type I dorsal dislocation of first metatarsophalangeal joint. Note that sesamoids are not fractured nor is intersesamoid ligament disrupted.

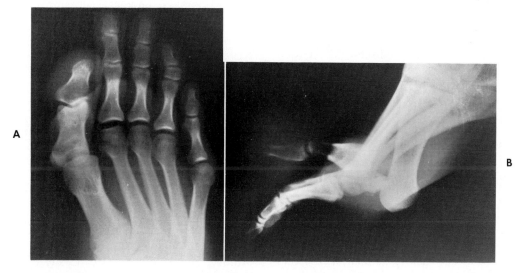

Fig. 24-129. A, Anteroposterior radiograph of Type I dislocation with slight medial displacement. Sesamoids are neither fractured nor separated on this view. **B,** Lateral radiograph of type I metatarsophalangeal joint dislocation. Both sesamoids are dorsal to first metatarsal head and there is marked plantar angulation of first metatarsal shaft.

tached to the base of the proximal phalanx, rides over the dorsum of the metatarsal head and locks the head in a plantar position (Fig. 24-129). The medial and lateral conjoined tendons (consisting of the medial head of the flexor hallucis brevis and abductor hallucis medially and the lateral head of the flexor hallucis brevis and the adductor hallucis laterally) come to rest tightly on either side of the metatarsal neck (Fig. 24-128, B). This is a so-called type I dislocation.[14] Such cases in the literature have been irreducible by closed manipulation.[7,12,14,18] Several authors have compared the type I dislocation to that of the complex metatarsophalangeal joint dislocation noted in the hand.[18,26]

With more dorsiflexion force, the intersesamoid ligament will rupture, resulting in wide separation of the sesamoids, (type IIA) or a transverse fracture of one or both sesamoids will occur (type IIB)[3,14] (Fig. 24-130). These are the so-called type II dislocations.[14] If the mechanism is a fall from a height, the sesamoid fracture may be caused by crushing force against the metatarsal condyles, which results in comminution of the sesamoid fracture.[21] If pure hyperextension is the force responsible for the dislocation, the fracture more often resembles an avulsion. In either situation, the more proximal fragment of the fractured sesamoid remains in a normal position in relationship with the adjacent sesamoid via the remaining intact intersesamoid ligament. The distal fragment widely separates from its proximal fragment, because it is not only forcibly separated from its attachment to the intersesamoid ligament but is also pulled distally into the joint space by its peripheral attachments at the base of the proximal phalanx. This fragment essentially acts as a loose body and may require removal.[8,16] In a situation in which there is rupture of the plantar plate through the intersesamoid ligament or through a fracture of one or both sesamoids, reduction is usually easily accomplished by closed means.

The importance in classifying these injuries as type I or type II injuries lies in being able to predict whether closed reduction will be successful.

MECHANISM OF INJURY
Hallux metatarsophalangeal dislocations

The hallux dislocation is usually the result of forces that hyperextend the great toe, causing displacement of the proximal phalanx onto the dorsum of the first metatarsal neck.[12,29] Hyperextension of the proximal phalanx of the hallux on the first metatarsal, such as occurs when the toes are forcibly dorsiflexed against the floorboard of an automobile, results in the metatarsal head being pushed through the plantar capsule between (1) the medial head of the flexor hallucis brevis, the abductor hallucis and the associated medial sesamoid, and (2) the lateral head of the

flexor hallucis brevis, adductor hallucis, and the lateral sesamoid. The plantar capsule is disrupted at its proximal attachment to the neck of the metatarsal, similar to the volar capsular avulsion noted in dorsal dislocation of the metacarpophalangeal joints in the hand.[26] Coker et al.[5] and Coker and Arnold[6] note that when one player lands on the back of the leg of another in pileups in a football game, such hyperextension of the metatarsophalangeal joint can occur. Changes in playing surfaces, the decreased support of the footgear used, and, finally, poor shoe fitting are reported as explaining an increased incidence of such metatarsophalangeal injuries noted in football today.[2,5,6]

Konkel and Muehlstein[16] suggest that in dislocations of the first metatarsophalangeal joint with a displaced fracture of the medial sesamoid, an alternative mechanism of injury is crushing of the medial sesamoid at the time the great toe is forced dorsally and dislocated. When the displacing force is relieved, the medial sesamoid returns to its normal position, leaving a displaced fragment in the joint. Jahss[14] stresses that in the pure hyperextension mechanism, any associated sesamoid fractures are avulsion fractures in nature, while comminution of the sesamoid suggests crushing against the metatarsal condyles caused by a fall from a height.[14,21]

Lesser metatarsophalangeal dislocation

Rao and Banzon[25] report that forcible dorsiflexion of the proximal phalanx over the metatarsal head is also the most common mechanism of injury in dislocations of the metatarsophalangeal joints of the lesser toes. This results in the metatarsal head being forced through the plantar fibrocartilaginous plate. Murphy[24] also documents forcible dorsiflexion as the mechanism of injury in this dislocation. In both of these patients there was an associated fracture of the second metatarsal neck confirming a similar mechanism[24,25] (see Fig. 24-132).

Jahss[15] has reported chronic lateral dislocations of the fifth metatarsophalangeal joint. The mechanism of injury in these cases is forced abduction, such as occurs when the small toe catches on a piece of furniture. Reports of lateral dislocations of the other toes are not present in the literature.

DIAGNOSIS
Clinical diagnosis

In dislocations of the first metatarsophalangeal joint the physical examination reveals marked distortion of the anatomic contour of the great toe (see Fig. 24-131). Swelling and tenderness are usually present, and the patient has an inability to walk or bear weight on the foot.[11] The most impressive finding is the prominence of the metatarsal head on the plantar aspect of the foot.[12,14,19] Pressure from the metatarsal head may re-

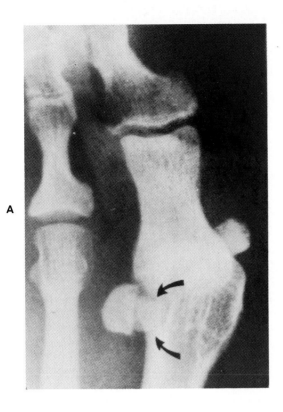

A

Fig. 24-130. A, Anteroposterior radiograph of type II metatarsophalangeal dislocation. Hallux metatarsophalangeal joint is dislocated and medial sesamoid is fractured. Arrows denote displaced fragment of *medial* sesamoid. (From Jahss, M.H.: Foot Ankle, **1:**15-21, 1980. © 1980, American Orthopaedic Foot Society.) **B,** Type II dislocations. Type IIA: intersesamoid ligament is ruptured. Type IIB: transverse fracture of medial sesamoid is noted. Proximal fragment remains in its normal relationship to adjacent sesamoid via intact intersesamoid ligament. Distal fragment is separated from proximal fragment and remains attached to base of proximal phalanx.

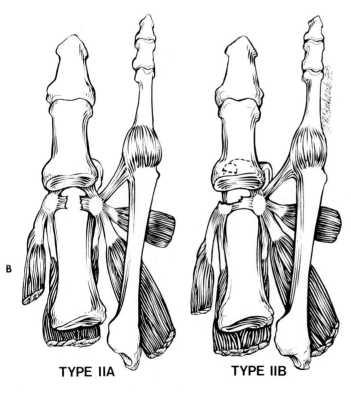

B   **TYPE IIA**   **TYPE IIB**

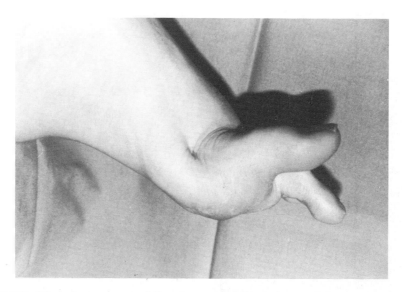

Fig. 24-131. Clinical appearance of first metatarsophalangeal joint dislocation. Notice skin dimple, which suggests irreducibility.

sult in blanching of the plantar skin.[18] The proximal phalanx rests on the dorsum of the metatarsal head in extension with slight outward deviation.[12,18] If there is a lateral component to the dislocation there will be an increase in the interdigital space between the toes.[11] The distal phalanx of the great toe is usually flexed and the extensor tendons relaxed.

Rao and Banzon[25] report that the important clinical findings in dislocations of the lesser metatarsophalangeal joints include swelling and hyperextension deformity with corresponding prominences on the sole of the foot. Murphy[24] reports that swelling of the forefoot and shortening of the involved toe are also important clinical findings. Again, a palpable tender bony prominence on the sole of the forefoot representing the displaced metatarsal head is a classic finding.

Jahss,[15] mentions abduction deformity with widening of the interdigital space as the classic clinical finding in lateral dislocation of the fifth metatarsophalangeal joint.

Radiographic diagnosis

Hallux metatarsophalangeal dislocations. Anteroposterior, lateral, and oblique views of the metatarsophalangeal joints are essential in confirming the diagnosis. Garcia and Parkes[10] believe the injury is best visualized radiographically on the lateral and oblique views of the foot. Giannestras and Sammarco[11] stress that anteroposterior radiographs demonstrate a double density of the proximal phalanx overlying the metatarsal head in a pure dorsal dislocation. In evaluating the radiographs, it is important to specifically analyze each sesamoid. Fractures of the sesamoid that may be associated with

these injuries need to be identified before reduction. Additionally, careful evaluation of postreduction radiographs is essential to rule out the presence of a fracture fragment within the joint.[8,12,16] Finally, careful evaluation of these radiographs is necessary to classify the injury as type I or type II. If there is frank separation of the sesamoids to either side of the metatarsal head on the anteroposterior radiograph there is a complete disruption of the intersesamoid ligament and a type II injury. Additionally, if fracture of the sesamoids is present, it can be seen on anteroposterior and oblique views, and this also represents a type II lesion (Fig. 24-130). As mentioned by Jahss,[14] these are usually reducible by closed methods. If, however, the sesamoids are not separated or fractured on the anteroposterior view, and on the lateral view they are seen riding dorsal to the metatarsal head, a type I dislocation, which is usually irreducible by closed means, is present (Fig. 24-129). It is important to note that the involved metatarsal is plantar flexed at the tarsometatarsal joint in this injury (Fig. 24-129, *B*). According to Giannikas et al.[12] a lateral radiograph demonstrating the head of the first metatarsal depressed into the sole of the foot and the proximal phalanx resting on the dorsum of the head of the metatarsal is the most important view.

Lesser metatarsophalangeal dislocations. Murphy[24] emphasizes that in dislocations of the lesser metatarsophalangeal joints, the anteroposterior radiograph may be diagnostic. He stresses the finding of widening of the metatarsophalangeal joint on the anteroposterior view. The plantar location of the metatarsal head may be visualized on the lateral radiograph. However, over-

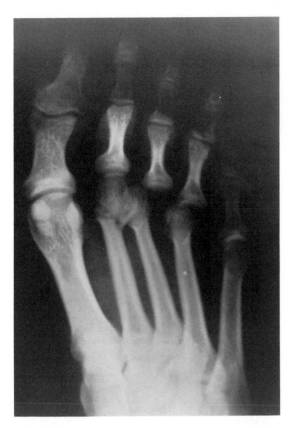

Fig. 24-132. Anteroposterior radiograph of dislocations of third and fourth metatarsophalangeal joints. Joint spaces are widened, and phalanges are displaced laterally with respect to metatarsals. (Reprinted with permission from Rao, J.P., and Banzon, M.T.: Clin. Orthop. **145**:224-226, 1979.)

lap of metatarsal heads may obscure this finding. Rao and Banzon[25] demonstrated widening of the metatarsophalangeal joints of the third and fourth digits with lateral displacement of the phalanges with respect to the metatarsals as findings suggesting dislocation of these joints (Fig. 24-132).

TREATMENT
Hallux metatarsophalangeal dislocations

Dislocations of the metatarsophalangeal joint of the hallux can initially be approached by closed reduction. The closed reduction is first attempted with the patient under local anesthesia.[10] This can be augmented by intravenous analgesia.[10,11] The method of manipulation includes hyperextension of the phalanx with plantar angulation of the metatarsal so the inferior edge of the articular surface of the phalanx contacts the superior aspect of the articular surface of the metatarsal head.[4,10,20] Traction and then direct plantar pressure and flexion of the phalanx are used to complete the reduction.[4,10,20] Following reduction, most dislocations

are stable.[4,20] As emphasized by DeLuca and Kenmore[8] it is essential to obtain adequate postreduction radiographs to identify loose bony fragments remaining in the metatarsophalangeal joint, which may require subsequent surgical excision. After a stable reduction, Garcia and Parkes[10] recommend immobilization for 2 to 3 weeks by the use of a dorsal metallic splint to prevent extension of the metatarsophalangeal joint. The patient is allowed to begin weight bearing within the limits of pain.[11] Moseley[20] believes that a metatarsal bar to protect the foot from plantar pressure during the early postreduction period is all that is necessary. Chapman recommends the use of minimal external fixation by strapping following reduction.[4] Coker et al.[5] and Coker and Arnold[6] recommend the use of a 0.5 mm thick spring steel splint within the shoe extending from just anterior to the heel to the forward edge of the inner sole to protect the metatarsophalangeal joint from further hyperextension.

If following reduction there is even a slight tendency toward redislocation, a walking cast extending to the tip of the toes should be applied.[11] Giannestras and Sammarco[11] emphasize that in dislocations with a component of lateral displacement, the damage to the collateral ligaments may prevent a stable closed reduction. In this instance, a percutaneous Kirschner wire across the joint is used to help maintain the reduction.[11]

If closed reduction using a local anesthetic is unsuccessful, a second attempt with the patient under general anesthesia is warranted.[7] If this attempt at closed reduction is unsuccessful, a complex or irreducible dislocation requiring open reduction is present.[11] Open reduction may also be necessary if the dislocation is irreducible by closed means and the postreduction radiographs reveal an intraarticular loose body in the metatarsophalangeal joint that must be removed.[8] Daniel et al.[7] recommend a dorsomedial approach to the metatarsophalangeal joint through which a Z-plasty tenotomy is performed on the extensor hallucis longus tendon. The metatarsophalangeal joint capsule is opened via an inverted L-shaped capsulotomy. Following this arthrotomy, manipulative reduction is performed under direct vision. Wright[29] also recommends the use of a medial approach to the first metatarsophalangeal joint to perform this open reduction.

Salamon et al.[26] compare this dislocation of the metatarsophalangeal joint to the complex dislocation of the index finger and recommend the use of a plantar approach for the best visualization of the pathologic anatomy and the most direct means of reduction. Giannikas et al.[12] also recommend the use of a plantar incision, transverse in nature, under the first metatarsophalangeal joint.

Lewis and DeLee[18] recommend the use of a dorsal

incision in the web space between the first and second metatarsal heads to surgically reduce this dislocation. The advantages of the dorsal approach include the avoidance of an incision over the plantar aspect of the foot with the attendant risk of a painful plantar scar, better visualization of the pathologic anatomy, and decreased risk of damage to the plantar digital nerves. These authors also emphasize the importance of surgically releasing both heads of the adductor hallucis and the deep transverse metatarsal ligament from the lateral sesamoid to allow enough mobility to easily reduce the plantar fibrocartilaginous plate from its location dorsal to the neck of the metatarsal.

Following surgical reduction, these dislocations are usually stable.[18,26,29] Wright[29] recommends the use of a splint for 2 weeks to allow soft tissue healing, followed by progressive weight bearing in a good shoe. Daniel et al.[7] recommend non-weight bearing for a short period followed by progressive weight bearing within the limits of pain. The total period of cast immobilization is 3 to 4 weeks. Following cast removal, they recommend hydrotherapy and an exercise program to regain the range of motion.[7] Lewis and DeLee[18] recommend the use of a short leg cast for 2 weeks followed by weight bearing in a shoe. It is essential to begin early hydrotherapy and toe exercises to restore range of metatarsophalangeal motion.[7,18] Although Wright[29] recommends the use of a toe splint for 4 to 6 weeks following cast removal to prevent an extension contracture, other authors have not found this to be necessary.[18]

Lesser metatarsophalangeal dislocations

In dislocations of the lesser metatarsophalangeal joints, closed reduction is attempted first.[24,25] Rao and Banzon[25] attempted closed reduction by hyperextension of the phalanx, pressure against the base of the phalanx, and then flexion. They were able to reduce 1 of 3 lesser toe dislocations by this method. Murphy,[24] however, found a dislocation of the second metatarsophalangeal joint to be irreducible by this method. If the manipulation is unsuccessful, open surgical reduction is performed. Rao and Benzon[25] used a dorsal incision between the dislocated third and fourth metatarsophalangeal joints. They found this provided excellent exposure of the plantar fibrocartilaginous plate, which was interposed between the metatarsal head and the base of the phalanges. Once the surgical exposure was obtained, they again attempted a manipulative reduction, which was unsuccessful. They found that release of the dorsal capsule and deep transverse metatarsal ligament was necessary for successful reduction.

Like dislocation of the first metatarsophalangeal joint following closed or open reduction, these dislocations are usually stable.[24,25] Following reduction, Rao and

Benzon[25] protected the dislocations in a short leg walking cast for 6 weeks. Rao and Benzon[25] and Murphy[24] found at follow-up that their patients were able to dorsiflex their toes without pain and that radiographs showed no evidence of degenerative arthritis of the metatarsophalangeal joint.

Jahss[15] mentions abduction instability at the metatarsophalangeal joint following inadequate treatment of lateral metatarsophalangeal joint dislocations of the fifth metatarsophalangeal joint. The instability is demonstrated by abduction of the fifth toe on weight bearing. Such abduction instability is quite symptomatic, as it results in catching the fifth toe on the sock, shoe, etc., and may require later reconstructive surgery.[15] He recommends adequate immobilization of this joint following a lateral dislocation to allow the medial joint capsule to heal.

RESULTS

Usually no permanent disability results following these dislocations.[11] Lewis and DeLee[18] report restoration of essentially a normal range of motion to the metatarsophalangeal joint following this dislocation. Garcia and Parkes[10] also report in the majority of instances there is no permanent disability following this injury. They do caution that occasionally a patient may return 4 to 5 years after the injury with symptoms of early osteoarthritis of the first metatarsophalangeal joint, as evidenced by the slight restriction of motion often noted in patients with hallux rigidus.[10] Garcia and Parkes[10] stress that in dislocations that remain unreduced the long extensors and flexors of the toe produce a clawing deformity, which leads to severe metatarsalgia and plantar callosities beneath the involved metatarsal head. In this instance, radiographic evidence of degenerative arthritis is present, and clinically the patients are seen with restricted joint motion. Reconstructive surgery of the metatarsophalangeal joint is then necessary.

AUTHOR'S PREFERRED METHOD
OF TREATMENT
Hallux metatarsophalangeal dislocations

I have found Jahss' classification[15] most helpful in predicting reducibility of dislocations of the first metatarsophalangeal joint. Radiographs clearly demonstrating both sesamoids are essential before closed reduction is attempted. Patients in whom the sesamoids are not separated on the anteroposterior view and are not fractured represent type I injuries in Jahss' classification and usually require an open reduction. I have also noted that the presence of a skin dimple located *medially* on the metatarsophalangeal joint may be associated with irreducibility by closed methods (Fig. 24-131).

Even in patients with type I dislocations I attempt a closed reduction. All type II dislocations initially undergo an attempted closed reduction.

I attempt the closed reduction first with the patient under local anesthesia, augmented by intravenous analgesia. Longitudinal traction, hyperextension of the metatarsophalangeal joint, and plantar pressure on the dorsal aspect of the base of the involved proximal phalanx are attempted in an effort to obtain a reduction. Postreduction radiographs are carefully evaluated to make certain that the reduction is anatomic and there are no intraarticular bone fragments that require surgical removal. If this attempt at closed reduction is unsuccessful, the patient is taken to the operating room. There a second attempt at closed reduction, using the same manipulation but with the patient under general anesthesia, is attempted.

If the closed reduction is successful, the foot is placed in a short leg walking cast that extends past the toes to prevent their hyperextension. Weight bearing is encouraged as soon as pain is tolerable. Cast immobilization is used for 2 to 3 weeks. Following this, a stiff-soled shoe with a metatarsal bar is recommended. After the cast is removed, toe flexion exercises and hydrotherapy are instituted in an effort to restore a complete range of metatarsophalangeal joint motion. In my experience, the most frequent disability following simple dislocation of this joint is loss of metatarsophalangeal joint motion.

If the second attempt at closed reduction is unsuccessful or if bony fragments are trapped in the joint, open reduction is performed through a *dorsal* incision placed between the first and second metatarsal heads. Following exposure of the joint, a second closed reduction is attempted to demonstrate the pathologic anatomy. In my experience, detachment of both heads of the adductor hallucis from the fibular sesamoid followed by transection of the deep transverse metatarsal ligament allows the return of fibrocartilaginous plate to the plantar aspect of the metatarsal head. Following this reduction, the joint is irrigated and documentation of articular cartilage damage to the metatarsal head and base of the proximal phalanx is made. The adductor and the deep transverse metatarsal ligaments are reattached to the lateral sesamoid. In my experience, these dislocations are stable following open reduction. The postoperative immobilization is similar to that following closed reduction.

Lesser metatarsophalangeal dislocations

I treat dislocations of the lesser toe metatarsophalangeal joints in a way similar to the method used for the hallux. Closed reduction is attempted first using the same hyperextension maneuver. If this is unsuccessful,

open reduction through a dorsal longitudinal incision placed adjacent to the involved metatarsophalangeal joint is preferred. After open reduction, a short leg walking cast with a toe plate is used for 2 weeks, followed by the use of a stiff-soled shoe. Range of motion exercises are begun after 3 weeks.

DISLOCATIONS OF INTERPHALANGEAL JOINTS

Dislocations of the interphalangeal joints of the toes are extremely unusual, those of the great toe being by far the most common.[9] Giannestras and Sammarco[11] report these dislocations are most commonly associated with other trauma to the foot. Anteroposterior, oblique, and lateral radiographs reveal loss of integrity of the interphalangeal joint. Care must be taken to evaluate the joint surfaces for associated fractures. This injury is often open and may be associated with comminuted fractures at the base of the distal phalanx.[11]

Eibel,[9] Laczay and Csapo,[17] and Murakawami and Tokuyasu[23] reported dislocations of the interphalangeal joint of the great toe with interposition of the plantar sesamoid. Muller[22] is credited by Eibel as first reporting this dislocation.[9] In Eibel's case[9] the interphalangeal joint was dislocated dorsally. He reported marked swelling dorsally and an open laceration on the plantar surface of the interphalangeal joint. Although closed reduction was successfully accomplished, it required considerable force, and the reduction was not stable. Postreduction radiographs revealed an osseous body within the interphalangeal joint, which proved to be an interphalangeal sesamoid. Following the open reduction, a splint was applied to the great toe for 3 weeks, following which ambulation was initiated. Recovery was reported to be complete at 5 weeks.

Interphalangeal joint dislocations of the lesser toes have been reported to occur following abduction stresses to the interphalangeal joints, particularly of the fifth toe.[15] These dislocations are usually stable if reduction is performed soon after the injury. If there is any sign of instability after reduction because of capsular damage, a Kirschner wire from the distal phalanx into the proximal phalanx may be necessary to hold the reduction. If such a pin is used, it usually remains in place for 3 weeks to allow the soft tissues to heal. If closed reduction is successful, simple taping to the adjacent digit is all the immobilization that is necessary.

AUTHOR'S PREFERRED METHOD OF TREATMENT

For interphalangeal joint dislocations of the hallux, I prefer closed reduction by traction, hyperextension, and plantar pressure on the distal phalanx. If the reduction is stable, the foot is placed in a short leg walking cast for 2 to 3 weeks, followed by a stiff-soled shoe or a stainless steel insert, as has been recommended by Coker et al.[5] and Coker and Arnold.[6] This is used for 4 to 6 weeks. If closed reduction is unsuccessful or unstable, careful analysis of radiographs is performed to detect an interphalangeal sesamoid or other incarcerated bone fragment preventing a stable reduction. An open reduction through a dorsal incision is then performed with removal of the offending sesamoid or fragment. Postoperative management is similar to that after closed reduction.

In the lesser toes, if the dislocation is stable, I prefer to tape the involved toe to the adjacent toe until swelling and pain have subsided. If the dislocation is unstable, a Kirschner wire across the interphalangeal joint is used for 3 weeks to provide stability.

Late complications following interphalangeal or distal interphalangeal dislocations are not common. If they do occur, however, I have found that excisional arthroplasty or arthrodesis usually results in pain relief.

REFERENCES

1. Blodgett, W.H.: Injuries of the forefoot and toes. In Jahss, M.H., editor: Disorders of the foot, vol. 2, Philadelphia, 1982, W.B. Saunders Co.
2. Bowers, K.D., Jr., and Martin, R.B.: Impact absorption, new and old Astroturf at West Virginia University. Med. Sci. Sports, 6:217, 1974.
3. Brown, T.I.S.: Avulsion fracture of the fibular sesamoid in association with dorsal dislocation of the metatarsophalangeal joint of the hallux. Clin. Orthop. 149:229-231, 1980.
4. Chapman, M.W.: Fractures and dislocations of the ankle and foot. In Mann, R.A., editor: DuVries' surgery of the foot, ed. 4, St. Louis, 1978, The C.V. Mosby Co.
5. Coker, T.P., Jr., and Arnold, J.A.: Sports injuries to the foot and ankle. In Jahss, M.H., editor: Disorders of the foot, vol. 2, Philadelphia, 1982, W.B. Saunders Co.
6. Coker, T.P., Jr., Arnold, J.A., and Weber, D.L.: Traumatic lesions of the metatarsophalangeal joint of the great toe in athletes, J. Arkansas Med. Soc. 74:309, 1978.
7. Daniel, W.L., Beck, E.L., Duggar, G.E., and Bennett, A.J.: Traumatic dislocation of the first metatarsophalangeal joint: a case report, J. Am. Podiatry Assoc. 66:97-100, 1976.
8. DeLuca, F.N., and Kenmore, P.I.: Bilateral dorsal dislocations of the metatarsophalangeal joints of the great toes with a loose body in one of the metatarsophalangeal joints, J. Trauma 15:737-739, 1975.
9. Eibel, P.: Dislocation of the interphalangeal joint of the big toe with interposition of a sesamoid bone, J. Bone Joint Surg. 36A:880-882, 1954.
10. Garcia, A., and Parkes, J.C.: Fractures of the foot. In Giannestras, N.J., editor: Foot disorders: medical and surgical management, ed. 2, Philadelphia, 1973, Lea & Febiger.
11. Giannestras, N.J., and Sammarco, G.J.: Fractures and dislocations in the foot. In Rockwood, C.A., Jr., and Green, D.P., editors: Fractures, vol. 2, Philadelphia, 1975, J.B. Lippincott Co.
12. Giannikas, A.C., Papachristou, G., Papavasiliou, N., Nikifordis, P., and Hartofilakidis-Garofalidis, G.: Dorsal dislocation of the first metatarsophalangeal joint, J. Bone Joint Surg. 57B:384-386, 1975.
13. Jahss, M.H.: LeLievre bunion operation. In America Academy of Orthopaedic Surgeons: Instructional Course Lectures, vol. 21, St. Louis, 1972, The C.V. Mosby Co.
14. Jahss, M.H.: Chronic and recurrent dislocations of the fifth toe, Foot Ankle 3:275-278, 1981.
15. Jahss, M.H.: Traumatic dislocations of the first metatarsophalangeal joint, Foot Ankle 1:15-21, 1980.
16. Konkel, K.F., and Muehlstein, J.H.: Unusual fracture-dislocation of the great toe: case report, J. Trauma 15:733-736, 1975.
17. Laczay, V., and Csapo, K.: Interphalangeal Luxation der Grobzehe mit Interposition eines Sesambeiwes, Fortschr. Rontgenstr. 116:571-572, 1972.
18. Lewis, A.G., and DeLee, J.C.: Type I complex dislocation of the first metatarsophalangeal joint: open reduction through a dorsal approach, J. Bone Joint Surg. 66A:1120, 1984.
19. McKinley, L.M., and Davis, G.L.: Locked dislocation of the great toe, J. La. State Med. Soc. 127:389-390, 1975.
20. Moseley, H.F.: Traumatic disorders of the ankle and foot, Clin. Symp. 17:30, 1965.
21. Mouchet, A.: Deux cas de luxation dorsale complete du gros orteil avec lesions des sesamoides, Rev. Orthop. 18:221-227, 1931.
22. Muller, G.M.: Dislocation of sesamoid of hallux, Lancet 1:789, 1944.
23. Murakawami, Y., and Tokuyasu, Y.: A case of dislocation of the first toe with the sesamoid bone interfering with orthopaedic manipulation, Orthop. Surg. (Tokyo) 22:751-753, 1971.
24. Murphy, J.L.: Isolated dorsal dislocation of the second metatarsophalangeal joint, Foot Ankle, 1:30-32, July 1980.
25. Rao, J.P., and Banzon, M.T.: Irreducible dislocation of the metatarsophalangeal joints of the foot, Clin. Orthop., 145:224-226, November-December 1979.
26. Salamon, P.B., Gelberman, R.H., and Huffer, J.M.: Dorsal dislocation of the metatarsophalangeal joint of the great toe: a case report, J. Bone Joint Surg. 56A:1073-1075, 1974.
27. Sarrafian, S.K.: Anatomy of the foot and ankle: topographical, functional and descriptive, Philadelphia, 1983, J.B. Lippincott Co.
28. Wilson, J.L., editor: Watson-Jones fractures and joint injuries, ed. 5, New York, 1976, Longman.
29. Wright, P.E.: Dislocations. In Edmonson, A.S., and Crenshaw, A.H., editors: Campbell's operative orthopaedics, vol. 1, ed. 6, St. Louis, 1980, The C.V. Mosby Co.

Index

Page numbers in *italics* indicate illustrations or boxed material. Page numbers followed by *t* indicate tables.